AF807109

Prepectoral Breast Reconstruction

Raghavan Vidya • Hilton Becker
Editors

Prepectoral Breast Reconstruction

Current Trends and Techniques

Springer

Editors
Raghavan Vidya
Birmingham University
The Royal Wolverhampton NHS Trust
Wolverhampton, UK

Hilton Becker
Charles E. Schmidt College of Medicine
Florida Atlantic University
Boca Raton, FL, USA

ISBN 978-3-031-15589-5 ISBN 978-3-031-15590-1 (eBook)
https://doi.org/10.1007/978-3-031-15590-1

© The Editor(s) (if applicable) and The Author(s), under exclusive license to Springer Nature Switzerland AG 2023, corrected publication 2023
This work is subject to copyright. All rights are solely and exclusively licensed by the Publisher, whether the whole or part of the material is concerned, specifically the rights of translation, reprinting, reuse of illustrations, recitation, broadcasting, reproduction on microfilms or in any other physical way, and transmission or information storage and retrieval, electronic adaptation, computer software, or by similar or dissimilar methodology now known or hereafter developed.
The use of general descriptive names, registered names, trademarks, service marks, etc. in this publication does not imply, even in the absence of a specific statement, that such names are exempt from the relevant protective laws and regulations and therefore free for general use.
The publisher, the authors, and the editors are safe to assume that the advice and information in this book are believed to be true and accurate at the date of publication. Neither the publisher nor the authors or the editors give a warranty, expressed or implied, with respect to the material contained herein or for any errors or omissions that may have been made. The publisher remains neutral with regard to jurisdictional claims in published maps and institutional affiliations.

This Springer imprint is published by the registered company Springer Nature Switzerland AG
The registered company address is: Gewerbestrasse 11, 6330 Cham, Switzerland

Foreword

Prepectoral breast reconstruction has been one of the most important new trends in plastic surgery over the last several years, and Drs. Raghavan Vidya and Hilton Becker's textbook is the definitive extant textbook on the subject.

There is some irony to the way this technique has evolved to become such a solid fixture in the armamentarium of reconstructive surgeons. When Cronin and Gerow placed their first implant in 1962[1], enterprising plastic surgeons immediately transposed this cosmetic procedure to the breast cancer realm and the natural extrapolation was made to a prepectoral direct-to-implant reconstruction. However, driven by concerns of vascularity and issues related to contour irregularity and aesthetic outcome, the field of prosthetic breast reconstruction detoured to subpectoral—and two staged—prosthetic reconstruction, and this permutation became the dominant form of prosthetic reconstruction for decades.

But recent issues related to functional and aesthetic outcomes have spurred a resurgent interest in revisiting prepectoral reconstruction. The advent of pectoral muscle release with lower pole dermal matrix reconstitution can exacerbate animation deformity and heighten soft tissue contour irregularity. This coupled with increased use of the nipple sparing and prophylactic mastectomies has created a need to better balance *form* and *function* with prosthetic breast reconstruction. Expectations for a more aesthetic and more functionally congruent breast reconstruction have stimulated a renewed interest in moving the prosthesis from an anatomically unnatural position under the muscle to a position more aligned with the original anatomic defect, namely over the muscle. Even as this prepectoral approach has been revisited, refinements in the mastectomy technique itself (with concomitantly more robust flaps) have allowed this renaissance of the prepectoral technique. Pioneers such as Dr. Becker and Dr. Vidya have led the way in creating new paradigms of clinical use of this approach and so it is very a propos that they co-edit this important compilation of the current thought in prepectoral breast reconstruction.

Indeed, from the very first chapter, Dr. Becker delineates the raison d'etre of prepectoral reconstruction, illuminating the whys and wherefores of its contemporaneous popularity. Before prepectoral direct-to-implant breast reconstruction became vogue, Dr. Becker had already glimpsed beyond the

[1]Cronin, TD and Gerow FJ. Augmentation Mammoplasty: A New "Natural Feel" Prosthesis. Excerpta Medica International Congress 66(1963): 41–9.

event horizon of prosthetic breast reconstruction. He invented and developed some of the core technology platforms (Spectrum implant, Becker Implant, *Mentor Corporation, Santa Barbara, USA*) and associated techniques that facilitated the introduction of this approach to the mainstream.

The textbook itself is very logically structured with initial chapters detailing the intersection of oncology and prepectoral indications. Then there are several chapters on the technology platforms that are so critical to the success of this procedure including varying types of dermal matrices and synthetic mesh. Next follows the technical aspects of diverse surgical approaches that may used. Indeed prior to the resurgence of prepectoral reconstruction, we had variegated technique modifications with fat grafting, direct-to-implant, meshless/meshful permutations. This textbook artfully combines these pre-existing surgical trends with the novel interface of the prepectoral approach to provide a very modern, cutting-edge overview of these near-future trends. Additionally, prepectoral reconstruction has increasingly been seen as a way to obviate the traditional distortion and displacement seen with subpectoral prosthetic reconstruction in the setting of radiation. Drs. Vidya and Becker's textbook responsively surveys the planning, technique, and divergent outcomes seen with this novel approach.

There are 25 chapters in this book, and in each of the chapters is ensconced high level pearls for understanding and optimally executing the prepectoral strategy. The authors of these chapters are the same authors who have published and presented extensively over the last decade on prepectoral breast reconstruction—as such, this textbook collates their deep experience so that the reader may accelerate along the learning curve. As plastic surgeons we must constantly innovate in the creative space of reconstruction; however, to do so we must learn from our past and learn from each other. Drs. Raghavan Vidya and Hilton Becker's book *Prepectoral Breast Reconstruction* provides a complete telling of both elements so we can forge a better path into the future for ourselves and for our patients.

December 2022

John Kim MD, FACS
Professor, Division of Plastic and Reconstructive Surgery
Department of Surgery
Northwestern University Feinberg School of Medicine
Northwestern Medicine
Chicago, IL, USA

Preface

Breast cancer is the commonest female cancer globally, and surgery remains one of the main modality forms of treatment. Increase in understanding of the biology has led to advances in treatment. Breast surgery has moved from mutilating surgery of Halsted to oncoplastic and oncoaesthteic surgery combining principles of oncological surgery with restoration of body image.

Breast reconstruction has evolved from complex autologous reconstruction to simple implant-based techniques. The latest in breast reconstructive surgery is the technique of prepectoral breast reconstruction with preservation of normal anatomy. Historically, subcutaneous implant-based reconstructions were associated with poor cosmetic outcome including rippling and visible implant contours. Hence there was a subsequent paradigm shift toward submuscular implant-based breast reconstructions. However over recent years due to problems like animation and prolonged postoperative pain as well as the development of new meshes and implants, prepectoral implant-based reconstructions have once again gained popularity. As techniques have been advancing, there has been a need to provide a concise update on prepectoral breast reconstruction.

This book aims to provide a comprehensive review on prepectoral breast reconstruction with particular emphasis on current trends and techniques. We are grateful for the valuable contribution from this esteemed group of pioneers in the field as well as the early pioneers who preceded us.

The journey to publish this book started more than two years ago and was impacted by the Covid-19 pandemic; nevertheless the dedication and effort of all the contributing authors enabled to complete the book along with the help of the publisher and the editors to whom we are indebted and thankful.

Wolverhampton, UK — Raghavan Vidya
Boca Raton, FL, USA — Hilton Becker

Acknowledgments

As a plastic surgery resident in South Africa, I was fascinated by the way the local Africans were performing tissue expansion on their ears using serial earrings .I was therefore totally receptive to the concept of tissue expansion and particularly the Radovan expanders for breast reconstruction.

I contacted Dr. Radovan who sent me one of his expanders which I used successfully. The expanders were initially placed in the prepectoral plane following modified radical mastectomy.

The submuscular placement of breast implants was advocated as a means of reducing capsular contracture and to add additional coverage to the implant. I found the Radovan expander to be of particular value when total muscular coverage was performed, where the implant could be placed tension free and then slowly expanded postoperatively.

In several cases when it became time to remove the injection port of the Radovan expander, patients were satisfied with their results and did not want to remove the injection port. This led me to develop a saline expander with a detachable injection port and subsequently a double lumen with a silicone outer shell (the Becker 50/50).

Having performed submuscular reconstruction for several years I noticed patients with complaints related to animation deformity, discomfort, and pain. It was at this time that Dr. Loren Eskanazi, who was using the Becker 50/50, informed me that she was placing her implants above the muscle. I saw this as an excellent solution and was indebted to her for going out on a limb. I was, however, concerned about having an incision over the implant; I therefore utilized a dermal flap as well as ADM as a protective layer. I then started performing prepectoral placement of the implant and replacement of submuscular implants to the prepectoral position. I immediately noticed the improvement in those three symptoms and in the overall cosmetic results.

While doing a second residency at the Medical College of Virginia, I was fortunate enough to spend some time doing wound healing with Professor Robert Diegelman. My research revolved around tissue regeneration which I have applied to developing a synthetic, biological scaffold.

I am indebted to my coauthor Dr. Raghavan Vidya firstly for inviting me to the Innovations and Advances in Breast Surgery at the University of Wolverhampton UK in June 2017 where we both presented our experiences on prepectoral breast reconstruction and discussed the need for a book, and for all her input and expertise in bringing this book to fruition.

I am grateful to my referring surgeons and all our contributors for their excellent chapters that will be of immense interest to readers.

My gratitude goes out to my parents who encouraged me to pursue a career in medicine, to my family for supporting me, and to my wife Janet who works as my first assistant and whose help with these surgeries was a major contribution to this project.

With gratitude to the editors at Springer Verlag.

Hilton Becker

Having my roots and initial years of surgical training in India, I was always fascinated with the art and science of plastic surgery, which aimed to restore function and body image. My interest and passion was furthered, and I developed a lifelong sense of purpose alongside the professional knowledge during my years at the renowned Stanley Medical College, with an institutional history of over 300 years and an exemplary set of dedicated and deeply learned faculty such as Prof. CMK Reddy and Prof. Venkataswami. Prof. Nitynanth and Prof. Palanivel instilled in me a determination to pursue nothing less than excellence in surgery during my Master's in General Surgery. I found inspiring mentors during my research stint in Edinburgh breast unit such as Dr. Udi Chetty who instilled an interest in breast surgery and Prof. Mike Dixon who inspired confidence in me often saying "*less is more*." I understood the key concepts of integrating oncological safety with plastic techniques during my oncoplastic fellowship guided by Mr. F Fatah and Mr. G Sterne, each of whom set such exemplary standards which inspire me to this day.

During my early years of surgical practice, I observed that submuscular implant-based reconstructions were very popular, but the muscle had to be disrupted and patients presented with animation deformity and pain. Historically, subcutaneous implant-based reconstructions were associated with high failure rate and poor cosmesis. However, with the innovation of preshaped matrix along with the collaborative work with Dr. Giorgio Berna, Mr. Simon Cawthorn, Prof. J Masia, and other European surgeons we could demonstrate that prepectoral breast reconstruction was the way forward. The incorporation of the technique promoted preservation of anatomy, received good feedback with high patient satisfaction, and mitigated the need for destruction of chest wall musculature. The technique was audited in the UK, Europe, and gradually gained popularity in the Western world.

We have been teaching this technique to colleagues and trainees through cadaveric and live courses. Although the technique is a proven success and continues to further evolve, there is no concise book that explains its concepts. Therefore, I joined with Prof. Becker and eminent global authors to share their techniques and experience in day-to-day clinical practice.

As I glance over the completed manuscript, I feel indebted to thank my family members including my father, late Mr. Raghavan, my mother Annapoorani, my sister Chitra, and brother-in-law Vaidyanthan for always encouraging me to share knowledge and promote innovation. My sincere thanks to my husband Dr. S Venkatachalam and my son Abhinav without whose support and sacrifice (time), this would not be possible.

I would like to thank all the authors who contributed to this book detailing their brilliant surgical techniques. My special thanks to my teachers who have taught me from my school Holy Angles Convent and Adarsh Vidyalaya, India. Finally, my heartfelt and sincere gratitude to my patients and author colleagues without whose participation and efforts this book would not take its current form. Special thanks to Springer Verlag for their support to publish the book.

Raghavan Vidya

Contents

About the Editors

Raghavan Vidya MS, MD, FRCS, is a Senior lecturer at Birmingham University and Consultant Oncoplastic breast surgeon at the Royal Wolverhampton NHS Trust. She graduated from the University of Madras, India, followed by postgraduate training in General Surgery. She completed her MD (Research) on aromatase inhibitors from the University of Edinburgh and higher surgical training in Wessex and West Midlands. Dr. Vidya is a faculty in several national and international meetings and has more than 120 peer-reviewed publications. She has introduced and mentored new innovations including muscle-sparing implant-based breast reconstruction. She produced the report of Future of Surgery of the Royal College of Surgeons as a national member of Association of Breast Surgeons (ABS) Academic Group. She is the lead for the Royal College of Surgeons (RCS) International Surgical Training Programme (ISTP) in Breast Surgery. She is Associate Director of West Midlands Genomic Medicine Service Alliance (GMSA). Dr. Vidya has founded the Virtual Global Breast Hub, to bring together global experts on a single platform. She is actively involved in clinical trials and has a special interest in Oncoplastic Breast Surgery, new technology, and advances in breast surgery. She is an active member of Association of Breast Surgery UK (ABS), European Society of Surgical Oncology (ESSO), Breast Surgery International (BSI), Asian and Indian Society of Breast Surgery.

Hilton Becker is an Adjunct Professor of Surgery at the Charles E. Schmidt College of Medicine, Florida Atlantic University, Boca Raton, Florida and serves as a voluntary faculty member at the Department of Plastic and Reconstructive Surgery at the Cleveland Clinic, Florida.

Dr. Becker received his medical degree from the University of Witwatersrand Johannesburg, South Africa, where he completed his internship and residency in general surgery and plastic surgery. He was elected as a fellow of the Royal College of Surgeons, Edinburgh, Scotland before completing a second residency in plastic surgery at the Medical College of Virginia, USA. He has been engaged in plastic surgery practice since 1981 and is certified by the American Board of Plastic Surgery. A member of numerous regional and national medical societies (American Society of Plastic Reconstructive Surgeons, American Society for Aesthetic Plastic Surgery, American College of Surgeons, and the Royal College of Surgeons-Edinburgh, the International Society of Aesthetic Plastic Surgery, and honorary member of the Association of Plastic Reconstructive Surgeons of Southern Africa).

Dr. Becker also has extensive experience in surgical lecturing and teaching and has published over 100 articles and chapters in surgical textbooks. He is a reviewer for the journal Plastic and Reconstructive Surgery, the Aesthetic Surgery Journal, and the European Journal of Plastic Surgery. He has multiple medical patents on medical devices including the Becker adjustable breast implant, the Becker basket liposuction cannula, and the cutting cannula. He has recently developed the Micronizer a device which reduces the size of fat particles facilitating injection into mastectomy flaps.

List of Videos

Evolution of Pre-Pectoral Breast Reconstruction

1

Hilton Becker, Raghavan Vidya, Oscar Adrian Vazquez, and Simon Cawthorn

1.1 Introduction

In the past few decades, breast reconstructive and plastic surgeons have continued to evolve and develop new techniques in implant-based breast reconstruction. Simultaneous innovations and advancements in implants and biological mesh have enabled successful pre-pectoral or muscle-sparing reconstruction. Reviewing the circle of evolution and timeline from pre-pectoral reconstruction to submuscular reconstruction and back to pre-pectoral implant-based reconstruction renders a thorough understanding of the complications and issues that led to biomedical innovations and advancements in surgical technique to strive for the best cosmetic outcome with minimal morbidity. We review the history of pre-pectoral breast reconstruction.

The original version of the chapter has been revised. A correction to this chapter can be found at https://doi.org/10.1007/978-3-031-15590-1_26

H. Becker
Department of Surgery, Charles E. Schmidt College of Medicine, Boca Raton, FL, USA

Atlantic University, Boca Raton, FL, USA
e-mail: Hilton@beckermd.com

R. Vidya (✉)
Breast Department, The Royal Wolverhampton NHS Trust, Wolverhampton, UK
e-mail: Raghavan.Vidya@nhs.net

O. A. Vazquez
General Surgery, PGY-3, University of Florida, USA

S. Cawthorn
Breast Care Centre, Southmead Hospital, Bristol, UK

1.2 Breast Implants

Breast implants date back to 1951, with the first experiment done by Grindlay and Clagett studying the Ivalon sponge made of polyvinyl alcohol (Beverly Hills Surgical Supply Company) in vivo [1]. Modifications were made to the Ivalon sponge by Pangman, resulting in a new Compound Ivalon Polyethylene prosthesis. Complication profile comprising of significant capsular contracture, breast firmness, and a loss of breast volume was similar with all modifications of the sponges and was seen within a year of implantation [2]. The popularity of breast augmentation surgery declined progressively until 1963 when the silicone gel implant was introduced by Cronin and Gerow [3]. Arion Laboratories then released saline-filled implants in 1965 [4]. With the advent of breast implants, breast reconstruction became possible. Implants were initially placed above the muscle and beneath the mastectomy skin flap in the subcutaneous or "pre-pectoral" space. The complication rate was high, limiting their use [5].

In 1982, Radovan described the use of tissue expansion for breast reconstruction (Radovan expander) [6]. Then, in 1984, Becker developed the adjustable breast implant based on the Radovan concept. Having a detachable injection

© The Author(s), under exclusive license to Springer Nature Switzerland AG 2023, corrected publication 2023
R. Vidya, H. Becker (eds.), *Prepectoral Breast Reconstruction*,
https://doi.org/10.1007/978-3-031-15590-1_1

port meant that the implant could function as a tissue expander and then be converted into a saline implant [7]. The second generation of this implant had an outer lumen of silicone [8]. Tissue expanders with an integral injection port were then developed with gradual skin expansion to replace the tissue lost from mastectomies. This sparked the use and popularity of breast reconstruction using tissue expanders. Since then, several have detailed the use of different textures, sizes, and shapes of tissue expanders. The first breast reconstructions using tissue expanders involved placement of the expander in a subcutaneous pocket, beneath the mastectomy skin, but over the pectoralis major muscle. This subcutaneous approach was a quick and easy technique and preserved the integrity of the pectoralis muscle. However, it was associated with several complications, the most reported being implant malposition, rippling/wrinkling, implant exposure following skin breakdown, and capsular contracture [6].

Pre-pectoral breast reconstruction fell out of favor in the 1970s because it was associated with high rates of postoperative infection, scar tissue buildup, and occasional breast implant exposure. In 1981, the first description of a total submuscular coverage with the partial elevation of the serratus anterior was described in the literature [9]. As the modified radical mastectomy and preservation of the pectoralis major muscle became more common, it was theorized that submuscular breast reconstruction provided an extra layer of tissue for implant coverage. It is believed that implants were placed beneath the muscle due to inadequate soft tissue coverage after mastectomy, because of large mastectomy incisions, and to protect the implant [10].

The advent of Acellular Dermal Matrix (ADM) greatly facilitated the use of the submuscular plane resulting in the most common form of breast reconstruction [11]. Total muscular coverage resulted in tightness and flattening of the implant. It also limited the size of the implant that could be used. In some cases, the lower fascia could not be elevated in contiguity with the muscle flap and in these cases, surgeons would detach the muscle and suture it back into position. This suturing technique was not very stable, so some surgeons resorted to various meshes to secure the muscle flap.

Surgeons started becoming aware of the complications of submuscular placement, particularly animation deformity. This eventually led to surgeons considering the pre-pectoral space again to prevent animation deformity, lessen the pain from the submuscular placement, and avoid chest tightness and muscle spasms [12, 13]. One of the first reports of pre-pectoral breast reconstruction was that of Eskenazi, who reported using an adjustable breast implant placed above the muscle [14]. Since pre-pectoral implant placement was not the standard of care, surgeons proceeded with caution. On an interesting note, a surgeon in the US was sued for pre-pectoral placement, with the allegation being that this was not the standard of care. The surgeon prevailed, which resulted in more interest in this technique.

1.3 Acellular Dermal Matrix (ADM)

The creation of ADM, thanks to advances in biomechanical engineering, provided the means to create a larger pocket under the muscle, which allowed for a larger immediate implant reconstruction to be carried out with a better cosmetic outcome due to improved symmetry and lower pole fullness. This approach was justified by evidence that the ADM prevented capsular contraction over the lower pole of the implant in the subcutaneous plane. The technique required division of the lower insertion of the pectoralis major muscle and suturing of a rectangular piece of ADM graft (up to 20 cm wide and 10 cm long) onto the lower edge of the divided muscle. An appropriately sized and shaped implant was then placed under the muscle, and the ADM was sewn onto the chest wall just above the inframammary fold resulting in the one-stage implant reconstruction. The ADM-enhanced subpectoral implant reconstruction was performed simultaneously as the mastectomy achieved good symmetry with modest ptosis and better projection. However, despite the improved cosmesis, the extensive dissection to elevate the pectoralis major muscle and part of the serratus anterior from their ribcage attachments resulted in the loss of function and damage to the lateral cutaneous branches of the intercostal nerves. This resulted in acute and chronic pain [15]. Additionally, there was a tendency for distortion of the breast shape on muscle contraction resulting in animation deformity of the breast [16].

An Italian company (Decomed) specializing in tissue grafts for surgical reconstruction suggested the next logical step was to preserve the pectoralis muscle, wrap the entire implant in ADM, and place it in the subcutaneous plane. This was done because the ADM was not associated with capsular contracture. This is due to its incorporation into the subcutaneous tissue around the lower pole of a predominantly subpectoral implant. The silicone implant placement on the muscle and not under it wrapped completely in an ADM mesh envelope would give better shape, appearance, and comfort outcomes while lowering the risk of delayed capsular contraction. The shaped ADM mesh was named Braxon, described as a brassiere (B.R.A.) wrapped (X) in ADM and placed on (ON) the muscle.

Berna et al. published the first study of mastectomy with Braxon ADM-assisted immediate pre-pectoral implant reconstruction. They compared a pre-shaped porcine ADM (0.9 mm thick), which required washing out the chemical preservatives in the ADM before implantation, to a thinner ADM (0.6 mm thick), which was chemical preservative-free and only needed rehydration in 25 procedures, with an average follow-up of 14 months [17]. The thinner and chemical-free ADM was chosen (Braxon). The reported implant explantation rate was 12% with the 0.9 mm thick ADM and 0% using the thinner and chemical-free ADM.

In 2017, Vidya et al. published a study showing that pre-pectoral breast reconstruction is safe, feasible, and has good short-term outcomes [18]. The largest multicenter retrospective analysis of the first pre-pectoral breast reconstruction with Braxon ADM has collected the experience of 30 European centers with 1450 procedures collected in 6 years since 2014 [19]. Complications led to implant loss in nearly 6.5% of the cases. Diabetes, smoking, implant weight, and immunosuppression influenced complications. Capsular contracture was associated with postoperative radiotherapy but was low at 2.1%. With the innovation of the first complete implant ADM wrap, what has followed is a transition back to pre-pectoral reconstruction at the time of mastectomy without the postoperative morbidity of pain and capsular contraction. As the switch from submuscular to pre-pectoral reconstruction occurs globally, many other innovative methods to prevent capsular contraction have yet to be thoroughly evaluated.

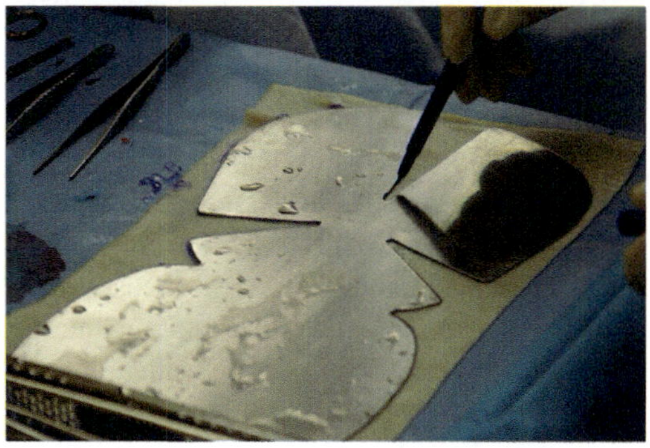

The first pre-shaped Braxon mesh 0.9 mm thick

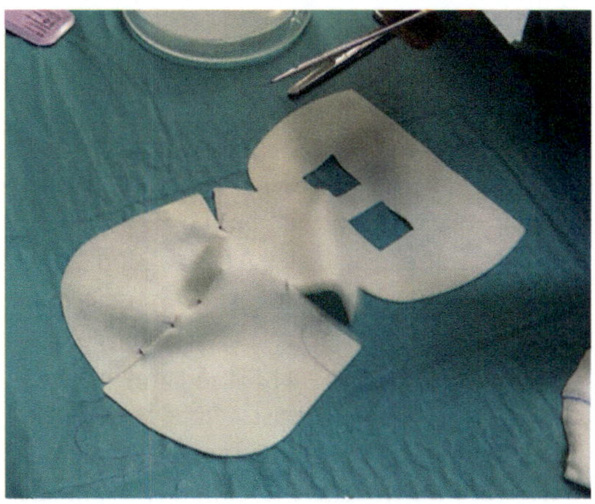

The second pre-shaped Braxon mesh 0.6 mm thick

1.4 Mesh (ADMs) with Implants

Pre-pectoral breast augmentation started becoming more popular and used the fascia that could offer sufficient support for the implant. The elimination of animation in these patients further stimulated interest in the pre-pectoral plane. As opposed to the augmentation patient, in the reconstructive patient, the fascia is absent, and, hence, anterior placement of ADM was found to be a suitable replacement for the fascia. This use of ADM for soft tissue coverage led to pre-pectoral breast reconstruction becoming a more viable alternative [20]. With the advent of skin and nipple-sparing mastectomies, surgeons began performing their mastectomies through inframammary or vertical incisions. With the vertical incision, there was concern about an incision directly above the ADM. One solution offered was de-epithelialization of a portion of the lateral flap, which was tucked under the medial flap since it provided an additional layer above the ADM. In pre-pectoral breast reconstructions, ADMs give some degree of tissue support. The handling of ADM in pre-pectoral breast reconstruction can be achieved either with an anterior wrap method where the ADM is sutured to the upper end/border of the breast pocket, followed by the medial and lateral edges. The implant and the ADM are then sutured inferiorly to allow a snug fit in the breast pocket [21]. The second method allows wrapping the ADM around the implant. This technique was initially described by Sbitany et al. [22]. The ADM is cut to the size of the implant/expander and is sutured to the inframammary fold (IMF). Following this, an implant/expander is placed on the surface of the pectoralis muscle, and the ADM is completely wrapped. The technique has shown higher rates of implant loss, flap necrosis, capsular contracture, rippling, and seroma [23]. A study by Vidya et al. (2017) on 100 breasts demonstrated that pre-pectoral breast reconstruction is safe and feasible, with excellent short-term outcomes, including cosmesis and patient satisfaction [18].

In 2015, Becker proposed that an immediate single-stage pre-pectoral breast reconstruction with a smooth saline adjustable implant, using a vertical incision, in conjunction with mesh/matrix support, can be performed with excellent esthetic outcomes and minimal complications. As pre-pectoral placement resulted in an incision directly over the implant, surgeons used de-epithelialized flaps or a meshed ADM to protect the implant [24]. The vertical incision for mastectomy allowed a portion of the lateral flap to be de-epithelialized, resulting in a more secure water-tight closure. Some considerations were the increased risk of mesh seroma, infection, cost, and longer surgery time [25].

To reduce the rate of seroma formation, the ADM is meshed or fenestrated, allowing for more rapid integration and improved fluid drainage [24]. In Comparison to non-meshed ADM, meshed ADM results in decreased fluid drainage and a shorter time to drain removal [26]. In a study in 2019, types of meshes described by Vidya et al. have ideal properties like minimal inflammation response, faster integration, easy malleability, high strength, and cost-effective [27]. ADM can be fenestrated or formally meshed to increase conformability [28].

Due to the high cost of ADM and increased risk of seroma and infection, surgeons have looked at using synthetic mesh. A study from 2014 by Casella et al. showed that a subcutaneous two-stage reconstruction with a titanium-coated polypropylene synthetic mesh proved safe and feasible. Patient satisfaction was excellent after 14 months of median follow-up from final implant placement [28]. Other meshes used include absorbable mesh (Vicryl) and long-term absorbable mesh (T.I.G.R. Phasix) [12, 29]. A new mesh recently being investigated is a fine monofilament P.D.S. mesh (Durasorb), with the initial studies being encouraging [30].

1.5 Direct-to-Implant Pre-Pectoral Breast Reconstruction

Two-stage implant-based reconstruction remains the most common method of breast reconstruction. A tissue expander or adjustable implant is placed initially and replaced with a fixed volume implant at a second stage. Initially, mastectomies resulted in a shortage of overlying skin necessitating tissue expansion; however, current skin-sparing mastectomy techniques result in sufficient skin availability [31]. In 2019, Jones proposed a single-stage, pre-pectoral direct-to-implant breast reconstruction to be a state-of-the-art breast reconstruction technique and found it safe and reproducible [32].

Pre-pectoral reconstruction was initially performed with optimal flaps, using spy software to verify circulation. This has enabled immediate pre-pectoral breast reconstruction with silicone implants. Polyurethane foam-covered silicone gel-filled breast implants were introduced in the 1970s but were withdrawn from the US market in 1991 due to concerns about possible toxicity. However, they remain popular in other parts of the world. A study in 2006 by Handel showed that these implants resulted in a long-term reduction in the risk of capsular contracture and appeared to have a safety profile similar to other silicone gel-filled devices [33]. A recent study in 2015 by Castel showed an inverse correlation between the amount of polyurethane coating on the implant and the occurrence of capsular contracture [34]. Roy de Vita pioneered the use of polyurethane-coated implants for pre-pectoral reconstruction [35].

1.6 Fat Grafting

Fat has historically been used to treat step-off deformities caused by a marked delineation between the native chest wall and the implant [36]. It has also been commonly used during implant placement after tissue expansion, where delayed fat grafting with injection into the subcutaneous plane superficial to the implant capsule is advantageous. There is some evidence that fat grafting improves chest wall healing and may reverse damage to the soft tissue by stabilizing it during tissue expansion [37].

In suboptimal patients with radiation exposure, thin/fragile skin flaps, significant ptosis, and obesity, immediate single-stage pre-pectoral breast reconstruction is a viable alternative to subpectoral implant placement or delayed procedures. By using a spacer initially, vascular compromise can be averted [38]. Air partially fills the adjustable Breast implant, which then functions as a spacer, preventing the flap from adhering to the underlying muscle and avoiding pressure on the skin flap, particularly the inferior pole where saline accumulates. Contraction results in thickening and elevation of the flap, eliminating the need for skin excision and reducing the need for an acellular dermal matrix. Further, the air is added during the follow-up office visits. Air is then replaced with normal saline when the desired breast size is achieved [31].

A study in 2020 found that in patients with large and ptotic breasts, nipple-sparing mastectomy with pre-pectoral breast reconstruction and immediate mastopexy showed promising results. However, adequate preoperative planning and intraoperative flap assessment are necessary to minimize complications [39].

1.7 Evolution of Pre-Pectoral Breast Reconstruction Timeline

Topic	Author	Year
Pre-Pectoral Saline-filled Tissue Expander [6]	Radovan	1982
Pre-Pectoral Immediate Breast Reconstruction with Becker 50 Implants [14]	Eskenazi	2007
Pre-Pectoral Immediate Breast Reconstruction Using Pre-Shaped Braxon Mesh [17]	Berna	2014
TiLoop Bra Mesh Pre-Pectoral vs Subcutaneous Reconstruction [29]	Casella	2014
Vertical Incision Immediate Pre-Pectoral Reconstruction with Dermal Flap [25]	Becker	2015
Pre-Pectoral Reduction Dermal Flap with ADM [52]	Caputo	2016
Pre-Pectoral Implant-based Reconstruction: Rationale and Indications [40]	Sigalove	2017
Full-Implant Coverage Technique with Braxon [27]	Vidya	2017
Pre-Pectoral Immediate Breast Reconstruction: A Safe Alternative [22]	Sbitany	2017
Air-filled Tissue Expander in Pre-Pectoral Reconstruction [38]	Becker	2017
Pre-pectoral breast reconstruction (review) [21]	Ter Louw	2017
Immediate Pre-Pectoral DTI Reconstruction with Indocyanine Angiography [41]	Jones	2017

Topic	Author	Year
Pre-Pectoral Reconstruction with Bovine ADM [24]	Scheflan	2018
Pre-Pectoral Breast Reconstruction with Vicryl Absorbable Mesh Pocket [12]	Gfrerer	2018
Pre-Pectoral Reconstruction and Tissue Contraction with Underfilled Expander [31]	Becker	2018
Direct-to-Implant Pre-Pectoral Breast Reconstruction [32]	Jones	2019
Direct-to-Implant Polyurethane Pre-Pectoral Breast Reconstruction [35]	de Vita	2019
Review of complications in pre-pectoral reconstruction (review) [13]	Wagner	2019
Pre-Pectoral Breast Reconstruction with Spacer in Sub-Optimal Patients [42]	Becker	2019
Direct-to-Implant Pre-Pectoral Reconstruction Risks [43]	Nealon	2020

1.8 Radiation

Postmastectomy radiotherapy is a risk factor for implant-based reconstruction. It leads to capsular contracture and reconstruction failure [44, 45]. Some studies have quoted higher rates of capsular contracture in the subpectoral group compared to pre-pectoral breast reconstruction following radiotherapy (52.2 versus 16.1%) [45]. With delayed reconstruction, migration of the expander is higher in the dual plane than in the pre-pectoral group following postmastectomy radiation. It occurs due to radiation-induced fibrosis and contraction of the pectoralis major muscle, which causes displacement which is not seen in Pre-pectoral breast reconstruction.

1.9 Benefits of Pre-Pectoral Breast Reconstruction

The most clinical benefit of pre-pectoral breast reconstruction appears to be the significantly lower associated pain with lower use of intravenous and oral postoperative opioids and analgesics [28, 40]. Several early retrospective articles appear to show such an advantage. This seems directly related to the lower dissection associated with this technique, especially as it relates to the lack of need for submuscular dissection and rearrangement of soft tissues. Given the current healthcare climate surrounding increased opioid abuse and its present crisis, the decreased use of these medications should benefit patient safety and the overall social environment [46]. Early studies surrounding pre-pectoral breast reconstruction appear to show a benefit of decreased length of hospital stay from approximately 2–3 days to 1–2 days on average [40, 47]. Several authors have shown a significant decrease in actual operative time when looking at the specific varied techniques of pre-pectoral breast reconstruction outlined earlier in this supplement. This probably results from the ability to prepare the tissue expander or implant with the ADM in some instances on the back table while the mastectomy is still taking place. In addition, preparing a subpectoral pocket also contributes to decreased surgical time. Long-term benefits include the absence of animation deformity, reduced chest wall discomfort and pain, and fewer adverse effects on shoulder movement and joint problems [48].

1.10 Complications Specific to Pre-Pectoral Breast Reconstruction

Capsular contracture is the most typical complication following the procedure and accounts for nearly 9% of a recent review of pre-pectoral breast reconstruction complications. The capsular contracture rate with ADM decreased to around 2% compared to 12% in the non-ADM group. ADM is also associated with a condition referred to as red breast syndrome, which accounts for nearly 6–7%. This is characterized by erythema directly overlying the ADM and is thought to be secondary to lymphedema and lymphatic obstruction. The use of ADM correlated with a higher implant loss rate, infection, and mastectomy skin flap necrosis [13]. Red Breast Syndrome is usually treated conservatively and tends to settle with time. However, prolonged red breast syndrome is sometimes treated with ADM removal and the implant [49].

Flap or nipple necrosis can present with a complication in pre-pectoral breast reconstruction and is usually due to direct pressure on thin compromised skin flaps, impairing the perfusion, and with this overlying soft tissue, coverage loss can result in reconstruction failure [43]. This can be prevented by using intraoperative viability techniques to check skin circulation using indocyanine green tissue perfusion assessment.

Infection is often a concern during implant-based breast reconstruction and can lead to implant loss. This can be treated with antibiotics, minimal theater personnel, and cavity washings. The large subcutaneous pocket left before reconstruction opens up the possibility for hematoma or seroma formation postoperatively. Adequate hemostasis and drain placement help mitigate these risks [13].

Implant rippling, usually noticed at the upper pole, given thinner, soft tissue coverage, can be seen more commonly in pre-pectoral reconstruction as compared to submuscular reconstruction. However, newer implants with a full shell volume show less rippling [22]. In two-stage pre-pectoral reconstruction, the tissue expanders or adjustable implants should ideally be underfilled to the anticipated final implant size to reduce complications such as rippling. The rippling effect can be avoided or reduced by using fat grafting to the upper pole of the mastectomy flap and/or by using ADM or synthetic mesh [47]. Sometimes it is vital to counsel patients undergoing immediate, direct-to-implant pre-pectoral reconstruction that they may need a second procedure such as fat grafting to cover the implant and reduce rippling and implant visibility.

1.11 Conclusion

Breast reconstruction has evolved from the traditional submuscular to the new pre-pectoral implant-based or muscle-sparing reconstruction. With the realization of the complications associated with submuscular implant placement, pre-pectoral breast reconstruction has evolved with several modified techniques and procedures, leading to the current pre-pectoral success. The invention of breast implants has allowed for breast augmentation and breast reconstruction.

References

1. Grindlay JH, Waugh JM. Plastic sponge which acts as a framework for living tissue. Arch Surg. 1951;63:288–97. https://doi.org/10.1001/archsurg.1951.01250040294003.
2. Pangman WJ, Wallace RM, Hills B. The use of plastic prosthesis in breast plastic and other soft tissue surgery. West J Surg Obstet Gynecol. 1955;63:503–12.
3. Cronin T, Gerow FG. Augmentation mammaplasty: a new natural feel prosthesis. Transact III Internat Congr Plast Surg. 1964;51(2):41–9. https://doi.org/10.1016/S0039-6109(16)39388-4.
4. Arion HG. Retromammary prosthesis. C R Soc Fr Gynecol. 1965;5
5. Peters W. The evolution of breast implants. Can J Plast Surg. 2002;10(5):223–36.
6. Radovan C. Breast reconstruction after mastectomy using the temporary expander. Plast Reconstr Surg. 1982;69(2):195–208. https://doi.org/10.1097/00006534-198202000-00001.
7. Becker H. Breast reconstruction using an inflatable breast implant with detachable reservoir. Plast Reconstr Surg. 1984;73(4):678–83. https://doi.org/10.1097/00006534-198404000-00031. PMID: 6709750
8. Becker H. The expandable mammary implant. Plast Reconstr Surg. 1987;79(4):631–7.
9. Apfelberg DB, Laub DR, Maser MR, Lash H. Submuscular breast reconstruction—indications and techniques. Ann Plast Surg. 1981;7(3):213–21.
10. Glasberg SB, Light D. AlloDerm and Strattice in breast reconstruction: a comparison and techniques for optimising outcomes. Plast Reconstr Surg. 2012;129:1223–33. https://doi.org/10.1097/PRS.0b013e31824ec429.
11. Bloom JA, Patel K, Cohen S, Chatterjee A, Homsy C. Prepectoral breast reconstruction: an overview of the history, technique, and reported complications. Open Access Surg. 2020;13:1–9. https://doi.org/10.2147/OAS.S201298.
12. Gfrerer L, Liao EC. Technique refinement in prepectoral implant breast reconstruction with vicryl mesh pocket and acellular dermal matrix support. Plast Reconstr Surg Glob Open. 2018;6(4):e1749. https://doi.org/10.1097/GOX.0000000000001749. Published 2018 Apr 9
13. Wagner RD, Braun TL, Huirong Z, Winocour S. A systematic review of complications in prepectoral breast reconstruction. J Plast Reconstr Aesthet Surg. 2019;72(7):1051–9. https://doi.org/10.1016/j.bjps.2019.04.005.

14. Eskenazi LB. New options for immediate reconstruction: achieving optimal results with adjustable implants in a single stage. Plast Reconstr Surg. 2007;119:28–37.
15. Ducic I, Seiboth LA, Iorio ML. Chronic postoperative breast pain: danger zones for nerve injuries. Plast Reconstr Surg. 2011;127:41–6.
16. Spear SL, Schwartz J, Dayan JH, Clemens MW. Outcome assessment of breast distortion following submuscular breast augmentation. Aesthet Plast Surg. 2009;33:44–8.
17. Berna G, Cawthorn SJ, Papaccio G, Balestrieri N. Evaluation of a novel breast reconstruction technique using the Braxon® acellular dermal matrix: a new muscle-sparing breast reconstruction. ANZ J Surg. 2014;87(6):493–8. https://doi.org/10.1111/ans.12849. Epub 2014 Sep 29
18. Vidya R, Masia J, Cawthorn S, et al. Evaluation of the effectiveness of the prepectoral breast reconstruction with Braxon dermal matrix: first multicenter European report on 100 cases. Breast J. 2017;23(6):670–6. https://doi.org/10.1111/tbj.12810.
19. Masià J, iBAG Working Group. The largest multicentre data collection on prepectoral breast reconstruction: The iBAG study. J Surg Oncol. 2020;122(5):848–60.
20. Antony AK, Poirier J, Madrigano A, Kopkash KA, Robinson EC. Evolution of the surgical technique for "breast in a day" direct-to-implant breast reconstruction: transitioning from dual-plane to prepectoral implant placement. Plast Reconstr Surg. 2019;143(6):1547–56. https://doi.org/10.1097/PRS.0000000000005627.
21. Ter Louw RP, Nahabedian MY. Prepectoral breast reconstruction. Plast Reconstr Surg. 2017;140:51S–9S. https://doi.org/10.1097/PRS.0000000000003942.
22. Sbitany H, Piper M, Lentz R. Prepectoral breast reconstruction: a safe alternative to submuscular prosthetic reconstruction following nipple-sparing mastectomy. Plast Reconstr Surg. 2017;140(3):432–43. https://doi.org/10.1097/PRS.0000000000003627.
23. Nadeem R. Prepectoral implant-based breast reconstruction complete acellular dermal matrix wrap or anterior circumferential cover. Breast J. 2018;24(2):223–4. https://doi.org/10.1111/tbj.12881. Epub 2017 Aug 1. PMID: 28763153
24. Scheflan M, Grinberg-Rashi H, Hod K. Bovine acellular dermal matrix in immediate breast reconstruction: a retrospective, observational study with SurgiMend. Plast Reconstr Surg. 2018;141:1e–10e.
25. Becker H, Lind JG 2nd, Hopkins EG. Immediate implant-based prepectoral breast reconstruction using a vertical incision. Plast Reconstr Surg Glob Open. 2015;3(6):e412. https://doi.org/10.1097/GOX.0000000000000384. Published 2015 Jul 8
26. Fabrizio T, Serio S, Massariello D, Vestita M, Simeon V. The meshed biological matrix in immediate, definitive breast reconstruction. J Plast Reconstr Aesthet Surg. 2019;72(1):137–71. https://doi.org/10.1016/j.bjps.2018.09.004. Epub 2018 Sep 23. PMID: 30291046
27. Vidya R, Iqbal FM. A guide to prepectoral breast reconstruction: a new dimension to implant-based breast reconstruction. Clin Breat Cancer. 2017;17(4):266–71. https://doi.org/10.1016/j.clbc.2016.11.009. Epub 2017 Jan 9. P.M.I.D.: 28190760
28. Vidya R, Berna G, Sbitany H, et al. Prepectoral implant-based breast reconstruction: a joint consensus guide from U.K., European and U.S.A. breast and plastic reconstructive surgeons. Ecancermedicalscience. 2019, 13:927. Published 2019 May 7. https://doi.org/10.3332/ecancer.2019.927.
29. Casella D, Bernini M, Bencini L, et al. TiLoop® bra mesh used for immediate breast reconstruction: comparison of retro pectoral and subcutaneous implant placement in a prospective single-institution series. Eur J Plast Surg. 2014;37(11):599–604. https://doi.org/10.1007/s00238-014-1001-1.
30. Becker H, Lind JG. The use of synthetic mesh in reconstructive, revision, and cosmetic breast surgery. Aesthetic Plast Surg. 2013;37:914–21. https://doi.org/10.1007/s00266-013-0171-8.
31. Becker H, Zhadan O. Tissue contraction-a new paradigm in breast reconstruction. Plast Reconstr Surg Glob Open. 2018;6(7):e1865. Published 2018 Jul 13. https://doi.org/10.1097/GOX.0000000000001865.
32. Jones G, Antony AK. Single-stage, direct-to-implant prepectoral breast reconstruction. Gland Surg. 2019;8(1):53–60. https://doi.org/10.21037/gs.2018.10.08.
33. Handel N, Gutierrez J. Long-term safety and efficacy of polyurethane foam-covered breast implants. Aesthet Surg J. 2006;26(3):265–74. https://doi.org/10.1016/j.asj.2006.04.001. P.M.I.D.: 19338905
34. Castel N, Soon-Sutton T, Deptula P, Flaherty A, Parsa FD. Polyurethane-coated breast implants revisited: a 30-year follow-up. Arch Plast Surg. 2015;42(2):186–93. https://doi.org/10.5999/aps.2015.42.2.186. Epub 2015 Mar 16. PMID: 25798390; PMCID: PMC4366700
35. De Vita R, Buccheri EM, Villanucci A, Pozzi M. Breast reconstruction actualized in nipple-sparing mastectomy and direct-to-implant, prepectoral polyurethane positioning: early experience and preliminary results. Clin Breast Cancer. 2019;19(2):e358–63. https://doi.org/10.1016/j.clbc.2018.12.015. Epub 2018 Dec 27. P.M.I.D.: 30691930
36. Kanchwala SK, Glatt BS, Conant EF, Bucky LP. Autologous fat grafting to the reconstructed breast: the management of acquired contour deformities. Plast Reconstr Surg. 2009;124(2):409–18. https://doi.org/10.1097/PRS.0b013e3181aeeadd. P.M.I.D.: 19644255
37. Hammond DC, O'Connor EA, Scheer JR. Total envelope fat grafting: a novel approach in breast reconstruction. Plast Reconstr Surg. 2015;135(3):691–4. https://doi.org/10.1097/PRS.0000000000000968.
38. Becker H, Zhadan O. Filling the spectrum expander with air-a new alternative. Plast Reconstr Surg Glob Open. 2017;5(10):e1541. Published 2017 Oct 25. https://doi.org/10.1097/GOX.0000000000001541.

39. Manrique OJ, Arif C, Banuelos J, Abu-Ghname A, Martinez-Jorge J, Tran NV. Prepectoral breast reconstruction in nipple-sparing mastectomy with immediate mastopexy. Ann Plast Surg. 2020;85(1):18–23. https://doi.org/10.1097/SAP.0000000000002136. P.M.I.D.: 31855861
40. Sigalove S, Maxwell GP, Sigalove NM, Storm-Dickerson TL, Pope N, Rice J, Gabriel A. Prepectoral implant-based breast reconstruction: rationale, indications, and preliminary results. Plast Reconstr Surg. 2017;139(2):287–94. https://doi.org/10.1097/PRS.0000000000002950. P.M.I.D.: 28121858
41. Jones G, Yoo A, King V, et al. Prepectoral immediate direct-to-implant breast reconstruction with anterior AlloDerm coverage. Plast Reconstr Surg. 2017;140(6S):31S–8S. https://doi.org/10.1097/PRS.0000000000004048.
42. Becker H, Mathew PJ. Immediate prepectoral breast reconstruction in suboptimal patients using an air-filled spacer. Plast Reconstr Surg Glob Open. 2019;7(10):e2470. https://doi.org/10.1097/GOX.0000000000002470. PMID: 31772895; PMCID: PMC6846304
43. Nealon KP, Weitzman RE, Sobti N, Gadd M, Specht M, Jimenez RB, Ehrlichman R, Faulkner HR, Austen WG Jr, Liao EC. Prepectoral direct-to-implant breast reconstruction: safety outcome endpoints and delineation of risk factors. Plast Reconstr Surg. 2020;145(5):898e–908e. https://doi.org/10.1097/PRS.0000000000006721. PMID: 32332523
44. Elswick SM, Harless CA, Bishop SN, Schleck CD, Mandrekar J, Reusche RD, Mutter RW, Boughey JC, Jacobson SR, Lemaine V. Prepectoral implant-based breast reconstruction with postmastectomy radiation therapy. Plast Reconstr Surg. 2018;142(1):1–12. https://doi.org/10.1097/PRS.0000000000004453. P.M.I.D.: 29878988
45. Sinnott CJ, Persing SM, Pronovost M, Hodyl C, McConnell D, Young AO. Impact of postmastectomy radiation therapy in prepectoral versus subpectoral implant-based breast reconstruction. Ann Surg Oncol. 2018;25(10):2899–908. https://doi.org/10.1245/s10434-018-6602-7.
46. Glasberg SB. The economics of Prepectoral breast reconstruction. Plast Reconstr Surg. 2017;140:49S–52S. https://doi.org/10.1097/PRS.0000000000004051.
47. Salibian AA, Frey JD, Choi M, Karp NS. Subcutaneous implant-based breast reconstruction with acellular dermal matrix/mesh: a systematic review. Plast Reconstr Surg Glob Open. 2016;4(11):e1139.
48. Kim SE. Prepectoral breast reconstruction. Yeungnam Univ J Med. 2019;36(3):201–7. https://doi.org/10.12701/yujm.2019.00283.
49. Nahabedian MY. Prosthetic breast reconstruction and red breast syndrome: demystification and a review of the literature. Plast Reconstr Surg. 2019;7(5):e2108. https://doi.org/10.1097/GOX.0000000000002108.

2 Anatomy of the Breast

Robert D. Rehnke

2.1 Introduction

Historically, there have been different sources of wisdom and knowledge. *Archival* wisdom, truth handed down by respected sages such as Hippocrates and Galen were responsible for most of the medical knowledge before the Renaissance, and they were not questioned. Andreas Vesalius is thought of as the father of modern medicine because he studied human anatomy by looking for himself. In 1543, he published his work in the book, De Humani Corporis Fabrica Libri Septem [1]. This sort of empirical knowledge, gained by observation and experience, became the scientific basis of modern medicine. The knowledge possessed by surgeons is a combination of all of the above: patriarchal wisdom handed down to us from schooling and books; and first-hand empirical knowledge we develop by observation and experience. We need both to confront a topic as complicated as human anatomy. We observe through the lens of a paradigm, in order to make sense of the overwhelming raw data the human body presents. The following description of breast anatomy is analyzed through a new paradigm called the superficial fascia system of the breast. This chapter will be a combination of archival knowledge, referencing text and journal articles, and empirical knowledge I have gained over the last 30 plus years, supported be video evidence from my operating room.

Verbally describing anatomy is a complex and difficult task. This introduction uses an analogy to describe the organizing anatomic principles of breast anatomy, which can act as a support structure for more detailed information. Breast organization is like down pillow, with its feathers (the cells of ectodermal origin) contained in a zippered casing (the corpus mammae with its capsule), held within a "superficial fascia pillow-case" lying on a mattress covered by a sheet. The incased corpus mammae is located inside of a cloth pillowcase, which represents the layers of superficial fascia that surround it. The pillow in the pillowcase lies on the mattress, which is the chest muscles covered by a "sheet" of deep fascia. The frame of the bed, which holds up the mattress is the rib cage. Video 2.1 demonstrates this analogy.

Supplementary Information The online version contains supplementary material available at https://doi.org/10.1007/978-3-031-15590-1_2. The videos can be accessed individually by clicking the DOI link in the accompanying figure caption or by scanning this link with the SN More Media App.

R. D. Rehnke (✉)
Private Practice Plastic Surgery, The Center for Surgical Excellence, St. Petersburg, FL, USA

© The Author(s), under exclusive license to Springer Nature Switzerland AG 2023
R. Vidya, H. Becker (eds.), *Prepectoral Breast Reconstruction*,
https://doi.org/10.1007/978-3-031-15590-1_2

2.2 The Superficial Fascia System of the Breast

2.2.1 The Basic Body Segment

At the beginning of the third week after conception, the embryonic disk forms in the blastula stage and has three layers: ectoderm, mesoderm, and endoderm—the so-called germ layers [2]. By the end of the third week, the embryonic disc now resembles a tubular structure with the same three germ layers, with a cephalic end, caudal end, dorsal side (with neural tube), and ventral side (with a primitive foregut, midgut, and hindgut). About this time, the mesoderm forms paired plates that lie on either side of the dorsal longitudinal embryonic axis. This mesoderm then becomes segmented into mesodermic somites, running from the cephalic to caudal poles. If not for the rapidly growing brain and heart, the embryo would look like a worm. It is from this abstracted basic tubular form that the concept of a "basic body segment" can be derived and is useful in understanding anatomic arrangements. As differentiation takes place, limbs and organs form according to their position along the segmented tube. For instance, the breasts develop from cells inhabiting the ventral surface of the cephalic end of the basic body segment. On the large-scale perspective, the thorax is tubular. In a more myopic view, it seems that the anterior chest wall and breast start as a flat plane. Didactic knowledge of how embryonic tissues develop can inform us about the arrangement of the adult organ; while empirical knowledge of the adult breast informs us about previously unseen embryonic development. In this case, it is helpful to remember that the abdomen and thorax derive from the same basic body segment pattern, making many structures in the chest analogues of structures in the abdomen—which is a simpler version of the thorax. For instance, the chest is like the abdominal wall but has a boney sternum at its ventral midline instead of the linea alba. On either side of the abdominal midline are the paired rectus abdominis muscles, which in the chest are the pectoral muscles (with their insertions pulled out into the upper extremity). Finally, the analogues of the oblique muscles of the abdomen have ribs interspersed among them in the chest.

Soft tissue between the skin and deep muscle fascia, in the abdomen and chest, is arranged in stacked horizontal layers or lamina, which are prevented from shearing apart by vertical cutaneous ligaments, sometimes called the retinacula cutis or superficial retinaculum. In the breast, these retinacula cutis are known as "Cooper's ligaments" [3]. We are all familiar with the more famous horizontal layers of superficial fascia in the abdomen, named Camper's and Scarpa's fascia. The anterior and posterior lamella superficial fascia in the chest are analogs of these layers [4]. What is not widely known is that there are multiple stacked horizontal layers of superficial fascia. Their arrangement can be described as a fractal, since the same primary organization of tissue and cells can be seen in the same, self-similar subsets or patterns, as illustrated in successive magnifications, at the mesoscopic level. Depending on location in the body, specific layers are thicker, due to functional needs, and have names. While in other areas of the body, these layers go unnoticed, ignored, and unknown [5]. This arrangement of sheets of fascia and cells arranged in horizontal layers, held together by a vertical retinaculum (whose fibers run at 90 degrees to the horizontal planes), is reminiscent of quilted fabric. This concept of the superficial fascia was first described by Vesalius when he described the superficial fascia system as the "fleshy membrane." Vesalius stated that the fleshy membrane ran throughout the body between skin and muscle. In the chest, it contained the breast gland. He introduced the topic of the breast with the statement, "We could now show the *fabric* of the breast…" [1].

The renaissance mind comprehended the human anatomy as a continuous interwoven fabric, unlike our nineteenth and twentieth century reductionist concepts. It would take Sir Astley

Cooper's seminal text on breast anatomy, published in 1842, to describe the superficial fascia system in greater detail. Cooper described, "the skin covered with hairs; fat and ligamenta suspensoria placed beneath it; the anterior and posterior fascia with the gland between them…". These ligamenta suspensoria that Cooper described were the vertical retinaculum, which were later named, "Cooper's ligaments." His atlas still contains some of the most accurate illustrations of the breast [6]. He, however, failed to describe or illustrate the perimeter of these fascial boundaries of the breast and how exactly they attach to the deep fascia and chest.

[The superficial fascia system of the breast describes a biologic tensegrity system. Orthopedic surgeon, Stephen Levin first conceived of *biotensegrity* to explain nature's design of the musculoskeletal system. Biotensegrity has taken nearly 40 years to catch on, but it is an accurate approximation of breast construction, and also goes a long way to describing the physics and geometry of self-organizing biologic systems {see *Constructal Law:* (https://www.youtube.com/watch?v=tgEBTPee9ZM).}

Buckminster Fuller, who invented the geodesic dome, coined the term tensegrity in the 1950s, as a system characterized by a continuous network of tension, acting on a discontinuous set of compressible elements. Tensegrity sounds complicated until one realizes that tensegrity systems are all around us; for instance, bubble wrap is a continuous tensioned network of plastic, which acts on a discontinuous set of compressible air bubbles. Levin, in the 1980s, suggested that tensegrity did a better job of explaining the musculoskeletal system than did classical mechanics. The superficial fascia system, with its tensioned, stacked horizontal sheets of fascia and vertical retinaculum, acting on a discontinuous set of fat lobules, almost exactly approximates bubble wrap. It provides not only a similar protective function, but also thermal, metabolic, paracrine, and regenerative functions. In the twenty-first century, Scarr has used tensegrity models to explain the physics of biologic structures [7], a concept first described by D'Arcy Thompson in 1917 [8]. {Guimberteau presented his model of tensegrity at the loose areolar connective tissue level, which he called a multimicrovacuolar collagenic dynamic system (https://www.youtube.com/watch?v=eW0lvOVKDxE).}].

2.2.2 The Corpus Lamina

One of the essential layers of the superficial fascia is the corpus lamina (Fig. 2.1). We described it as a layer of horizontal superficial fascia which runs between Cooper's anterior and posterior layer. It is the layer in which the breast gland, or corpus mammae, develops. It is the target within the embryonic mammary fat pad, into which the invaginating ectodermal cells migrate. As the female breast develops, this two-dimensional sheet of fascia expands into a three-dimensional macroscopic structure, whereas the undeveloped male breast remains relatively two dimensional, See Video 2.2. The corpus lamina continues beyond the breast as a two-dimensional sheet of superficial fascia, seen after a mastectomy or breast reduction removes the three-dimensional corpus mammae Video 2.3.

This intermediate layer of superficial fascia is also present in the abdomen, as the basic body segment reasoning would predict, but is easy to miss without careful dissection, see Video 2.4. Plate II of Cooper's book, "*On the Anatomy of the Breast*" which shows the development of the female breast [6], clearly illustrates the transition between the early embryonic breast bud and the developing corpus mammae. The immature corpus resembles a turned over shiitake mushroom, with the stem pointing up towards the areola, before maturing into the adult form, which is three dimensionally expanded into the familiar frustoconical shape, caused by the branching growth of the ductal lobular system, reminiscent of inflorescence seen in plant growth. The overlying SFS and skin round out the shape into the convex, hemispherical shape, of the young adult breast, see Video 2.5. Further growth and enlargement, followed by involution, seen in the multiparous woman, lead to a less projecting corpus, and relaxed SFS / skin envelope, which accounts for the breast ptosis of maturity.

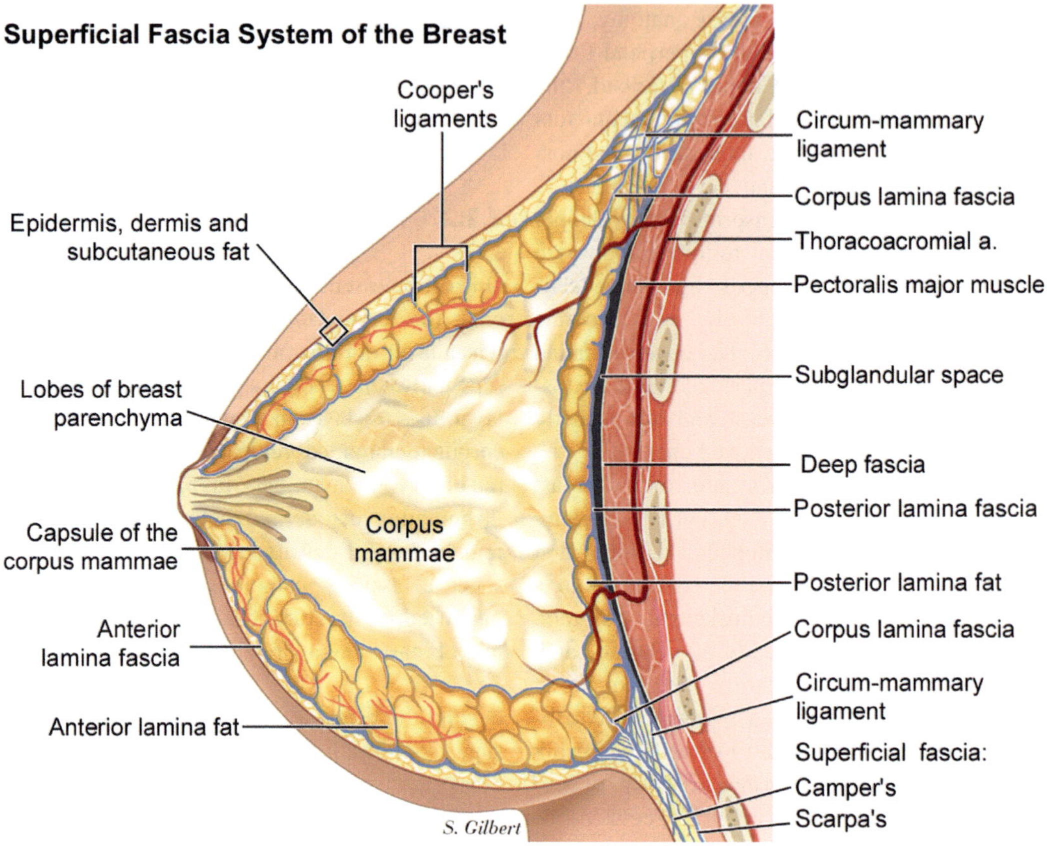

Fig. 2.1 The superficial fascia of the breast, showing the important layers: anterior, posterior, and corpus lamina. (Courtesy of Susan Gilbert, 2020, All rights retained)

2.2.3 Anterior and Posterior Lamina

The SFS is composed of the anterior and posterior lamella fascia, with the corpus lamina in between. The anterior lamella fat layer and posterior lamella fat layer lie on either side of the corpus mammae (Figs. 2.2 and 2.3). The superficial retinaculum is a system of fascial fibers that runs from the posterior lamella fascia, up through the stacked sheets of horizontal superficial fascia. Its wispy fibers are seen as one dissects through the posterior lamella fat; by the time it has passed through the corpus mammae and exited out its anterior surface, it has taken on a three-dimensional cupped shape, like an egg carton. The lobules of anterior lamella fat sit, like eggs, in this retinaculum known as Cooper's ligaments. They continue on at 90 degrees, passing through the delicate anterior lamella fascia, and insert into the dermis. Some Cooper's ligaments are more developed than others and have dense bases that fuse with extensions of the anterior capsule of the corpus mammae, known as peripheral pyramidal processes [9]. Within their bases lie the most peripherally situated end terminal ductal lobular units of the breast parenchyma. Between the anterior lamella fascia and the skin is an even layer of subcutaneous fat, roughly two to three millimeters thick. The anterior lamella fat layer varies in thickness between individuals, depending on the person's percent body fat. It, however, is always thicker at the peripheral base of the breast and gradually decreases in thickness as it approaches the edge of the areola. There is no fat under the nipple-areola, where the corpus mammae breaks through an opening in the anterior lamella fat, called the anterior lamellar annulus, and penetrates the nipple, see Video 2.6. The

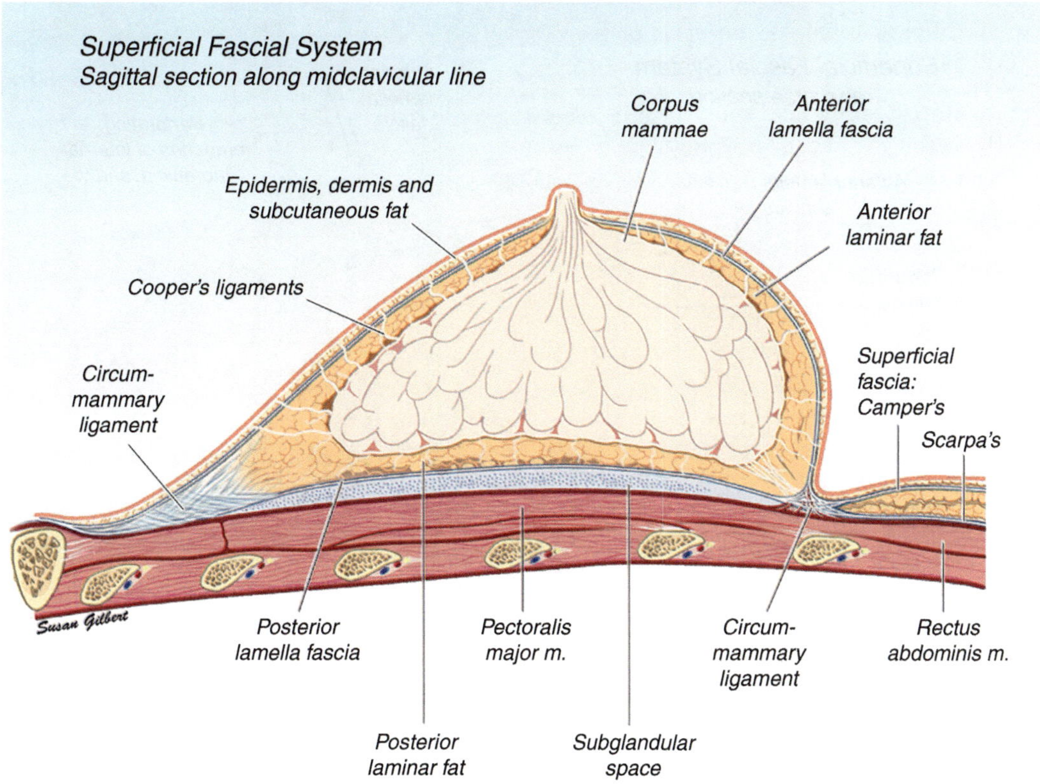

Fig. 2.2 Sagittal view of anterior and posterior superficial fascia and fat layers. (Courtesy of Susan Gilbert, 2020, All rights retained)

15–20 lactiferous ducts gather here, amongst dense connective tissue, and enlarge in collecting sinuses before narrowing again and penetrating the nipple skin. When one performs skin and nipple-sparing mastectomy, a surgical plane can be sharply dissected between the corpus mammae and smooth muscle fibers on the deep surface of the areolar dermis. The lactiferous ducts, however, must be transected, distal to the sinuses, in order to release the corpus from the overlying skin envelope (Fig. 2.4). The dense, white capsule of the corpus mammae, with its anterior surface of pyramidal processes and Cooper's ligaments, is distinct from the adjacent yellow anterior and posterior lamella fat (Fig. 2.5).

The deep surface of the capsule of the corpus is smooth in comparison, and if one is not attentive, the superficial retinaculum entering its deep surface will not be seen. In the larger, involuted breast of some older women, the capsule is not as noticeable, and once cut through, it can be hard to delineate anterior or posterior lamina fat from the stromal fat within the corpus mammae. In such difficult cases, it is easy to see the breast as one globe of fat without its anatomic compartments. All of the parts are most assuredly there, just nuanced. Usually, the deep surface of the capsule is thicker, and the peripheral edges are more distinct, with a nubby "live edge" of peripheral pyramidal processes. Frequently, dissection in the posterior lamella fat (assisted by traction and counter traction) enters one of the horizontal planes of superficial fascia, allowing for a clean separation which exposes the intact and bare deep capsule of the corpus mammae. Deep to the posterior lamella fat layer (which is quite thin in comparison to the anterior lamella fat layer) is the posterior lamella fascia. The posterior lamella fascia is much thicker and more robust than the anterior lamella fascia. The comparable thickness is reminiscent of the thickness of Camper's and Scarpa's fascia, in the abdomen. Between the

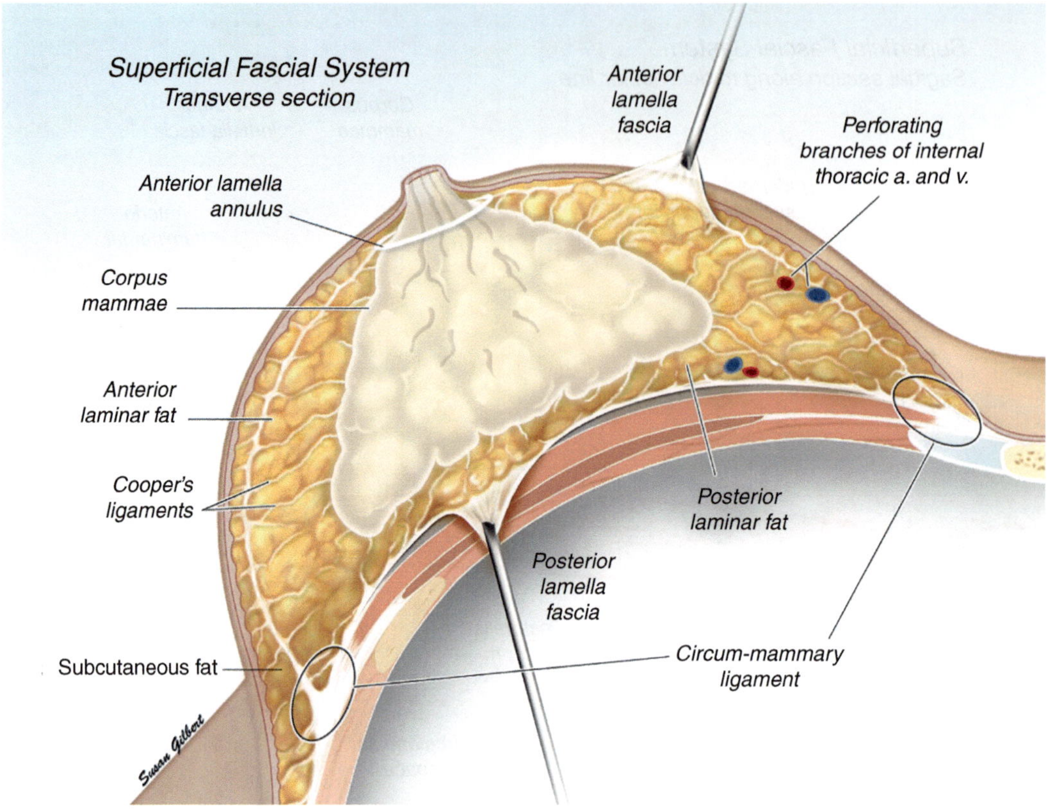

Fig. 2.3 Axial view of anterior and posterior superficial fascia and fat layers. (Courtesy of Susan Gilbert, 2020, All rights retained)

posterior lamella fascia and deep fascia of the pectoralis major, lies the retro-mammary space or bursa. It is a potential space known as a fascial cleft, which allows for some shearing movement of the breast over the underlying chest wall. In all but the most obese women, there is no fat present in this deep, loose areolar connective tissue, unlike the abdomen (below Scarpa's fascia), where it is a region of localized fat storage.

2.2.4 Circum-mammary Ligament

The superficial fascia system fuses to the underlying deep fascia compartment, at certain *zones of adhesion* [10]. This concept, seen throughout the body, is credited to Lockwood. He said it "is responsible for the topographic landmarks, where localized fatty deposits create bulges adjacent to thin tight connections responsible for the creases, folds, and valleys of the soft tissue" [11, 12]. Abdominal creases and folds in the inguinal region always separate the trunk and lower extremity, no matter the degree of obesity. The semi-lunar lines, abdominal midline, and inscriptions over the rectus muscles, commonly known as a "six-pack," are only seen in very thin, muscular people. Careful reflection in the chest shows the semi-lunar line of the abdomen extends along the lateral border of the breast, and the midline of the abdomen continues to define the cleavage between the breast. The crease below the breast, known as the inframammary fold, is an inscription that separates the rectus from the pectoralis. Faintest of these adhesions is the inscription above the breast, which indicates the separation between the sternocostal head of the pectoralis major from the sternoclavicular pectoral head. Above this upper breast inscription, supernumerary breast development can rarely take place along the path of the "milk line" running to the axilla, see Video 2.7. As the breast enlarges and

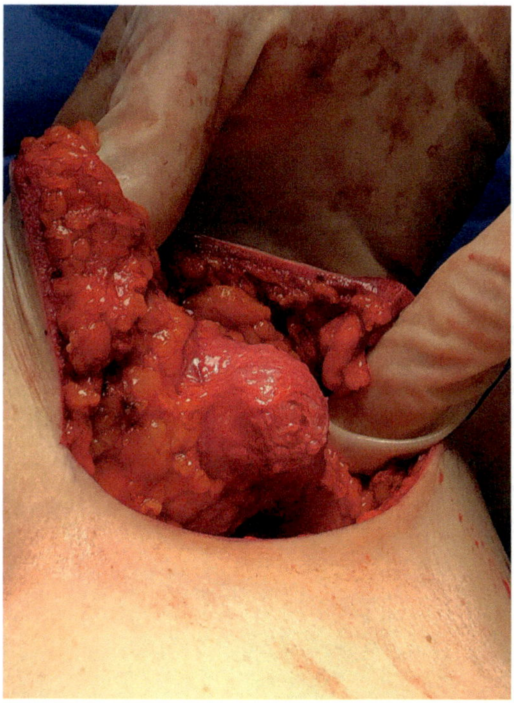

Fig. 2.4 View of the Anterior Lamella Annulus, from an inverted "T" incision, at the completion of resection of the corpus mammae. Note the absence of subcutaneous fat and exposure of smooth muscle, deep to the areolar dermis. The stumps of the lactiferous ducts are seen centrally penetrating the everted nipple. (Courtesy of Robert Rehnke, 2020, All rights retained)

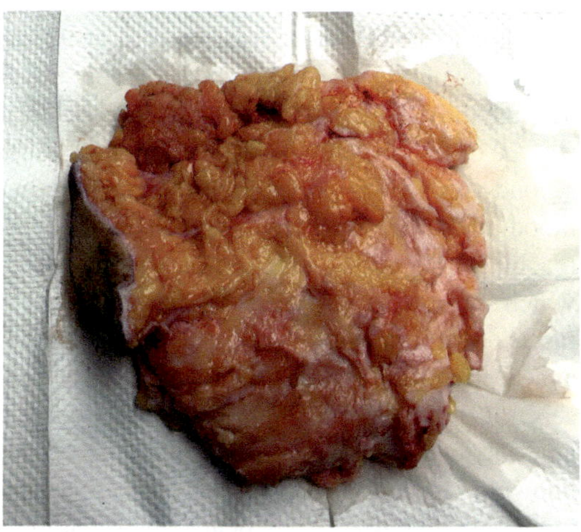

Fig. 2.5 Mastectomy specimen seen after resection of the entire corpus mammae, through an elliptical excision of skin, anterior lamella fascia and fat, over the region of the tumor, in the upper, outer quadrant of the right breast. Note the uneven anterior surface, due to Copper's ligaments, and the rough, natural edge peripherally. (Courtesy of Robert Rehnke, 2020, All rights retained)

matures, this rhomboidal zone of adhesion between the superficial and deep fascia becomes curvilinear and teardrop-shaped, with the sharp tail end pointing to the axilla (Fig. 2.6).

We have called this circular zone of adhesion, the circum-mammary ligament [4]. These findings have been confirmed by a cadaver dissection study published by Gaskin, Peoples, and McGhee [13]. It is not uniform in thickness, like a hula hoop, but instead varies in diameter like an old truck tire inner tube (Fig. 2.7). It is the border wall surrounding the corpus mammae and has depth and thickness, like the end zone of an American football field, not the linear plane of its goal line. The interface between the corpus mammae and the circum-mammary ligament (both of which also are composed of dense white collagen fibers) can be distinguished when distracting forces of traction and counter traction are applied. The white fibers of the corpus capsule are denser and opaque, and can be distinguished from the CML fibers, which run in curved loops interlaced with fat. Sir Astley Cooper described the attachment as "ligamentous or *fascial loops* which connect the breast to the aponeurosis of the pectoralis major muscle" [6]. So, seen in its entirety, the circum-mammary ligament surrounds the corpus mammae, as a zone of densely packed retinaculum cutis, with fat in between the fibers, which have been curved into loops by the expanding, developing corpus mammae, see Video 2.8. It is here, in this zone of adhesion, as in other regions of the body, that neuro-vascular and lymphatic channels pass on their way to the soft tissue envelope, which surrounds the breast gland (Fig. 2.8, b).

2.2.5 Circulation of the Breast

There are multiple sources of blood supply to the breast, which anastomose with each other in a richly collateralized system supplying the nipple-areola. Surgeons will find it useful to categorize the blood supply to the breast as a superficial system and a deep system of vessels (Fig. 2.9). Three primary sources in the superficial system, which provides arterial circulation to the soft tissue envelope and skin over the breast gland, are the internal thoracic artery (internal mammary

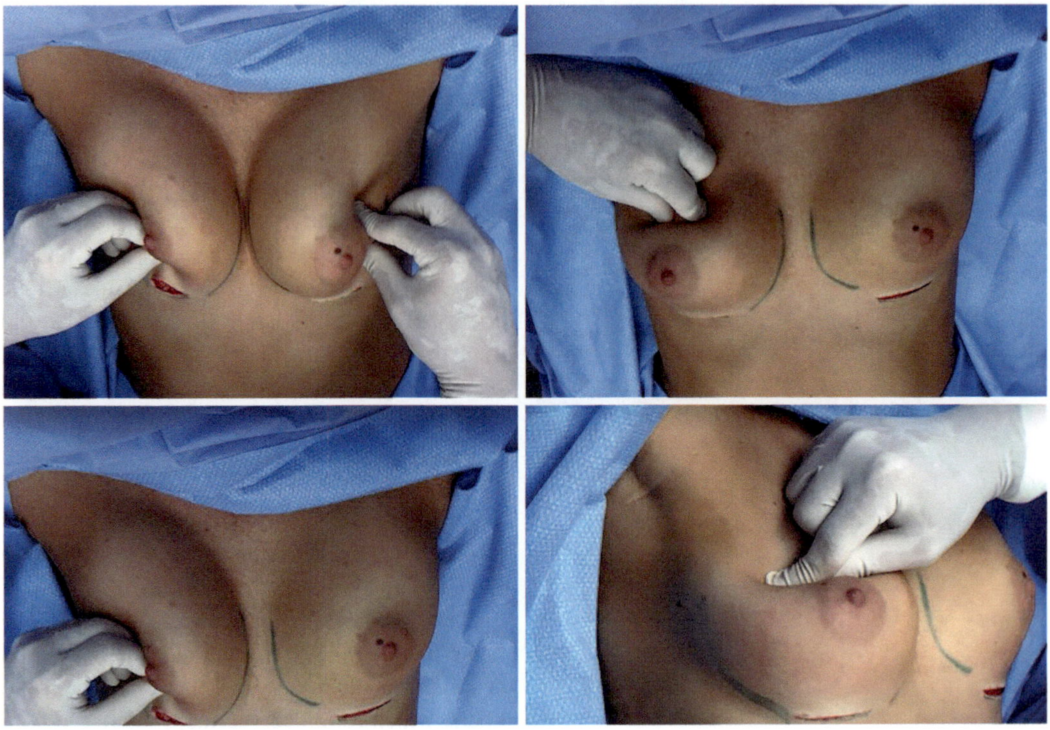

Fig. 2.6 The circum-mammary ligament forms a tear drop zone of adhesion between the skin and chest wall. (Courtesy of Robert Rehnke, 2020, All rights retained)

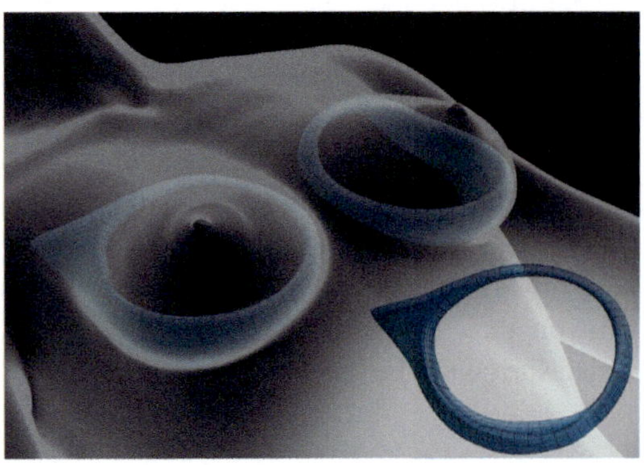

Fig. 2.7 Illustration showing the relative thickness of the circum-mammary ligament. (Courtesy of David Killpack, 2015, All rights retained)

artery) and its intercostal perforators (2nd, 3rd, and sometimes fourth), lateral thoracic artery, with branches supplying the inferior lateral aspect of the breast region, and the anterior intercostal branches of the intercostal arteries, especially at the inferior medial aspect of the breast, see Video 2.9. The deep system is made up of branches of the fifth anterior intercostal, and thoraco-acromial artery, Video 2.10. which runs in the deep substance of the pectoralis major muscle and sends perforators, upward at 90° to the plane of the chest, to penetrate and travel through the posterior lamina fat and into the deep surface of the corpus mammae (at the level of the second and fifth ribs). They continue, supplying blood to the lobes of the parenchyma, before reaching the nipple-areola anastomotic ring, which surrounds it just below the anterior lamella fascia. In this peri-areola region, the superficial and deep systems connect. The superficial vessels travel in the anterior lamella fat, between the anterior lamella fascia and corpus mammae, known as the segmental blood supply to the nipple-areola [14].

The veins of the breast can also have a superficial set, which runs just beneath the anterior lamella superficial fascia, in transverse and vertical patterns. The transverse type converges towards the edge of the sternum and join with the

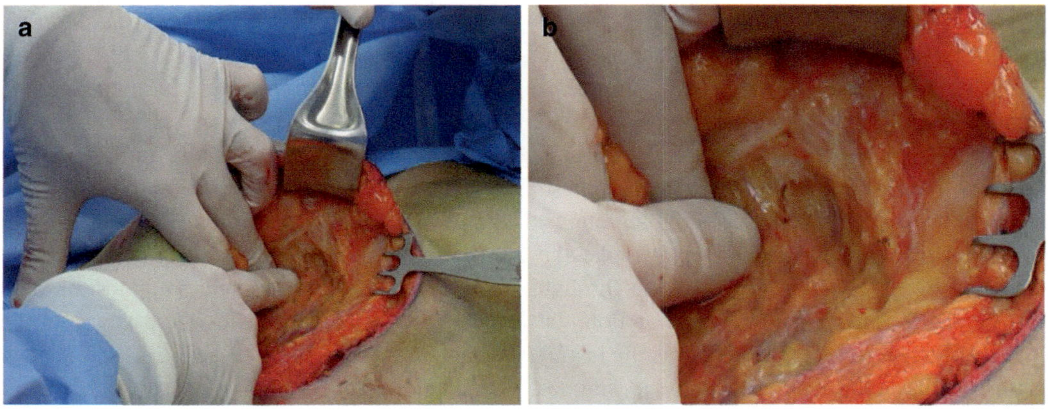

Fig. 2.8 (**a**) Inside look at the medial circum-mammary ligament, along the parasternal attachments; (**b**) Close up of the medial circum-mammary ligament showing, from top to bottom, the intercostal artery, vein, nerve, and lymphatics. (Courtesy of Robert Rehnke, 2020, All rights retained)

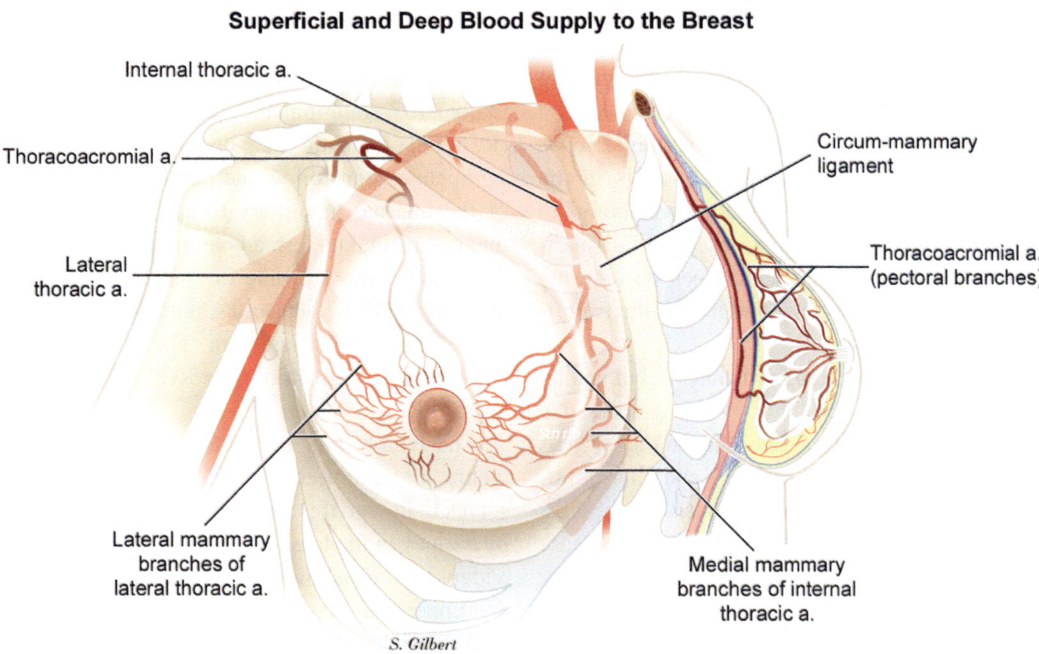

Fig. 2.9 Circulation to the breast and nipple. (Courtesy of Susan Gilbert, 2020, All rights retained)

internal mammary perforator veins and empty into the internal mammary vein. The vertical type drains the upper breast and chest, with the lower neck, into the supra sternal notch region, where they empty into the anterior jugulars. The deep veins of the breast run parallel to the branches of the arteries off of the axillary artery and drain into axillary and innominate veins [15].

2.2.6 Lymphatic System of the Breast

Most surgery texts have an inordinate amount of attention paid to the lymphatic system of the breast. This is because the early theory of breast cancer development and spread, called the "permeation theory," suggested that cancerous tumors grew and spread incrementally, millimeter by millimeter until they encroached on ever more extensive anatomic territories. As they grew, they invaded nearby lymphatics, which they fill and thrombose with tumor cells. It would then gain access to lymph node basins in the axilla, chest, and neck as it spread to surrounding structures, like the pectoral muscles, and organs like the liver and lungs. Hematogenous spread through veins and arteries was felt to be rare and only at the end of advanced disease. This was the justification of the "radical" mastectomy techniques for surgical care of breast cancer. It called for the removal of the entire breast gland, its overlying skin, the pectoral muscles below, and the en-bloc resection of the axillary contents. Since cancer was felt to spread primarily through the lymphatics, a detailed knowledge of this system was mandatory, so as not to leave lymphatic channel or node behind—what Halstead referred to as a "complete operation." As better anatomic knowledge was attained, like Grey's findings in the 1940s that deep breast lymphatic connections to the pectoral muscles were inconsequential, modified radical mastectomy techniques became the standard of care for the second half of the twentieth century.

The permeation theory was later debunked by rival theories on the biology of cancer, like Bernard Fisher's alternative cancer theory. His laboratory research in the 1960s, and later multicentered, randomized clinical trials in the 70s, showed that "breast cancer is a systemic disease with complex host-tumor inter-relationships… that the bloodstream is of considerable importance in tumor dissemination, and positive lymph node involvement with cancer is an indicator of a host-tumor relationship that permits the development of metastases rather than the instigator." [16]. This led to an evolution of breast conservation therapies and ever less- radical mastectomies. An excellent historical review, of the anatomy of the lymphatic system of the breast, is available in the text by Haagensen [15], but the most succinct summary is seen in Morris's Human Anatomy: "The lymphatics of the mammae are extremely numerous, forming rich and freely anastomosing plexuses." There is a rich plexus in the skin of the areola and nipple that empties mainly into a subareolar plexus. Deep lymphatics arise in the spaces around the alveoli in all parts of the gland. They anastomose freely with the cutaneous lymphatics and most of these converge toward the nipple where they join the subareolar plexus. From these plexuses, the main lymphatic channels pass outward to communicate with the pectoral, subscapular, axillary, and central nodes of the axilla. Metastases or infection from the mammary gland are therefore most likely to be transmitted to the axillary nodes.

There are three subsidiary or secondary lymphatic channels of the breast: (1) Grozman's path passes directly backward through the pectorals major to communicate with lymph nodes (Rotter's) beneath the pectoralis major. (2) Lymphatics that follow the perforating branches of the internal mammary to communicate with the mediastinal nodes and pleural lymphatics. (3) The paramammary route of Gerota, which may account for liver metastases and skin metastases in the upper abdominal wall. The lymphatics of the skin also anastomose across the front of the chest" [2].

The lymph drainage of the corpus mammae, where all carcinomas of the breast originate, seems to flow to this subareolar plexus, described by Sappey in the late nineteenth century [15], see Video 2.11. He showed that the skin of the chest and upper abdomen, lateral to the midline, drains to the ipsilateral axillary lymph nodes. Because the breast gland is embryonically derived from the chest skin, it makes sense that the corpus mammae would drain first into Sappey's plexus, then along with the rest of the skin's lymphatics into the axilla. The secondary lymphatic channels mentioned above appear to be draining the mesodermal elements of the breast. Because of the rich anastomotic connections between the two systems, rarely the secondary routes can also be a path for cancerous metastases. In any case, complete axillary lymphadenectomy has changed to lymph node sampling or sentinel lymph node biopsy. This approach removes the first lymph node in the axillary drainage of the breast, for prognostic purposes, and as a guide on decisions to prescribe adjuvant therapies.

2.2.7 Innervation of the Breast

The thoracic intercostal nerves, both lateral cutaneous branches, and anterior cutaneous branches supply their particular aspects of the breast. These lateral branches run within the portion of the circum-mammary ligament that lies over the anterior axillary line. The medial branches run with the internal thoracic perforators in the parasternal circum-mammary ligament (Fig. 2.8). Also, the skin of the upper breast region receives enervation from the supraclavicular nerves of the cervical plexus. The branches of the fourth and fifth lateral intercostal nerves innervate the nipple-areola.

2.3 Summary

The superficial fascia system of the breast is composed of stacked sheets of fascia, with vertical ligaments running from the deepest layer up through to the dermis, where it anchors and prevents shearing forces from pulling apart soft tissue form. The circum-mammary ligament is the teardrop-shaped zone of adhesion around the perimeter of the breast, which forms when the corpus mammae expand in an intermediate layer of superficial fascia, known as the corpus lamina. The corpus is sandwiched between layers of fat: a thinner deep layer, the posterior lamina, and a thicker anterior lamina between the anterior surface of the corpus and the skin. In the breast, the vertical retinaculum is more developed and resembles an egg crate carton, with large anterior lamella lobules of fat resting in between these vertical ligaments known as Cooper's ligaments. The entire system is packaged in a fascial containment of anterior lamella fascia and posterior lamella fascia. There is an opening in this system, below the nipple-areola, where there is no subcutaneous or anterior lamella fat, called the anterior lamella annulus (Fig. 2.10). All of this soft tissue system lays on top of a musculoskeletal foundation (Figs. 2.11 and 2.12). The size, shape, and contours of the underlying boney foundation have a great deal to do with the variation in the shape of the breast, as well as why some breasts are better supported than others and avoid breast sagging, or ptosis, with aging. The inherent quality and strength of the collagen and elastic fibers of the superficial fascia explain why breast with a given size and mass vary in their sagging. Understanding the superficial fascia system is integral to surgeries of the breast.

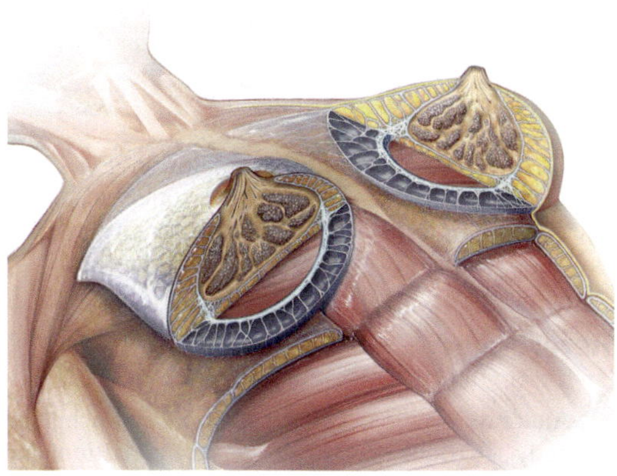

Fig. 2.10 Illustration of the superficial fascia system of the breast. (Courtesy of David Killpack, 2015, All rights retained)

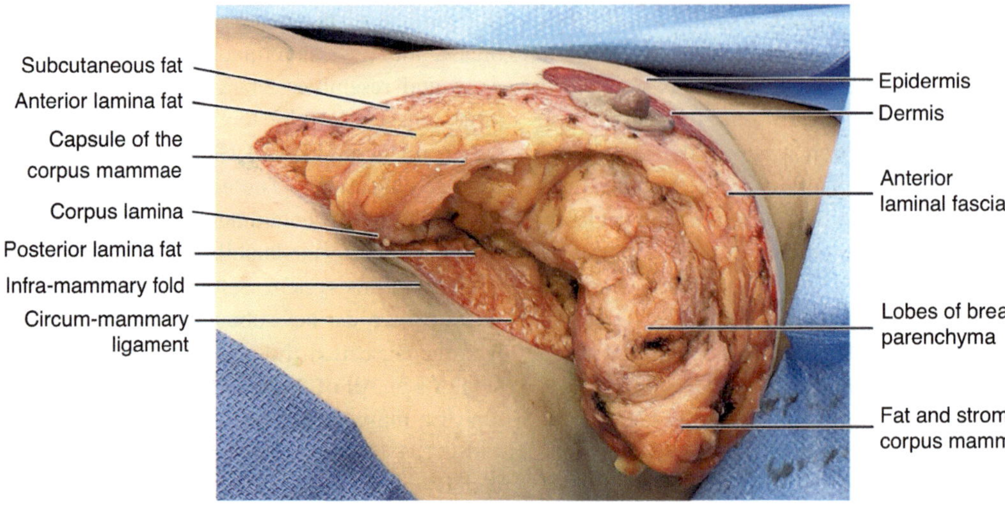

Fig. 2.11 Picture from a superior pedicle, breast reduction. (Courtesy of Susan Gilbert, 2020, All rights retained)

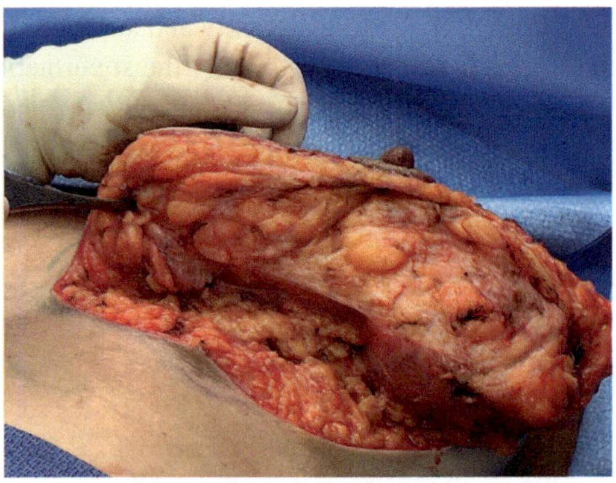

Fig. 2.12 The same breast, as shown in Fig. 2.11, retracted to show the capsule of the corpus mammae. (Courtesy of Susan Gilbert, 2020, All rights retained)

References

1. Andreas Vesalius, On the fabric of the human body. In Book V: The organs of nutrition and generation, transl. William Frank Richardson in collaboration with John Burd Carman, Novato, CA, Norman Publishing, 2007, pp. xix, 257, illus (hardback 978-0-930405-88-5). Medical History. 2009;53(1):153.
2. Schaeffer JP, Arey LB. Morris' human anatomy: a complete systematic treatise. JAMA. 1942;120(11):869.
3. Bland KI, Klimberg VS, Copeland EM, Gradishar WJ. The breast: comprehensive management of benign and malignant diseases. 5th ed. Philadelphia, PA: Elsevier; 2018.
4. Rehnke RD, Groening RM, Buskirk ERV, Clarke JM. Anatomy of the superficial fascia system of the breast. Plast Reconstr Surg. 2018;142(5):1135–44.
5. Abu-Hijleh MF, Roshier AL, Al-Shboul Q, Dharap AS, Harris PF. The membranous layer of superficial fascia: evidence for its widespread distribution in the body. Surg Radiol Anat. 2006;28(6):606–19.
6. Cooper A. On the anatomy of the breast. Longman, Orme, Green, Brown, and Longmans: London; 1840.
7. Scarr G. Biotensegrity: the structural basis of life. 2nd ed. Pencaitland: Handspring Publishing; 2018.
8. Thompson DAW. On growth and form. D'Arcy Wentworth Thompson. Am Nat. 1942;76(767):614–6.
9. Stiles HJ. The surgical anatomy of the breast and axillary lymphatic gland. Edinburgh: Oliver and Boyd; 1892.
10. Rohrich RJ, Smith PD, Marcantonio DR, Kenkel JM. The zones of adherence: role in minimizing and preventing contour deformities in liposuction. Plast Reconstr Surg. 2001;107(6):1562–9.
11. Lockwood TE. Superficial fascial system (SFS) of the trunk and extremities. Plast Reconstr Surg. 1991;87(6):1009–18.
12. Lockwood T. Reduction mammaplasty and mastopexy with superficial fascial system suspension. Plast Reconstr Surg. 1999;103(5):1411–20.
13. Gaskin KM, Peoples GE, Mcghee DE. The attachments of the breast to the chest wall: a dissection study. Plastic Reconstr Surg. 2020;146(1):11e–22e.
14. Deventer PVV. The blood supply to the nipple-areola complex of the human mammary gland. Aesthet Plast Surg. 2004;28(6):393–8.
15. Haagensen CD. Diseases of the breast.... 2nd ed. Philadelphia, PA: Saunders; 1971.
16. Fisher B, Anderson SJ. The breast cancer alternative hypothesis: is there evidence to justify replacing it? J Clin Oncol. 2010;28(3):366–74.

Understanding Breast Cancer Oncology: The Need for Mastectomy and Axillary Staging

3

Kate R. Pawloski and Audree B. Tadros

3.1 Introduction

In the era of multidisciplinary breast cancer management, less extensive surgery compared with the maximally invasive interventions of the early- to mid-twentieth century is both feasible and oncologically sound. Most patients with early-stage tumors are candidates for breast-conserving surgery with whole-breast radiation (BCT) or mastectomy and can expect excellent survival with either option. Increasing utilization of systemic therapy prior to surgery has afforded the opportunity for patients with locally advanced tumors, considered "inoperable" by historical standards, to successfully undergo surgery with curative intent. Similarly, management of the axilla has evolved in recent decades, incorporating sentinel lymph node biopsy as the standard approach to axillary staging for patients who present with clinically negative axillae. In this chapter, we discuss the surgical management of breast cancer and its evolution over time, focusing on considerations in the multidisciplinary management of patients treated with mastectomy.

K. R. Pawloski · A. B. Tadros (✉)
Breast Service, Department of Surgery, Memorial Sloan Kettering Cancer Center, New York, NY, USA
e-mail: tadrosa@mskcc.org

3.2 Surgical Treatment of Breast Cancer: Historical Perspective

Until the mid-twentieth century, the Halsted radical mastectomy with en bloc resection of the breast and overlying skin, pectoralis muscles, and axillary contents (levels I-III) represented the primary treatment for all stages of breast cancer [1]. In the latter half of the twentieth century, adjuvant chemotherapy and radiotherapy were routinely incorporated into breast cancer treatment and reduced both locoregional and systemic recurrence. As imaging modalities for breast cancer screening improved and surveillance became routine, tumors were increasingly detected at early stages while still confined to the breast; these represent the most common presentation of breast cancer today [2, 3]. Advances in screening and early diagnosis established the need to investigate the feasibility and oncologic safety of less radical surgery for breast cancer.

The effect on overall survival of a more conservative approach, namely total mastectomy, was first rigorously tested in the landmark National Surgical Adjuvant Breast and Bowel Project (NSABP) B-04 randomized clinical trial [4]. From 1971 to 1974, 1665 women were

© The Author(s), under exclusive license to Springer Nature Switzerland AG 2023
R. Vidya, H. Becker (eds.), *Prepectoral Breast Reconstruction*,
https://doi.org/10.1007/978-3-031-15590-1_3

randomized to receive either radical or total mastectomy with and without axillary radiation. Radical mastectomy included en bloc resection of the breast and overlying skin, pectoralis muscle, and axillary contents (levels I-III), while total mastectomy spared the pectoralis and axillary nodes. The B-04 trial provided the first evidence that the anatomic extent of mastectomy does not affect overall survival at 25 years of follow-up in women with or without axillary nodal metastases. There was no difference in disease-free survival or locoregional recurrence-free survival for women with clinically positive or negative nodes, respectively, signaling that local control is feasible with less radical surgery. These findings led to a significantly reduced morbidity for patients undergoing mastectomy.

For patients with early-stage breast cancer, the oncologic safety of breast conservation therapy (BCT) was established by the NSABP B-06 and Milan trials. These trials demonstrated equivalent overall survival and disease-free survival for patients with stage I-II breast cancer treated with modified radical mastectomy, lumpectomy with axillary lymph node dissection (ALND), and lumpectomy with ALND followed by whole-breast irradiation, respectively, at 20 years of follow-up. The ipsilateral breast tumor recurrence (IBTR) at 20 years of follow-up, however, was significantly lower among patients receiving whole-breast irradiation following lumpectomy compared with those who did not (14.3% vs. 39.2%, $P < 0.001$) [4, 5].

Rates of IBTR differ according to regional lymph node status and clear margins in the excision specimen. For invasive cancers excised with a margin of "no ink on tumor," the rates of IBTR are 5% and 9% in patients with clinically negative and positive axillary nodes, respectively [6, 7], and are not significantly reduced by excision of wider margins [8]. For ductal carcinoma in situ (DCIS) treated with BCT, IBTR is minimized by a margin width of 2 mm and is not significantly reduced by use of more liberal margins [9]. If negative margins cannot be obtained after re-excision(s), mastectomy is ultimately required for local control.

3.3 Indications for Mastectomy

While BCT is an excellent option for many patients with early-stage breast cancer, mastectomy is still indicated for cases of multiple ipsilateral tumors or T4 disease, defined as a tumor of any size with direct extension to the chest wall and/or the skin (with ulceration or skin nodules) or inflammatory breast cancer (IBC) [10] (Fig. 3.1.). Other indications traditionally associated with the need for mastectomy include unfavorable tumor-to-breast ratio, high-risk genetic mutation carriers (i.e., *BRCA1* or *BRCA2*), prior radiation to the breast or chest wall, or, if other contraindications to radiation exist, including pregnancy. While mastectomy is the primary surgical therapy rendered in these clinical scenarios, several caveats exist that may allow for successful BCT in select circumstances.

One condition traditionally considered a contraindication to BCT is the presence of multiple ipsilateral tumors in separate quadrants of the breast, or multicentric disease, due to concern for high locoregional recurrence rates, reported at up to 40% in historical retrospective studies [11–13]. The results from the ACOSOG Z11102 (Alliance) prospective trial demonstrated that appropriately selected patients with multicentric tumors can successfully opt for BCT via at least one excision in the ipsilateral breast without compromising the cosmetic result [14, 15], but longer follow-up data is required to determine the local recurrence risk. Although BCT is a feasible option for multicen-

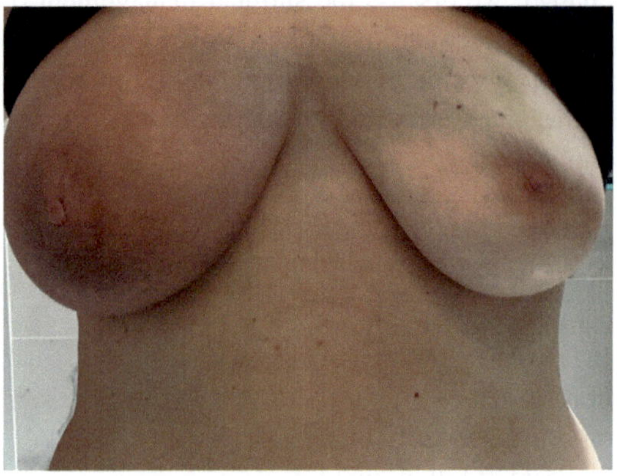

Fig. 3.1. Inflammatory breast cancer

tric breast cancer, rates of conversion to mastectomy after inability to obtain clear margins by re-excision have been reported at 7.1% for invasive cancer of any histologic subtype and 12.5% for invasive lobular carcinoma in at least one site [14]. Following neoadjuvant chemotherapy, patients with multicentric disease have higher rates of local recurrence compared with those with unifocal cancers at 3 years (9.6% vs. 7.1%; $P = 0.002$); however, these rates do not differ by surgical therapy or in those with a pathologic complete response [16]. Mastectomy remains the standard recommendation for those with extensive multicentric disease with intervening areas of DCIS between invasive tumor foci. Mastectomy is also preferred for patients with multiple ipsilateral breast cancers who prefer to minimize the risk of multiple surgical interventions.

For locally advanced breast cancer, the use of systemic chemotherapy prior to surgery, i.e., neoadjuvant chemotherapy (NAC), has led to increased opportunities for successful BCT where previously contraindicated. For patients who are ineligible for BCT because the clinically estimated tumor size is large relative to breast size, conversion rates from BCT-ineligible to BCT-eligible up to 75% have been reported after NAC [17–20]. For well-selected patients with an unfavorable tumor-to-breast ratio and who desire breast conservation, the probability of successful BCT is high enough to warrant consideration of this approach, provided that systemic chemotherapy is otherwise indicated. Patients with an unfavorable tumor-to-breast ratio who would not be considered good candidates for BCT include those for whom a lumpectomy would result in unacceptable cosmetic outcome and those who fail to adequately downstage after receipt of systemic therapy.

Salvage mastectomy was historically considered the standard of care for ipsilateral breast tumor recurrence (IBTR) after BCT due to concerns regarding the oncologic safety of repeat BCT and the risks associated with repeat radiation. Rates of IBTR following BCT have been reported at 9–20% in prospective trials with up to 20 years of follow-up [4, 5, 21–23]. While no randomized clinical trials have directly compared salvage mastectomy to repeat BCT and reirradiation for IBTR, 10-year equivalence in overall survival has been reported in retrospective series (65.7% vs. 58.0%; P = ns), with similarly equivalent cause-specific survival (73.1% vs. 61.1%; P = ns) observed at the same timepoint [24, 25]. Importantly, patients with IBTR who were selected for repeat BCT in these studies had tumors of lower grade, smaller size, and favorable biology, highlighting the importance of selecting patients with lower risk of recurrence for repeat BCT. Mastectomy remains the standard option for IBTR in young patients with high-risk breast cancer who were previously treated with BCT [26]. For patients undergoing repeat BCT and reirradiation, the risks and benefits of reconstruction following mastectomy should be discussed given the increased risk of post-surgical complications in the previously irradiated breast [27].

Another indication for mastectomy is risk reduction for patients with *BRCA1* or *BRCA2* mutations, in whom this strategy has been associated with a 90–95% reduction in lifetime breast cancer risk [28, 29]. Mutations in *BRCA1* and *BRCA2* are found in 1 in 300 individuals in the general population and are most frequent in the Ashkenazi Jewish population (1 in 40 individuals). For patients with *BRCA1* and *BRCA2* mutations, the cumulative breast cancer risk is 72% (95% CI 65–79%) and 69% (95% CI 61–77%) at the age of 80 years, respectively, with most incident cases occurring in young patients (age 30–40 years for *BRCA1* and 40–50 years for *BRCA2*) [30]. The cumulative risk for contralateral breast cancer after a first breast cancer diagnosis is higher for *BRCA1* carriers compared with *BRCA2* carriers (40% vs. 26%; $P = 0.001$); nonetheless, bilateral risk-reducing surgery should be considered for patients with *BRCA1* and *BRCA2* mutations. The National Comprehensive Cancer Network (NCCN) recommends the consideration of risk-reducing mastectomy versus high-risk imaging surveillance in a multidisciplinary setting for patients with genetic mutations conferring a high risk for breast cancer [31]. There is insufficient data on moderate penetrance genetic mutations to recommend risk-reducing mastectomy.

3.4 Types of Mastectomies

The most appropriate surgical technique for mastectomy depends on oncologic factors, patient preference, and surgeon experience. In the modern era, the most commonly performed types of mastectomies include the total (simple) mastectomy for patients who do not undergo immediate reconstruction, as well as skin-sparing mastectomy and nipple-sparing mastectomy for patients who elect for immediate reconstruction. Rates of local recurrence vary according to the extent of the mastectomy, with incrementally higher rates observed as more native tissue is preserved. The overall rate of local recurrence is low enough to justify the option of skin- or nipple-sparing mastectomy for many patients, provided their individual risk profiles show that they are suitable candidates.

Total mastectomy represents the first definitive departure from the maximally invasive procedures of the early twentieth century [32, 33]. Total mastectomy involves complete excision of the breast parenchyma, overlying skin and nipple–areolar complex with preservation of the pectoral muscles. As most of the skin overlying the breast is excised with this procedure, reconstruction is not performed in the immediate setting following a total mastectomy. Indications for total mastectomy include IBC or other T4 tumors for which local control requires excision of the overlying skin envelope. Several retrospective studies have suggested that immediate reconstruction is safe in well-selected T4 patients after NAC [34, 35], but postoperative complication rates are higher in these patients compared with those who do not undergo reconstruction (31.3% vs. 2.6%; $P = 0.006$) [35]. Postoperative complications that require re-operation, coupled with possible delays in adjuvant radiation, support the use of total mastectomy for patients with T4 tumors, especially those with IBC, regardless of successful downstaging post-NAC.

Skin-sparing mastectomy (SSM) preserves the skin envelope, which permits immediate reconstruction using implant-based or tissue-transfer techniques and thereby enhances the final aesthetic result. In SSM, all glandular tissue is removed through a small peri-areolar incision while preserving the maximum possible amount of skin and the inframammary fold [36, 37]. The nipple–areola complex is traditionally included in SSM but may be reconstructed after implant-based or autologous reconstruction (Figs. 3.2 and 3.3). The same incision or a separate incision can be used for the appropriate axillary procedure

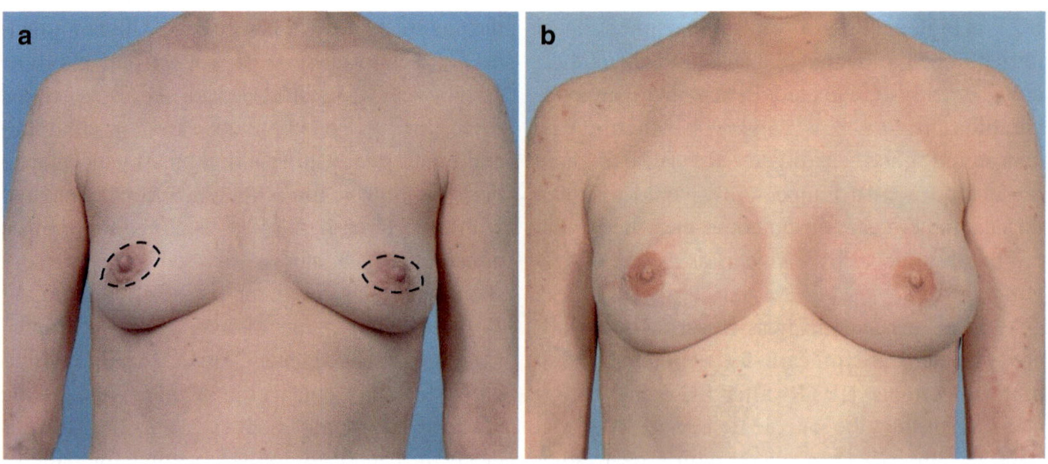

Fig. 3.2 Bilateral skin-sparing mastectomies with pre-pectoral implant-based reconstruction and nipple tattooing. (**a**) Preoperative baseline (**b**) Cosmetic result at 11 months post-reconstruction

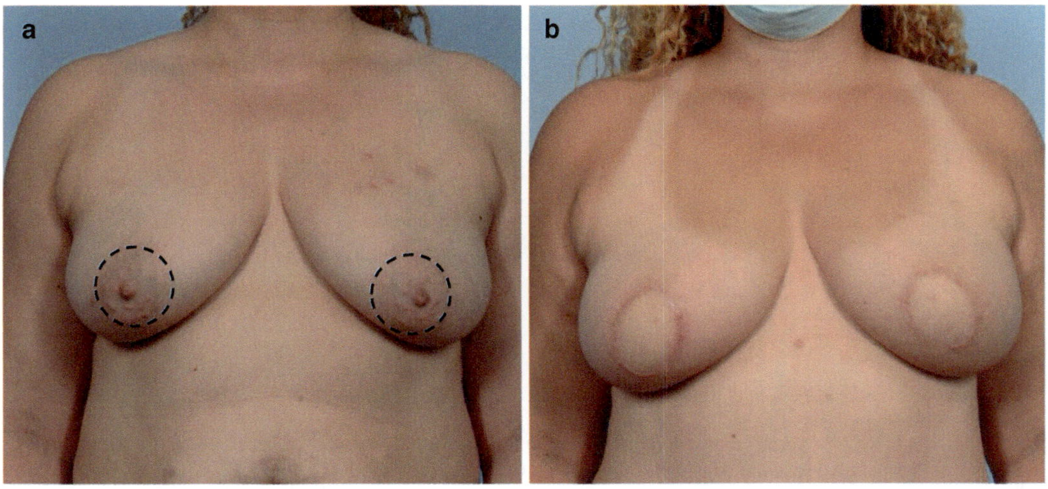

Fig. 3.3 Bilateral skin-sparing mastectomies via circum-areolar incisions with autologous reconstruction. (**a**) Preoperative baseline (**b**) Cosmetic result at 6 months post-reconstruction

based on clinical stage. Ideal candidates for SSM include patients without contraindications to immediate reconstruction, such as IBC or other T4 tumors with skin or dermal lymphatic involvement.

SSM and total mastectomy have not been directly compared in prospective trials, but the oncologic safety of SSM has been demonstrated in retrospective series including patients with stage 0-III disease. Early studies that evaluated the risk of LR after SSM and immediate reconstruction in well-selected populations reported rates of 4.0–6.2%, comparable to conventional (non-skin-sparing) mastectomy [38–41]. In a contemporary study of 1810 patients that compared outcomes after SSM vs. conventional mastectomy, LR rates of 0.2% and 1.6% were reported in patients with stage 0-IIA and IIB-III disease, respectively, at a median follow-up of 53 months after SSM [42]. Excellent LR control was attributed to the high proportion of patients who received adjuvant therapy compared with previous studies [40, 41, 43–47]. Neither adjusted disease-free survival (DFS) nor overall survival (OS) differed between patients who had SSM vs. conventional mastectomy after controlling for clinical TNM stage.

In the appropriately selected patient, SSM is a safe option that provides cosmetically superior results compared with total mastectomy. A multidisciplinary approach between an experienced breast surgeon, plastic surgeon, and colleagues in radiation and medical oncology is important to ensure appropriate patient selection and to determine the optimal sequence of reconstruction and adjuvant treatment.

Nipple-sparing mastectomy (NSM) is a type of skin-sparing mastectomy that preserves the skin envelope including the nipple-areolar complex (Figs. 3.4 and 3.5). NSM is associated with improved psychosocial well-being and quality of life compared with conventional mastectomy, largely due to excellent cosmetic results [48, 49]. To date, the NCCN suggests that NSM can be offered to patients for prophylactic indications as well as for breast carcinoma, provided that the nipple margin, a section of retroareolar tissue, is pathologically assessed and free of tumor, ideally with a tumor-to-nipple distance of ≥1 cm [50]. Eligibility criteria vary by institution, but characteristics of an ideal candidate for NSM generally include small breast size without breast ptosis, low BMI, and not smoking [51]. Contraindications to NSM include clinical evidence of nipple involvement by tumor, including Paget's disease, or preoperative imaging findings suggestive of nipple or skin involvement, including a tumor-to-nipple distance of less than 1 cm or the presence of calcifications within 1 cm of the nipple-areolar complex suggesting an extensive intraductal

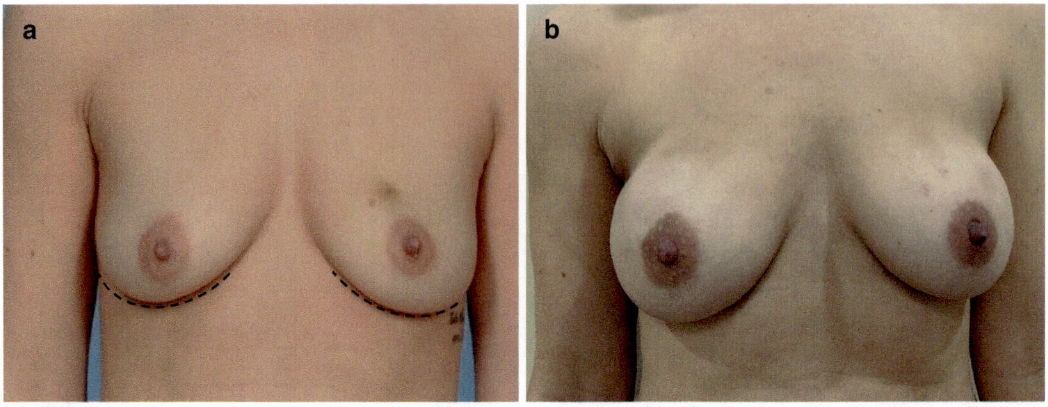

Fig. 3.4 Bilateral nipple-sparing mastectomies via inframammary incisions with pre-pectoral implant-based reconstruction. (**a**) Preoperative baseline (**b**) Cosmetic result at 10 months post-reconstruction

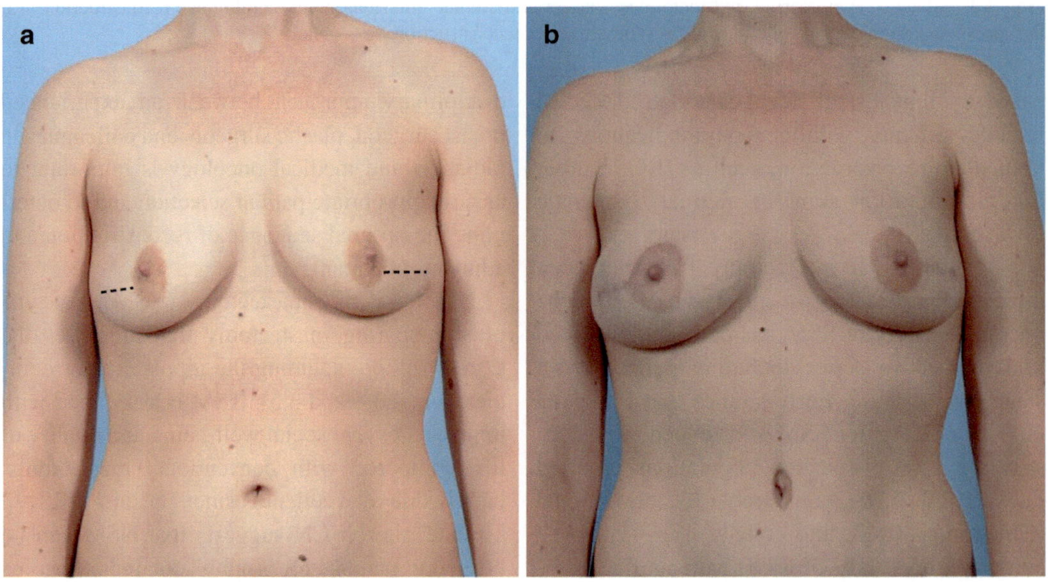

Fig. 3.5 Bilateral nipple-sparing mastectomies with autologous reconstruction. (**a**) Preoperative baseline (**b**) Cosmetic result at 6 months post-reconstruction

component extending to the nipple [52]. Relative contraindications include prior radiation, smoking, and large breast cup size (C or above), which may be associated with an increased risk of nipple necrosis after reconstruction.

As indications have expanded over time, therapeutic NSM is increasingly performed [53–57], and large studies support its oncologic efficacy. In a systematic review and meta-analysis of patients treated with mastectomy for invasive breast cancer (*n* = 2207), the majority of whom had stage I–II breast cancer, a non-statistically significant LR risk difference of 0.4% was reported between NSM and modified radical mastectomy/SSM. Rates of LR after NSM were 5.4%, 1.4%, and 11.4% at <3 years, 3–5 years and >5 years, respectively, and rates of nipple-areolar recurrence were 2.1%, 1.5%, and 3.4% at these time points [58]. In a large, contemporary series that evaluated outcomes after NSM for T1–3 breast cancer in the upfront setting, the 5-year cumulative incidence of cancer recurrence at the nipple-areolar complex was 3.5%, and 3.4% for LR in the skin or chest wall outside the nipple-areolar complex, at a median follow-up of 85 months [59]. Ten-year rates of distant disease-free survival and overall survival, respectively, were similarly high in patients with and without cancer recurrence at the nipple-areolar complex.

NSM is increasingly offered to patients with locally advanced breast cancer treated with NAC. In 2015, 10.7% of patients with stage III breast cancer were treated with NSM and immediate reconstruction, which was largely driven by patients who received NAC and were successfully downstaged [60]. Further investigation is needed to evaluate the long-term oncologic safety of NSM in the neoadjuvant setting. Evidence suggests that postoperative complications following NSM after NAC are low and have no impact on initiation of adjuvant therapy [61], but additional data to support this finding is awaited.

The use of prophylactic NSM in high-risk patients (i.e., *BRCA1* or *BRCA2* mutation carriers and those with strong family history of breast cancer or atypia) is also likely to increase in response to a growing body of evidence suggesting that rates of LR and postoperative complications are low [62, 63]. Long-term follow-up data after NSM is also needed to determine survival outcomes in this population.

While the indications for NSM have expanded over time, caution should be applied for patients at the highest risk for locoregional and systemic recurrence including those with T4 tumors or in whom occult disease in the nipple cannot be reliably ruled out by clinical exam or imaging. The likelihood and impact of complications requiring re-operation, reported at 9.4% following therapeutic NSM in a contemporary review, should be considered when determining the appropriateness of this procedure for an individual patient [53].

3.5 Post-mastectomy Radiation Therapy

Following mastectomy, many patients with pathologically negative axillary nodes do not require radiation, although it remains indicated for those at highest risk for locoregional recurrence (LRR). The goal of post-mastectomy radiation therapy (PMRT) is to sterilize any residual disease in the chest wall to reduce the risk of LRR and systemic recurrence. The National Comprehensive Cancer Network (NCCN) recommends PMRT for tumors >5 cm, or if margins are positive in node-negative disease [50]. PMRT is also routinely offered to patients with at least 4 positive lymph nodes, based on evidence that the most important predictor of LRR after mastectomy is a high axillary nodal burden [64, 65]. The application of PMRT in patients with limited axillary nodal metastases (1–3 lymph nodes) varies by institution, but should be guided by the presence of high-risk features, including larger metastases, young age, larger tumor size, higher grade, presence of LVI, and HER2-positive or triple-negative receptor status [66]. The American Society of Clinical Oncology (ASCO), American Society for Radiation Oncology (ASTRO), and Society of Surgical Oncology (SSO) recommend multidisciplinary management to determine the benefit of PMRT in patients with 1–3 nodal metastases [67]. The role of regional nodal irradiation for clinically node-positive patients who downstage to clinically node-negative after receipt of NAC is discussed later in this chapter.

3.6 Management of the Axilla in Early-stage Breast Cancer

Invasive breast cancer prognosis is informed by the presence or absence of metastases in the axillary lymph nodes. Surgical treatment of the axilla has evolved in recent decades as selective staging techniques have been adopted. Sentinel lymph node biopsy (SLNB) has replaced axillary lymph node dissection (ALND) as the standard approach to assess axillary nodal status in patients with invasive early-stage, clinically node-negative breast cancer. For patients with DCIS treated with mastectomy, SLNB may be performed in patients at increased risk for upgrade to invasive carcinoma at final pathology [68].

Selective axillary staging is based on the principle that the entire breast drains to a limited number of axillary nodes, i.e. the "sentinel lymph nodes (SLNs)," the status of which predict tumor involvement of non-SLNs. The SLNB procedure involves identification of the SLNs by injection of blue dye (isosulfan blue, methylene blue, or patent blue), radioactive colloid (technetium-99 m), or both (i.e. "dual mapping"). Intradermal or retroareolar injection of blue dye is recommended for patients undergoing mastectomy [69]. When technetium-99 m is used, SLNs are intraoperatively identified using a gamma probe to identify "hot spots" of increased radioactivity. The node with the highest absolute count, as well as all nodes with absolute counts >10% of this value, are considered SLNs. SLNB identifies 98.3% of positive nodes in patients with multiple SLNs [70]. A success rate of 96% and a false-negative rate (FNR, negative SLN with positive non-SLNs at ALND) of 7% have been reported in the upfront surgical setting [71].

The NSABP B-04 trial [4] provided the first evidence that routine ALND for patients with clinically negative nodes does not confer a survival advantage. The B-04 trial randomized 1079 patients with clinically negative axillary nodes to radical mastectomy, total mastectomy without ALND with postoperative axillary radiation, or total mastectomy without ALND unless the patient developed clinically positive nodes, as well as an additional 586 patients with clinically positive nodes to radical mastectomy or total mastectomy with radiation. At 20 years, overall survival was equivalent between treatment arms for node-negative and node-positive patients and even among those with positive nodes, there was no significant disease-free survival advantage for ALND compared with radiation and no axillary surgery. These results critically established that residual nodal metastases are not associated with decreased survival, suggesting that ALND and its associated morbidity [72], including lymphedema, shoulder dysfunction, motor and sensory neuropathies, and axillary web syndrome, can be spared without compromising oncologic outcomes.

The feasibility of lymphatic mapping and selective lymphadenectomy in breast cancer was first reported in 1994 by Giuliano and colleagues following evidence for its use in melanoma [73, 74]. Proof of concept was first established by the European Institute of Oncology (Milan) [75] and NSABP B-32 [76] randomized clinical trials, which compared survival and axillary recurrence rates following SLNB with or without ALND. (Table 3.1) Both trials found comparable overall

Table 3.1 Randomized clinical trials of sentinel lymph node biopsy for early-stage, clinically node-negative breast cancer with negative sentinel lymph nodes. Survival estimated by Kaplan-Meier methods

Study	Treatment arm	*n*	Overall survival (95% CI)[a]	*P*	Disease-free survival (95% CI)[a]	*P*	Axillary recurrence as first event	*P*
NSABP B-32	SLNB + ALND	1975	91.8% (90.4–93.3%) Unadjusted HR vs. SLNB alone: 1.20 (0.96–1.50)	0.12	82.4% (80.5–84.4%) Unadjusted HR vs. SLNB alone: 1.05 (0.90–1.22)	0.54	8	0.22
	SLNB alone[b]	2011	90.3% (88.8–91.8%)		81.5% (79.6–83.4%)		14	
Milan	SLNB + ALND	257	89.7% (85.5–93.8%)	0.15	88.8% (84.6–92.9%)	0.52	0	0.17
	SLNB alone[b]	259	93.5% (90.3–96.8%)		89.9% (85.9–93.9%)		2	

[a]8-year outcomes reported for NSABP B-32 and 10-year for Milan
[b]Backup ALND performed if SLN was positive

Table 3.2 Randomized clinical trials of sentinel lymph node biopsy for early-stage, clinically node-negative breast cancer with positive sentinel lymph nodes

Study	Treatment arm	Number with positive SLNs[a]	Number undergoing mastectomy	Median follow-up	10-year OS	10-year DFS (%)	Axillary recurrence (%)
IBCSG 23-01	SLNB	469	44	9.7 years	–	76.8	1.7
	ALND	465	42		–	74.9	0.4
AMAROS	ALND	744	127	10 years	93.3%	86.9	1.8
	Axillary RT	681	121		92.5%	82.7	0.9
Z-0011	SLNB	446	0	9.3 years	86.3%	80.2	1.1
	ALND	445	0		83.6%	78.2	0.5

[a]Patients with SLN micrometastases only included in IBCSG 23-01; SLN macro- and micrometastases included in AMAROS and Z-0011

survival (OS), disease-free survival (DFS), and low rates of axillary recurrence after extended follow-up. Results from these landmark trials established that SLNB without routine ALND can safely inform prognosis in patients with clinically node-negative breast cancer. Additional evidence supports the finding that late axillary recurrence after negative SLNB is uncommon. In a retrospective cohort of 1529 patients treated between 1997 and 2000 with a median of 3 SLNs retrieved, the incidence of axillary recurrence as a first event was 0.9% (13/1529) at median follow-up of 10.8 years, with a cumulative incidence of 0.9% (95% CI 0.5–1.6) at 15 years. Of the 13 patients with an axillary recurrence, 7 (62%) experienced recurrence within the first 5 years of surgery [77].

Subsequent prospective investigation has informed management of the axilla in clinically node-negative patients with limited SLN disease, which varies according to type of surgery. Patients treated with mastectomy with 1–2 SLN micrometastases (≤2 mm) may be spared ALND based on evidence from the IBCSG 23-01 trial [78]. (Table 3.2) If SLN macrometastases or micrometastases are identified, results of the AMAROS trial support omission of ALND in patients who received nodal radiation [79]. Both trials included mostly patients undergoing BCT, with subsets undergoing mastectomy. Neither reported differences in DFS or axillary recurrence after 10 years of follow-up. For patients who are eligible for breast-conserving surgery and whole-breast irradiation (BCT), the results of these trials and the landmark ACOSOG Z0011 trial [80] have provided evidence that patients with 1–2 positive SLNs of any size can be safely spared ALND and its associated morbidity.

The results from IBCSG 23-01 and AMAROS indicate that patients with early-stage, clinically node-negative breast cancer undergoing mastectomy with limited SLN involvement can safely avoid ALND and its associated morbidity if they are candidates for adjuvant systemic therapy [81–83]. Importantly, however, not all patients undergoing mastectomy with positive SLNs require axillary radiation outside of a clinical trial. Multidisciplinary management of the axilla with consideration of omission of ALND in patients with 1–2 positive SLNs receiving post-mastectomy radiation therapy is recommended.

3.7 Downstaging the Axilla

The aim of preoperative systemic therapy is to downstage inoperable breast cancer, and indications for NAC have expanded over time [84]. Currently, the NCCN recommends NAC for patients with IBC, T4 tumors, or N2-N3 disease, with ALND regardless of response to NAC. In patients with early-stage breast cancer and clinical N1 disease, however, NAC may lead to clinical downstaging of the axilla. In this case, SLNB may be offered and if no evidence of residual carcinoma is identified, the patient can be spared the morbidity of ALND. The likelihood of axillary downstaging is highest among the HER2+ and HR−/HER2− (triple-negative) subtypes.

In the last 10 years, SLNB in the neoadjuvant setting has been the subject of significant investigation. Several large prospective trials have evaluated the false-negative rate of SLNB in patients treated with NAC who were clinically node-positive at presentation and underwent routine ALND to identify the proportion who had residual axillary disease [85–88]. The identification rate of SLNB in these studies was high (79.5–92.7%), with FNRs ranging from 11.9 to 14.2%, which were reduced to <10% by retrieval of ≥3 SLNs and by use of the dual tracer technique (radiolabeled colloid and blue dye).

The ACOSOG Z1071 trial evaluated the FNR of SLNB in patients with clinical T0–4, biopsy-proven N1–2 tumors, of whom 84% converted to cN0 after NAC, although this was not required for eligibility (Table 3.3). Among the 649 patients in whom ≥2 SLNs were identified, the FNR was 12.6%, which exceeded the prespecified benchmark (10%), preventing recommendation of SLNB as an alternative to ALND after NAC. Similarly, the SENTinel NeoAdjuvant (SENTINA) trial was a prospective 4-arm, multi-institutional study that evaluated the FNR of SLNB in patients with clinically positive nodes (cN+) at presentation who were required to have converted to clinically node-negative (cN0) after NAC, representing 83% of the original cohort. Approaches found to reduce the FNR in both trials included dual tracer mapping and retrieval of ≥3 SLNs; Z1071 also supported excision of the preoperatively clipped metastatic node. Current NCCN guidelines support the use of SLNB after NAC in patients who convert to cN0 and in whom at least 3 SLNs are identified using dual tracer [50].

To date, evidence suggests that 41% of patients treated with NAC who achieve nodal pathologic complete response (pCR) can avoid ALND [89]. Rates of nodal pCR vary according to tumor subtype but are highest among those patients with HR−/HER2− and HER2+ tumors (70–80%), with the lowest rates observed in those with HR+/HER2− disease (0–50%) [90–96]. For patients who achieve a nodal pCR after NAC, either by SLNB or ALND if indicated, whether regional nodal irradiation (RNI) improves invasive breast cancer-recurrence free survival (IBC-RFS), invasive breast cancer-recurrence free survival (IBC-RFS) will be addressed by the NSABP B-51 randomized clinical trial [97]. In this ongoing study, patients with cT1-3, biopsy-proven N1 breast cancer with nodal pCR are randomized to receive comprehensive chest and RNI or no radiation if treated with mastectomy. Patients undergoing lumpectomy are randomized to whole-breast radiation with a boost to the lumpectomy cavity with or without RNI.

Contrary to the upfront surgical setting, ALND is indicated after NAC for patients with ≥1 positive SLN macro- or micrometastasis [50]. The

Table 3.3 Comparison of false-negative rates (FNR) of sentinel lymph node biopsy after neoadjuvant chemotherapy reported by the ACOSOG Z1071 and SENTINA trials

Study characteristic	Z1071	*P*	SENTINA	*P*
Overall FNR	12.6%[a]		14%	
FNR according to technical modifications of SLNB procedure				
1 SLN retrieved	31%	–	24%	Ref
2 SLNs retrieved	21%	Ref	19%	0.008*
≥3 SLNs retrieved	9.1%	0.007	4.9%	
Single tracer mapping	20%	Ref	16%	Ref
Dual tracer mapping	10.8%	0.052	8.6%	0.145
Proportion with ≥3 SLNs retrieved[b]	57%		27%	

**P*-value for odds ratio per additional sentinel node
[a]FNR in patients with ≥2 SLNs retrieved
[b]2 SLNs required in Z1071 study protocol; no prespecified number of SLNs in SENTINA

benefit of comprehensive RNI in this clinical scenario is presently undefined but will be further elucidated by results of the prospective ALLIANCE A011202 trial [98]. Patients with cT1–3, N1 breast cancer with a positive SLN after NAC are randomized to comprehensive breast or chest wall radiation and RNI with or without ALND, with the primary aim of estimating IBC-RFS in those with residual, undissected axillary disease. If non-inferiority with radiation is reached, the need for ALND in patients with residual nodal disease after NAC may be diminished.

Based on the most recent evidence, patients with limited axillary nodal metastases at clinical presentation no longer routinely require ALND in the upfront surgical setting or after a favorable response to NAC, which represents a significant achievement in the multimodal treatment of breast cancer. Looking forward, further de-escalation of axillary surgery is likely to continue across different subgroups of patients as rigorous, prospective evidence accumulates.

3.8 Summary with Tips

The oncologic safety of BCT has been established for early-stage breast cancer, and evidence suggests that it may be offered to patients with locally advanced tumors who downstage following NAC. Total mastectomy without reconstruction remains the standard of care for patients with a heavy disease burden in the breast, including those with T4 tumors and skin involvement and IBC, for whom local control is contingent upon complete excision of the skin envelope and all glandular tissue. Although most patients with newly diagnosed breast cancer are candidates for BCT, many choose to undergo mastectomy to minimize the risk of local recurrence. In this clinical scenario, options for mastectomy with immediate reconstruction should be discussed, provided there are no contraindications. Skin-sparing mastectomy and nipple-sparing mastectomy are excellent options with superior cosmesis for patients who are willing to accept a slightly higher risk of local recurrence compared with total mastectomy.

Axillary staging has dramatically evolved in the twenty-first century with the routine incorporation of SLNB for staging and prognosis. SLNB is indicated in the upfront surgical setting for clinically node-negative patients, and more recently is performed for patients with clinical N1 disease who downstage to clinically node-negative with NAC. While many patients can safely avoid ALND in the modern era, it is routinely performed in the post-NAC setting for patients who fail to downstage or for those with SLN metastases of any size.

References

1. Halsted WS. I. The results of radical operations for the cure of carcinoma of the breast. Ann Surg. 1907;46(1):1–19.
2. Welch HG, Prorok PC, O'Malley AJ, Kramer BS. Breast-cancer tumor size, overdiagnosis, and mammography screening effectiveness. N Engl J Med. 2016;375(15):1438–47.
3. Cancer Facts & Figures 2020 Atlanta: American Cancer Society; 2020 [Available from: https://www.cancer.org/research/cancer-facts-statistics/all-cancer-facts-figures/cancer-facts-figures-2020.html.
4. Fisher B, Jeong JH, Anderson S, Bryant J, Fisher ER, Wolmark N. Twenty-five-year follow-up of a randomized trial comparing radical mastectomy, total mastectomy, and total mastectomy followed by irradiation. N Engl J Med. 2002;347(8):567–75.
5. Veronesi U, Cascinelli N, Mariani L, et al. Twenty-year follow-up of a randomized study comparing breast-conserving surgery with radical mastectomy for early breast cancer. N Engl J Med. 2002;347(16):1227–32.
6. Wapnir IL, Anderson SJ, Mamounas EP, et al. Prognosis after ipsilateral breast tumor recurrence and locoregional recurrences in five National Surgical Adjuvant Breast and Bowel Project node-positive adjuvant breast cancer trials. J Clin Oncol. 2006;24(13):2028–37.
7. Anderson SJ, Wapnir I, Dignam JJ, et al. Prognosis after ipsilateral breast tumor recurrence and locoregional recurrences in patients treated by breast-conserving therapy in five National Surgical Adjuvant Breast and Bowel Project protocols of node-negative breast cancer. J Clin Oncol. 2009;27(15):2466–73.
8. Moran MS, Schnitt SJ, Giuliano AE, et al. Society of Surgical Oncology-American Society for Radiation Oncology consensus guideline on margins for breast-conserving surgery with whole-breast irradiation in

stages I and II invasive breast cancer. Ann Surg Oncol. 2014;21(3):704–16.
9. Morrow M, Van Zee KJ, Solin LJ, et al. Society of Surgical Oncology-American Society for Radiation Oncology-American Society of Clinical Oncology Consensus Guideline on Margins for Breast-Conserving Surgery With Whole-Breast Irradiation in Ductal Carcinoma In Situ. J Clin Oncol. 2016;34(33):4040–6.
10. AJCC. Cancer Staging Manual. Chicago, IL: American Joint Committee on Cancer; 2018.
11. Wilson LD, Beinfield M, McKhann CF, Haffty BG. Conservative surgery and radiation in the treatment of synchronous ipsilateral breast cancers. Cancer. 1993;72(1):137–42.
12. Kurtz JM, Jacquemier J, Amalric R, et al. Breast-conserving therapy for macroscopically multiple cancers. Ann Surg. 1990;212(1):38–44.
13. Leopold KA, Recht A, Schnitt SJ, et al. Results of conservative surgery and radiation therapy for multiple synchronous cancers of one breast. Int J Radiat Oncol Biol Phys. 1989;16(1):11–6.
14. Rosenkranz KM, Ballman K, McCall L, et al. The feasibility of breast-conserving surgery for multiple ipsilateral breast cancer: an initial report from ACOSOG Z11102 (alliance) trial. Ann Surg Oncol. 2018;25(10):2858–66.
15. Rosenkranz KM, Ballman K, McCall L, et al. Cosmetic outcomes following breast-conservation surgery and radiation for multiple ipsilateral breast cancer: data from the alliance Z11102 study. Ann Surg Oncol. 2020;27(12):4650–61.
16. Ataseven B, Lederer B, Blohmer JU, et al. Impact of multifocal or multicentric disease on surgery and locoregional, distant and overall survival of 6,134 breast cancer patients treated with neoadjuvant chemotherapy. Ann Surg Oncol. 2015;22(4):1118–27.
17. Petruolo O, Sevilimedu V, Montagna G, Le T, Morrow M, Barrio AV. How often does modern neoadjuvant chemotherapy downstage patients to breast-conserving surgery? Ann Surg Oncol. 2020;28(1):287–94.
18. Golshan M, Cirrincione CT, Sikov WM, et al. Impact of neoadjuvant chemotherapy in stage II-III triple negative breast cancer on eligibility for breast-conserving surgery and breast conservation rates: surgical results from CALGB 40603 (Alliance). Ann Surg. 2015;262(3):434–9. discussion 8-9
19. Golshan M, Cirrincione CT, Sikov WM, et al. Impact of neoadjuvant therapy on eligibility for and frequency of breast conservation in stage II-III HER2-positive breast cancer: surgical results of CALGB 40601 (Alliance). Breast Cancer Res Treat. 2016;160(2):297–304.
20. Golshan M, Loibl S, Wong SM, et al. Breast conservation after neoadjuvant chemotherapy for triple-negative breast cancer: surgical results from the brightness randomized clinical trial. JAMA Surg. 2020;155(3):e195410.
21. van Dongen JA, Voogd AC, Fentiman IS, et al. Long-term results of a randomized trial comparing breast-conserving therapy with mastectomy: European Organization for Research and Treatment of Cancer 10801 trial. J Natl Cancer Inst. 2000;92(14):1143–50.
22. Poggi MM, Danforth DN, Sciuto LC, et al. Eighteen-year results in the treatment of early breast carcinoma with mastectomy versus breast conservation therapy: the National Cancer Institute Randomized Trial. Cancer. 2003;98(4):697–702.
23. Arriagada R, Lê MG, Rochard F, Contesso G. Conservative treatment versus mastectomy in early breast cancer: patterns of failure with 15 years of follow-up data. Institut Gustave-Roussy Breast Cancer Group. J Clin Oncol. 1996;14(5):1558–64.
24. Yoshida A, Takahashi O, Okumura Y, et al. Prognosis after mastectomy versus repeat lumpectomy in patients with ipsilateral breast cancer recurrence: a propensity score analysis. Eur J Surg Oncol. 2016;42(4):474–80.
25. Alpert TE, Kuerer HM, Arthur DW, Lannin DR, Haffty BG. Ipsilateral breast tumor recurrence after breast conservation therapy: outcomes of salvage mastectomy vs. salvage breast-conserving surgery and prognostic factors for salvage breast preservation. Int J Radiat Oncol Biol Phys. 2005;63(3):845–51.
26. Montagne L, Hannoun A, Hannoun-Levi JM. Second conservative treatment for second ipsilateral breast tumor event: a systematic review of the different re-irradiation techniques. Breast. 2020;49:274–80.
27. Cordeiro PG, Snell L, Heerdt A, McCarthy C. Immediate tissue expander/implast breast reconstruction after salvage mastectomy for cancer recurrence following lumpectomy/irradiation. Plast Reconstr Surg. 2012;129(2):341–50.
28. Carbine NE, Lostumbo L, Wallace J, Ko H. Risk-reducing mastectomy for the prevention of primary breast cancer. Cochrane Database Syst Rev. 2018;4(4):Cd002748.
29. Domchek SM, Friebel TM, Singer CF, et al. Association of risk-reducing surgery in BRCA1 or BRCA2 mutation carriers with cancer risk and mortality. JAMA. 2010;304(9):967–75.
30. Kuchenbaecker KB, Hopper JL, Barnes DR, et al. Risks of breast, ovarian, and contralateral breast cancer for BRCA1 and BRCA2 mutation carriers. JAMA. 2017;317(23):2402–16.
31. NCCN Guidelines Version 1.2020 Breast Cancer Risk Reduction. National Comprehensive Cancer Network; 2020.
32. Maddox WA, Carpenter JT Jr, Laws HL, et al. A randomized prospective trial of radical (Halsted) mastectomy versus modified radical mastectomy in 311 breast cancer patients. Ann Surg. 1983;198(2): 207–12.
33. Staunton MD, Melville DM, Monterrosa A, Thomas JM. A 25-year prospective study of modified radical mastectomy (Patey) in 193 patients. J R Soc Med. 1993;86(7):381–4.
34. Wang M, Chen H, Wu K, Ding A, Zhang P, Zhang M. Post-mastectomy immediate breast reconstruction is oncologically safe in well-selected T4 locally advanced breast cancer: a large population-based

study and matched case-control analysis. Breast Cancer Res Treat. 2019;176(2):337–47.
35. Simpson AB, McCray D, Wengler C, et al. Immediate reconstruction in inflammatory breast cancer: challenging current care. Ann Surg Oncol. 2016;23(Suppl 5):642–8.
36. Freeman BS. Subcutaneous mastectomy for benign breast lesions with immediate or delayed prosthetic replacement. Plast Reconstr Surg Transplant Bull. 1962;30:676–82.
37. Toth BA, Lappert P. Modified skin incisions for mastectomy: the need for plastic surgical input in preoperative planning. Plast Reconstr Surg. 1991;87(6):1048–53.
38. Downes KJ, Glatt BS, Kanchwala SK, et al. Skin-sparing mastectomy and immediate reconstruction is an acceptable treatment option for patients with high-risk breast carcinoma. Cancer. 2005;103(5):906–13.
39. Foster RD, Esserman LJ, Anthony JP, Hwang ES, Do H. Skin-sparing mastectomy and immediate breast reconstruction: a prospective cohort study for the treatment of advanced stages of breast carcinoma. Ann Surg Oncol. 2002;9(5):462–6.
40. Medina-Franco H, Vasconez LO, Fix RJ, et al. Factors associated with local recurrence after skin-sparing mastectomy and immediate breast reconstruction for invasive breast cancer. Ann Surg. 2002;235(6):814–9.
41. Newman LA, Kuerer HM, Hunt KK, et al. Presentation, treatment, and outcome of local recurrence afterskin-sparing mastectomy and immediate breast reconstruction. Ann Surg Oncol. 1998;5(7):620–6.
42. Yi M, Kronowitz SJ, Meric-Bernstam F, et al. Local, regional, and systemic recurrence rates in patients undergoing skin-sparing mastectomy compared with conventional mastectomy. Cancer. 2011;117(5):916–24.
43. Carlson GW, Page A, Johnson E, Nicholson K, Styblo TM, Wood WC. Local recurrence of ductal carcinoma in situ after skin-sparing mastectomy. J Am Coll Surg. 2007;204(5):1074–8. discussion 8-80
44. Garwood ER, Moore D, Ewing C, et al. Total skin-sparing mastectomy: complications and local recurrence rates in 2 cohorts of patients. Ann Surg. 2009;249(1):26–32.
45. Kroll SS, Khoo A, Singletary SE, et al. Local recurrence risk after skin-sparing and conventional mastectomy: a 6-year follow-up. Plast Reconstr Surg. 1999;104(2):421–5.
46. Spiegel AJ, Butler CE. Recurrence following treatment of ductal carcinoma in situ with skin-sparing mastectomy and immediate breast reconstruction. Plast Reconstr Surg. 2003;111(2):706–11.
47. Vaughan A, Dietz JR, Aft R, et al. Scientific Presentation Award. Patterns of local breast cancer recurrence after skin-sparing mastectomy and immediate breast reconstruction. Am J Surg. 2007;194(4):438–43.
48. Romanoff A, Zabor EC, Stempel M, Sacchini V, Pusic A, Morrow M. A comparison of patient-reported outcomes after nipple-sparing mastectomy and conventional mastectomy with reconstruction. Ann Surg Oncol. 2018;25(10):2909–16.
49. Wei CH, Scott AM, Price AN, et al. Psychosocial and sexual well-being following nipple-sparing mastectomy and reconstruction. Breast J. 2016;22(1):10–7.
50. NCCN Guidelines Version 5.2020 Breast Cancer. National Comprehensive Cancer Network; 2020.
51. Tousimis E, Haslinger M. Overview of indications for nipple sparing mastectomy. Gland Surg. 2018;7(3):288–300.
52. Moo TA, Sanford R, Dang C, Morrow M. Overview of breast cancer therapy. PET Clin. 2018;13(3): 339–54.
53. Valero MG, Muhsen S, Moo TA, et al. Increase in utilization of nipple-sparing mastectomy for breast cancer: indications, complications, and oncologic outcomes. Ann Surg Oncol. 2020;27(2):344–51.
54. Agarwal S, Agarwal S, Neumayer L, Agarwal JP. Therapeutic nipple-sparing mastectomy: trends based on a national cancer database. Am J Surg. 2014;208(1):93–8.
55. Krajewski AC, Boughey JC, Degnim AC, et al. Expanded indications and improved outcomes for nipple-sparing mastectomy over time. Ann Surg Oncol. 2015;22(10):3317–23.
56. de Alcantara FP, Capko D, Barry JM, Morrow M, Pusic A, Sacchini VS. Nipple-sparing mastectomy for breast cancer and risk-reducing surgery: the Memorial Sloan-Kettering Cancer Center experience. Ann Surg Oncol. 2011;18(11):3117–22.
57. Moo TA, Pinchinat T, Mays S, et al. Oncologic outcomes after nipple-sparing mastectomy. Ann Surg Oncol. 2016;23(10):3221–5.
58. De La Cruz L, Moody AM, Tappy EE, Blankenship SA, Hecht EM. Overall survival, disease-free survival, local recurrence, and nipple-areolar recurrence in the setting of nipple-sparing mastectomy: a meta-analysis and systematic review. Ann Surg Oncol. 2015;22(10):3241–9.
59. Wu ZY, Kim HJ, Lee JW, et al. Breast cancer recurrence in the nipple-areola complex after nipple-sparing mastectomy with immediate breast reconstruction for invasive breast cancer. JAMA Surg. 2019;154(11):1030–7.
60. Wong SM, Chun YS, Sagara Y, Golshan M, Erdmann-Sager J. National patterns of breast reconstruction and nipple-sparing mastectomy for breast cancer, 2005-2015. Ann Surg Oncol. 2019;26(10):3194–203.
61. Bartholomew AJ, Dervishaj OA, Sosin M, et al. Neoadjuvant chemotherapy and nipple-sparing mastectomy: timing and postoperative complications. Ann Surg Oncol. 2019;26(9):2768–72.
62. Valero MG, Moo TA, Muhsen S, et al. Use of bilateral prophylactic nipple-sparing mastectomy in patients with high risk of breast cancer. Br J Surg. 2020; https://doi.org/10.1002/bjs.11616.
63. Heemskerk-Gerritsen BA, Menke-Pluijmers MB, Jager A, et al. Substantial breast cancer risk reduction and potential survival benefit after bilateral mastectomy when compared with surveillance in healthy

BRCA1 and BRCA2 mutation carriers: a prospective analysis. Ann Oncol. 2013;24(8):2029–35.
64. Recht A, Gray R, Davidson NE, et al. Locoregional failure 10 years after mastectomy and adjuvant chemotherapy with or without tamoxifen without irradiation: experience of the Eastern Cooperative Oncology Group. J Clin Oncol. 1999;17(6):1689–700.
65. Overgaard M, Jensen MB, Overgaard J, et al. Postoperative radiotherapy in high-risk postmenopausal breast-cancer patients given adjuvant tamoxifen: Danish Breast Cancer Cooperative Group DBCG 82c randomised trial. Lancet. 1999;353(9165):1641–8.
66. Morrow M, Van Zee KJ, Patil S, et al. Axillary dissection and nodal irradiation can be avoided for most node-positive Z0011-eligible breast cancers: a prospective validation study of 793 patients. Ann Surg. 2017;266(3):457–62.
67. Recht A, Comen EA, Fine RE, et al. Postmastectomy Radiotherapy: An American Society of Clinical Oncology, American Society for Radiation Oncology, and Society of Surgical Oncology Focused Guideline Update. Ann Surg Oncol. 2017;24(1):38–51.
68. Lyman GH, Temin S, Edge SB, et al. Sentinel lymph node biopsy for patients with early-stage breast cancer: American Society of Clinical Oncology clinical practice guideline update. J Clin Oncol. 2014;32(13):1365–83.
69. Valero MG, Golshan M. Management of the axilla in early breast cancer. Cancer Treat Res. 2018;173:39–52.
70. Chung A, Yu J, Stempel M, Patil S, Cody H, Montgomery L. Is the "10% rule" equally valid for all subsets of sentinel-node-positive breast cancer patients? Ann Surg Oncol. 2008;15(10):2728–33.
71. Kim T, Giuliano AE, Lyman GH. Lymphatic mapping and sentinel lymph node biopsy in early-stage breast carcinoma: a metaanalysis. Cancer. 2006;106(1):4–16.
72. Norton S. Chapter 104. Lymphedema. In: Kuerer HM, editor. Kuerer's Breast Surgical Oncology. New York: McGraw-Hill; 2010. p. 1067–80.
73. Giuliano AE, Kirgan DM, Guenther JM, Morton DL. Lymphatic mapping and sentinel lymphadenectomy for breast cancer. Ann Surg. 1994;220(3):391–8. discussion 8-401
74. Krag DN, Weaver DL, Alex JC, Fairbank JT. Surgical resection and radiolocalization of the sentinel lymph node in breast cancer using a gamma probe. Surg Oncol. 1993;2(6):335–9. discussion 40
75. Veronesi U, Paganelli G, Viale G, et al. A randomized comparison of sentinel-node biopsy with routine axillary dissection in breast cancer. N Engl J Med. 2003;349(6):546–53.
76. Krag DN, Anderson SJ, Julian TB, et al. Sentinel-lymph-node resection compared with conventional axillary-lymph-node dissection in clinically node-negative patients with breast cancer: overall survival findings from the NSABP B-32 randomised phase 3 trial. Lancet Oncol. 2010;11(10):927–33.
77. Matsen C, Villegas K, Eaton A, et al. Late axillary recurrence after negative sentinel lymph node biopsy is uncommon. Ann Surg Oncol. 2016;23(8):2456–61.
78. Galimberti V, Cole BF, Zurrida S, et al. Axillary dissection versus no axillary dissection in patients with sentinel-node micrometastases (IBCSG 23-01): a phase 3 randomised controlled trial. Lancet Oncol. 2013;14(4):297–305.
79. Donker M, van Tienhoven G, Straver ME, et al. Radiotherapy or surgery of the axilla after a positive sentinel node in breast cancer (EORTC 10981-22023 AMAROS): a randomised, multicentre, open-label, phase 3 non-inferiority trial. Lancet Oncol. 2014;15(12):1303–10.
80. Giuliano AE, Hunt KK, Ballman KV, et al. Axillary dissection vs no axillary dissection in women with invasive breast cancer and sentinel node metastasis: a randomized clinical trial. JAMA. 2011;305(6): 569–75.
81. Galimberti V, Cole BF, Viale G, et al. Axillary dissection versus no axillary dissection in patients with breast cancer and sentinel-node micrometastases (IBCSG 23-01): 10-year follow-up of a randomised, controlled phase 3 trial. Lancet Oncol. 2018;19(10):1385–93.
82. Solá M, Alberro JA, Fraile M, et al. Complete axillary lymph node dissection versus clinical follow-up in breast cancer patients with sentinel node micrometastasis: final results from the multicenter clinical trial AATRM 048/13/2000. Ann Surg Oncol. 2013;20(1):120–7.
83. Rutgers E, Donker M, Poncet C, et al. Abstract GS4-01: Radiotherapy or surgery of the axilla after a positive sentinel node in breast cancer patients: 10 year follow up results of the EORTC AMAROS trial (EORTC 10981/22023). Cancer Res. 2019;79(4 Supplement):GS4-01-GS4-.
84. King TA, Morrow M. Surgical issues in patients with breast cancer receiving neoadjuvant chemotherapy. Nat Rev Clin Oncol. 2015;12(6):335–43.
85. Boughey JC, Suman VJ, Mittendorf EA, et al. Sentinel lymph node surgery after neoadjuvant chemotherapy in patients with node-positive breast cancer: the ACOSOG Z1071 (Alliance) clinical trial. JAMA. 2013;310(14):1455–61.
86. Kuehn T, Bauerfeind I, Fehm T, et al. Sentinel-lymph-node biopsy in patients with breast cancer before and after neoadjuvant chemotherapy (SENTINA): a prospective, multicentre cohort study. Lancet Oncol. 2013;14(7):609–18.
87. Boileau JF, Poirier B, Basik M, et al. Sentinel node biopsy after neoadjuvant chemotherapy in biopsy-proven node-positive breast cancer: the SN FNAC study. J Clin Oncol. 2015;33(3):258–64.
88. Classe JM, Loaec C, Gimbergues P, et al. Sentinel lymph node biopsy without axillary lymphadenectomy after neoadjuvant chemotherapy is accurate and safe for selected patients: the GANEA 2 study. Breast Cancer Res Treat. 2019;173(2):343–52.
89. Montagna G, Mamtani A, Knezevic A, Brogi E, Barrio AV, Morrow M. Selecting node-positive patients for axillary downstaging with neoadjuvant chemotherapy. Ann Surg Oncol. 2020;27(11):4515–22.

90. Pilewskie M, Morrow M. Axillary nodal management following neoadjuvant chemotherapy: a review. JAMA Oncol. 2017;3(4):549–55.
91. Boughey JC, McCall LM, Ballman KV, et al. Tumor biology correlates with rates of breast-conserving surgery and pathologic complete response after neoadjuvant chemotherapy for breast cancer: findings from the ACOSOG Z1071 (Alliance) Prospective Multicenter Clinical Trial. Ann Surg. 2014;260(4):608–14. discussion 14-6
92. Zhang GC, Zhang YF, Xu FP, et al. Axillary lymph node status, adjusted for pathologic complete response in breast and axilla after neoadjuvant chemotherapy, predicts differential disease-free survival in breast cancer. Curr Oncol. 2013;20(3):e180–92.
93. Kim JY, Park HS, Kim S, Ryu J, Park S, Kim SI. Prognostic nomogram for prediction of axillary pathologic complete response after neoadjuvant chemotherapy in cytologically proven node-positive breast cancer. Medicine (Baltimore). 2015;94(43):e1720.
94. Mamtani A, Barrio AV, King TA, et al. How often does neoadjuvant chemotherapy avoid axillary dissection in patients with histologically confirmed nodal metastases? results of a prospective study. Ann Surg Oncol. 2016;23(11):3467–74.
95. T ALT, AlSayed A, Alawadi S, et al. A multicenter prospective phase II trial of neoadjuvant epirubicin, cyclophosphamide, and 5-fluorouracil (FEC100) followed by cisplatin-docetaxel with or without trastuzumab in locally advanced breast cancer. Cancer Chemother Pharmacol. 2016;77(1):147–53.
96. Diego EJ, McAuliffe PF, Soran A, et al. Axillary staging after neoadjuvant chemotherapy for breast cancer: a pilot study combining sentinel lymph node biopsy with radioactive seed localization of pre-treatment positive axillary lymph nodes. Ann Surg Oncol. 2016;23(5):1549–53.
97. Standard or Comprehensive Radiation Therapy in Treating Patients With Early-Stage Breast Cancer Previously Treated With Chemotherapy and Surgery. National Library of Medicine; 2013.
98. Alliance A011202: A Randomized Phase III Trial Comparing Axillary Lymph Node Dissection to Axillary Radiation in Breast Cancer Patients (cT1-3 N1) Who Have Positive Sentinel Lymph Node Disease After Receiving Neoadjuvant Chemotherapy. National Library of Medicine; 2019.

4 Oncological Safety and Technical Advances in Skin and Nipple-Sparing Mastectomy

Paolo Veronesi, Francesca Magnoni, and Antonio Toesca

4.1 Introduction

Skin-sparing mastectomy (SSM) and nipple-sparing mastectomy (NSM) represent a significant evolution of the basic modified-radical mastectomy (MRM). The increasing trend towards breast-conservative surgery, thanks to the introduction of new surgical techniques where the skin and/or nipple–areolar complex (NAC) are preserved, is better accepted by breast cancer (BC) patients [1].

Professor Umberto Veronesi introduced the term "conservative mastectomy" to define SSM and NSM, to emphasize the aesthetic appearance and not just the technical side of surgical procedure, as the final objective of the breast surgical approach: "…Conservative mastectomy might initially seem a contradiction in terms; however, if we regard conservation as the maintenance of body image the expression is appropriate…" [1]. Conservative mastectomy became therefore a significant improvement in quality of life for women with BC. The evolution of breast surgery in favor of body image and the consequent psychological advantages, progressed contextually to scientific research aimed at confirming the oncological safety of the conservative surgical approach.

P. Veronesi (✉)
IEO, European Institute of Oncology, IRCCS, Division of Breast Cancer Surgery, Milan, Italy

Department of Oncology and Hemato-Oncology, Faculty of Medicine, University of Milan, Milan, Italy
e-mail: paolo.veronesi@ieo.it

F. Magnoni · A. Toesca
IEO, European Institute of Oncology, IRCCS, Division of Breast Cancer Surgery, Milan, Italy

4.2 History of Conservative Mastectomy

The growing affirmation of conservative mastectomy has significantly impacted the surgical management of women with breast cancer over the last two decades, with NSM progressively prevailing as the preferred alternative to SSM. Many studies have described the increased patient satisfaction and improved aesthetic outcomes with NSM when performed with immediate reconstruction [2–5].

Mastectomy is usually indicated for women with multicentric or locally advanced disease. Rates of this procedure vary among breast cancer centers and countries [1]. The growth in mastectomy rates is partly attributable to the evolution and widespread use of breast reconstructive surgery and improved accuracy in breast imaging. The high sensitivity of breast MRI, and an increase in its use as a diagnostic method, has allowed additional disease foci to be identified in 16% of women, with no differences in local recurrence or survival [6]. Thus, breast MRI has

© The Author(s), under exclusive license to Springer Nature Switzerland AG 2023
R. Vidya, H. Becker (eds.), *Prepectoral Breast Reconstruction*,
https://doi.org/10.1007/978-3-031-15590-1_4

increased diagnostic rates of multifocal and multicentric tumors in screening and staging [7]. However, the results from the randomized COMICE trial demonstrated a limited role of MRI in decision making between conservative treatment or mastectomy [8]. Having said this, preoperative breast MRI seems to play a role in the BC patients' preference for mastectomy compared to those who don't undergo the procedure (43% vs 28%) [1, 9, 10].

In women with large or multicentric invasive cancers, with extensive intraductal component, or multicentric pure ductal carcinoma in situ, SSM or NSM become mandatory [1]. In particular, patients with multicentric cancers who have small or medium-size breasts, mastectomy is often unavoidable to order to guarantee clear margins. Conservative mastectomy allows the complete removal of all mammary tissue, including all the ducts in cases of nipple–areola complex (NAC) conservation in NSM, with a much appreciated aesthetic outcome. In this context, reconstructive techniques, used during immediate breast reconstruction, aim to create a natural looking breast, and minimize the patient's psychological distress [1].

The preservation of the NAC is crucial for a natural looking breast, improving patients' post-mastectomy quality of life when compared with non-NSM [11–13]. However, the oncological safety of nipple preservation is still under debate [1]. Skin-envelope preservation in SSM does not have negative oncological implications, as equivalent recurrence rates compared with a standard total mastectomy were reported [14–22], and it is considered a mastectomy standard procedure without increased risk of local recurrence [23].

In NSM, the removal of the nipple-areolar ducts is mandatory [24], preserving only the epidermis and the dermis behind at the nipple. Even so oncological concerns for possible future local recurrence still remain, due to the potential for a small amount of residual ductal tissue behind the nipple [25]. Preoperative clinical involvement of the NAC and positive retro-areolar margins are the main contraindications for NSM. Frozen sections for intraoperative assessment of the NAC have become routine in clinical practice, with a specificity and positive predictive value of 100% and a negative predictive value of 83% [1].

Another significant development in recent decades has been the discovery of genetic mutations, such as germline BRCA mutations. The identification of such individuals with elevated breast cancer risk has increased the rate of prophylactic unilateral or bilateral mastectomy and the desire for NSM [26]. The goal of the prophylactic mastectomy is to achieve maximum risk reduction by completely removing all the breast gland. Moreover, reconstructive surgery allows an aesthetically positive outcome. On the basis of current evidence and updated recommendations [27], these aims can be reached through NSM with immediate reconstruction, which allows to preserve skin and the nipple–areola complex, obtaining good oncological and aesthetic results [26, 27].

4.3 Surgical Technique

SSM and NSM require a double-time approach, the gland dissection and the reconstructive surgery, preserving NAC in NSM. SSM was first described in 1991 by Toth and Lappert [28] who aimed to maximize skin preservation in order to improve cosmetic outcome and enable reconstruction. The procedure involves removing the entire mammary gland and NAC through a small ellipse of skin that encircles the NAC, while preserving the skin envelope and the natural inframammary fold [23, 29].

NSM was first described by Freeman [30] and preserves the skin envelope and the NAC, while all glandular breast tissue is removed. Preserving the skin envelope in either SSM and NSM facilitate immediate breast reconstruction, using implant-based or tissue-transfer techniques [23]. Technically, it is important to completely and precisely remove all the breast parenchyma, with respect to the anatomical limits, while saving the skin envelope and the inframammary folds enabling better immediate breast reconstruction.

The breast surgeon must ensure that all the glandular tissue is removed and that the skin flaps are meticulously prepared, identifying Cooper's ligaments within the fascia superficialis, between the gland and the subcutaneous fat, and carefully dissecting within this generally avascular plan. The aim is to find the correct balance between the amount of subcutaneous fat that is removed without compromising vascularization and increasing the risk of flap necrosis [31].

Likewise, the retro-areolar dissection is technically challenging by the need to completely remove all ducts while protecting the nipple vascularization [32]. During the dissection of the gland from the pectoralis muscle, the fascia should be preserved if there is no cancer involvement [1]. For large-breasted women, this dissection is challenging, and skin reduction might be necessary to achieve a normal-looking breast shape with good ptosis [33, 34].

Various types of skin incision are used, depending on the tumor location and breast type [31]. The upper outer linear skin incision is the most commonly used, but surgical approaches can be personalized in relation to various clinical features and different skin incisions for NSM have been proposed in the literature. According to the breast size, areola size, different types of breast ptosis, other "non-standard" surgical incisions have been documented. In particular, a retrospective study by Corso and Colleagues analyzed 117 surgical procedures performed in 100 patients with BC [35], specifically: (1) hemi-periareolar incision, used for cup A-B-sized breasts with no ptosis and medium–large areolas, (2) round block approach or complete periareolar incision, used for cup A-B-sized breasts with ptosis grade I-II and small areolas; this procedure is particularly suitable when there is excessive breast tissue in small-ptosis breasts, (3) vertical incision pattern, used for cup C-D-sized breasts with ptosis grade II-IV, (4) wise pattern, used for cup D-sized breasts with ptosis grade III-IV. No significant associations between clinical and pathological data, complications, pre- and post-surgery satisfactions, and specific characteristics, such as ptosis and breast size were identified, confirming these approaches as the heterogeneous, safe and effective evolutions of conventional NSM [35].

Breast reconstruction is offered by breast surgeons trained in oncoplastic surgery or by dedicated teams of breast surgeons and reconstructive surgeons [36–38].

Considering the growing need to personalize the surgical technique, robotic mastectomy has been introduced as an alternative to open surgery, to perform precise dissection in areas that are remote from skin incision [39]. Robotic nipple-sparing mastectomy (RNSM) was developed in order to allow for enhanced visualization of tissue planes and better access to areas that are difficult to reach through conventional open nipple-sparing mastectomy incisions. With a mid-axillary line incision of the breast, the aim of robotic mastectomy was to achieve superior technical and cosmetic results while maintaining the same oncologic principles of the standard mastectomy (i.e., anatomic dissection planes and removal of breast en-bloc) [40, 41]. Additionally, the robotic approach was intentionally planned as it should cause less vascular damage in the nipple–areolar complex.

Robotic mastectomy was first described in 2015 [40] and since then the advantages and disadvantages of this new approach have been studied in prospective and randomized trials [41, 42]. Its feasibility and safety were consistently reported with low complication rates and no local failure at short-term follow-up [43–45]. During the 15th St Gallen International Breast Cancer Conference, robotic mastectomy was recognized as an option in selected patients [46]. Furthermore, several opinion manuscripts [47–51] and an international protocol [52] are ongoing to confirm long-term follow-up.

To access the long-term results of robotic mastectomy, a prospective randomized controlled trial comparing robotic mastectomy with the open classical technique was carried out and we are awaiting the publication of the results [42].

RNSM was reported by several pioneer surgeons. However, Korea Robot-Endoscopy Minimal Access Breast Surgery Study Group (KoREa-BSG) reported early experiences with 11 surgeons at eight institutions with appropriate training [53]. They showed rapid learning curve stabilization, especially in 2nd generation surgeons, who learned from the pioneer surgeon. As any new surgical procedures, RNSM needs an appropriate training protocol. Pivotal elements of training are understanding conventional NSM (CNSM), dry lab for robotic surgical systems, cadaveric lab, supervision of an experienced surgeon.

Meanwhile an analysis of perioperative data was concluded in 2019 [54]. Between June 2014 and January 2019, 94 consecutive procedures prospectively studied for the treatment or prevention of breast cancer. In all cases, the operation was technically successful and very low complication rates were recorded. Complications of re-operations and loss of implant occurred in only 4 cases (4%) and other minor complications requiring only observation occurred in an additional 13% of patients. This rate is acceptable and similar to our larger single-center experience with open nipple-sparing mastectomy and reconstructions [55, 56].

The technical advantages of the robotic approach compared to the standard open technique are related to enhanced visualization as well as incision placement. The robotic arms and camera allow for superior vision of tissue planes and higher precision dissections, as the robotic arms allow access at angles that are not possible with the retractors used in open surgery. The robot also allows for incision placement outside of the breast in the mid-axillary line. This has cosmetic benefit but more importantly, may have vascular advantages. The vascular supply to the nipple after NSM relies on small vessels that traverse subcutaneous tissue from larger branching vessels of the internal mammary, anterior intercostal and lateral thoracic arteries with less reliance on branches from the axillary artery or posterior intercostal branches [57]. Regarding cosmetic outcomes, Toesca et al. [58] reported a phase III, open label, single center, randomized controlled trial (RCT) involving women with breast cancer or with *BRCA1/2* mutation, which compares RNSM and CNSM for the first time. Primary endpoints were surgical complications and quality of life, and secondary endpoints were oncologic outcomes. All self-reported outcome scores in satisfaction with breasts and psychosocial, physical, and sexual well-being were significantly higher in RNSM than CNSM groups ($p <$ 0.0001, <0.0001, 0.0005, <0.0001, respectively). Results remained stable 12 months after RNSM ($p = 0.12$, 0.93, and 1.00, respectively) whereas they significantly decreased after CNSM ($p = 0.02$, 0.005, 0.02, respectively). The overall Body Image Scale questionnaire score was significantly better in RNSM than CNSM (20.7 ± 13.8 versus 9.9 ± 5.1 in the RNSM versus CNSM, $p < 0.0001$). Regarding oncological outcome, this RCT reported no local recurrence at median follow-up of 28.6 months [58].

In explorative analysis of oncologic follow-up of RCT with median follow-up of 42.0 months, there was no significant difference for disease free survival (DFS) and overall survival between RNSM and CNSM ($p = 0.910$ and $p = 0.760$, respectively). RNSM had no nipple recurrence whereas, CNSM had one nipple recurrence (data presented at ACOI National Italian Congress 18–21 Sept. 2022). We acknowledge that, because the present RCT started enrolling patients in 2017, follow up of oncologic outcome is still relatively short. However, the result of no local recurrence with median follow-up of 42.0 months in the RNSM group is encouraging. Oncologic outcomes from the international pooled analysis, the SORI study, showed similar results [59]. Nevertheless, we need RCT with primary endpoint of DFS to confirm RNSM is not inferior to CNSM in terms of long-term oncologic outcomes with high level of evidence. KoREa-BSG is planning a RCT for evaluating DFS as primary endpoint of RNSM in the near future. Early data suggest that the procedure is safe but larger trials should continue to study this approach.

In terms of prepectoral reconstruction, to ensure the integrity of skin flap perfusion, close collaboration between the general and plastic surgeons is mandatory to minimize aggressive mastectomies, although, a correct superficial layer must be maintained for oncological reasons. To reduce the incidence of skin flap or NAC necrotic complications, patient eligibility for mastectomy and immediate prepectoral implant reconstruction should follow objective assessment for tissue perfusion. The clinician should consider that prior breast irradiation and active smoking can compromise skin perfusion. Also, obese and immunocompromised individuals are at increased risk of complications. Furthermore, candidates for immediate prepectoral implant reconstruction should also have adequate fat depots for fat grafting, as it is integral to the prepectoral approach [60].

4.4 Complications

Complications after conservative mastectomies include flap necrosis, hematoma, seroma, wound dehiscence, implant loss, and prosthesis loss [31, 61]. Several risk factors for complications, specifically after NSM, have been identified in multiple studies including incision type, adjuvant chemotherapy/radiation, initial tumor size, lymph node involvement, and tobacco use [4, 31, 62].

NAC necrosis in NSM is also relatively common [31], therefore survival of the NAC is one of the most important issues to consider when performing conservative mastectomy [1]. Findings from study conducted at the European Institute of Oncology [63] demonstrated that comorbidities, smoking, type of incision, flap thickness, and type of reconstruction all influenced the NAC necrosis rate in NSM.

In their pooled analysis, Headon et al. [64] reviewed 12,358 NSMs to investigate complications and oncological safety. They found that the complication rate associated with NSMs was comparable to that of skin sparing and total mastectomy, although there was an additional risk of postoperative necrosis of the nipple. The overall complication rate was 22.3%, and the nipple necrosis rate was 5.9%: both decreased over time and were correlated with surgical expertise. Large breast volume, ptotic breast, smoking, prior radiotherapy, and periareolar incision were confirmed as predisposing factors for nipple necrosis [63].

A large, single-center study of 1989 patients who underwent NSM and reconstruction for BC at European Institute of Oncology assessed the oncological outcomes and nipple necrosis rate of NSM [56]. In this wide series, 1711 patients had invasive cancer and 278 ductal carcinoma in situ. In patients with in situ disease, NAC necrosis was 2.2% and 3.5% in those with invasive disease, demonstrating that NAC necrosis rate was slightly lower than previously reported by Headon and Colleagues [56].

4.5 Oncological Safety: Review to Date

A recent study from the National Cancer Database of the American College of Surgeons and the American Cancer Society highlighted an increasing trend towards NSM in patients with advanced disease, particularly in those who received neoadjuvant chemotherapy. However, they specified that there is still insufficient evidence to demonstrate that this surgical procedure is oncologically safe [65]. The nipple–areola complex is considered to be at risk of local recurrence and, therefore, its preservation is strictly correlated with the oncological safety of conservative mastectomy [1] Findings from two large, multicenter, randomized trials underlined that mastectomy had similar long-term survival to wide local excision with radiotherapy, suggesting that the nipple–areola complex is not a risk factor for OS [66, 67].

A study conducted at European Institute of Oncology on 934 women undergoing conservative mastectomy between 2002 and 2007 [68, 69], revealed that at a median follow-up of 50 months, the 5-year OS was 96.4%: 95.5% for women with invasive cancer and 100% for women with ductal carcinoma in situ. The 5-year cumulative incidence of breast-related events for invasive cancer was 14.7%. The high survival rates of this cohort are comparable with those of SSM, total mastectomy, and quadrantectomy with adjuvant radiotherapy, suggesting that conservative mastectomy combines safety with good cosmesis [66, 70].

Further studies reported the oncological safety of skin-envelope preservation, with a local recurrence rate (LRR) of SSM similar to that of modified-radical mastectomy (5–6%) [71, 72]. A meta-analysis of 9 studies involving 3739 patients reported that rates of local recurrence in SSM did not differ significantly from the non-SSM group, while the SSM group had a lower proportion of distant relapses compared to the non-SSM group [19].

In this perspective, the main issue has become whether preservation of the nipple amplifies the LRR [1].

Several prospective trials are underway to evaluate oncological safety of NSM. Currently, the US National Comprehensive Cancer Network (NCCN) recommends NSM in patients who are carefully selected by an expert multidisciplinary team, according to specific clinical parameters, such as early stage, biologically favorable features, absence of nipple discharge, and Paget's disease [73].

These recommendations have been consolidated by multiple studies. Several analyses reported a NAC involvement in BC patients undergoing NSM ranging from 8% to 33% [23, 72, 74, 75].

In 2012, Veronesi et al. conducted a literature review of conservative mastectomy and found NAC involvement in 0–18% of cases [1]. The LRR reported was 0–20.8%, and these recurrences presented mostly on the skin envelope [1]. Gerber and colleagues [72] analyzed 3 groups of patients who underwent either modified-radical mastectomy, SSM, or NSM: LRR was 8%, 6%, and 5%, respectively, and OS was similar between groups after 59 months of follow-up.

To date, many studies, with follow-ups ranging from 10 to 101 months, have demonstrated low rates of LRR in conservative mastectomy [69, 72, 76].

Specifically, long follow-up studies reported LRRs after SSM ranging from 5.5 to 6.2% over 25–78.1 months [22, 77], while LRRs with NSM from 0 to 4.6% over 10–60 months [76–82].

Oncological outcomes of NSM were evaluated in a large series of patients with invasive or in situ breast cancer treated at the European Institute of Oncology [56]: results from a median follow-up of nearly 8 years demonstrated that NSM is oncologically safe for selected patients. Local recurrences occurred in 5.3% of patients with invasive cancer and in 4% of patients with in situ disease. NAC recurrence occurred in 1.8% of patients, with an OS at 5 years of 96.1% in women with invasive cancer and 99.2% in women with in situ disease.

A recent study by Wu et al. [83], in a cohort of 944 patients undergoing 962 NSM for invasive breast cancer, 39 had NAC recurrences. However, there was no difference in distant metastasis-free survival and OS between those with a NAC recurrence and those without it. Several factors were associated with NAC recurrence, including multifocality or multicentricity, negative hormone receptor status, high histologic grade, and an extensive intraductal component [83]. The authors pointed out the excellent prognosis after appropriate treatment for the NAC recurrences [84].

Further, a recent systematic review of 14 studies including 3015 mastectomies found no significant differences between the NSM and SSM groups for LRR (3.9% vs 3.3%; $P = 0.45$) or mortality ($P = 0.34$) [85].

An early study, published in 2009, from the Memorial Sloan Kettering Cancer Center (MSKCC) on its first experience with NSMs, mostly performed as prophylactic surgery in risk-reducing setting [86], could not draw conclusions on the oncological safety of the procedure due to the small sample size. However, more recent published findings from a retrospective study on 467 therapeutic NMSs performed at MSKCC for invasive breast cancers, DCIS and phyllodes tumors [23] demonstrated the significant increase in NSMs performed for BC respect to before 2011 (58% vs.77%; $P < 0.001$). Authors reported low postoperative complications and recurrence rates: at a median follow-up of 39.4 months (range 0.4–150), four of 449 patients in that series developed LRR, and none of those recurrences involved the nipple–areolar complex.

Another very recent study consolidates the oncologic safety of NSM for appropriately selected patients. A retrospective review of a cohort of 322 patients who underwent 588 NSMs (83% bilateral, 17% unilateral), including 399 (68%) for BC revealed a low LRR rate, of which 50% had triple negative biology and/or lymph node involvement. None of the recurrences involved the NAC [61].

Encouraging and newsworthy results on outcomes deriving from very recent retrospective studies [87, 88] confirm the pressing need to verify the oncological safety of NSM with greater appropriateness and more extensive indications, such as in the case of previous neoadjuvant chemotherapy (NACT) [87] or of a disease located close to the nipple [88].

Wu and co-workers [87] analyzed among 1226 therapeutic NSM procedures, 319 NSMs in 310 patients after neoadjuvant chemotherapy. During a mean follow-up of 63 ± 22 months, 38 cases had LRR, including 6 cases of NAC recurrence. The 5-year cumulative LRR and NAC recurrence rates were 11.0% and 1.9%, respectively. The 5-year OS in the whole population studied was 91.3%. Significantly, following multivariate analysis, post-NACT Ki67 > 10% (hazard ratio, 4.245; 95% confidence interval, 1.865–9.663; $P = 0.001$) resulted as an independent risk factor for LRR and represented the only significant risk factor for NAC recurrence. In their report, Kim et al. investigated the role on outcome of the distance between tumor and NAC. In 47.4% of 251 NSMs, the tumor-to-nipple distance was ≤2 cm and in 27.5% was ≤1 cm. During a mean follow-up period of 68.0 months, the LRR was 4.4%, of which 0.4% in the retained NAC and OS rate at 5 years was 98.0% in patients with invasive cancer and 100% in patients with in situ disease [88].

4.6 Cosmesis and Psychological Benefit

The aesthetic implication of NSM is closely correlated with the psychological state of the woman and her sexual and relational well-being. Studies have shown that the preservation of NAC in NSM, compared to its deferred reconstruction after SSM, leads to a better acceptance of the mastectomy and is associated with a significantly better self-esteem and satisfaction with the physical image [89], even if nipple sensation is largely or completely lost in most cases [31].

Yueh and colleagues [90] noted good aesthetic results and high patient satisfaction in a series of ten women; however, nipple sensitivity score was low (2.8, scale 0–10). These results are in accordance with findings of Petit et al. [68] reporting a median satisfaction rating for the cosmetic result of 8 (scale 0–10), with a sensitivity score for the NAC of 2 (scale 0–10), with some improvement in sensitivity after 1 year in only 15% of women. Djohan and colleagues [91] reported reasonable sensitivity of the NAC in 67 of 141 patients, with lower satisfaction in women with large breasts, high body-mass index, and greater expansion volumes.

A 2016 review by Sisco et al. [92] documented a varied sensory outcome in NSM, with normal sensation self-reported in the range 10–43%.

4.7 Conclusion

Professor Umberto Veronesi's axiom "from maximum tolerable treatment to minimum effective treatment" [93] represents a significant shift and the constant trend towards progressively conservative approaches in breast surgery. Conservative mastectomy is a clear example of this tendency, and scientific research is dedicating efforts to validate its oncological safety in clinical practice. As emerged in literature here reported, NSM followed by immediate and personalized reconstruction represents an oncologically safe procedure, both in surgical treatment for breast cancer and in risk-reducing procedure for BRCA mutation carriers or women with strong family history of breast cancer, if defined by an expert multidisciplinary team adhering to specific selection criteria.

Nevertheless, further long-term follow-up studies are needed to consolidate the safety of the procedure in selected patients with breast cancer.

4.8 Summary with Tips

- The development of new techniques for mastectomy, which enable the preservation of the skin and/or the nipple–areola complex (NAC), has led to an improvement in the acceptance of breast cancer.

- Skin-sparing mastectomy (SSM) and nipple-sparing mastectomy (NSM) represent a significant evolution from modified-radical mastectomy, symbolizing the growing propensity towards breast-conservative surgery.
- Professor Umberto Veronesi introduced the term "conservative mastectomy" to define SSM and NSM, in which the concept of "body image" was as much a priority as the technical side of the surgery. Conservative mastectomy resulted in considerable benefit in terms of well-being for the breast cancer patient.
- Over the last 2 decades, NSM has emerged as the preferred choice over SSM, thanks to improved cosmetic outcomes and increased patient satisfaction when NSM is carried out with immediate reconstruction, in both oncological and risk reducing settings.
- SSM and NSM require a procedure that takes twice the time in order to complete the gland dissection followed by reconstruction, preserving NAC in NSM.
- New skin incisions have been developed and applied in clinical practice for NSM, depending on the tumor site and the breast type.
- Robotic mastectomy has been recently introduced as an alternative to open surgery, given the rising exigency to personalize the surgical technique.
- Skin and in particular nipple preservation during mastectomy have prompted in-depth discussion on the oncological safety of conservative mastectomy.
- As documented by extensive studies, the indication for NSM with immediate and personalized reconstruction should be discussed by a multidisciplinary specialized panel, in accordance with specific clinical criteria.

Further studies are needed to consolidate oncologic safety and extend the clinical indications for NSM.

Acknowledgments We acknowledge Linda Ann Cairns for her support in editing the draft of this chapter and Maria Grazia Villardita for her editorial assistance.

Conflict of Interest The authors declare that they have no conflict of interest.

References

1. Veronesi U, Stafyla V, Petit JY, Veronesi P. Conservative mastectomy: extending the idea of breast conservation. Lancet Oncol. 2012;13(7):e311–7. https://doi.org/10.1016/S1470-2045(12)70133-X.
2. Moyer HR, Ghazi B, Daniel JR, Daniel JR, Gasgarth R, Carlson GW. Nipple-sparing mastectomy: technical aspects and aesthetic outcomes. Ann Plast Surg. 2012;68:446e450.
3. Frey JD, Alperovich M, Levine JP, Choi M, Karp NS. Does smoking history confer a higher risk for reconstructive complications in nipplesparing mastectomy? Breast J. 2017;23:415e420.
4. Radovanovic Z, Radovanovic D, Golubovic A, Ivkovic-Kapicl T, Bokorov B, Mandic A. Early complications after nipple-sparing mastectomy and immediate reconstruction with silicone prosthesis: results of 214 procedures. Scand J Surg. 2010;99:115e118.
5. Wengler CA, Valente SA, Al-Hilli Z, Woody NM, Muntean JH, Abraham J, et al. Determinants of short and long term outcomes in patients undergoing immediate breast reconstruction following neoadjuvant chemotherapy. J Surg Oncol. 2017;116:797e802.
6. Houssami N, Ciatto S, Macaskill P, Lord SJ, Warren RM, Dixon JM, et al. Accuracy and surgical impact of magnetic resonance imaging in breast cancer staging: systematic review and meta-analysis in detection of multifocal and multicentric cancer. J Clin Oncol. 2008;26:3248–58.
7. Corso G, Magnoni F, Provenzano E, Girardi A, Iorfida M, De Scalzi AM, et al. Multicentric breast cancer with heterogeneous histopathology: a multidisciplinary review. Future Oncol. 2020;16(8):395–412. https://doi.org/10.2217/fon-2019-0540.
8. Turnbull L, Brown S, Harvey I, Olivier C, Drew P, Napp V, et al. Comparative eff ectiveness of MRI in breast cancer (COMICE) trial: a randomised controlled trial. Lancet. 2010;375:563–71.
9. Barchie MF, Clive KS, Tyler JA, Sutcliffe JB, Kirkpatrick AD, Bell LM, et al. Standardized pretreatment breast MRI-accuracy and influence on mastectomy decisions. J Surg Oncol. 2011;104:741–5.
10. Miller BT, Abbott AM, Tuttle TM. The influence of preoperative MRI on breast cancer treatment. Ann Surg Oncol. 2012;19:536–40.
11. Weber WP, Haug M, Kurzeder C, Bjelic-Radisic V, Koller R, Reitsamer R, et al. Oncoplastic breast consortium consensus conference on nipple-sparing mastectomy. Breast Cancer Res Treat. 2018;172(3):523–37. https://doi.org/10.1007/s10549-018-4937-1.
12. Bailey CR, Ogbuagu O, Baltodano PA, Simjee UF, Manahan MA, Cooney DS, et al. Quality-of life

outcomes improve with nipple-sparing mastectomy and breast reconstruction. Plast Reconstr Surg. 2017;140(2):219–26.
13. Metcalfe KA, Cil TD, Semple JL, Xuan Li LD, Bagher S, Zhong T, et al. Long-term psychosocial functioning in women with bilateral prophylactic mastectomy: does preservation of the nipple-areolar complex make a difference? Ann Surg Oncol. 2015;22(10):3324–30.
14. Eldor L, Spiegel A. Breast reconstruction after bilateral prophylactic mastectomy in women at high risk for breast cancer. Breast J. 2009;15(Suppl 1):S81–9.
15. Lostumbo L, Carbine NE, Wallace J. Prophylactic mastectomy for the prevention of breast cancer. Cochrane Database Syst Rev. 2010;(11):CD002748. https://doi.org/10.1002/14651858.CD002748.pub3.
16. Morrow M, Mehrara B. Prophylactic mastectomy and the timing of breast reconstruction. Br J Surg. 2009;96(1):1–2.
17. Peled AW, Irwin CS, Hwang ES, Ewing CA, Alvarado M, Esserman LJ. Total skin-sparing mastectomy in BRCA mutation carriers. Ann Surg Oncol. 2014;21(1):37–41.
18. Peled AW, Foster RD, Stover AC, et al. Outcomes after total skin-sparing mastectomy and immediate reconstruction in 657 breasts. Ann Surg Oncol. 2012;19(11):3402–9.
19. Lanitis S, Tekkis PP, Sgourakis G, Dimopoulos N, Al Mufti R, Hadjiminas DJ. Comparison of skin-sparing mastectomy versus non-skin-sparing mastectomy for breast cancer: a meta-analysis of observational studies. Ann Surg. 2010;251(4):632–9.
20. Kroll SS, Schusterman MA, Tadjalli HE, Singletary SE, Ames FC. Risk of recurrence after treatment of early breast cancer with skin-sparing mastectomy. Ann Surg Oncol. 1997;4(3):193–7.
21. Kroll SS, Khoo A, Singletary SE, Ames FC, Wang BG, Reece GP, et al. Local recurrence risk after skin-sparing and conventional mastectomy: a 6-year follow-up. Plast Reconstr Surg. 1999;104(2):421–5.
22. Newman LA, Kuerer HM, Hunt KK, Kroll SS, Ames FC, Ross MI, et al. Presentation, treatment, and outcome of local recurrence after skin-sparing mastectomy and immediate breast reconstruction. Ann Surg Oncol. 1998;5(7):620–6.
23. Valero MG, Muhsen S, Moo TA, Zabor EC, Stempel M, Pusic A, et al. Increase in utilization of nipple-sparing mastectomy for breast cancer: indications, complications, and oncologic outcomes. Ann Surg Oncol. 2020;27(2):344–51. https://doi.org/10.1245/s10434-019-07948-x.
24. Tokin C, Weiss A, Wang-Rodriguez J, Blair SL. Oncologic safety of skin-sparing and nipple-sparing mastectomy: a discussion and review of the literature. Int J Surg Oncol. 2012;2012:921821. https://doi.org/10.1155/2012/921821.
25. De La Cruz L, Moody AM, Tappy EE, Blankenship SA, Hecht EM. Overall survival, disease-free survival, local recurrence, and nipple-areolar recurrence in the setting of nipple-sparing mastectomy: a meta-analysis and systematic review. Ann Surg Oncol. 2015;22(10):3241–9. https://doi.org/10.1245/s10434-015-4739-1.
26. Jakub JW, Peled AW, Gray RJ, Greenup RA, Kiluk JV, Sacchini V, et al. Oncologic safety of prophylactic nipple-sparing mastectomy in a population with BRCA mutations. JAMA Surg. 2018;153:123.
27. Corso G, Magnoni F. Hereditary breast cancer: translation into clinical practice of recent American Society of Clinical Oncology, American Society of Radiation Oncology, and Society of Surgical Oncology recommendations [published online ahead of print, 2020 Sep 3]. Eur J Cancer Prev. 2020;10.1097/CEJ.0000000000000624. https://doi.org/10.1097/CEJ.0000000000000624.
28. Toth BA, Lappert P. Modified skin incisions for mastectomy: the need for plastic surgical input in preoperative planning. Plast Reconstr Surg. 1991;87(6):1048–53.
29. Carlson GW. Skin sparing mastectomy: anatomic and technical considerations. Am Surg. 1996;62(2):151–5.
30. Freeman BS. Subcutaneous mastectomy for benign breast lesions with immediate or delayed prosthetic replacement. Plast Reconstr Surg Transplant Bull. 1962;30:676–82.
31. Galimberti V, Vicini E, Corso G, Morigi C, Fontana S, Sacchini V, et al. Nipple-sparing and skin-sparing mastectomy: review of aims, oncological safety and contraindications. Breast. 2017;34 Suppl 1(Suppl 1):S82–4. https://doi.org/10.1016/j.breast.2017.06.034.
32. Franceschini G, Masetti R. What the surgeons should know about the bilateral prophylactic mastectomy in BRCA mutation carriers. Eur J Breast Health. 2019;15:135–6.
33. Larson DL, Basir Z, Bruce T. Is oncologic safety compatible with a predictably viable mastectomy skin flap? Plast Reconstr Surg. 2011;127:27–33.
34. Nava MB, Ottolenghi J, Pennati A, Spano A, Bruno N, Catanuto G, et al. Skin/nipple sparing mastectomies and implant-based breast reconstruction in patients with large and ptotic breast: oncological and reconstructive results. Breast. 2012;21(3):267–71. https://doi.org/10.1016/j.breast.2011.01.004.
35. Corso G, De Lorenzi F, Vicini E, Pagani G, Veronesi P, Sargenti M, et al. Nipple-sparing mastectomy with different approaches: surgical incisions, complications, and cosmetic results. Preliminary results of 100 consecutive patients at a single center. J Plast Reconstr Aesthet Surg. 2018;71(12):1751–60. https://doi.org/10.1016/j.bjps.2018.07.022.
36. Petit J, Rietjens M, Garusi C. Breast reconstructive techniques in cancer patients: which ones, when to apply, which immediate and long term risks? Crit Rev Oncol Hematol. 2001;38:231–9.
37. Masetti R, Di Leone A, Franceschini G, Magno S, Terribile D, Fabbri MC, et al. Oncoplastic techniques in the conservative surgical treatment of

breast cancer: an overview. Breast J. 2006;12(5 suppl 2):S174–80.
38. Kollias J, Davies G, Bochner MA, Gill PG. Clinical impact of oncoplastic surgery in a specialist breast practice. ANZ J Surg. 2008;78:269–72.
39. Toesca A, Peradze N, Galimberti V, et al. Robotic nipple-sparing mastectomy and immediate breast reconstruction with implant: first report of surgical technique. Ann Surg. 2017;266(2):e28–30. Epub 2015
40. Toesca A, Manconi A, Peradze N, et al. 1931 preliminary report of robotic nipple-sparing mastectomy and immediate breast reconstruction with implant. Eur J Cancer. 2015;51(3):S309.
41. Toesca A, Peradze N, Manconi A, Manconi A, Intra M, Gentilini O, et al. Robotic nipple-sparing mastectomy for the treatment of breast cancer: feasibility and safety study. Breast. 2017;31:51–6.
42. NIH U.S. National Library of Medicine. ClinicalTrials.gov https://clinicaltrials.gov/ct2/show/NCT03440398.
43. Lai HW, Wang CC, Lai YC, Chen CJ, Lin SL, Chen ST, et al. The learning curve of robotic nipple sparing mastectomy for breast cancer: an analysis of consecutive 39 procedures with cumulative sum plot. Eur J Surg Oncol. 2019;45(2):125–33. https://doi.org/10.1016/j.ejso.2018.09.021.
44. Lai HW, Chen ST, Lin SL, Chen CJ, Lin YL, Pai SH, et al. Robotic nipple-sparing mastectomy and immediate breast reconstruction with gel implant: technique, preliminary results and patient-reported cosmetic outcome. Ann Surg Oncol. 2019;26(1):42–52. https://doi.org/10.1245/s10434-018-6704-2. Epub 2018 Aug 14
45. Sarfati B, Honart JF, Leymarie N, Rimareix F, Al Khashnam H, Kolb F. Robotic da Vinci xi-assisted nipple-sparing mastectomy: first clinical report. Breast J. 2018;24(3):373–6. https://doi.org/10.1111/tbj.12937. Epub 2017 Dec 18
46. Morigi C. Highlights from the 15th St Gallen international breast cancer conference 15-18 March, 2017, Vienna: tailored treatments for patients with early breast cancer. Ecancermedicalscience. 2017;11:732.
47. Margenthaler JA. Robotic mastectomy-program malfunction? JAMA Surg. 2020;155(6):461–2.
48. Kopkash K, Sisco M, Poli E, Seth A, Pesce C. The modern approach to the nipple-sparing mastectomy. J Surg Oncol. 2020;122:29–35.
49. Selber JC. Robotic nipple-sparing mastectomy: the next step in the evolution of minimally invasive breast surgery. Ann Surg Oncol. 2019;26(1):10–1.
50. Struk S, Qassemyar Q, Leymarie N, Honart J-F, Alkhashnam H, De Fremicourt K, et al. The ongoing emergence of robotics in plastic and reconstructive surgery. Ann Chir Plast Esthet. 2018;63(2):105–12.
51. Toesca A, Peradze N, Manconi A, Nevola Teixeira LF. Reply to the letter to the editor "Robotic-assisted Nipple Sparing Mastectomy: a feasibility study on cadaveric models" by Sarfati B. et al. J Plast Reconstr Aesthet Surg. 2017;70(4):558–60.
52. NIH U.S. National Library of Medicine. ClinicalTrials.gov (https://clinicaltrials.gov/ct2/show/NCT04108117).
53. Ryu JM, Kim JY, Choi HJ, Ko B, Kim J, Cho J, et al. Robot-assisted nipple-sparing mastectomy with immediate breast reconstruction: an initial experience of the Korea Robot-endoscopy Minimal Access Breast Surgery Study Group (KoREa-BSG). Ann Surg. 2022;275(5):985–91. https://doi.org/10.1097/SLA.0000000000004492.
54. Toesca A, Invento A, Massari G, Girardi A, Peradze N, et al. Update on the feasibility and Progress on robotic breast surgery. Ann Surg Oncol. 2019;26:3046. https://doi.org/10.1245/s10434-019-07590-7.
55. Botteri E, Gentilini O, Rotmensz N, Veronesi P, Ratini S, Fraga-Guedes C, et al. Mastectomy without radiotherapy: outcome analysis after 10 years of follow-up in a single institution. Breast Cancer Res Treat. 2012;134(3):1221–8.
56. Galimberti V, Morigi C, Bagnardi V, Corso G, Vicini E, Kahler Ribeiro Fontana S, et al. Oncological outcomes of nipple-sparing mastectomy: a single-center experience of 1989 patients. Ann Surg Oncol. 2018;25(13):3849–57. https://doi.org/10.1245/s10434-018-6759-0.
57. Dm O'D, Prescher A, Pallua N. Vascular reliability of nipple-areola complex-bearing pedicles: an anatomical microdissection study. Plast Reconstr Surg. 2007;119(4):1167–77.
58. Toesca A, Sangalli C, Maisonneuve P, Massari G, Girardi A, Baker JL, et al. A randomized trial of robotic mastectomy versus open surgery in women with breast cancer or BrCA mutation. Ann Surg. 2022;276(1):11–9. https://doi.org/10.1097/SLA.0000000000004969. Epub 2021 Jun 9
59. Prospective Study of MAstectomy With Reconstruction Including Robot Endoscopic Surgery (MARRES). https://clinicaltrials.gov/ct2/show/NCT04585074. Accessed 12 Jan 2023.
60. Sigalove S, Maxwell GP, Sigalove NM, Storm-Dickerson TL, Pope N, Rice J, Gabriel A. Prepectoral implant-based breast reconstruction: rationale, indications, and preliminary results. Plast Reconstr Surg. 2017;139(2):287–94. https://doi.org/10.1097/PRS.0000000000002950.
61. Mergenthaler JA, Gan C, Yan Y, Cyr AE, Tenenbaum M, Hook D, et al. Oncologic safety and outcomes in patients undergoing nipple-sparing mastectomy. J Am Coll Surg. 2020;230(4):535–41. https://doi.org/10.1016/j.jamcollsurg.2019.12.028.
62. Colwell AS, Tessler O, Lin AM, Liao E, Winograd J, Cetrulo CL, et al. Breast reconstruction following nipple-sparing mastectomy: predictors of complications, reconstruction outcomes, and 5-year trends. Plast Reconstr Surg. 2014;133:496e506.
63. Lohsiriwat V, Rotmensz N, Botteri E, Intra M, Veronesi P, Martella S, et al. Do clinicopathological

features of the cancer patient relate with nipple areolar complex necrosis in nipple-sparing mastectomy? Ann Surg Oncol. 2013;20(3):990e6. https://doi.org/10.1245/s10434-012-2677-8.
64. Headon HL, Kasem A, Mokbel K. The oncological safety of nipple-sparing mastectomy: a systematic review of the literature with a pooled analysis of 12,358 procedures. Arch Plast Surg. 2016;43(4):328e38. https://doi.org/10.5999/aps.2016.43.4.328.
65. Wong SM, Chun YS, Sagara Y, Golshan M, Erdmann-Sager J. National patterns of breast reconstruction and nipple-sparing mastectomy for breast cancer, 2005-2015. Ann Surg Oncol. 2019;26:3194–203.
66. Fisher B, Anderson S, Bryant J, Margolese RG, Deutsch M, Fisher ER, et al. Twenty-year follow-up of a randomized trial comparing total mastectomy, lumpectomy, and lumpectomy plus irradiation for the treatment of invasive breast cancer. N Engl J Med. 2002;347:1233–41.
67. Salgarello M, Visconti G, Barone-Adesi L. Nipple-sparing mastectomy with immediate implant reconstruction: cosmetic outcomes and technical refinements. Plast Reconstr Surg. 2010;126:1460–71.
68. Petit JY, Veronesi U, Orecchia R, Rey P, Martella S, Didier F, et al. Nipple sparing mastectomy with nipple sparing areola intraoperative radiotherapy: one thousand and one cases of five years experience at the European Institute of Oncology of Milan (EIO). Breast Cancer Res Treat. 2009;117:333–8.
69. Petit JY, Veronesi U, Orecchia R, Curigliano G, Rey PC, Botteri E, et al. Risk factors associated with recurrence after nipple-sparing mastectomy for invasive and intraepithelial neoplasia. Ann Oncol. 2012;23(8):2053–8.
70. Veronesi U, Cascinelli N, Mariani L, Greco M, Saccozzi R, Luini A, et al. Twenty-year follow-up of a randomized study comparing breast-conserving surgery with radical mastectomy for early breast cancer. N Engl J Med. 2002;347:1227–32.
71. Yi M, Kronowitz SJ, Meric-Bernstam F, Feig BW, Symmans WF, Lucci A, et al. Local, regional and systemic recurrence rates in patients undergoing skin sparing mastectomy compared with conventional mastectomy. Cancer. 2011;117:916–24.
72. Gerber B, Krause A, Dieterich M, Kundt G, Reimer T. The oncological safety of skin sparing mastectomy with conservation of the nipple-areola complex and autologous reconstruction: an extended follow-up study. Ann Surg. 2009;249:461–8.
73. National Comprehensive Cancer Network (NCCN). NCCN guidelines version 6.2020. Invasive breast cancer. https://www.nccn.org/professionals/physician_gls/pdf/breast.pdf. Accessed 12 December 2020.
74. Crowe JP, Patrick RJ, Yetman RJ, Djohan R. Nipple-sparing mastectomy update: one hundred forty-nine procedures and clinical outcomes. Arch Surg. 2008;143(11):1106–10. (discussion 10)
75. Lagios MD, Gates EA, Westdahl PR, Richards V, Alpert BS. A guide to the frequency of nipple involvement in breast cancer. a study of 149 consecutive mastectomies using a serial subgross and correlated radiographic technique. Am J Surg. 1979;138(1):135–42.
76. de Alcantara FP, Capko D, Barry JM, Morrow M, Pusic A, Sacchini VS. Nipple-sparing mastectomy for breast cancer andrisk-reducing surgery: the memorial Sloan-Kettering cancer center experience. Ann Surg Oncol. 2011;18(11):3117–22.
77. Carlson GW, Styblo TM, Lyles RH, Jones G, Murray DR, Staley CA, et al. The use of skin sparing mastectomy in the treatment of breast cancer: the Emory experience. Surg Oncol. 2003;12(4):265–9.
78. Orzalesi L, Casella D, Santi C, Cecconi L, Murgo R, Rinaldi S, et al. Nipple sparing mastectomy: surgical and oncological outcomes from a national multicentric registry with 913 patients (1006 cases) over a six year period. Breast. 2016;25:75–81.
79. Coopey SB, Tang R, Lei L, Freer PE, Kansal K, Colwell AS, et al. Increasing eligibility for nipplesparing mastectomy. Ann Surg Oncol. 2013;20(10):3218–22.
80. Krajewski AC, Boughey JC, Degnim AC, Jakub JW, Jacobson SR, Hoskin TL, et al. Expanded indications and improved outcomes for nipple-sparing mastectomy over time. Ann Surg Oncol. 2015;22(10):3317–23.
81. Boneti C, Yuen J, Santiago C, et al. Oncologic safety of nipple skin-sparing or total skin-sparing mastectomies with immediate reconstruction. J Am Coll Surg. 2011;212(4):686–93. (discussion 93–5)
82. Lohsiriwat V, Martella S, Rietjens M, Botteri E, Rotmensz N, Mastropasqua MG, et al. Paget's disease as a local recurrence after nipple-sparing mastectomy: clinical presentation, treatment, outcome, and risk factor analysis. Ann Surg Oncol. 2012;19(6):1850–5.
83. Wu ZY, Kim HJ, Lee JW, Chung IY, Kim JS, Lee SB, et al. Breast cancer recurrence in the nipple-areola complex after nipple-sparing mastectomy with immediate breast for invasive breast cancer. JAMA Surg. 2019;154:1030e1037.
84. Wu ZY, Ko B. Recurrence at nipple-areola complex and safety of nipple-sparing mastectomy-reply. JAMA Surg. 2020;155(4):365. https://doi.org/10.1001/jamasurg.2019.5478.
85. Agha RA, Al Omran Y, Wellstead G, Sagoo H, Barai I, Rajmohan S, et al. Systematic review of therapeutic nipple-sparing versus skin-sparing mastectomy. BJS Open. 2019;3:135e145.
86. Garcia-Etienne CA, Cody Iii HS, Disa JJ, Cordeiro P, Sacchini V. Nipple-sparing mastectomy: initial experience at the memorial Sloan-Kettering cancer center and a comprehensive review of literature. Breast J. 2009;15(4):440–9.
87. Wu ZY, Kim HJ, Lee JW, Chung IY, Kim JS, Lee SB, et al. Oncologic outcomes of nipple-sparing mastectomy and immediate reconstruction after neoadjuvant chemotherapy for breast cancer. Ann Surg. 2020; https://doi.org/10.1097/SLA.0000000000003798. Online ahead of print

88. Kim S, Lee S, Bae Y, Lee S. Nipple-sparing mastectomy for breast cancer close to the nipple: a single institution's 11-year experience. Breast Cancer. 2020;27(5):999–1006. https://doi.org/10.1007/s12282-020-01104-0.
89. Didier F, Radice D, Gandini S, Bedolis R, Rotmensz N, Maldifassi A, et al. Does nipple preservation in mastectomy improve satisfaction with cosmetic results, psychological adjustment, body image and sexuality? Breast Cancer Res Treat. 2009;118(3):623e33. https://doi.org/10.1007/s10549-008-0238-4.
90. Yueh JH, Houlihan MJ, Slavin SA, Lee BT, Pories SE, Morris DJ. Nipple-sparing mastectomy: evaluation of patient satisfaction, aesthetic results, and sensation. Ann Plast Surg. 2009;62:586–90.
91. Djohan R, Gage E, Gatherwright J, Pavri S, Firouz J, Bernard S, et al. Patient satisfaction following nipple-sparing mastectomy and immediate breast reconstruction: an 8-year outcome study. Plast Reconstr Surg. 2010;125:818–299.
92. Sisco M, Yao KA. Nipple-sparing mastectomy: a contemporary perspective. J Surg Oncol. 2016;113(8):883e90. https://doi.org/10.1002/jso.24209.
93. Veronesi U, Stafyla V, Luini A, Veronesi P. Breast cancer: from "maximum tolerable" to "minimum effective" treatment. Front Oncol. 2012;2:125. https://doi.org/10.3389/fonc.2012.00125.

5 Prepectoral Breast Reconstruction: Selection Criteria and Patient Considerations

Hani Sbitany, Sharat Chopra, Raghavan Vidya, and Hilton Becker

5.1 Introduction

With nearly one million new breast cancer cases diagnosed worldwide yearly, around 55,900 new breast cancers are diagnosed alone in the United Kingdom [1]. With further advances in treating these patients with synthetic (Vicryl®, Titanium or TIGR® Mesh) and biological material, i.e., Acellular Dermal Matrix (ADM) for implant-based reconstructions, the traditional post-pectoral implant-based reconstruction has given way to less traumatic and minimally invasive prepectoral breast reconstruction. The prepectoral space is a space between the breast skin envelope and chest wall muscle [2] and is used to place the ADM and implant. This technique involves the placement of a breast implant above the pectoralis major and serratus muscles, thereby leaving the chest wall muscles in their original anatomic locations [3]. Prepectoral reconstruction avoids irradiation-induced fibrosis and tightening of the chest wall, resulting in impaired upper arm strength and range of motion, thus avoiding implant mispositioning. The advantage of this technique includes early discharge from hospitals due to reduced postoperative pain, avoidance of animation deformities, higher patient satisfaction rates, and superior aesthetic outcomes [4–6].

With careful patient selection and a thorough surgical technique, prepectoral breast reconstruction can be performed with minimal morbidity and high patient satisfaction. With the proximity of the breast implant to the mastectomy skin flaps and relatively less vascularized coverage, the surgeon/ clinician must assess preoperative and intraoperative risk factors to ensure good outcomes. This article discusses preoperative, intraoperative, and postoperative essential considerations that should help optimize prepectoral breast reconstruction outcomes.

H. Sbitany (✉)
Plastic and Reconstructive Surgery, Mount Sinai West Medical Center, New York, NY, USA
e-mail: hani.sbitany@mountsinai.org

S. Chopra
Honorary Lecturer Cardiff University, Cardiff & Vale University Health Board, Breast Centre, University Hospital Llandough, Cardiff, Wales, UK

R. Vidya
The Royal Wolverhampton N.H.S. Trust, Wolverhampton, UK
e-mail: Raghavan.vidya@nhs.net

H. Becker
Department of Surgery, Clinic of Plastic Surgery, Florida Atlantic University, Boca Raton, FL, USA

Weston, USA
e-mail: Hilton@beckermd.com

© The Author(s), under exclusive license to Springer Nature Switzerland AG 2023

R. Vidya, H. Becker (eds.), *Prepectoral Breast Reconstruction*,
https://doi.org/10.1007/978-3-031-15590-1_5

5.2 Preoperative Selection Considerations

5.2.1 Patient Criteria

Prepectoral implant reconstruction should be considered in anyone who would generally be suitable for an implant breast reconstruction (Fig. 5.1).

Relative Contraindications to a prepectoral breast reconstruction generally include obesity (BMI-over 35), patients with poorly controlled diabetes mellitus, immunocompromised, and active smokers. These comorbidities often result in compromised blood perfusion of flaps, increasing the risk of mastectomy flap necrosis and implant extrusion. Other contraindications include poor skin quality, which can be due to inherent deficiency of collagen in the skin or secondary to radiation to the chest wall following breast cancer treatment or in cases of Hodgkin's lymphoma [7]. Delayed radiation tissue changes in the breast lead to skin fibrosis, ultimately leading to more complications such as higher capsular contracture rates, implant failures, and poor cosmesis [8]. Above such, patients would be suitably treated with autologous reconstruction.

In contrast, patients receiving postmastectomy radiation therapy (PMRT) can be considered for prepectoral reconstruction. Although the risk of complications after prepectoral reconstruction with PMRT is more, it is comparable to complete submuscular breast reconstruction receiving PMRT [9]. Thus, prepectoral reconstruction should be considered in these subsets of patients.

The use of prepectoral breast reconstruction in delayed reconstruction settings has also been studied with some success. It is believed that the mastectomy flaps have adapted to vascular change over time, thereby increasing the likelihood of reconstructive success. Another subset of patients that benefit from delayed prepectoral reconstruction is those that have undergone postpectoral implant reconstruction and have developed significant muscle pain and tightness or animation deformity. These patients often tend to have complete resolution of their symptoms, including animation deformity [10].

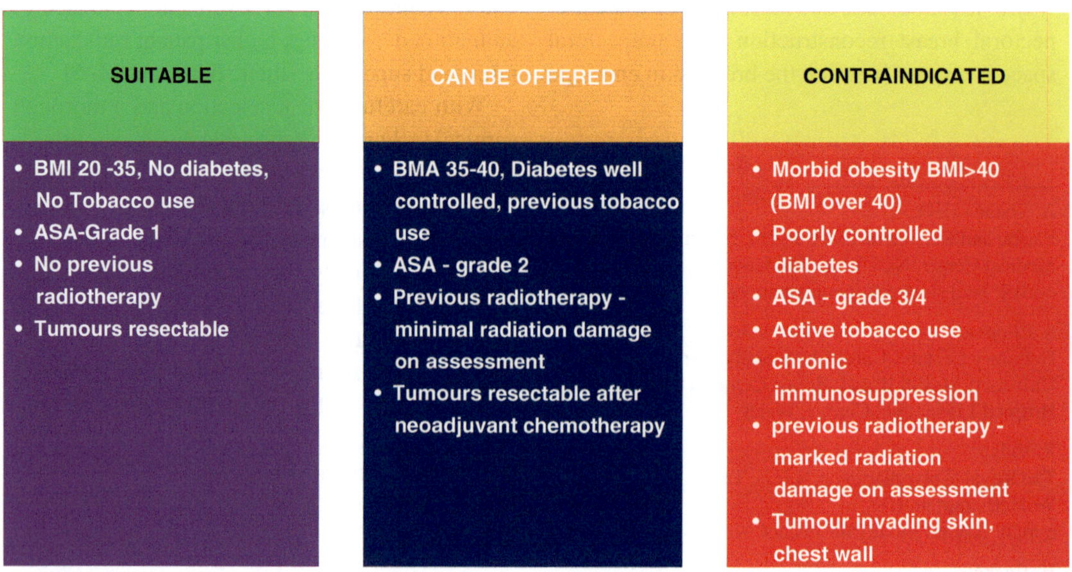

Fig. 5.1 Preoperative selection Considerations

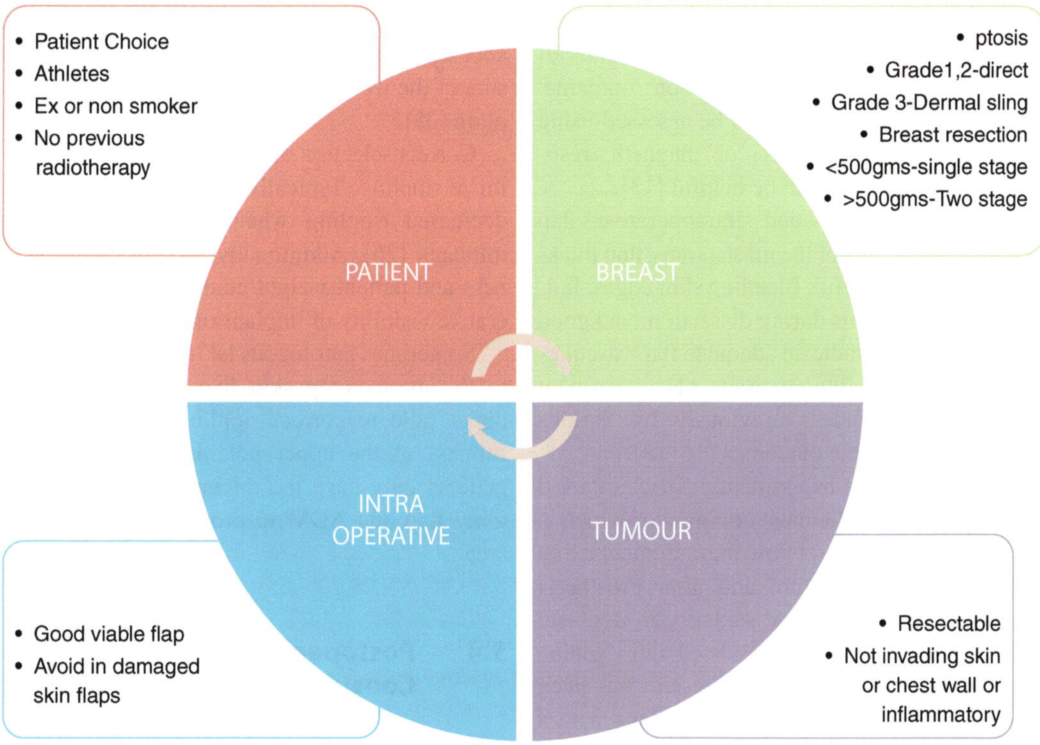

Fig. 5.2 Prepectoral Breast Reconstruction: Selection Criteria and Patient Considerations

5.2.2 Tumor-Specific Considerations

In addition to the above, tumor location and histology should be assessed before mastectomy and reconstruction. Tumors that invade the chest wall or are close to the pectoralis muscle should be considered a contraindication to prepectoral reconstruction, as these patients have a higher risk of tumor recurrence [7, 11]. These patients could potentially benefit from a post-pectoral implant reconstruction that might not prevent a local recurrence but could enable early detection through easier palpation/examination.

The other oncologic considerations not suitable for prepectoral breast reconstruction include patients with inflammatory breast cancer or stage IV breast cancer, aggressive axillary disease, or a non-resectable disease. These patients often require aggressive adjuvant therapy that may make them poor candidates for prepectoral reconstruction.

Figure 5.2 demonstrates selection criteria and patient considerations for prepectoral breast reconstruction.

5.3 Intraoperative Considerations

5.3.1 Intraoperative Assessment of Mastectomy Flaps

A poorly vascularized skin flap may result in skin necrosis, poor tissue healing, and subsequent infection, leading to implant extrusion. The appropriate assessment of skin flap vascularity is vital to the operation's success. It can be done through a careful clinical evaluation or by using devices to assess flap vascularity, intraoperatively.

Ideal patient selection [7] is the most crucial step whilst considering prepectoral implant reconstruction. A good patient's skin elasticity, previous radiotherapy to the skin and other factors negatively impacting such as diabetes mellitus, high body mass index, and smoking status all adversely affect the reconstruction outcome. Breast skin thickness can also be assessed using digital mammography [12] or magnetic resonance imaging which can be helpful [13].

Visual inspection and intraoperative flap assessment [14, 15] of the mastectomy flap thickness can also be useful. Bleeding skin edges, failure to expose dermis during dissection, and good capillary refill all indicate adequate flap vascularity. Intraoperative blood/ tissue pH assessment for flaps was studied previously by various authors with variable outcomes [16–18].

Tissue perfusion assessment devices are used at various centers, the most common of which is angiography with blood flow measurement using indocyanine green before and after prosthesis placement to assess flap vascularity in doubtful cases. The use of a laser-assisted indocyanine green fluorescent angiography system has been in use to check the viability of the flaps with a higher degree of sensitivity and specificity [19–21].

Preoperative incision planning over skin flaps is essential to avoid compromising flap vascularity which would ultimately lead to poor cosmesis. Incisions placed on the outer edge/lateral aspect or in the inframammary fold can usually avoid such complications [22]. Incisions around the nipple should be best avoided as they can damage the blood supply.

5.3.2 Cosmetic Considerations

Rippling is a common cosmetic problem with prepectoral reconstruction. The rate varies from 0 to 35% through the literature [10, 23, 24] more commonly seen with a saline implant than with a silicone implant. Several techniques are used to minimize such complications. Sometimes underfilling the expander by 100 cc during initial expander placement might be helpful. This helps with the final implant placement which can fit in a tighter pocket and could reduce the potential for implant mobility. In thin individuals with a body mass index <21, the base pocket size should be kept smaller than the implant for adequate closure of the wound to minimize postoperative rippling [25].

Correct selection of an implant can often minimize rippling. Typically, silicone implants have decreased rippling when compared to saline implants [26]. Additionally, suitable flap thickness and patient weight could influence postoperative visibility of implant rippling [25, 26].

Sometimes autologous fat transfer can be used to the mastectomy skin flap, especially in the upper pole to correct rippling [27]. Providing fullness in the upper pole is critical as these patients only have the thickness of the mastectomy flap and ADM to provide volume in this area.

5.4 Postoperative Considerations

5.4.1 Infection

With no muscle coverage in prepectoral breast reconstruction, skin breakdown is likely to lead to exposure to ADM and subsequent implant extrusion. These patients with a suspected infection should be closely followed. Hence it is important to treat suspected infection carefully with oral antibiotics and closely monitored in a outpatient setting. However if patient demonstrates threatened implant exposure then hospital admission is required with intravenous antibiotics, urgent surgical debridement, threatened skin excision, implant removal if needed. Postoperative surgical site infection in the context of prior implant placement needs immediate operative management due to the risk of biofilm formation. They are a major threat in the context of surgical site infection and difficult to eradicate in spite of long-term antibiotics [28, 29].

Earlier study by the senior author in 51 patients (84 breasts), noted a 5% rate of cellulitis with 2.4% rate of infections requiring a washout during a follow up period of 11.1 + 5.8 months [10].

A retrospective review of 54 patients who underwent two-stage prepectoral implant-based breast reconstruction with postmastectomy radiation therapy found the infection rate was higher in the irradiated breast than in non-irradiated one (18.8% vs 7.7%, respectively) [30].

In another group of patients who underwent prepectoral implant reconstruction without mesh, De vita et al. reported no infection in their retrospective review of 34 nipple-sparing prepectoral implant reconstructions with polyurethane over a 4-month follow-up period [31]. However, in a similar study by Singla et al., he reported an infection rate of 15% (Minor 11.5% and Major 3.8%) [32]. This rate could perhaps be related to the study's seroma rate (15.3%) with its tendency to get superficial cellulitis/ infection.

5.5 Conclusion

As the demand for breast reconstruction increases, newer and novel breast reconstruction methods are being used to provide both cosmesis and oncological safety. With an increase in subcutaneous mastectomy, the role of prepectoral implant-based reconstruction has gained even more popularity. The prepectoral breast reconstruction with an implant following mastectomy using synthetic mesh or Acellular Dermal Matrix (ADM) provides an adequate soft tissue coverage to the implant under the skin with near comparable outcomes to subpectoral implant-based reconstruction. However, obtaining optimal results depends on various preoperative, intraoperative, and postoperative strategies. Patient selection remains one of the main factors in minimizing potential risks and complications, with oncologic factors playing a significant role in discussions, especially during the multidisciplinary meetings before offering or contemplating a prepectoral reconstruction. Intraoperatively, a suitable mastectomy technique with an assessment of the viability of mastectomy flap perfusion both by clinical examination and with perfusion devices, such as indocyanine green laser angiography, can be critical for reconstructive success.

Prepectoral reconstruction offers numerous benefits, including eliminating animation deformity, decreased pain, creating a breast pocket with ADM, high patient satisfaction, and good cosmesis. Following the methods and considerations mentioned above, a surgeon can minimize the risk of complications and provide adequate reconstruction to the patient.

References

1. Cancer Research U.K. Breast Cancer Statistics, Available at: http://www.cancerresearchuk.org/health-professional/cancer-statistics/statistics-by-cancer-type/breast-cancer. Accessed: October 25, 2021.
2. Vidya R, Iqbal FM. Breast anatomy: Time to classify the subpectoral and prepectoral spaces. Clin Anat. 2017;30(4):434–5. https://doi.org/10.1002/ca.22878. Epub 2017 April 8. P.M.I.D.: 28318062
3. Becker H, Lind JG 2nd, Hopkins EG, et al. Immediate implant-based prepectoral breast reconstruction using a vertical incision. Plast Reconstr Surg Glob Open. 2015;3(6):e412.
4. Sigalove S, Maxwell GP, Sigalove NM, et al. Prepectoral implant-based breast reconstruction: rationale, indications, and preliminary results. Plast Reconstr Surg. 2017;139(2):287–94.
5. Becker H, Fregosi N. The impact of animation deformity on quality of life in post-mastectomy reconstruction patients. Aesthet Surg J. 2017;37(5):531–6.
6. Gabriel A, Sigalove S, Sigalove NM, et al. Prepectoral revision breast reconstruction for treatment of implant-associated animation deformity: a review of 102 reconstructions. Aesthet Surg J. 2018;38(5):519–26.
7. Vidya R, Berna G, Sbitany H, Nahabedian M, Becker H, Reitsamer R, Rancati A, Macmillan D, Cawthorn S. Prepectoral implant-based breast reconstruction: a joint consensus guide from U.K., European and U.S.A. breast and plastic reconstructive surgeons. Ecancermedicalscience. 2019;13:927. https://doi.org/10.3332/ecancer.2019.927. PMID: 31281424; PMCID: PMC6592711
8. Barry M, Kell MR. Radiotherapy and breast reconstruction: a meta-analysis. Breast Cancer Res Treat. 2011;127(1):15–22. https://doi.org/10.1007/s10549-011-1401-x. Epub 2011 February 20. P.M.I.D.: 21336948
9. Sbitany H, Gomez-Sanchez C, Piper M, et al. Prepectoral breast reconstruction in the setting of postmastectomy radiation therapy: an assessment of clinical outcomes and benefits. Plast Reconstr Surg. 2019;143(1):10–20.
10. Sbitany H, Piper M, Lentz R. Prepectoral breast reconstruction: a safe alternative to submuscular prosthetic reconstruction following nipple-sparing mastectomy.

Plast Reconstr Surg. 2017;140(3):432–43. https://doi.org/10.1097/PRS.0000000000003627.
11. Buchanan CL, Dorn PL, Fey J, et al. Locoregional recurrence after mastectomy: incidence and outcomes. J Am Coll Surg. 2006;203(4):469–74.
12. Rancati AO, Angrigiani CH, Hammond DC, et al. Direct to implant reconstruction in nipple-sparing mastectomy: patient selection by preoperative digital mammogram. Plast Reconstr Surg Glob Open. 2017;5(6):e1369. https://doi.org/10.1097/GOX.0000000000001369.
13. Frey JD, Salibian AA, Choi M, Karp NS. Mastectomy flap thickness and complications in nipple-sparing mastectomy: objective evaluation using magnetic resonance imaging. Plast Reconstr Surg Glob Open. 2017;5(8):e1439. https://doi.org/10.1097/GOX.0000000000001439.
14. Pafitanis G, Raveendran M, Myers S, Ghanem AM. Flowmetry evolution in microvascular surgery: a systematic review. J Plast Reconstr Aesthet Surg. 2017;70(9):1242–51. https://doi.org/10.1016/j.bjps.2017.05.010.
15. Jeon FHK, Varghese J, Griffin M, Butler PE, Ghosh D, Mosahebi A. Systematic review of methodologies used to assess mastectomy flap viability. BJS Open. 2018;2(4):175–84. https://doi.org/10.1002/bjs5.61.
16. Raskin DJ, Erk Y, Spira M, Melissinos EG. Tissue pH monitoring in microsurgery: a preliminary evaluation of continuous tissue pH monitoring as an indicator of perfusion disturbances in microvascular free flaps. Ann Plast Surg. 1983;11(4):331–9. https://doi.org/10.1097/00000637-198310000-00013.
17. Dunn RM, Kaplan IB, Mancoll J, Terzis JK, Trengove-Jones G. Experimental and clinical use of pH monitoring of free tissue transfers. Ann Plast Surg. 1993;31(6):539–45. https://doi.org/10.1097/00000637-199312000-00011.
18. Warner KG, Durham-Smith G, Butler MD, Attinger CE, Upton J, Khuri SF. Comparative response of muscle and subcutaneous tissue pH during arterial and venous occlusion in musculocutaneous flaps. Ann Plast Surg. 1989;22(2):108–16. https://doi.org/10.1097/00000637-198902000-00005. PMID: 2735706
19. Mirhaidari SJ, Beddell GM, Orlando MV, Parker MG, Pedersen JC, Wagner DS. A prospective study of immediate breast reconstruction with laser-assisted indocyanine green angiography. Plast Reconstr Surg Glob Open. 2018;6(9):e1774. https://doi.org/10.1097/GOX.0000000000001774.
20. Phillips BT, Lanier ST, Conkling N, et al. Intraoperative perfusion techniques can accurately predict mastectomy skin flap necrosis in breast reconstruction: results of a prospective trial. Plast Reconstr Surg. 2012;129:778e–88e. https://doi.org/10.1097/PRS.0b013e31824a2ae8.
21. Mattison GL, Lewis PG, Gupta SC, et al. S.P.Y. imaging use in postmastectomy breast reconstruction patients: preventative or overly conservative? Plast Reconstr Surg. 2016;138:15e–21e. https://doi.org/10.1097/PRS.0000000000002266.
22. Frey JD, Salibian AA, Levine JP, Karp NS, Choi M. Incision choices in nipple-sparing mastectomy: a comparative analysis of outcomes and evolution of a clinical algorithm. Plast Reconstr Surg. 2018;142:826e–35e. https://doi.org/10.1097/PRS.0000000000004969.
23. Downs RK, Hedges K. An alternative technique for immediate direct-to-implant breast reconstruction-a case series. Plast Reconstr Surg Glob Open. 2016;4(7):e821.
24. Casella D, Bernini M, Bencini L, et al. TiLoop® Bra mesh used for immediate breast reconstruction: comparison of retropectoral and subcutaneous implant placement in a prospective single-institution series. Eur J Plast Surg. 2014;37:599–604.
25. Salibian AH, Harness JK, Mowlds DS. Staged suprapectoral expander/implant reconstruction without acellular dermal matrix following nipple-sparing mastectomy. Plast Reconstr Surg. 2017;139(1):30–9. https://doi.org/10.1097/PRS.0000000000002845.
26. Isaac KV, Murphy BD, Beber B, et al. The reliability of anthropometric measurements used preoperatively in aesthetic breast surgery. Aesthet Surg J. 2016;36(4):431–7.
27. Sbitany H. Important considerations for performing prepectoral breast reconstruction. Plast Reconstr Surg. 2017;140(6S Prepectoral Breast Reconstruction):7S–13S. https://doi.org/10.1097/PRS.0000000000004045. PMID: 29166342
28. Vidya R, Masià J, Cawthorn S, et al. Evaluation of the effectiveness of the prepectoral breast reconstruction with Braxon dermal matrix: first multicenter European report on 100 cases. Breast J. 2017;23(6):670–6. https://doi.org/10.1111/tbj.12810.
29. Chopra S, Al-Ishaq Z, Vidya R. The journey of prepectoral breast reconstruction through time. World J Plast Surg. 2021;10(2):3–13. https://doi.org/10.29252/wjps.10.2.3. PMID: 34307092; PMCID: PMC8290458
30. Elswick SM, Harless CA, Bishop SN, et al. Prepectoral implant-based breast reconstruction with postmastectomy radiation therapy. Plast Reconstr Surg. 2018;142(1):1–12. https://doi.org/10.1097/PRS.0000000000004453.
31. De Vita R, Buccheri EM, Villanucci A, Pozzi M. Breast reconstruction actualized in nipple-sparing mastectomy and direct-to-implant, prepectoral polyurethane positioning: early experience and preliminary results. Clin Breast Cancer. 2019;19(2):e358–63. https://doi.org/10.1016/j.clbc.2018.12.015.
32. Singla A, Singla A, Lai E, Caminer D. Subcutaneously placed breast implants after a skin-sparing mastectomy: do we always need A.D.M.? Plast Reconstr Surg Glob Open. 2017;5(7):e1371. https://doi.org/10.1097/GOX.0000000000001371. PMID: 28831335; PMCID: PMC5548558

6 Skin and Nipple-Sparing Mastectomy with Axillary Staging in Prepectoral Breast Reconstruction

Marios-Konstantinos Tasoulis and Gerald Gui

6.1 Introduction

In the era of multimodality management of breast cancer, breast conserving surgery has been shown to be a safe approach to treat early-stage disease [1, 2]. Analysis of temporal trends has demonstrated a significant increase in the uptake of breast conservation with a reduction in mastectomy rates [3]. Advances in oncoplastic techniques [4] and use of primary systemic therapies [5] may, at least in part, explain this trend. Where possible, breast conservation often provides the most natural and sensate breast that tolerates radiotherapy. However, mastectomy will always be an important tool in the surgical armamentarium. The commonest oncologic indications leading to a recommendation for a mastectomy despite early detection are multicentric disease across multiple quadrants, a failure to secure clear margins at initial breast conservation and local recurrence despite previous breast conservation surgery with radiotherapy. Increased availability of genetic testing and understanding of risk conferred by inheritable predisposition have also seen an increase in the practice of risk-reducing mastectomies.

M.-K. Tasoulis · G. Gui (✉)
Breast Surgery Unit, The Royal Marsden NHS Foundation Trust, London, UK
e-mail: Marios.Tasoulis@rmh.nhs.uk; Gerald.Gui@rmh.nhs.uk

With the evolution and adoption of more conservative surgical techniques shown to confer equivalent oncological outcomes [6–10], skin and nipple-sparing mastectomy has gained significant popularity and is now considered standard of care for the majority of patients requiring removal of the totality of the breast tissue. Apart from the oncological safety, this approach lends itself well to immediate breast reconstruction utilizing the preserved skin envelope to maximum benefit. Native skin confers natural breast covering, avoiding the patchwork appearance of donor site tissue, whilst nipple preservation where possible, conserves breast identity. Maintaining the nipple–areolar complex (NAC) retains the character of the breast and allows women to relate more readily with their breast reconstruction.

The majority of patients who have a skin-sparing mastectomy subsequently undergo nipple reconstruction [11]. The long-term results of nipple reconstruction have some limitations, the more common being a loss of projection, an inability to mimic the rugosity conferred by the smooth muscle of the areolar and the presence of Montgomery's tubercles [11]. These may be further compounded by the use of radiotherapy. In order to improve the aesthetic outcomes, 3-D nipple tattooing has been employed and has been shown to produce promising results although radiotherapy and fading of the micropigmentation may lead to subsequent revisions [12, 13].

© The Author(s), under exclusive license to Springer Nature Switzerland AG 2023

R. Vidya, H. Becker (eds.), *Prepectoral Breast Reconstruction*,
https://doi.org/10.1007/978-3-031-15590-1_6

Whilst nipple reconstruction may result in high levels of patient satisfaction, these are inferior to the level of satisfaction achieved when the NAC is retained [14].

Despite advances in autologous breast reconstruction, implant-based reconstruction (IBR) is the most commonly used method to recreate the breast mound following a mastectomy [15]. As surgical techniques are refined, there has been an increasing trend over the last decade to place the implant in the pre-pectoral plane [16] as opposed to sub-pectoral placement which was traditionally considered the standard method for IBR. Skin and nipple-sparing mastectomy and pre-pectoral breast reconstruction (PPBR) are often combined with axillary staging.

6.2 Skin and Nipple-sparing Mastectomy with Pre-Pectoral Breast Reconstruction: Surgical Planning

Table 6.1 Pre-operative parameters in the surgical planning of nipple and skin-sparing mastectomy for pre-pectoral breast reconstruction

General	Patient BMI and body habitus Level of activity, e.g., work, leisure, and sports Comorbidities: smoking, diabetes, hypertension, coagulopathy
Oncologic	Therapeutic or risk-reducing Unilateral or bilateral Size of cancer including distribution of malignant microcalcifications Proximity of tumor to skin and distance from nipple Previous or planned radiotherapy Locally advanced disease and inflammatory breast cancer
Local tissue	Breast size, shape, ptosis Skin quality including tissue elasticity Characteristics of trunk and hips Pre-existing scars Contralateral breast properties and symmetrization requirements
Patient choice	Understanding of benefits, risks, and complications Expectations Secondary procedures and maintenance surgery Informed consent

The planning of skin and nipple-sparing mastectomy and PPBR begins during the pre-operative consultation. A number of parameters should be taken into consideration. These are summarized in Table 6.1. The attributes of the existing breast form, the breast to match, patient height and weight, and the soft tissues of the trunk should be taken into account and considered in detail with the patient's input. The surgeon should take measurements of the sternal notch to nipple distance, nipple to inframammary fold (IMF) distance, midline to nipple distance, transverse breast width, vertical breast height, and projection. All these measurements along with pre-operative medical photographs form an essential part of the patient's medical record.

The breast width may be assessed either with the use of a caliper or a tape, measuring the projected distance between the lateral edge of the breast plate to the medial border of the breast (Fig. 6.1a). Similarly, the breast height can be measured as the projected distance between the IMF and uppermost point of the breast contour (Fig. 6.1b). The breast projection is measured as the distance between the chest wall or posterior breast margin and the site of maximum breast projection which frequently corresponds to the nipple. A vertical line dropped from the sternal notch may be used as an indicator of the posterior breast margin (Fig. 6.1c). The breast height and in particular the width play an important role in implant selection as they will determine the dimensions of the implant that would fit in the breast pocket following the mastectomy. The breast projection is also a significant consideration that is taken into account along with patient preferences during the pre-operative consultation to select the implants. For a given breast footprint, the projection is the third dimension that determines volume and forms the view unique to the patient when she looks down at the reconstructed breast(s) and the cleavage that is formed.

Apart from the dimensions of width, height, and projection that determine the reconstructed breast volume, the implant shape whether round or anatomical contributes to breast form. The relationship between the selected implant and the

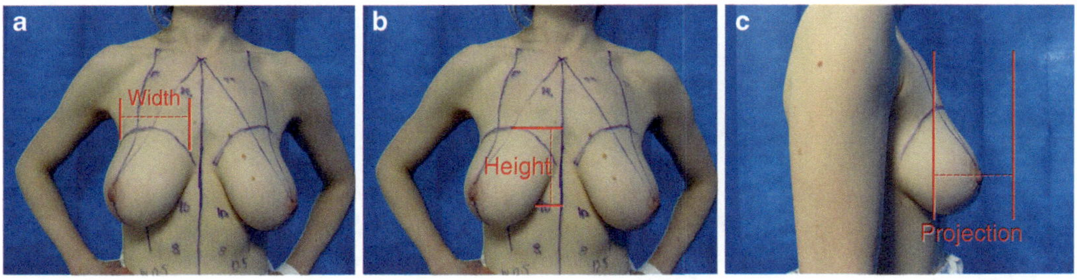

Fig. 6.1 Demonstration of pre-operative marking and measurement of (**a**) breast width, (**b**) breast height, and (**c**) breast projection

perceived reconstructed breast form is complex and goes beyond the simple measurements of height, width, and projection. The characteristics of the upper pole and the nipple to IMF distance differ in principle between anatomical and round implants. The cohesivity and form-stable properties of silicone gel versus saline filled (dual chamber or saline alone) implants are additional parameters to consider to optimize the reconstructive outcome. This is an important part of the surgical planning and forms part of the implant selection and shared decision-making process with the patient. For example, women who prefer a fuller breast with upper pole convexity may favor a round implant, while an anatomical implant may result in a more natural breast contour with more volume in the lower pole. The slope of this contour in the part of the breast above the bra, the "social aspect," is determined by implant projection. The elastomer properties influence tethering to the anterior mastectomy flap, with texturing deliberately causing adhesion to minimize rotation as opposed to smooth implants that are associated with less tissue adhesion. Round implants are available in both smooth and textured surfaces, and this is an additional parameter that may influence the choice of shape. There is increasing data to suggest a potential association between the implant texture and the risk of developing breast implant associated anaplastic large cell lymphoma (BIA-ALCL) [17, 18]. Although this risk appears to be small [17], it may be an important factor for women to decide against a textured surface and opt instead for a round implant.

In women where the desired reconstruction has a similar width and height, the gains of anatomical or round implants are likely to be less apparent, the immediate post-operative characteristics being driven by the projection and upper pole slope. In the middle term, the breast form is primarily dependent on the soft tissue maintaining pliability overlying the implant and the stability of the pocket allowing the implant to sit comfortably in the position it was placed at the end of the surgery. This is the reason why one-stage implant breast reconstruction, including PPBR, requires a stable and tension free pocket to be created at the index operation; if a stable pocket cannot be created following the mastectomy, a two-stage approach is necessary.

6.3 Pre-Operative Marking

Pre-operative assessment and skin marking are performed with the patient upright, sitting or standing, using a measuring tape and a surgical marker pen. Key anatomical landmarks including the sternal notch, midline, breast meridian, and IMF should be marked. The breast meridian is marked from a fixed point on the clavicle, either 5 cm from the medial end or the midclavicular point, projected caudally to include the nipple, extending to intersect the IMF and beyond. In addition, it may be useful to draw the breast contour including the superior breast takeoff and the IMF in order to define the borders of resection and control the "pocket" which is particularly important for IBR and especially PPBR (Fig. 6.2).

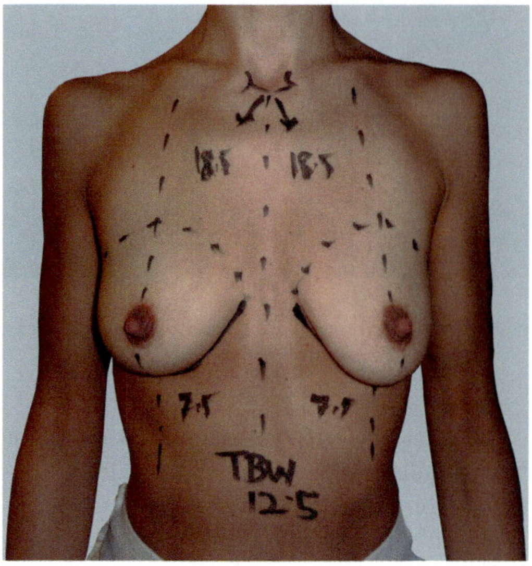

Fig. 6.2 Demonstration or pre-operative markings with the patient standing. Markings include sternal notch, midline, breast meridians, inframammary fold, and breast contour. Measurements demonstrate sternal notch—nipple distance, nipple—midline distance and transverse breast width

It is important to mark both breasts, even when planning to perform unilateral mastectomy in order to try to optimize symmetry.

6.4 Intraoperative Set-up

For surgery, the patient is placed in the supine position with both arms abducted at the shoulder. Preparation and draping should include both breasts regardless of whether the plan is for unilateral or bilateral mastectomy. Skin preparation extends from the base of the neck to the upper abdomen, to exclude the umbilicus in implant reconstruction. Positioning and draping should enable the patient to adopt a sitting position as required during surgery. The operating table should allow intraoperative repositioning of the patient to compare shape, position, and dimensions of the breast, particularly if the aims of surgery are to provide a match to the contralateral side.

Fiber-optic lighting or headlamps are useful to visualize dissection, particularly with remote incisions such as through the IMF. Great care should be taken to avoid trauma by traction or diathermy injury to skin flaps. Insulated instruments are helpful when using diathermy dissection.

6.4.1 Skin-Sparing Mastectomy: Incision Placement

In planning a nipple-sacrificing mastectomy, the incision is usually designed to incorporate the NAC (Fig. 6.3). When used with an implant reconstruction, an ellipse encompassing the NAC usually results in a scar that lies horizontally in the equator of the breast (Figs. 6.3a, b and 6.4). An alternative approach is to design the elliptical incision to include the nipple but spare the areola. When used in the horizontal orientation, this can be extended as a lateral approach for the mastectomy (Fig. 6.5). This incision may also be orientated in a vertical fashion [19] (Fig. 6.3d) and be incorporated into a vertical access for the mastectomy or a mastopexy incision. In either case, the areolar part of the incision can be incorporated into the surgical planning for the nipple reconstruction. Vertical incisions to include the nipple, with or without NAC preservation may result in a less flat appearance around the equator of the reconstructed breast, but consideration and careful planning are required to avoid a scar which would be visible above the bra line (Fig. 6.6).

Pre-existing scars may need to be included in the mastectomy incision especially if the anterior margin is involved following previous breast conserving surgery or if the mastectomy is performed for local recurrence within the previous scar (Fig. 6.3e). Should the cancer encroach close to the overlying skin, the incision should be planned to encompass the involved area. Tethering as a result of tumor traction on the ligaments of Astley Cooper is not an indication for skin resection, unlike tumor involvement of the skin which makes the presentation locally advanced.

It is accepted that implant reconstruction may not achieve the natural ptosis of many breast forms. Where necessary, the mastectomy incision and planning of the reconstruction need to take

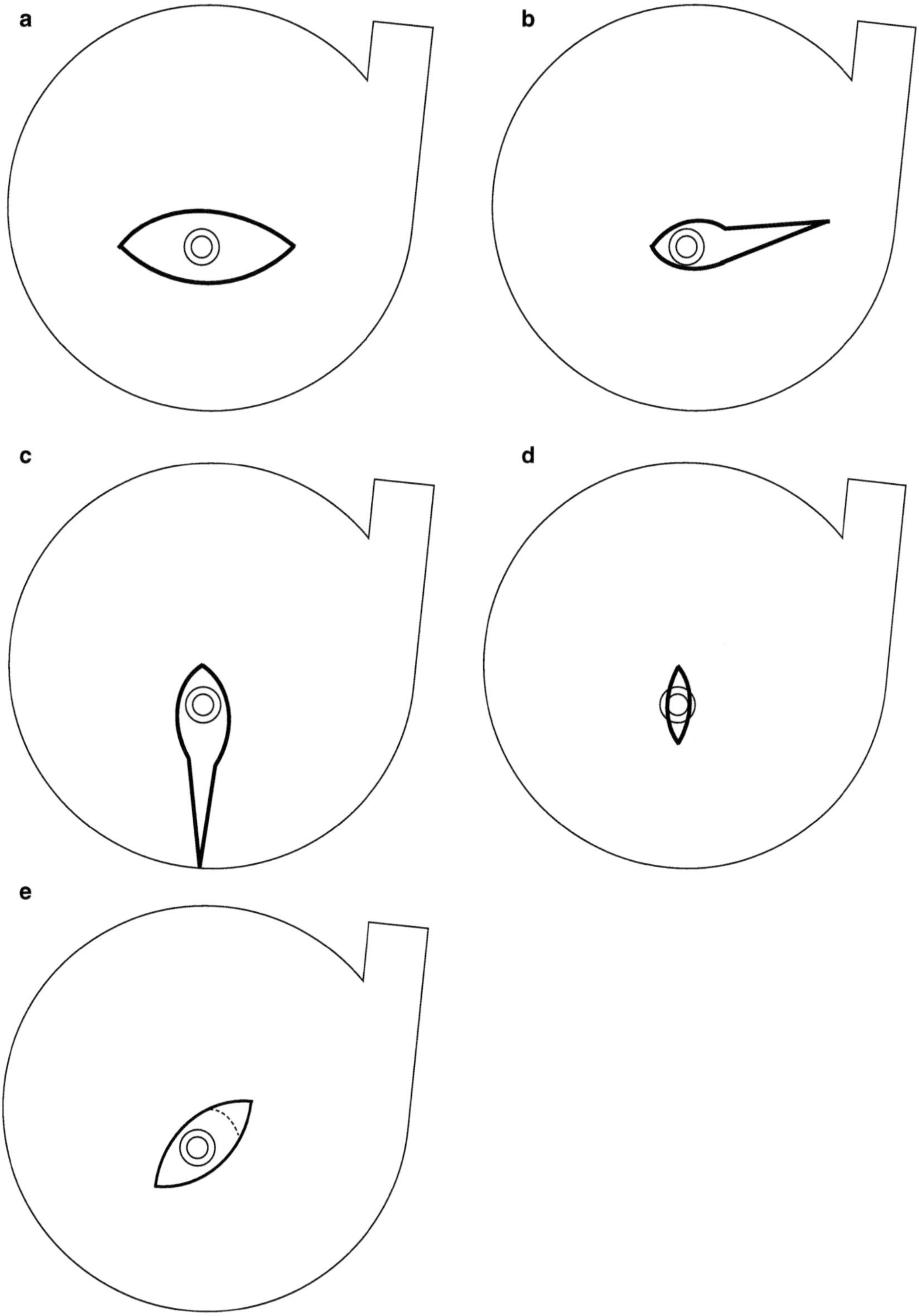

Fig. 6.3 Common incisions for skin-sparing mastectomy and pre-pectoral breast implant breast reconstruction. (**a**) Elliptical incision to include the nipple-areolar complex (NAC), (**b**) Elliptical incision to include the NAC with lateral extension, (**c**) Elliptical incision to include the NAC with vertical extension, (**d**) Elliptical incision to include the nipple but spare the areola, (**e**) Elliptical incision to include NAC and previous breast conserving surgery scar

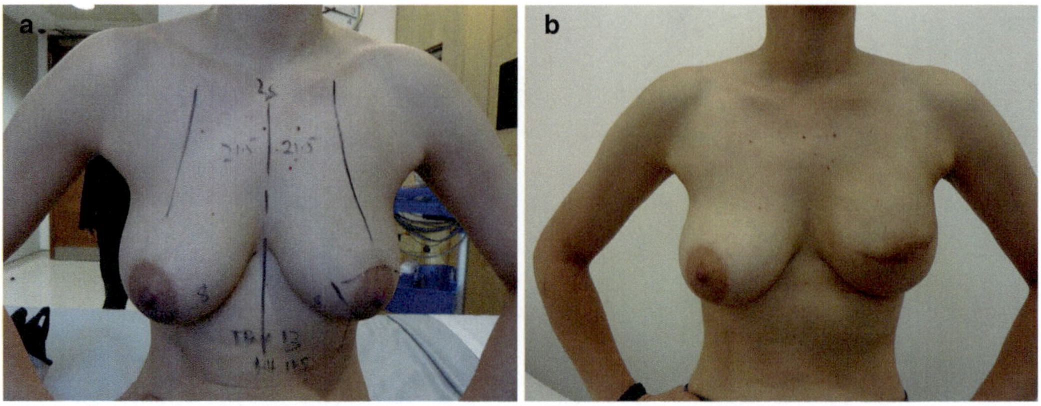

Fig. 6.4 Demonstration of pre-operative marking using a horizontal elliptical incision to encompass the nipple-areolar complex (**a**) and post-operative cosmetic outcome (**b**)

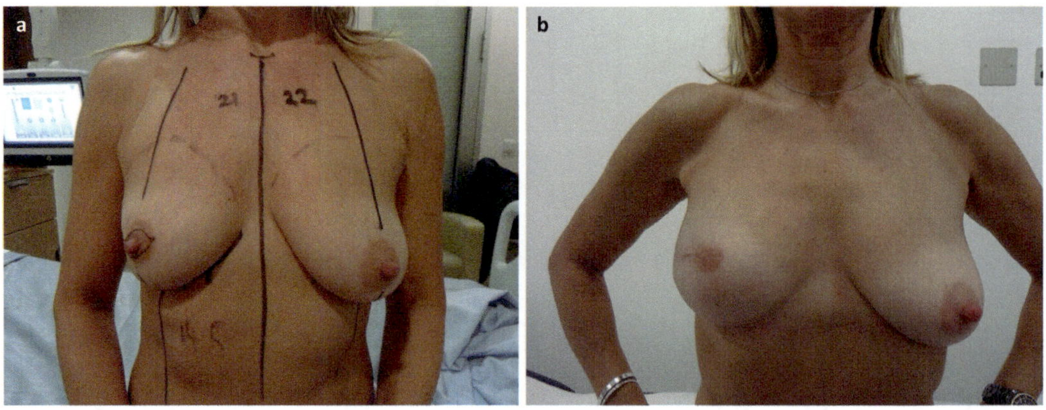

Fig. 6.5 Demonstration of pre-operative marking using a horizontal elliptical incision to include the nipple but spare the areola (**a**) and post-operative cosmetic outcome (**b**)

into account the need for subsequent optimization of symmetry with contralateral surgery as a secondary procedure (Fig. 6.6).

6.4.2 Nipple-Sparing Mastectomy: Incision Placement

Nipple-sparing mastectomy can be performed through a variety of surgical incisions (Fig. 6.7). One of the most widely used is through the IMF (Fig. 6.7a). This is frequently employed in patients with small or medium size breasts and can provide a good aesthetic outcome as it can be hidden within the IMF (Fig. 6.8). For larger volume breasts, lateral crease incisions may be used and can provide excellent access to the breast and may also facilitate access to the axilla when concurrent axillary surgery is required (Fig. 6.7b). The aesthetic benefits of the IMF and lateral crease incisions are that they avoid incisions on the breast mound itself [20]. The IMF incision in particular sits in the line of natural skin tension that heals well and has been shown to be associated with reduced risk of dehiscence particularly after radiotherapy [21] and also the lowest risk of ischemia and overall complication rates [22–24].

Radial incisions are also commonly performed with nipple-sparing mastectomy (Fig. 6.7c–e). A potential benefit is that if the nipple margin is subsequently found to be involved with cancer, the incision can be extended to excise the NAC

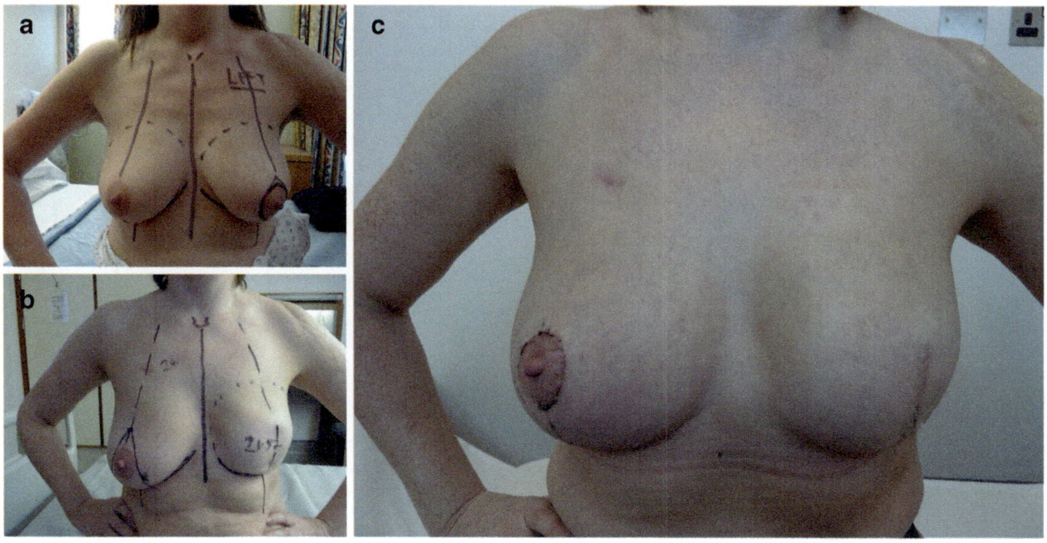

Fig. 6.6 (**a**) Pre-operative mastectomy marking using a vertical elliptical incision to encompass the nipple-areolar complex. (**b**) Pre-operative wise pattern marking for contralateral symmetrization surgery as secondary procedure. (**c**) Cosmetic outcome after bilateral surgery

without significant compromise of the skin envelope. The lateral radial incision (Fig. 6.7c) may be associated with low risk of nipple ischemia [25, 26]. Alternatively, a vertical radial incision may also be employed and is associated with a favorable complication profile [22] (Fig. 6.7d and e). This incision has a potential cosmetic advantage as it can be incorporated into the incision of any future secondary surgery if required, to resemble that of a mastopexy. Periareolar incisions (Fig. 6.7f–i), with or without radial extension, have also been described (Fig. 6.9) but may be associated with higher risk of nipple necrosis [24, 25] and complications [22, 23]. The same oncologic and reconstructive considerations discussed for skin-sparing mastectomy apply to nipple-sparing mastectomy. Particular attention is required where a recent peri- or circumareolar incision has been used, for example, as part of the original breast conservation procedure. Not only may the blood supply to the nipple be compromised but the formation of a second scar should avoid a bridge of tissue vulnerable to ischemia. A recent circumareolar scar may be a contraindication to preserve the NAC but a long-standing incision, after a previous breast conservation procedure or a mastopexy is not.

6.4.3 Raising the Skin Flaps and Removing the Breast

Following the incision, the skin and subcutaneous adipose tissue are gently lifted and the dissection plane is developed with the aim to remove maximal breast glandular tissue. This plane also referred to as the "oncoplastic" plane is defined by the suspensory ligaments of Cooper, between the limits of the breast parenchymal tissue and the subcutaneous adipose tissue (Fig. 6.10). Flap thickness will vary in every individual, and regular assessment of the dissection plane is advised during the surgery. Careful dissection is required to control the breast pocket, preserving the IMF and avoiding over-dissection into the subcutaneous non-breast tissue especially laterally. This is crucial for successful PPBR. The integrity of the vascular plexus in the subdermal plane must be preserved to maintain the blood supply to the mastectomy skin flaps. When the dissection

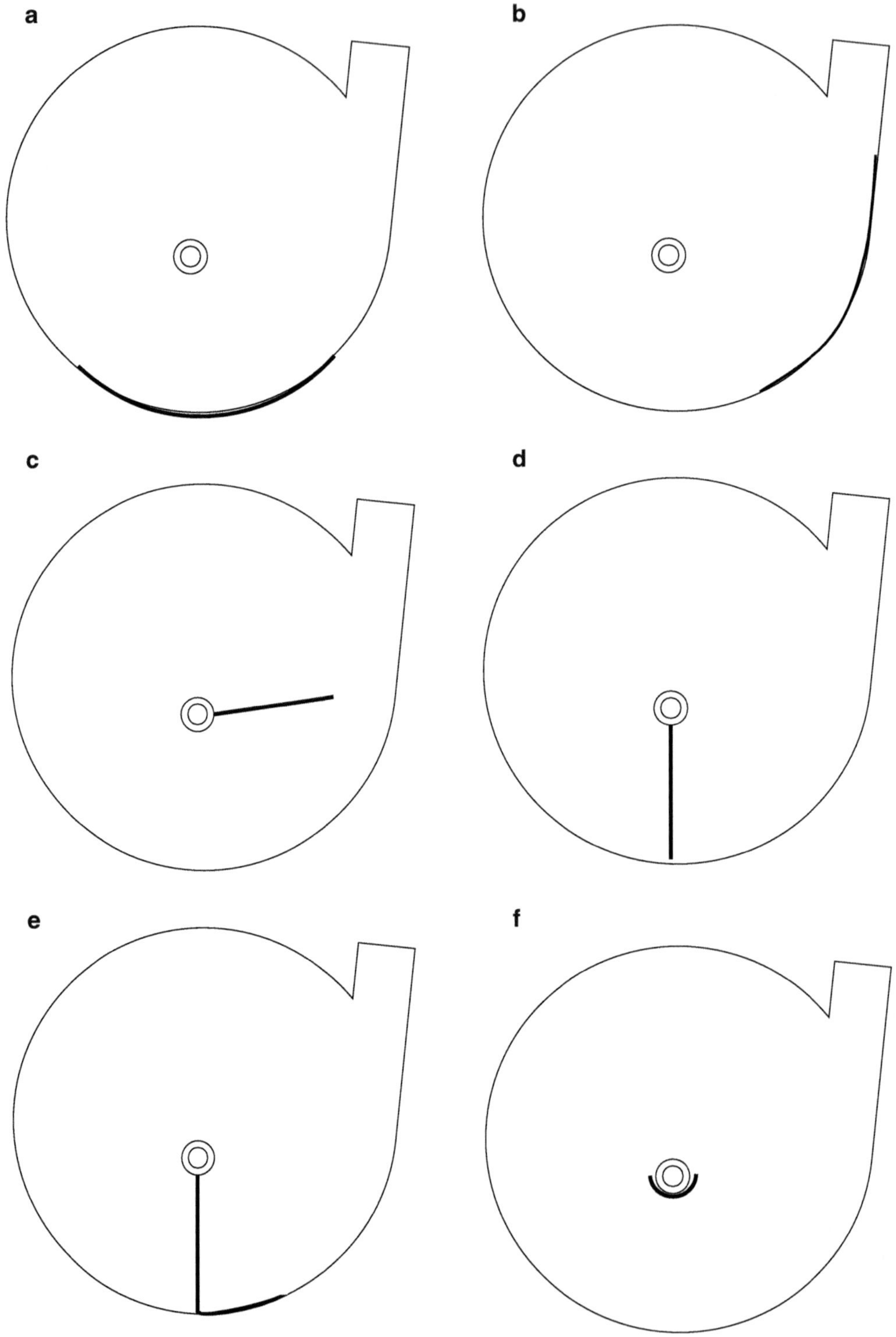

Fig. 6.7 Common incisions for nipple-sparing mastectomy and pre-pectoral implant breast reconstruction. (**a**) Inframammary fold incision, (**b**) Lateral mammary crease incision, (**c**) Radial lateral incision, (**d**) Radial vertical incision, (**e**) Radial vertical incision with lateral extension, (**f**) Periareolar incision, (**g**) Periareolar incision with lateral extension, (**h**) Periareolar incision with medial and lateral extension, (**i**) Periareolar incision with vertical extension

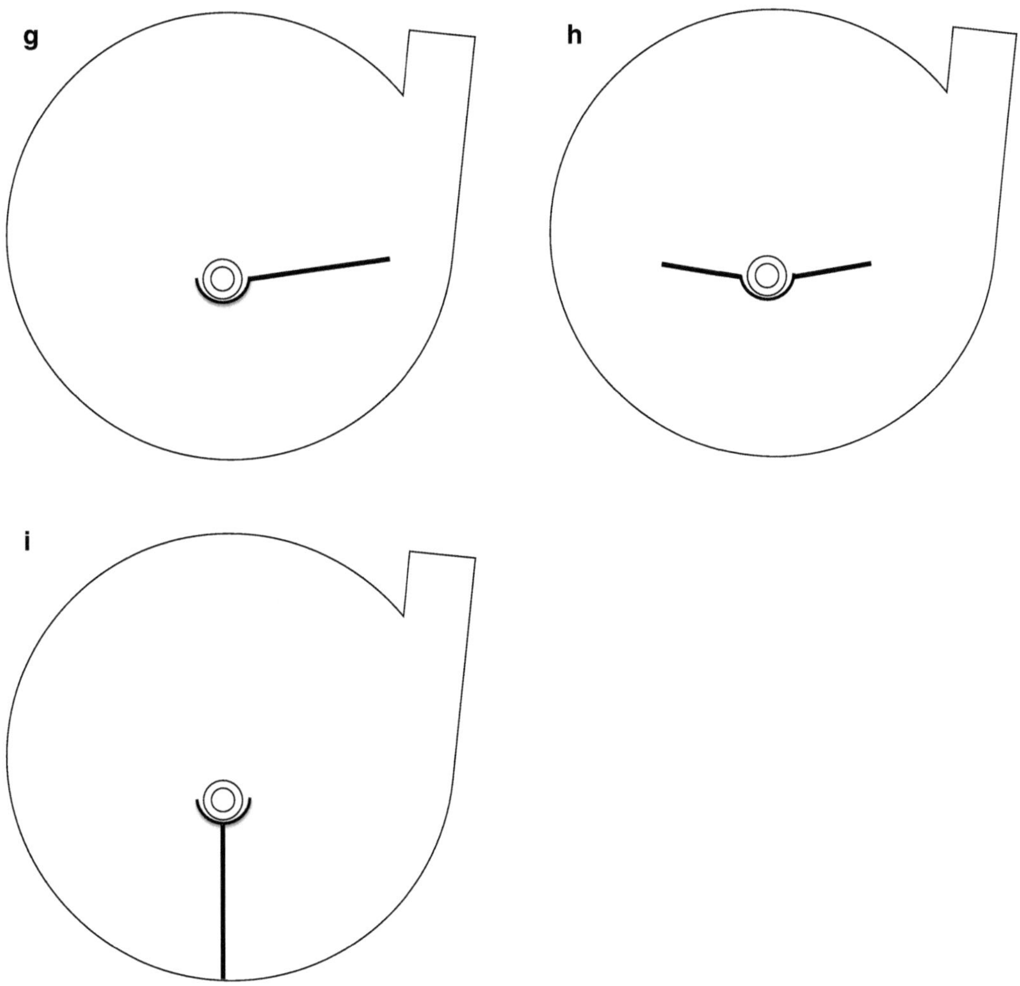

Fig. 6.7 (continued)

along the oncoplastic plane is complete, the breast gland can be dissected off the chest wall. It is important to avoid excessive flap traction throughout the mastectomy procedure to minimize potential injury. In the setting of nipple-sparing mastectomy, removal of the retroareolar tissue may be performed by coring or via nipple inversion. In case of oncological surgery, retroareolar cores are often subjected to intraoperative analysis to assess the presence of cancer and guide more surgery. The frozen section technique is the most frequently employed for intraoperative assessment and is associated with a false negative rate ranging between 1 and 9.2% [27–30]. A shared decision to use intraoperative assessment to determine nipple excision within the same surgery needs to be carefully considered with regard to patient consent. The possibility of needing to address a positive nipple margin at the primary surgery or at a subsequent operation highlights the importance of patient selection for nipple-sparing mastectomy and choice of incision. For example, an initial IMF incision in a patient eventually requiring excision of the NAC may result in awkward skin bridge at risk of ischemia, particularly in a small reconstructed breast. All these considerations should be discussed with the patient during the preoperative consultations as part of the shared decision-making and consenting process.

In nipple-sparing mastectomy, a retroareolar disc that inevitably contains a small amount of

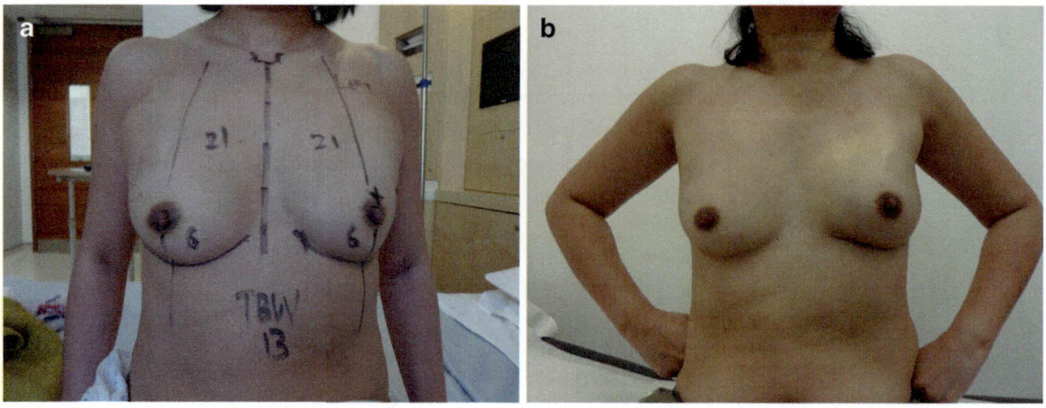

Fig. 6.8 Demonstration of pre-operative marking using an inframammary crease incision for nipple-sparing mastectomy (**a**) and post-operative cosmetic outcome (**b**)

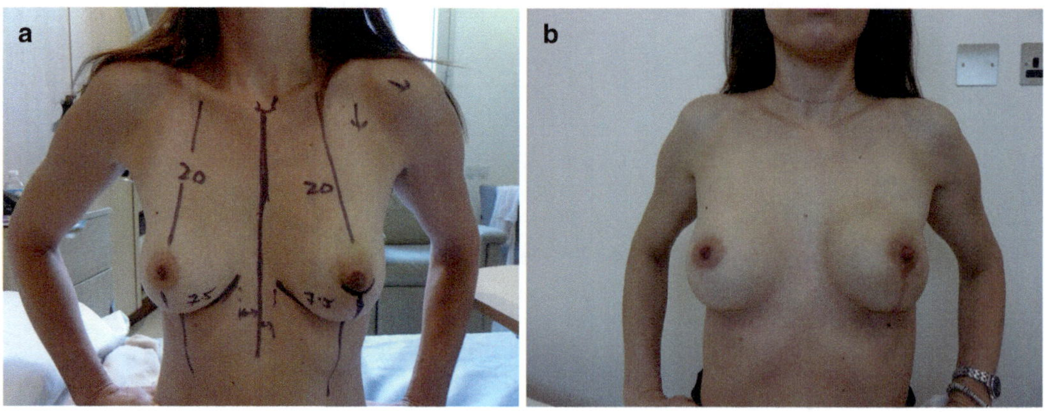

Fig. 6.9 Demonstration of pre-operative making using a periareolar incision with vertical radial extension (**a**) and post-operative cosmetic outcome (**b**)

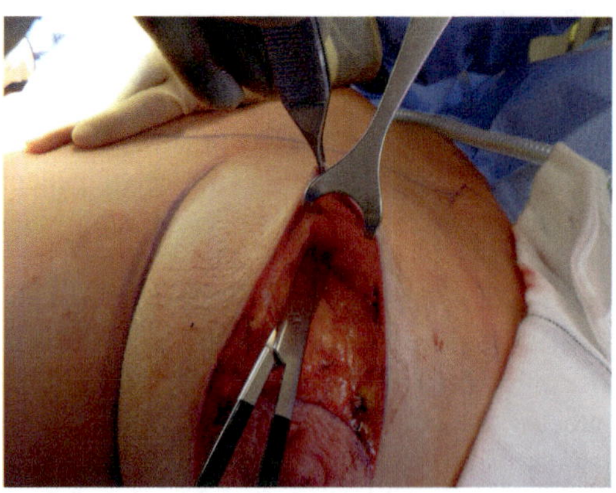

Fig. 6.10 The "oncoplastic" dissection plane

breast tissue is retained. The dominant blood supply to the nipple through perforators within the breast parenchyma arising from branches of the axillary artery (superior thoracic, thoracoacromial, lateral thoracic, and subscapular vessels), internal thoracic artery, and intercostal vessels is disrupted during a mastectomy. The nipple therefore becomes dependent on the cutaneous blood supply which reaches the nipple as the most distant point thought the subareolar plexus. It is essential to maintain this subareolar plexus which runs in the subdermal plain during the NAC dissection. Meticulous surgical technique should include the conscious effort to preserve anterior intercostal artery perforators, as branches arising from the axillary vessels are often interrupted in dissecting the axillary tail or during the axillary surgery (Fig. 6.11).

Equally important to NAC integrity is the venous outflow. Operative factors that can influence the venous outflow include skin tension at closure, size of the breast implant or volume of tissue expansion, and external pressure from the surgical dressings. Surgical incisions away from the nipple (e.g., lateral or IMF approaches) are less likely to compromise venous outflow than incisions in direct proximity to the nipple and the circumareolar region as post-operative swelling is more likely to occlude venous rather than arteriolar flow.

Various dissection techniques in performing a mastectomy have been described. These may include sharp dissection with scissors or scalpel or use of standard diathermy. Especially for nipple-sparing mastectomy, surgeons may choose to use sharp dissection around the NAC to avoid any potential thermal injury to the NAC vascular plexus. Another technique that is increasingly being used to raise the mastectomy skin flaps is hydrodissection [31–34]. This technique may be particularly useful in the era of nipple-sparing mastectomy when the mastectomy is performed through a remote incision such as the IMF as the procedure may be completed with minimal traction of the skin flaps. The use of infiltration during mastectomy should be distinguished from hydrodissection; in the latter, the hydrostatic pressure applied from infusion into the oncoplastic plane separates the subcutaneous fat, stretching the space around the superficial lamella and therefore the ligaments of Astley Cooper that traverse this space holding the breast parenchyma to skin structures. This technique is associated with lower intraoperative bleeding but is associated with a significant learning curve. Hydrodissection is an excellent tool to dissect the NAC from the retroareolar structures and can also be used to lift the submuscular plane.

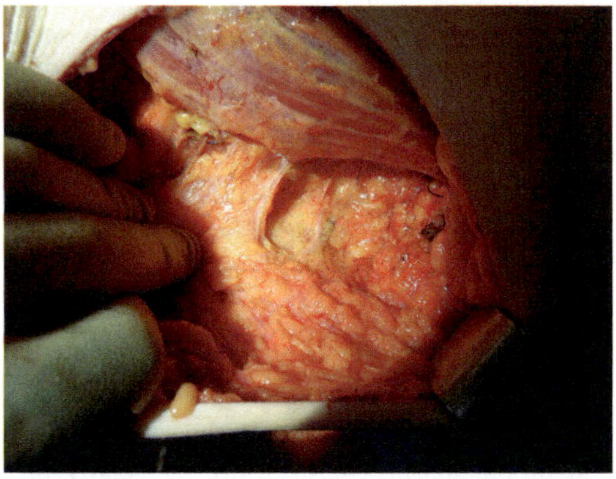

Fig. 6.11 Careful dissection to preserve lateral intercostal artery perforators and branches of the intercostal nerve

After mastectomy, meticulous hemostasis is essential but caution should be exercised to avoid needless compromise to the network of blood vessels within the skin flaps. Surgical drains may be inserted ensuring an adequate subcutaneous tunnel to avoid ascending infection. The exit point of the drain tubing should be distant from the dressings and at a comfortable point for the patient. The use of close-system, vacuum drains is most commonly employed but the practice especially with regard to the length of time they remain in situ is variable [35, 36]. Although drainless mastectomies have been described [37], there is paucity of data in the setting of skin and nipple-sparing mastectomy and PPBR.

Following completion of mastectomy and PPBR, a number of surgical dressings have been used to cover the incision(s). These include simple gauze dressings, waterproof film adhesive dressings (padded or unpadded), and special dressings (e.g., silver carboxymethylcellulose [38]) with an aim to reduce surgical site infections or negative-pressure dressings [39, 40]. There is no single dressing system, based on the existing literature, that has been found to be superior and the decision should therefore be individualized taking into consideration previous history of dressing sensitivity, risk factors, and patient parameters that include comfort and convenience.

6.4.4 Infection Prevention in Skin and Nipple-Sparing Mastectomy and Pre-Pectoral Breast Reconstruction

Surgical site infection (SSI) after mastectomy and PPBR may lead to other complications including implant infection and loss as well as prolonged hospital stay, the possible need for re-operation and multiple additional outpatient visits. Early implant complications often have a delayed impact and even if an implant reconstruction is salvaged, the risks of subsequent poor quality soft tissue and capsular contracture requiring further surgery are increased. It is therefore of paramount importance to try to prevent SSI. Despite its significant impact on successful PPBR, there is no gold standard protocol to reduce the risk of SSI. Several measures have been suggested including routine methicillin sensitive and resistant *Staphylococcus aureus* (MSSA and MRSA) screening and treatment, use of prophylactic antibiotics, alcoholic solution for surgical field preparation, use of laminar air flow, prevention of intraoperative hypothermia, minimization of staff movement during implantation, minimal implant manipulation, and double gloving. A set of these recommendations has been formatted into a practical checklist aimed to provide a simple tool for surgical teams to ensure adherence to SSI prevention measures [41].

6.4.5 Axillary Staging in the Setting of Skin and Nipple-Sparing Mastectomy and PPBR

Axillary surgery is routinely performed in patients undergoing skin and nipple-sparing mastectomy and PPBR for invasive or in situ breast cancer. Sentinel lymph node biopsy (SLNB) is standard of care for axillary staging in patients who are apparently node negative on clinical assessment and imaging. Although SLNB has also been described in the setting of risk-reducing surgery [42], in the era of MRI screening in carriers of high-risk breast cancer predisposition genes, the benefits versus adverse effects to this subgroup of patients should be viewed with caution. SLNB still carries a small but finite risk of lymphoedema, soft tissue complications, and persistent neuralgia. Axillary lymph node dissection (ALND) to treat the node positive axilla remains the usual standard of care.

6.4.6 Sentinel Lymph Node Biopsy

6.4.6.1 Sentinel Lymph Node Identification Technique

Several methods have been described for the identification of the sentinel lymph nodes. These include the use of a blue dye (isosulfan blue, methylene blue, or patent blue), a radioactive colloid (technetium-99m), or both (i.e., "dual technique") injected into the breast parenchyma close to the tumor or in the periareolar region [43, 44]. Each technique may be used based on availability and surgeon's preference but the dual technique is the preferred method especially in clinically node positive women with complete imaging response after neoadjuvant chemotherapy that undergo SLNB [45, 46]. Particularly in this setting, the use of targeted axillary dissection guided by the marking and localization for excision of the index, biopsy proven, metastatic axillary lymph node may result in lower false negative rates [47, 48]. Several methods of pre-operative marking of the clipped node have been described [49] including the use of wires [50], iodine seeds [47], or other wireless non-radioactive localizers [51–53]. Alternative techniques for SLNB include indocyanine green (ICG) with special infrared light used in the operating field [54–56] and superparamagnetic iron oxide (SPIO) with use of a handheld magnetic probe to identify the sentinel lymph nodes [56–59].

6.4.6.2 Incision

Sentinel lymph node biopsy in the setting of skin and nipple-sparing mastectomy in usually performed through a separate short incision most frequently placed in the lower hairline of the axilla. This is usually transverse or slightly oblique, and attention is required to avoid crossing the anterior axillary line. In selected patients,

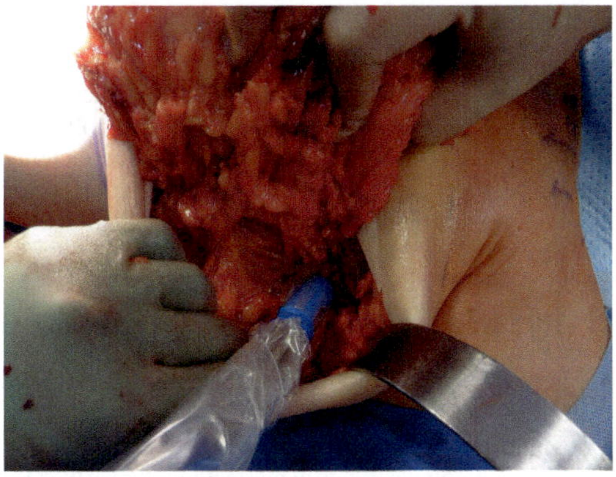

Fig. 6.12 Sentinel lymph node biopsy procedure through the mastectomy incision

the axillary procedure may be performed through the mastectomy incision (Fig. 6.12). Whilst access to the axilla can sometimes be combined with the surgical incision for the mastectomy, many surgeons prefer to keep the incisions separate. This may facilitate lateral breast pocket control and minimize skin flap retraction to optimize access to the axilla. Where there is a pre-existing axillary scar, the same incision may be utilized and can be extended as required for adequate access.

6.4.6.3 Surgical Technique

Careful blunt dissection is performed to identify the sentinel lymph node(s). Depending on the node identification method utilized, this may include the use of a handheld gamma probe, following radioisotope injection, to direct the dissection towards the radioactive node. If a "dual technique" is used (radioisotope and blue dye), the blue-stained lymphatic vessels are visualized and followed to the blue node. After harvesting the first sentinel lymph node which may be radioactive ("hot"), blue or both, the gamma probe is used again to search for additional radioactive nodes. If there are more blue-stained lymphatic vessels these may also be followed in search of additional blue nodes. As a rule of thumb, nodes with ≥10% of the radioactivity measured in the highest counting lymph node are also considered sentinel lymph nodes and removed. The same principles to identify the sentinel lymph node(s) are applied in the case of ICG or SPIO techniques, with the use of infrared light or a handheld magnetic probe to guide the dissection. The sentinel lymph node is most often located in the lower axilla alongside the lateral thoracic vein. In a clinically and radiologically node negative patient, there is rarely a need to sample more than four nodes at sentinel node biopsy.

6.4.7 Axillary Lymph Node Dissection

6.4.7.1 Incision

When ALND is indicated, usually a separate incision to that performed to access the breast cancer is performed, similar in fashion to the SLNB, but may need to be extended in length to facilitate access. Once again attention is required not to cross the anterior axillary line. As an alternative, a "lazy *S*" incision is an option to a transverse or oblique incision allowing excellent access and subsequent closure. In patients with history of previous axillary surgery, the existing scar can be utilized but it may require modification, repositioning, or revision. Axillary lymph node dissection could technically be performed through the mastectomy incision in selected cases (e.g., lateral breast crease or radial lateral mastectomy incision) but like in SLNB most surgeons prefer to keep the access separate for the same reasons.

6.4.7.2 Surgical Technique

When ALND is indicated for oncological reasons, this routinely involves dissection of the level I and II nodes unless otherwise indicated. The dissection typically starts by identifying key anatomical structures including the axillary vein, the long thoracic nerve, and the thoracodorsal bundle. The contents of the axilla are then removed dissecting the axillary fat while preserving the aforementioned key neurovascular structures. The intercostobrachial nerve(s) may also be preserved if technically and oncologically feasible. When the axilla is approached through the mastectomy incision, in addition to the intercostal nerve, lower lateral intercostal branches may be identified and preserved (Fig. 6.11) in an effort to maintain post-mastectomy sensation of the breast mound. After the ALND, careful palpation of the axilla is performed, and any remaining nodes should be excised. Particular attention is required to the interneural space, between the thoracodorsal bundle and the long thoracic nerve for retained lymphatic tissue.

6.5 Summary with Tips

- Pre-operative assessment and bilateral skin marking with the patient upright are the first step of skin and nipple-sparing mastectomy.
- Position the patient on the operating table to enable adoption of a sitting position to assess reconstruction outcome and symmetry.
- When performing a nipple-sparing mastectomy, IMF, lateral crease and radial incisions are associated with a lower risk of nipple necrosis.
- Careful assessment is required when selecting an incision in the setting of nipple-sparing mastectomy for breast cancer.
- Meticulous surgical technique, following the oncoplastic plane with the aim to remove maximum breast glandular tissue while maintaining viable skin flaps and preserving the skin blood supply, is of paramount importance. Avoid excessive skin flap retraction.
- Careful dissection of the NAC in nipple-sparing mastectomy is required to preserve the subareolar vascular plexus which is critical to avoid nipple ischemia and necrosis.
- Use of sharp dissection or hydrodissection may be particularly useful for NAC dissection especially when the mastectomy is performed through a remote incision.
- Axillary surgery is most frequently performed through a separate incision to the mastectomy although it may be feasible via the same incision in selected cases.

References

1. Fisher B, Anderson S, Bryant J, Margolese RG, Deutsch M, Fisher ER, et al. Twenty-year follow-up of a randomized trial comparing total mastectomy, lumpectomy, and lumpectomy plus irradiation for the treatment of invasive breast cancer. N Engl J Med. 2002;347(16):1233–41.
2. Veronesi U, Cascinelli N, Mariani L, Greco M, Saccozzi R, Luini A, et al. Twenty-year follow-up of a randomized study comparing breast-conserving surgery with radical mastectomy for early breast cancer. N Engl J Med. 2002;347(16):1227–32.
3. Kummerow KL, Du L, Penson DF, Shyr Y, Hooks MA. Nationwide trends in mastectomy for early-stage breast cancer. JAMA Surg. 2015;150(1):9–16.
4. Crown A, Wechter DG, Grumley JW. Oncoplastic breast-conserving surgery reduces mastectomy and postoperative re-excision rates. Ann Surg Oncol. 2015;22(10):3363–8.
5. Karakatsanis A, Tasoulis MK, Wärnberg F, Nilsson G, MacNeill F. Meta-analysis of neoadjuvant therapy and its impact in facilitating breast conservation in operable breast cancer. Br J Surg. 2018;105(5):469–81.
6. Simmons RM, Fish SK, Gayle L, La Trenta GS, Swistel A, Christos P, et al. Local and distant recurrence rates in skin-sparing mastectomies compared with non-skin-sparing mastectomies. Ann Surg Oncol. 1999;6(7):676–81.
7. Greenway RM, Schlossberg L, Dooley WC. Fifteen-year series of skin-sparing mastectomy for stage 0 to 2 breast cancer. Am J Surg. 2005;190(6):918–22.
8. Boneti C, Yuen J, Santiago C, Diaz Z, Robertson Y, Korourian S, et al. Oncologic safety of nipple skin-sparing or Total skin-sparing mastectomies with immediate reconstruction. J Am Coll Surg. 2011;212(4):686–93.
9. Smith BL, Tang R, Rai U, Plichta JK, Colwell AS, Gadd MA, et al. Oncologic safety of nipple-sparing mastectomy in women with breast cancer. J Am Coll Surg. 2017;225(3):361–5.
10. Wu Z-Y, Kim H-J, Lee J-W, Chung I-Y, Kim J-S, Lee S-B, et al. Breast cancer recurrence in the nipple-areola complex after nipple-sparing mastectomy with immediate breast reconstruction for invasive breast cancer. JAMA Surg. 2019;154(11):1030–7.
11. Paolini G, Firmani G, Briganti F, Sorotos M, Santanelli di Pompeo F. Guiding nipple-areola complex reconstruction: literature review and proposal of a new decision-making algorithm. Aesthet Plast Surg. 2021; https://doi.org/10.1007/s00266-020-02047-9.
12. Hammond JB, Teven CM, Bernard RW, Lucas HD, Casey WJ, Siebeneck ET, et al. 3D nipple-areolar tattoo: It's technique, outcomes, and utilization. Aesthet Plast Surg. 2021; https://doi.org/10.1007/s00266-020-01967-w.

13. Tomita S, Mori K, Yamazaki H. A survey on the safety of and patient satisfaction after nipple-areola tattooing. Aesthet Plast Surg. 2021; https://doi.org/10.1007/s00266-020-02018-0.
14. Satteson ES, Brown BJ, Nahabedian MY. Nipple-areolar complex reconstruction and patient satisfaction: a systematic review and meta-analysis. Gland Surg. 2017;6(1):4–13.
15. American Society of Plastic Surgery (ASPS): 2018 Plastic surgery statistics report; 2018
16. Tasoulis MK, Iqbal FM, Cawthorn S, MacNeill F, Vidya R. Subcutaneous implant breast reconstruction: time to reconsider? Eur J Surg Oncol. 2017;43(9):1636–46.
17. DeCoster RC, Lynch EB, Bonaroti AR, Webster JM, Butterfield TA, Evers BM, et al. Breast implant-associated anaplastic large cell lymphoma: an evidence-based systematic review. Ann Surg. 2021;273(3):449–58.
18. DeCoster RC, Clemens MW, Di Napoli A, Lynch EB, Bonaroti AR, Rinker BD, et al. Cellular and molecular mechanisms of breast implant-associated anaplastic large cell lymphoma. Plast Reconstr Surg. 2021;147(1):30e–41e.
19. Becker H, Lind JG 2nd, Hopkins EG. Immediate implant-based Prepectoral breast reconstruction using a vertical incision. Plast Reconstr Surg Glob Open. 2015;3(6):e412-e.
20. Kim JH, Chun YS, Park HK, Kim SE, Kim YW, Cheon YW. Inframammary fold incision can reduce skin flap necrosis in immediate breast reconstruction with implant and conjoined fascial flap. Ann Plast Surg. 2020;85(5):488–94.
21. Karunanayake M, Boghossian E, Govshievich A, Bernier C, Danino MA. A retrospective comparison study of the infra-mammary approach to the standard mastectomy scar in the 2nd stage of tissue expander to implant breast reconstruction. Ann Chir Plast Esthet. 2017;62(2):131–8.
22. Frey JD, Salibian AA, Levine JP, Karp NS, Choi M. Incision choices in nipple-sparing mastectomy: a comparative analysis of outcomes and evolution of a clinical algorithm. Plast Reconstr Surg. 2018;142(6):826e–35e.
23. Daar DA, Abdou SA, Rosario L, Rifkin WJ, Santos PJ, Wirth GA, et al. Is there a preferred incision location for nipple-sparing mastectomy? A systematic review and meta-analysis. Plast Reconstr Surg. 2019;143(5):906e–19e.
24. Park S, Yoon C, Bae SJ, Cha C, Kim D, Lee J, et al. Comparison of complications according to incision types in nipple-sparing mastectomy and immediate reconstruction. Breast (Edinburgh, Scotland). 2020;53:85–91.
25. Wijayanayagam A, Kumar AS, Foster RD, Esserman LJ. Optimizing the total skin-sparing mastectomy. Arch Surg. 2008;143(1):38–45.
26. Regolo L, Ballardini B, Gallarotti E, Scoccia E, Zanini V. Nipple sparing mastectomy: an innovative skin incision for an alternative approach. Breast (Edinburgh, Scotland). 2008;17(1):8–11.
27. Camp MS, Coopey SB, Tang R, Colwell A, Specht M, Greenup RA, et al. Management of positive subareolar/nipple duct margins in nipple-sparing mastectomies. Breast J. 2014;20(4):402–7.
28. D'Alonzo M, Pecchio S, Campisi P, De Rosa G, Bounous VE, Villasco A, et al. Nipple-sparing mastectomy: reliability of sub-areolar sampling and frozen section in predicting occult nipple involvement in breast cancer patients. Eur J Surg Oncol. 2018;44(11):1736–42.
29. Duarte GM, Tomazini MV, Oliveira A, Moreira L, Tocchet F, Worschech A, et al. Accuracy of frozen section, imprint cytology, and permanent histology of sub-nipple tissue for predicting occult nipple involvement in patients with breast carcinoma. Breast Cancer Res Treat. 2015;153(3):557–63.
30. Kneubil MC, Lohsiriwat V, Curigliano G, Brollo J, Botteri E, Rotmensz N, et al. Risk of Locoregional recurrence in patients with false-negative frozen section or close margins of Retroareolar specimen in nipple-sparing mastectomy. Ann Surg Oncol. 2012;19(13):4117–23.
31. Vargas CR, Koolen PG, Ho OA, Ricci JA, Tobias AM, Lin SJ, et al. Tumescent mastectomy technique in autologous breast reconstruction. J Surg Res. 2015;198(2):525–9.
32. Samper A, Blanch A. Improved subcutaneous mastectomy with hydrodissection of the subcutaneous space. Plast Reconstr Surg. 2003;112(2):694–5.
33. Folli S, Curcio A, Buggi F, Mingozzi M, Lelli D, Barbieri C, et al. Improved sub-areolar breast tissue removal in nipple-sparing mastectomy using hydrodissection. Breast (Edinburgh, Scotland). 2012;21(2):190–3.
34. Tasoulis MK, Agusti A, Karakatsanis A, Montgomery C, Marshall C, Gui G. The use of Hydrodissection in nipple- and skin-sparing mastectomy: a retrospective cohort study. Plast Reconstr Surg Glob Open. 2019;7(11):e2495.
35. Phillips BT, Wang ED, Mirrer J, Lanier ST, Khan SU, Dagum AB, et al. Current practice among plastic surgeons of antibiotic prophylaxis and closed-suction drains in breast reconstruction: experience, evidence, and implications for postoperative care. Ann Plast Surg. 2011;66(5):460–5.
36. Scomacao I, Cummins A, Roan E, Duraes EFR, Djohan R. The use of surgical site drains in breast reconstruction: a systematic review. J Plast Reconstr Aesthet Surg. 2020;73(4):651–62.
37. Baker E, Piper J. Drainless mastectomy: is it safe and effective? Surgeon. 2017;15(5):267–71.
38. Struik GM, Vrijland WW, Birnie E, Klem T. A randomized controlled trial on the effect of a silver

carboxymethylcellulose dressing on surgical site infections after breast cancer surgery. PLoS One. 2018;13(5):e0195715.
39. Nagata T, Miura K, Homma Y, Fukamizu H. Comparison between negative-pressure fixation and film dressing in wound management after tissue expansion: a randomized controlled trial. Plast Reconstr Surg. 2018;142(1):37–41.
40. Gabriel A, Sigalove SR, Maxwell GP. Initial experience using closed incision negative pressure therapy after immediate Postmastectomy breast reconstruction. Plast Reconstr Surg Glob Open. 2016;4(7):e819.
41. Barr SP, Topps AR, Barnes NL, Henderson J, Hignett S, Teasdale RL, et al. Infection prevention in breast implant surgery - a review of the surgical evidence, guidelines and a checklist. Eur J Surg Oncol. 2016;42(5):591–603.
42. Tasoulis MK, Hughes T, Babiera G, Chagpar AB. Sentinel lymph node biopsy in low risk settings. Am J Surg. 2017;214(3):489–94.
43. Ahmed M, Purushotham AD, Horgan K, Klaase JM, Douek M. Meta-analysis of superficial versus deep injection of radioactive tracer and blue dye for lymphatic mapping and detection of sentinel lymph nodes in breast cancer. Br J Surg. 2015;102(3):169–81.
44. Sadeghi R, Asadi M, Treglia G, Zakavi SR, Fattahi A, Krag DN. Axillary concordance between superficial and deep sentinel node mapping material injections in breast cancer patients: systematic review and meta-analysis of the literature. Breast Cancer Res Treat. 2014;144(2):213–22.
45. Boughey JC, Suman VJ, Mittendorf EA, Ahrendt GM, Wilke LG, Taback B, et al. Sentinel lymph node surgery after neoadjuvant chemotherapy in patients with node-positive breast cancer: the ACOSOG Z1071 (Alliance) clinical trial. JAMA. 2013;310(14):1455–61.
46. Kuehn T, Bauerfeind I, Fehm T, Fleige B, Hausschild M, Helms G, et al. Sentinel-lymph-node biopsy in patients with breast cancer before and after neoadjuvant chemotherapy (SENTINA): a prospective, multicentre cohort study. Lancet Oncol. 2013;14(7):609–18.
47. Caudle AS, Yang WT, Krishnamurthy S, Mittendorf EA, Black DM, Gilcrease MZ, et al. Improved axillary evaluation following neoadjuvant therapy for patients with node-positive breast cancer using selective evaluation of clipped nodes: implementation of targeted axillary dissection. J Clin Oncol. 2016;34(10):1072–8.
48. Boughey JC, Alvarado MD, Lancaster RB, Fraser Symmans W, Mukhtar R, Wong JM, et al. Surgical standards for Management of the Axilla in breast cancer clinical trials with pathological complete response endpoint. NPJ Breast Cancer. 2018;4(1):26.
49. Woods RW, Camp MS, Durr NJ, Harvey SC. A review of options for localization of axillary lymph nodes in the treatment of invasive breast cancer. Acad Radiol. 2019;26(6):805–19.
50. Balasubramanian R, Morgan C, Shaari E, Kovacs T, Pinder SE, Hamed H, et al. Wire guided localisation for targeted axillary node dissection is accurate in axillary staging in node positive breast cancer following neoadjuvant chemotherapy. Eur J Surg Oncol. 2020;46(6):1028–33.
51. Simons JM, Scoggins ME, Kuerer HM, Krishnamurthy S, Yang WT, Sahin AA, et al. Prospective registry trial assessing the use of magnetic seeds to locate clipped nodes after neoadjuvant chemotherapy for breast cancer patients. Ann Surg Oncol. 2021;28:4277.
52. Sun J, Henry DA, Carr MJ, Yazdankhahkenary A, Laronga C, Lee MC, et al. Feasibility of axillary lymph node localization and excision using radar reflector localization. Clin Breast Cancer. 2021; https://doi.org/10.1016/j.clbc.2020.08.001.
53. Laws A, Dillon K, Kelly BN, Kantor O, Hughes KS, Gadd MA, et al. Node-positive patients treated with neoadjuvant chemotherapy can be spared axillary lymph node dissection with wireless non-radioactive localizers. Ann Surg Oncol. 2020;27(12):4819–27.
54. Kedrzycki MS, Leiloglou M, Ashrafian H, Jiwa N, Thiruchelvam PTR, Elson DS, et al. Meta-analysis comparing fluorescence imaging with radioisotope and blue dye-guided sentinel node identification for breast cancer surgery. Ann Surg Oncol. 2021; https://doi.org/10.1245/s10434-020-09288-7.
55. Valente SA, Al-Hilli Z, Radford DM, Yanda C, Tu C, Grobmyer SR. Near infrared fluorescent lymph node mapping with Indocyanine green in breast cancer patients: a prospective trial. J Am Coll Surg. 2019;228(4):672–8.
56. Ahmed M, Purushotham AD, Douek M. Novel techniques for sentinel lymph node biopsy in breast cancer: a systematic review. Lancet Oncol. 2014;15(8):e351–62.
57. Alvarado MD, Mittendorf EA, Teshome M, Thompson AM, Bold RJ, Gittleman MA, et al. SentimagIC: a non-inferiority trial comparing superparamagnetic iron oxide versus technetium-99m and blue dye in the detection of axillary sentinel nodes in patients with early-stage breast cancer. Ann Surg Oncol. 2019;26(11):3510–6.
58. Karakatsanis A, Daskalakis K, Stålberg P, Olofsson H, Andersson Y, Eriksson S, et al. Superparamagnetic iron oxide nanoparticles as the sole method for sentinel node biopsy detection in patients with breast cancer. Br J Surg. 2017;104(12):1675–85.
59. Karakatsanis A, Christiansen PM, Fischer L, Hedin C, Pistioli L, Sund M, et al. The Nordic SentiMag trial: a comparison of super paramagnetic iron oxide (SPIO) nanoparticles versus Tc(99) and patent blue in the detection of sentinel node (SN) in patients with breast cancer and a meta-analysis of earlier studies. Breast Cancer Res Treat. 2016;157(2):281–94.

7 Importance of Tissue Perfusion and Assessment Methods of the Mastectomy Skin Flap

Nolan S. Karp and Ara A. Salibian

7.1 Background

Mastectomy flap quality remains one of the most important factors in determining the success (or failure) of alloplastic breast reconstruction. Multiple intrinsic and extrinsic risk factors have been identified for ischemic complications after mastectomy. However, poorly perfused mastectomy flaps can thwart the best reconstruction attempts in the most ideal candidates with the lowest risk profile.

The implications of mastectomy flap quality are magnified in prepectoral implant-based reconstruction. Prepectoral implant placement has recently "re-emerged" as a reconstructive technique that minimizes the morbidity of pectoralis muscle elevation and avoids complications such as animation deformity [1]. Mastectomy flap quality has a significant influence with regard to both reconstructive and aesthetic outcomes with prepectoral implant placement and moreover should determine whether prepectoral reconstruction is a feasible option.

N. S. Karp (✉)
Hansjörg Wyss Department of Plastic Surgery, NYU Langone Health, New York, NY, USA
e-mail: Nolan.Karp@nyumc.org

A. A. Salibian
Division of Plastic and Reconstructive Surgery, University of California, Davis, Sacramento, CA, USA

The absence of a vascularized layer of pectoralis muscle between the prosthesis and skin flaps begets more significant implications for any ischemia of the skin envelope. Full-thickness wounds or poor incisional healing can very rapidly progress to prosthesis exposure and explantation. Overly thinned mastectomy flaps can also result in poor aesthetic outcomes due to implant visibility, palpability, contour deformities, and rippling.

Mastectomy flap quality is an overarching term that is dependent on many variables including relative mastectomy flap thickness, maintenance of perfusion to the skin envelope, preservation of the anatomical elements superficial to the breast gland, and appropriate handling of the mastectomy flaps. Objectively assessing mastectomy flap quality is difficult, yet critical to making intraoperative decisions that influence the multiple aspects of surgical outcomes. Appropriate analysis can help mitigate the sequelae of ischemic complications and facilitate the delivery of optimal results.

The goal of optimizing mastectomy flap quality is providing an oncologically sound procedure while maximizing reconstructive and aesthetic outcomes by facilitating an anatomic dissection and tailoring the reconstructive choices to the mastectomy. This requires a team-based approach with the oncologic and plastic surgeon working together [2] during all components of the spectrum of care for these patients.

© The Author(s), under exclusive license to Springer Nature Switzerland AG 2023
R. Vidya, H. Becker (eds.), *Prepectoral Breast Reconstruction*,
https://doi.org/10.1007/978-3-031-15590-1_7

7.2 Anatomy

A thorough understanding of breast anatomy and blood supply to the skin envelope is paramount in preserving perfusion after mastectomy while performing an oncologically sound procedure [3]. The subcutaneous layer of breast fat is divided into a thinner superficial layer and thicker, deeper layer by the superficial layer of the superficial breast fascia [4]. The entirety of this subcutaneous layer is separated from the breast gland by a breast (pseudo) capsule that represents the anatomic plane of dissection during mastectomy (Fig. 7.1). This capsule does not maintain a consistent depth throughout the breast and therefore the subcutaneous layer varies in thickness.

The superficial perfusion of the breast and nipple–areolar complex is critical as this is all that remains after mastectomy. Preservation of the internal mammary artery perforators, in particular the dominant second perforator, is essential to maintain perfusion to the skin envelope. These vessels importantly run the subcutaneous fat of the breast and can therefore be protected if an anatomic dissection is maintained at the level of the breast capsule [5].

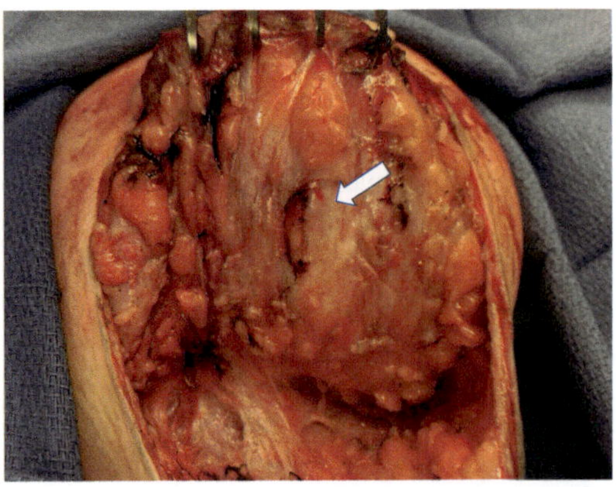

Fig. 7.1 The white breast capsule (*white arrow*) can be seen on the gland in the reduction mammoplasty patient, indicating the appropriate level of dissection between the superficial subcutaneous fat and the gland itself

7.3 Preoperative Planning

7.3.1 Patient-Specific Factors

Patient morphology and its implications for perfusion must be taken into consideration preoperatively. In particular, both ptosis [6] and higher mastectomy weights [7] have been associated with increased ischemic complications of the mastectomy skin envelope. We have specifically found mastectomy weights between 400 and 800 grams have a 2.6 times increased risk and those ≥800 grams a 5.1 times increased risk of complications in nipple-sparing mastectomy [7]. Increasing breast size and ptosis may correlate with a larger surface area of the skin envelope to be perfused and increasing distance from source vessels to the mastectomy flap edges that may further compromise perfusion.

In patients with ptosis and macromastia, the increased risk for ischemic complications should be discussed preoperatively. Skin reduction incisions typically in a wise pattern can be utilized in these patients [8, 9], though these incisions can often be complicated by skin necrosis at the T-point if there is any compromise in mastectomy flap vascularity and loss of the nipple–areola complex. Alternatively, staged breast reduction offers a means of controlling the skin envelope, optimizing the breast mound and nipple position, and potentially creating a vascular delay [10].

Assessment of the thickness of the subcutaneous layer of the breast is a useful practice to perform preoperatively. The thickness of this layer is inherently variable among patients and has been found to be thicker in patients with higher BMIs [11]. This thickness can be assessed on magnetic resonance imaging (Fig. 7.2) if already obtained for the oncologic workup, or can be even measured on bedside ultrasound. Preoperative assessment of the thickness of the subcutaneous layer and discussion with the oncologic surgeons

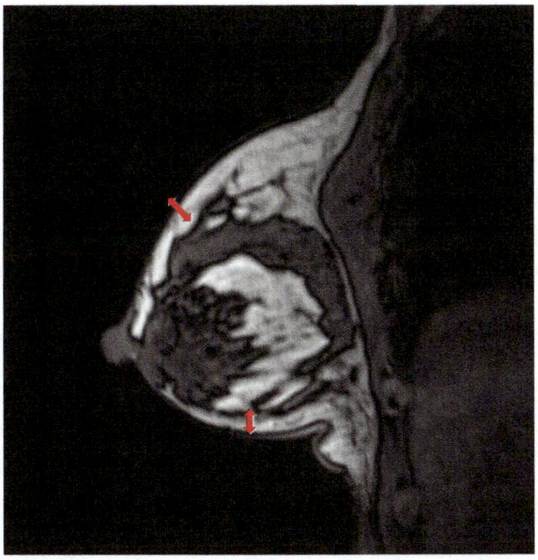

Fig. 7.2 The thickness of the skin and subcutaneous layer of the breast (*red arrows*) can be estimated on magnetic resonance imaging to serve as a guide for the mastectomy

solidifies a plan for the mastectomy and the expected mastectomy flap thickness that can then be used to make intraoperative decisions based on the residual thickness.

There are a multitude of additional potential risk factors for ischemic complications after mastectomy that must be taken into consideration during the preoperative evaluation. Certain patient comorbidities such as diabetes carry a higher risk of postoperative ischemic complications [12]. Extrinsic factors such as radiation [13] and tobacco use [14] should also be accounted for as these have known detrimental effects on perfusion and are associated with an increased risk of ischemic complications.

7.3.2 Nipple-Sparing Mastectomy

Nipple-sparing mastectomy allows for the optimization of aesthetic results after mastectomy and has been associated with improved patient satisfaction and quality of life [15]. However, particularly attention must be paid to mastectomy flap perfusion with nipple-sparing techniques as the entirety of the skin envelope is preserved. This can entail more difficult access for the breast surgeon, increased retraction of skin flaps, and the inability to resect compromised areas of skin. Patient selection, in addition to intraoperative techniques, is therefore key to the success of these procedures, particularly with prepectoral reconstruction.

Morphologic factors including breast size and ptosis are also important to consider as severe cases may serve as relative contraindications to nipple-sparing techniques when assessed in conjunction with other risk factors. It is important to evaluate all relevant risk factors to determine appropriateness of surgical options and what is an acceptable complication profile. We previously developed a risk-assessment model taking into account weighted contributions of 12 different risk factors to help estimate overall risk of complications after nipple-sparing mastectomy and immediate reconstruction [16]. Individualizing risk profiles for reach patient will allow for preoperative discussions that determine the optimal surgical plan and appropriately set patient expectations.

7.3.3 Incision Design

Incision choice has important implications for access for extirpation, perfusion of the mastectomy skin envelope, and aesthetic results. With regard to vascularity of the skin, it must be kept in mind that the farther the incision from the source vessels perfusing the skin envelope, the greater the watershed area at the incisional margin that is created. Incisions should therefore be designed to maximize perfusion (while taking other factors into account).

In cases of skin-sparing mastectomy and implant-based reconstruction, an elliptical incision is typically preferred. This incision is ideally centered equidistant from the four borders of the breast to optimize perfusion to all four quadrants (Fig. 7.3). Nipple-sparing mastectomy provides more choices for incision placement and more significant implications for each choice given the need to maintain perfusion to the nipple–areola complex.

The inframammary fold incision has been associated with a lower rate of ischemic complications [17] and has become the most widely used incision in nipple-sparing mastectomy (Fig. 7.4) [18]. It provides a concealed scar, wide access for the oncologic surgeon and minimal disruption of skin envelope perfusion [19]. However, it should be noted that in large breasts, visualization of the upper pole may be difficult for the extirpative surgeon which may result in increased traction on skin flaps. A counter incision can also be utilized to access the tail of the breast in these cases [20]. Lateral and vertical radial incisions similarly preserve perfusion to the nipple–areolar complex, though lateralization of the nipples can occur with lateral incisions [21]. Wise-pattern incisions allow for excellent oncologic access and can also offer skin reduction

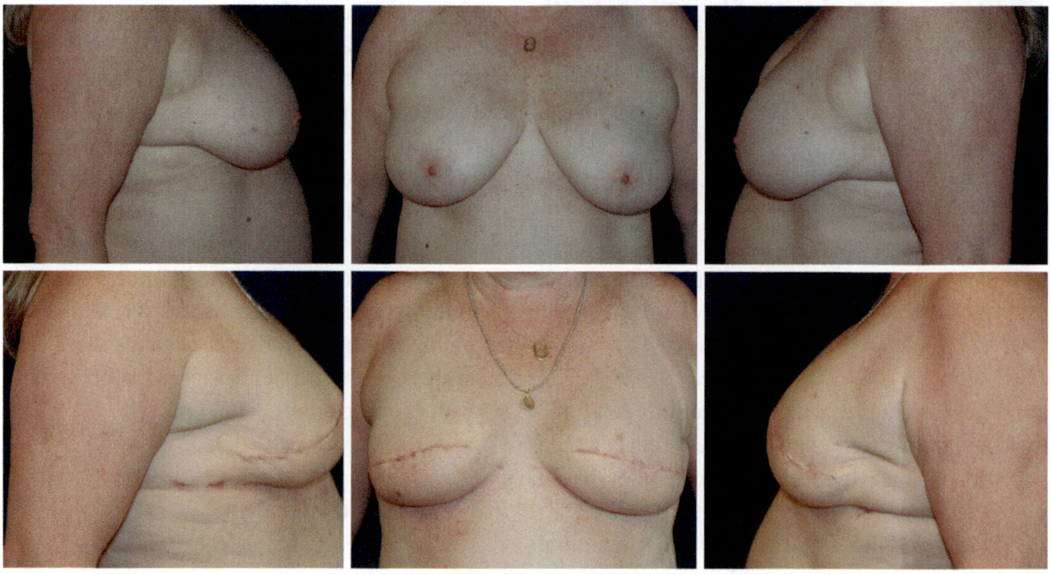

Fig. 7.3 Prepectoral reconstruction after skin-sparing mastectomy with a centered elliptical incision

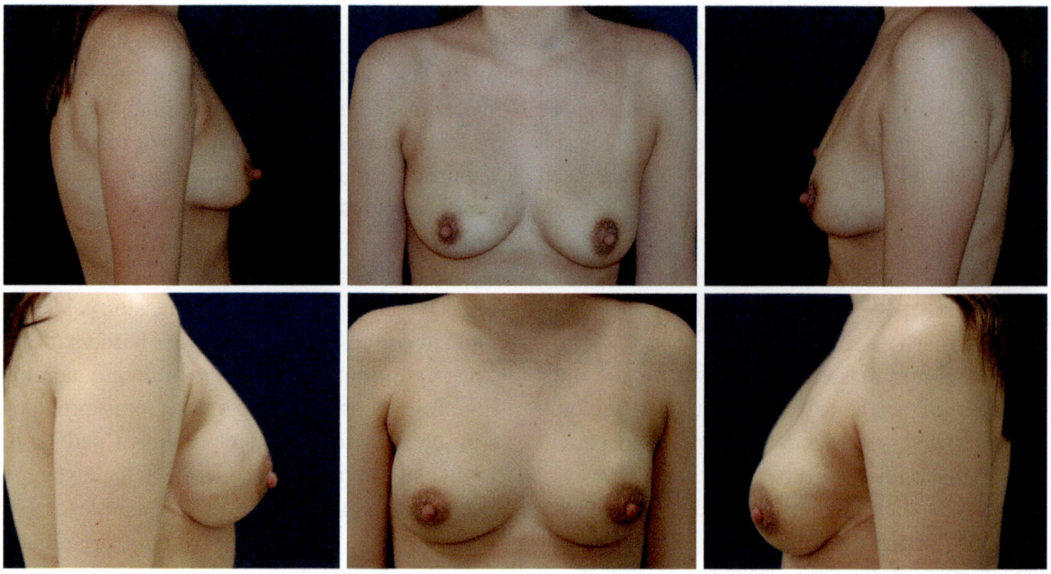

Fig. 7.4 Prepectoral reconstruction after nipple-sparing mastectomy with an inframammary fold incision

and nipple elevation, but have been associated with a higher rate of ischemic complications [17, 22]. Finally, periareolar incisions are generally avoided given the known increased risk of nipple–areola complex necrosis [17].

Choosing the desired incision should be completed in a process of shared decision-making that takes into account the patient's preferences, the oncologic surgeon's needs, and the implications of the incision on perfusion and the aesthetic result. Regardless of incision choice, it is paramount to counsel patients on the risks and benefits of each incision, and moreover all surgical decisions, and that no single perfect methods exists. Risks and benefits of each technique should be weighed as a team in and in coordination with the patient desires to arrive at the optimal surgical plan that is individualized for each patient.

7.4 Intraoperative Considerations

7.4.1 Mastectomy Flap Dissection

Mastectomy flap quality is rooted in mastectomy flap dissection. While multiple different dissection techniques exist, the appropriate plane of dissection should be a constant variable across all practices. This plane should aim to follow the layer of the breast capsule to leave the lobular subcutaneous tissue on the mastectomy flap (Fig. 7.5).

It is important to remember that the thickness of the subcutaneous layer is variable among patients and is also not constant throughout the breast. Imaging studies demonstrate that this layer consistently gets thicker moving from the nipple–areola complex to the periphery of the breast [23] and also has multiple variations along this plane. Therefore, the plane of dissection should not be maintained at a particular thickness, but should instead be adjusted to follow the breast capsule, changing thickness as needed to maintain an anatomic plane that preserves the subcutaneous fat but removes the gland below the capsule. Preoperative imaging can help estimate this tissue thickness to guide the depth of the mastectomy at different points in the breast mound.

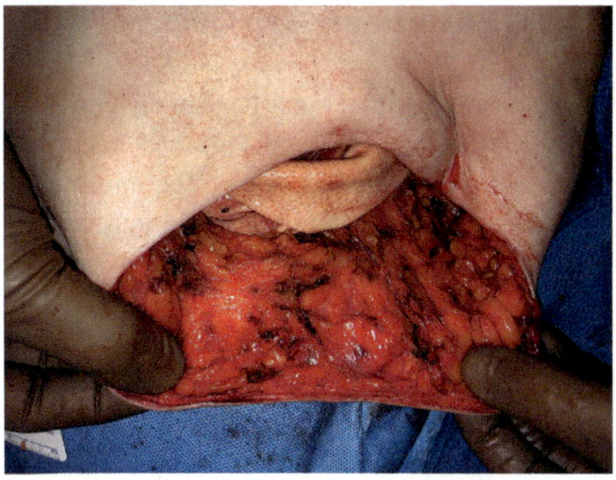

Fig. 7.5 The mastectomy should aim to preserve the lobular subcutaneous fat on the mastectomy while removing the breast gland by following the plane of the breast capsule

The superficial segmental perfusion of the skin envelope that travels through the subcutaneous tissue should be protected. It is of particular importance to preserve the second interspace internal mammary perforators, especially in nipple-sparing mastectomy. In addition, as there is no subcutaneous tissue behind the nipple and areola, the dissection must be transitioned to a subareolar plane under the nipple–areola complex.

Additional technical considerations during mastectomy can have significant implications for mastectomy flap viability. Retraction on skin flaps should be minimized and limited to only as needed for oncologic access. We prefer using a low-volume dilute epinephrine-containing solution to minimize bleeding and allow for sharp dissection of flaps. It is worthwhile to note that a recent meta-analysis of large volume tumescent techniques demonstrated that the use of tumescence may increase the risk of skin necrosis after mastectomy [24]. Electrocautery can be used judiciously for spot coagulation as needed to minimize thermal damage to the mastectomy flaps. A team effort in which the plastic surgeon is available and able to assist with the mastectomy often facilitates the best results.

7.4.2 Mastectomy Flap Quality

Assessment of mastectomy flap quality involves analysis of multiple different variables, including mastectomy flap thickness, by the breast and plastic surgeon in conjunction. Thin mastectomy flaps have been associated with an increased risk of ischemic complications [6, 14, 23]. In particular, an average postoperative flap thickness of less than 8.0 mm on magnetic resonance imaging has been found to be an independent predictor of ischemic complications [23]. Preoperative and intraoperative ultrasound can also be a useful and cost-effective tool to objectively assess the thickness of the subcutaneous tissue of the breast and of the residual mastectomy flaps. However, as thickness of the subcutaneous layer varies, it is the relative thickness of the flap that is more critical. We have previously found a significant difference in the percentage of postoperative to preoperative flap thickness in patients with ischemic complications (50% thickness) to those without ischemic complications (74% thickness) after nipple-sparing mastectomy [23]. While quantification of these values is helpful, the bottom line is that preservation of the subcutaneous fat during mastectomy, regardless of thickness, and therefore the superficial perfusion of the skin envelope is the goal.

Thin mastectomy flaps do not necessarily equate poor mastectomy flaps. Patients may inherently have a thinner subcutaneous layer of the breast and if this thin layer is preserved with a dissection at the breast capsule, then the viability and quality of the skin envelope are not compromised. For these reasons, preoperative assessment of subcutaneous tissue thickness with imaging modalities is useful to provide a baseline against which post-mastectomy thickness can be evaluated. Though thin mastectomy flaps may still be viable, thin flaps also have additional implications for aesthetic considerations, particularly in prepectoral reconstruction. Overly thin flaps may result in increased implant palpability and visibility, as well as accentuation of a superior pole step-off. The thickness of flaps should therefore be assessed intraoperatively not only to determine risk for ischemic complications, but also to aid in decision-making for the most appropriate implant plane and need for adjunctive techniques to provide the patient with the best aesthetic result.

Aside from thickness, there are multiple other methods for assessing the quality of mastectomy flaps, primarily focused on perfusion. We have found that clinical assessment of mastectomy flaps is a reliable and cost-efficient method. In addition to relative flap thickness, the flaps should be examined to look for preservation of subcutaneous fat as, areas of grossly visible dermis and electrocautery injury to the skin. Additional clinical factors include the presence of skin edge bleeding, capillary refill of the flaps, and skin bruising, though the use of epinephrine-containing solutions should be taken into account. We have previously found that the ischemic complications after immediate breast reconstruction correlate with intraoperative surgeon evaluation of mastectomy flaps [25]. In particular, these factors include visible flap mottling, visible dermis, capillary refill, methylene blue infiltration, bleed from flap edges, and flap thickness estimation, reinforcing the utility of clinical assessment.

Several adjunctive perfusion assessment tools can also be useful for evaluation of mastectomy flaps intraoperatively. These methods primarily utilized indocyanine green angiography to identify relative areas of ischemia or overall global ischemia. Indocyanine green angiography has been shown to reduce mastectomy flap necrosis in skin-sparing mastectomy compared to clinical assessment [26, 27], though determining the degree of hypoperfusion and the subsequent extent of intraoperative tissue excisions can be difficult. Reviews have determined that indocyanine or fluorescein angiography likely does not decrease mastectomy skin loss and may actually result in debriding healthy skin [28]. Other technologies such as light-based spectroscopy and near-infrared tissue oximetry have not been as well studied in mastectomy flap perfusion. In the end, tissue perfusion assessment technologies remain one method of evaluating mastectomy flap quality and should be used in conjunction with clinical analysis to determine appropriate intraoperative interventions.

7.5 Managing Compromised Flaps

7.5.1 Intraoperative Considerations

In cases with concern for compromised tissue perfusion intraoperatively, several decisions must be made depending on the suspected degree of tissue injury and the implications for the reconstruction. In skin-sparing or total mastectomies, grossly compromised skin should be excised without placing undue tension on the closure.

Management of ischemic mastectomy flaps is more challenging in nipple-sparing mastectomy as significant skin cannot be excised given preservation of the entire soft tissue envelope. Therefore, additional decisions regarding the reconstruction must be made. Immediate implant reconstructions have been found to have higher rates of ischemic complications compared to two-stage tissue expanders after nipple-sparing mastectomy as increased pressure on skin flaps likely worsens ischemia [29]. In cases of planned immediate implant reconstruction, consideration should be given to placement of tissue expanders at the initial operation if there is concern for mastectomy flap perfusion.

Similarly, tissue expanders should be underfilled (or not filled at all) if perfusion is compromised. Tissue expander type can also affect pressure on mastectomy flaps. Anatomical integral injection-port expanders tend to be bulkier than expanders with remote ports or adjustable implants [30, 31]. Under filling expanders with air places less pressure on the mastectomy skin, particularly the lower flap. In the worst-case scenario, reconstruction should be delayed to prevent likely complications secondary to full-thickness tissue injury and prosthesis exposure.

Plane of prosthesis placement is also an important consideration. Prepectoral reconstruction does not work under poorly perfused mastectomy flaps. Given the absence of a vascularized layer of pectoralis muscle, wound breakdown or major necrosis inherently is equivalent to prosthesis exposure. Patients should therefore always be counseled that total submuscular implant placement is a possibility, or if that is not desired, a delayed reconstruction, in the situation of a compromised skin envelope. It is important to remember that support materials such as acellular dermal matrix do not help in such cases. These matrices require juxtaposition to well-vascularized tissue to integrate. Placing a non-vascularized piece of cadaveric dermis under poorly perfused mastectomy flaps is equivalent to a foreign body under ischemic skin.

7.5.2 Postoperative Considerations

Postoperative skin envelope ischemia is a serious complication in prepectoral breast reconstruction. These cases require aggressive management and close follow-up to minimize the occurrence of prosthesis exposure, infection, and reconstructive failure. Postoperative mastectomy flap ischemia requires a comprehensive defensive approach to make all attempts to minimize tissue loss. In nipple-sparing mastectomy, prior radiation, immediate placement of implants, use of acellular dermal matrix, major infections and higher body mass index have been identified as risk factors for reconstructive failure after major ischemic complications. In prepectoral reconstruction, the goals are to carefully treat partial thickness necrosis to prevent its progression, and to rapidly identify and manage full-thickness injuries.

Care of partial thickness ischemia requires close follow-up and strict wound care. Treatment should be directed as minimizing the risk of infection and further tissue injury, while monitoring for progression to full-thickness necrosis. We prefer utilizing petroleum-based gauze or antibiotic ointments with nonadherent gauze dress changes. Adjunctive treatments such as nitroglycerin ointment and hyperbaric oxygen therapy can also be useful [32, 33].

In cases of full-thickness necrosis, the benefits of early, proactive treatment cannot be understated. Given the lack of a vascularized muscle layer between the implant and the skin, all wounds are serious matters. Early debridement of necrosis is paramount to allow for wound closure and minimize contamination of the implant pocket. With large areas of necrosis or if the wound edges are under tension, explantation and delay of reconstruction often serves the patient best to allow the tissues to heal.

7.6 Conclusions

The term mastectomy flap quality envelopes a myriad of different variables that can be summarized by relative thickness and perfusion of the skin envelope. The "high quality" mastectomy flap is one that has been dissected in the anatomic plane of the breast capsule to remove the gland while maintaining the full thickness of the subcutaneous layer to preserve the critical superficial perfusion. Mastectomy flap quality is the responsibility of both the oncologic and plastic surgeon and requires a team-oriented approached in the preoperative, intraoperative, and postoperative phases of care. Preoperative imaging can help guide a precise intraoperative dissection, while intraoperative assessment of flaps through both clinical and adjunctive methods should dictate the appropriate reconstructive choices to minimize complications and optimize both reconstructive and aesthetic outcomes in breast reconstruction patients.

References

1. Salibian AA, Frey JD, Choi M, Karp NS. Subcutaneous implant-based breast reconstruction with acellular dermal matrix/mesh: a systematic review. Plast Reconstr Surg Glob Open. 2016;4:e1139.
2. Storm-Dickerson T, Sigalove N. Prepectoral breast reconstruction: the breast Surgeon's perspective. Plast Reconstr Surg. 2017;140:43S–8S.
3. Vidya R, Iqbal FM. Breast anatomy: time to classify the subpectoral and prepectoral spaces. Clin Anat. 2017;30:434–5.
4. Rehnke RD, Groening RM, Van Buskirk ER, Clarke JM. Anatomy of the superficial fascia system of the breast: a comprehensive theory of breast fascial anatomy. Plast Reconstr Surg. 2018;142:1135–44.
5. Frey JD, Salibian AA, Choi M, Karp NS. The importance of tissue perfusion in reconstructive breast surgery. Plast Reconstr Surg. 2019;144:21S–9S.
6. De Vita R, Zoccali G, Buccheri EM, et al. Outcome evaluation after 2023 nipple-sparing mastectomies: our experience. Plast Reconstr Surg. 2017;139:335e–47e.
7. Frey JD, Salibian AA, Karp NS, Choi M. The impact of mastectomy weight on reconstructive trends and outcomes in nipple-sparing mastectomy: progressively greater complications with larger breast size. Plast Reconstr Surg. 2018;141:795e–804e.
8. Caputo GG, Marchetti A, Dalla Pozza E, et al. Skin-reduction breast reconstructions with prepectoral implant. Plast Reconstr Surg. 2016;137:1702–5.
9. Rusby JE, Gui GP. Nipple-sparing mastectomy in women with large or ptotic breasts. J Plast Reconstr Aesthet Surg. 2010;63:e754–5.
10. Spear SL, Rottman SJ, Seiboth LA, Hannan CM. Breast reconstruction using a staged nipple-sparing mastectomy following mastopexy or reduction. Plast Reconstr Surg. 2012;129:572–81.
11. Frey JD, Salibian AA, Choi M, Karp NS. Optimizing outcomes in nipple-sparing mastectomy: mastectomy flap thickness is not one size fits all. Plast Reconstr Surg Glob Open. 2019;7:e2103.
12. Matsen CB, Mehrara B, Eaton A, et al. Skin flap necrosis after mastectomy with reconstruction: a prospective study. Ann Surg Oncol. 2016;23:257–64.
13. Colwell AS, Tessler O, Lin AM, et al. Breast reconstruction following nipple-sparing mastectomy: predictors of complications, reconstruction outcomes, and 5-year trends. Plast Reconstr Surg. 2014;133:496–506.
14. Algaithy ZK, Petit JY, Lohsiriwat V, et al. Nipple sparing mastectomy: can we predict the factors predisposing to necrosis? Eur J Surg Oncol. 2012;38:125–9.
15. Didier F, Radice D, Gandini S, et al. Does nipple preservation in mastectomy improve satisfaction with cosmetic results, psychological adjustment, body image and sexuality? Breast Cancer Res Treat. 2009;118:623–33.
16. Frey JD, Salibian AA, Choi M, Karp NS. Putting together the pieces: development and validation of a risk-assessment model for nipple-sparing mastectomy. Plast Reconstr Surg. 2020;145:273e–83e.
17. Frey JD, Salibian AA, Levine JP, Karp NS, Choi M. Incision choices in nipple-sparing mastectomy: a comparative analysis of outcomes and evolution of a clinical algorithm. Plast Reconstr Surg. 2018;142:826e–35e.
18. Daar DA, Abdou SA, Rosario L, et al. Is there a preferred incision location for nipple-sparing mastectomy? A systematic review and meta-analysis. Plast Reconstr Surg. 2019;143:906e–19e.
19. Wagner JL, Fearmonti R, Hunt KK, et al. Prospective evaluation of the nipple-areola complex sparing mastectomy for risk reduction and for early-stage breast cancer. Ann Surg Oncol. 2012;19:1137–44.
20. Salibian AH, Harness JK, Mowlds DS. Inframammary approach to nipple-areola-sparing mastectomy. Plast Reconstr Surg. 2013;132:700e–8e.
21. Mori H, Uemura N, Okazaki M, Nakagawa T, Sato T. Nipple malposition after nipple-sparing mastec-

tomy and expander-implant reconstruction. Breast Cancer. 2016;23:740–4.

22. Munhoz AM, Aldrighi CM, Montag E, et al. Clinical outcomes following nipple-areola-sparing mastectomy with immediate implant-based breast reconstruction: a 12-year experience with an analysis of patient and breast-related factors for complications. Breast Cancer Res Treat. 2013;140:545–55.
23. Frey JD, Salibian AA, Choi M, Karp NS. Mastectomy flap thickness and complications in nipple-sparing mastectomy: objective evaluation using magnetic resonance imaging. Plast Reconstr Surg Glob Open. 2017;5:e1439.
24. Siotos C, Aston JW, Euhus DM, et al. The use of tumescent technique in mastectomy and related complications: a meta-analysis. Plast Reconstr Surg. 2019;143:39–48.
25. Frey JD, Salibian AA, Bekisz JM, et al. What is in a number? Evaluating a risk assessment tool in immediate breast reconstruction. Plast Reconstr Surg Glob Open. 2019;7:e2585.
26. Rinker B. A comparison of methods to assess mastectomy flap viability in skin-sparing mastectomy and immediate reconstruction: a prospective cohort study. Plast Reconstr Surg. 2016;137:395–401.
27. Liu EH, Zhu SL, Hu J, et al. Intraoperative SPY reduces post-mastectomy skin flap complications: a systematic review and meta-analysis. Plast Reconstr Surg Glob Open. 2019;7:e2060.
28. Khavanin N, Qiu C, Darrach H, et al. Intraoperative perfusion assessment in mastectomy skin flaps: how close are we to preventing complications? J Reconstr Microsurg. 2019;35:471–8.
29. Frey JD, Choi M, Salibian AA, Karp NS. Comparison of outcomes with tissue expander, immediate implant, and autologous breast reconstruction in greater than 1000 nipple-sparing mastectomies. Plast Reconstr Surg. 2017;139:1300–10.
30. Becker H, Zhadan O. Filling the Spectrum expander with air-a new alternative. Plast Reconstr Surg Glob Open. 2017;5:e1541.
31. Becker H, Mathew PJ. Immediate Prepectoral breast reconstruction in suboptimal patients using an air-filled spacer. Plast Reconstr Surg Glob Open. 2019;7:e2470.
32. Turin SY, Li DD, Vaca EE, Fine N. Nitroglycerin ointment for reducing the rate of mastectomy flap necrosis in immediate implant-based breast reconstruction. Plast Reconstr Surg. 2018;142:264e–70e.
33. Alperovich M, Harmaty M, Chiu ES. Treatment of nipple-sparing mastectomy necrosis using hyperbaric oxygen therapy. Plast Reconstr Surg. 2015;135:1071e–2e.

8 Meshes and Implants in Prepectoral Breast Reconstruction: Selecting the Right One

Kylie M. Edinger and Ahmed M. Afifi

8.1 Introduction

The methods of breast reconstruction are constantly evolving and changing, and these changes are largely driven by advancements in implant design and mesh development. In the 1970s, breast reconstruction was largely performed using prepectoral implant placement as submuscular techniques were not well described and understood [1]. In 1981, however, Gruber et al released a comparative study of submuscular and prepectoral breast reconstruction techniques which resulted in a cultural shift away from prepectoral reconstruction towards submuscular reconstruction [2]. Their study included a review of the literature and demonstrated a higher rate of capsular contracture , infection, implant malposition, and implant loss in prepectoral breast reconstruction compared to submuscular reconstruction. However, all the patients in the study underwent direct-to-implant reconstruction without tissue expansion, and none of the patients underwent reconstruction using mesh products. This highlights how imperative implant choice and the use of mesh are in successful prepectoral breast reconstruction. Even with today's advancements, prepectoral breast reconstruction performed without the proper choice of implant or supportive mesh would similarly fail. Simply stated, prepectoral breast reconstruction cannot exist without the proper use of implants and meshes.

It is likely the advent of acellular dermal matrix (ADM) that revived the interest in prepectoral reconstruction and made it a competitive alternative to submuscular breast reconstruction [3]. Biologic and synthetic meshes like ADM provide improved implant placement and pocket control, enhanced soft tissue coverage, less rippling, and possibly reduce the rates of capsular contracture. Meshes also allow the use of larger implants and initial expander fill volumes [4–6]. Today, over 50% of breast reconstruction in the United States is performed using ADM [7].

Choosing the best implant and mesh to use in prepectoral breast reconstruction is imperative to achieving a successful result. Although the decision between different profiles of breast implants may not be that consequential in submuscular reconstruction, these decisions are highly impactful in the results of prepectoral breast reconstruction and must be considered carefully. In the right hands and with the proper tools, prepectoral reconstruction can be highly successful, explaining its rapid acceptance by surgeons and patients (Fig. 8.1). A study by Marks et al in 2019 demon-

K. M. Edinger
Division of Plastic Surgery, University of Wisconsin, Madison, WI, USA

A. M. Afifi (✉)
Division of Plastic Surgery, University of Wisconsin, Madison, WI, USA

Division of Plastic Surgery, Cairo University, Cairo, Egypt

© The Author(s), under exclusive license to Springer Nature Switzerland AG 2023
R. Vidya, H. Becker (eds.), *Prepectoral Breast Reconstruction*,
https://doi.org/10.1007/978-3-031-15590-1_8

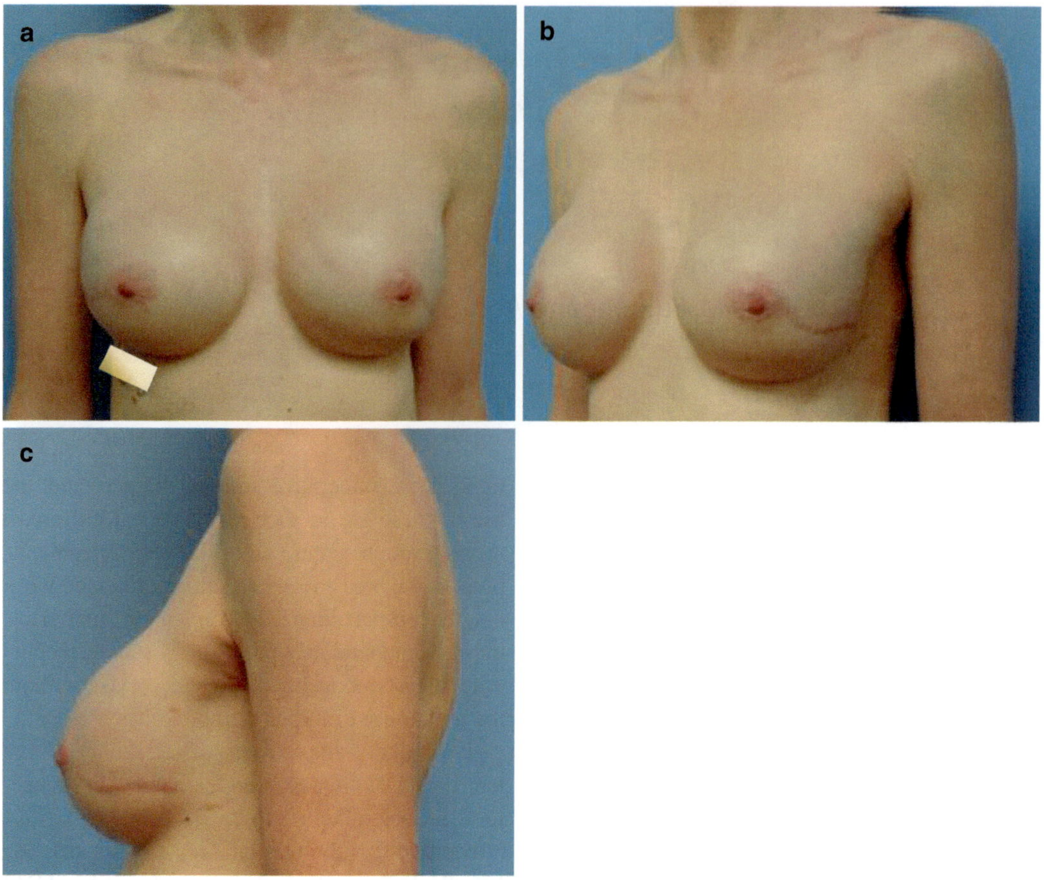

Fig. 8.1 Ideal prepectoral breast reconstruction patient, demonstrating the natural appearance that can be achieved with prepectoral breast reconstruction. Patient is viewed from the front (**a**), obliquely (**b**), and laterally (**c**)

strated that it has already surpassed submuscular reconstruction in popularity [8]. We expect this trend to continue as the surgical community gains more experience and as implants and meshes continue to evolve and improve.

8.2 Implant Selection

Choosing the right breast implant is one of the cornerstones to performing a successful prepectoral breast reconstruction. When it comes to selecting the appropriate breast implant, many factors including volume, shape, cohesivity, texture, width, and projection come into play. Breast implants are generally categorized according to three main manufacturing options: silicone vs saline, textured vs smooth, and round vs anatomic.

8.2.1 Silicone vs Saline

Both silicone and saline breast implants are comprised of an outer silicone elastomer shell. Saline implants are filled with sterile saline, whereas silicone breast implants are filled with a silicone gel of varying cohesivity. The higher the degree of crosslinking of the silicone gel, the more cohesive and firm the gel becomes. Highly cohesive breast implants have less rippling than lower cohesive breast implants, but they also come with less ptosis and a more rounded, unnatural appearance.

In the United States, most breast reconstructions are performed using silicone breast implants, with over 95% of alloplastic breast reconstruction surgery completed using silicone breast implants in 2019 compared to 5% using saline breast implants [9]. Breast reconstruction is usually performed using silicone implants because of the more natural feel and appearance that can be achieved with silicone over saline implants. Silicone implants are also utilized more commonly worldwide for both reconstruction and augmentation. In Europe, Latin America, and Asia, breast augmentation data show that silicone breast implants consume the majority of the breast implant markets worldwide over saline implants [10].

Saline and silicone breast implants have been shown to have a similar lifespan with time to implant failure averaging 8.4 years for saline implants compared to 8.1 years for silicone implants [11]. There are important differences, however, that make silicone the implant of choice in prepectoral breast reconstruction. In addition to silicone breast implants offering the advantage over saline of less rippling and a more natural appearance and feel, they also have a lower weight per volume. A 400 cc saline implant is on average only 25 g heavier than a silicone implant (attributed to the higher specific gravity of water compared to saline), but even a slightly heavier implant places more tension on incisions and increases the risk of wound breakdown and implant extrusion [12]. For the remainder of this chapter, we will be mostly focused on silicone implant reconstruction as it is by far the more common option and is what we use in our practice.

8.2.2 Textured vs Smooth

Texturing is a method by which breast implants are mechanically or chemically altered so their surface gains a rough, grippy texture. Texturing decreases rates of implant malpositioning and capsular contracture and is one of the most advantageous breast implant features in prepectoral breast reconstruction. Although this feature is not critical in submuscular reconstruction, it can be very beneficial in creating a successful prepectoral reconstruction. The method of texturing utilized varies by company, but is usually a chemical or mechanical process to roughen the silicone surface. Macro-texturing is a texturing process that results in larger and deeper texture pores than micro-texturing and has been shown to result in improved adherence to tissue and less migration than micro-texturing [13].

Allergan previously utilized a process known as the lost-salt technique, where the wet silicone shell was dipped in a salt mixture before curing, creating a gritty surface [1]. This macro-texturing method was banned in several countries and subsequently discontinued by the company after it was found to be associated with Breast Implant Associated Anaplastic Large Cell Lymphoma (BI-ALCL). Allergan no longer offers a textured implant, and all of their breast implants are now smooth. Mentor utilizes a mechanical stamping process where polyurethane stamps are imprinted into the wet silicone surface before it is cured in a micro-texturing technique [14]. Sientra does not disclose the specifics of its micro-texturing process. Mentor and Sientra utilize texturing methods that have not been found to have as strong of an association with ALCL as Allergan's previously macro-textured implants, but all textured implants have been declared a risk for developing BI-ALCL and should be used only after discussing this risk with patients.

Textured implants have fallen out of favor in the United States in recent years secondary to their correlation with BI-ALCL, but they are one of the best implant choices for prepectoral breast reconstruction. The FDA has not officially banned the use of textured implants, but most manufacturing companies have voluntarily discontinued production of textured implants at the FDA's recommendation. Although textured implants are still available and utilized globally, several countries have moved to ban macro-textured breast implants. France in particular banned both macro-textured and polyurethane textured breast implants in 2019 with the release of BI-ALCL data. Polyurethane textured implants were previously available in the United States from Surgitek until they were withdrawn from the market due to concerns of carcinogenicity of 2,4-toluenediamine (2,4-TDA), a breakdown product of polyurethane [15]. Although 2,4-TDA has only been shown to have carcinogenicity in animal models, polyurethane implants have been linked with BI-ALCL. Polyurethane implants remain widely popular throughout Europe.

In our practice after having treated several patients with ALCL ourselves, we do not use any textured devices and have switched exclusively to smooth implants and expanders. We commonly utilize shaped (anatomic) expanders with round implants. We hope that in the future we will know more about ALCL and that implant technology will continue to evolve and to develop safer shaped implants, but for now the risk of ALCL is one not worth taking in our practice.

8.2.3 Round vs Anatomic

Round implants have a round, spherical circumference, whereas anatomic implants are teardrop shaped with the intent of creating a more natural ptotic profile. Round implants can be either smooth or textured and filled with silicone or saline. Anatomic implants can also be silicone or saline filled, but most have a textured surface to minimize their risk of rotating and malpositioning on the chest wall. Motiva is currently the only company that produces smooth anatomic implants and has designed the implant with tabs to secure the implant into position on the chest wall [16]. Motiva breast implants are currently unavailable in the United States, but clinical safety trials are ongoing within the United States with hopes to start sales in North America soon.

Anatomic implants are especially useful in prepectoral breast reconstruction given that they achieve a more natural ptotic appearance with a gradual upper pole slope compared to traditional round implants. They are a powerful tool in prepectoral breast reconstruction, but are less commonly utilized in America as there are no smooth surfaced anatomic implants for sale in the US. With the anticipated release of smooth anatomic implants in the US, we predict that anatomic implants may gain popularity in prepectoral breast reconstruction. Although textured anatomic implants are less commonly utilized in the United States and Latin America, they are still heavily utilized in Europe and Asia [10].

8.2.4 Cohesivity

Cohesivity is an important factor to consider in prepectoral breast reconstruction, as implants with higher cohesivity have less rippling. Choosing the correct cohesivity of an implant is largely dependent on the thickness of the mastectomy skin flaps. If the flaps are thin, a more cohesive implant will decrease rippling. If the mastectomy skin flaps are thick, then less cohesive implants can be utilized for a more natural appearance with less upper pole fullness [4]. Highly cohesive implants have a more augmented appearance with a less gradual slope between the chest wall and upper breast pole. If a more gradual upper pole transition between the chest wall and implant is desired, fat grafting can be utilized to soften this transition. Fat grafting can also be used to decrease rippling with implants, although the patient and surgeon need to have realistic expectations regarding the amount of improvement in rippling that can be achieved with fat grafting. Implants with high cohesivity have also been anecdotally associated with higher rates of implant flipping (also known as anterior posterior malposition, where the posterior surface of the implant is facing the breast skin and nipple) in prepectoral breast reconstruction [17]. In our practice, we prefer moderately cohesive implants as they provide a nice balance of decreasing rippling while providing a natural shape and acceptable rates of flipping (Figs. 8.2 and 8.3).

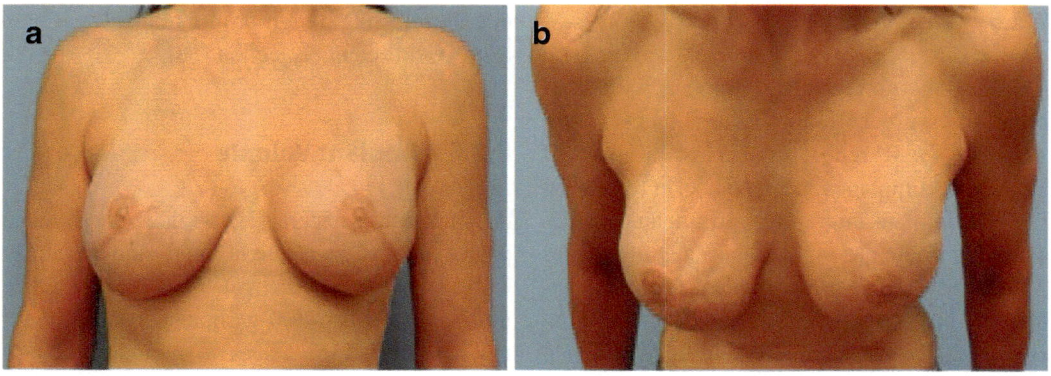

Fig. 8.2 Photograph of a patient who underwent breast reconstruction with a regular implant on the right, and a highly cohesive implant on the left (the right implant was ruptured in an accident and urgently replaced with a regular implant). Photograph (**a**) demonstrates how while upright the two implants are comparable. Photograph (**b**) demonstrates significantly more rippling in the lower cohesive implant on the right, demonstrating the value of highly cohesive implants in prepectoral breast reconstruction

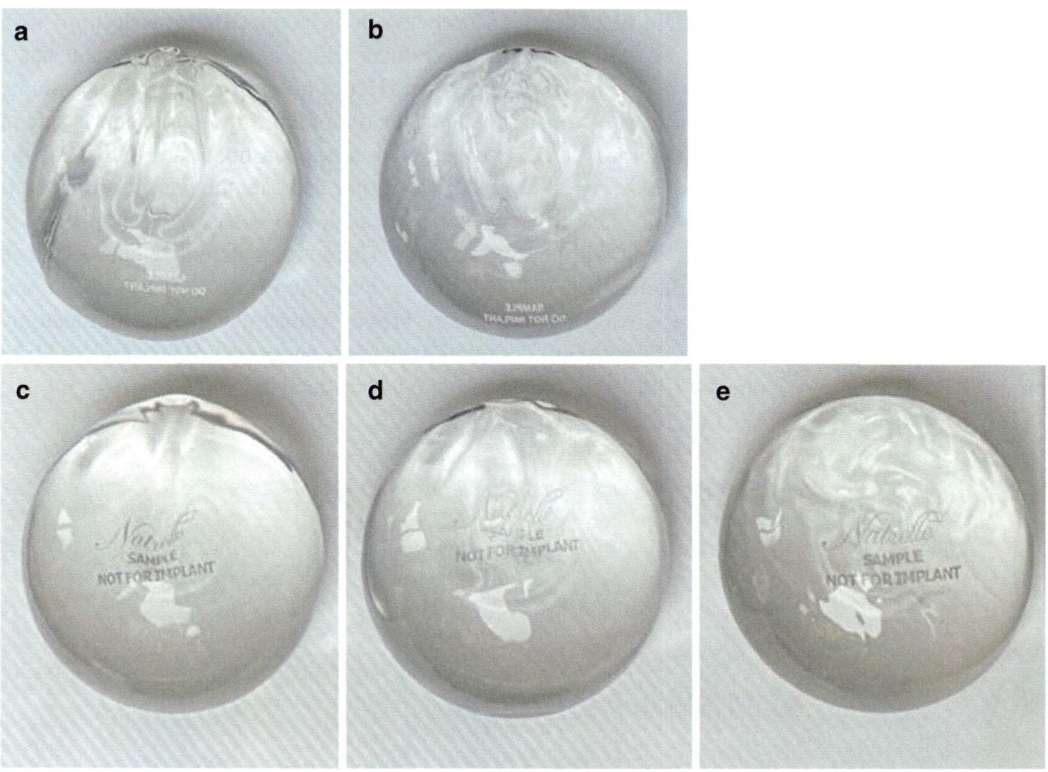

Fig. 8.3 Photograph of implants of varying cohesivity to demonstrate the degree of rippling between the cohesivities. Sientra's higher cohesive implant- HSC+ (**a**), Sientra's lower cohesive implant- HSC (**b**), Allergan's highest cohesive implant- SCX (**c**), Allergan's middle cohesive implant- SSX (**d**), Allergan's lowest cohesive implant- SRX (**e**)

8.2.5 Base Width

Choosing the correct breast implant width and projection is crucial for prepectoral breast reconstruction, as it relies on a hand-in-glove fit between the implant and tissue pocket to prevent rippling, implant migration, and implant malpositioning. There are typically a range of profiles offered for silicone breast implants (low, moderate, and high) depending on the manufacturing company. To select an implant for any given patient, the surgeon and patient must together determine the desired projection, implant width, and volume; only two of these three metrics in any combination must be decided on to find the implant that best fits the patient. Base width is the most important factor to consider in prepectoral breast reconstruction to ensure a tight fit of the implant in the pocket, and is what we start with for choosing expanders or implants.

Breast base width should be measured from the anterior axillary line to the medial breast, and an implant with a corresponding base width should be selected to achieve a hand-in-glove fit. In round implants, base width and height will be equal. For patients with wide chest diameters and shoulders, wider base width implants are a better choice, but it is important that you do not compromise projection. For patients with concave chests, selecting a high-profile implant will help achieve sufficient projection [18].

8.2.6 Implant Volume

As implant size increases, so does the demand placed on the breast tissue and skin envelope. Vidya et al suggest that patients with breast volumes greater than 500 g should undergo breast reconstruction in 2 stages to minimize risk of reconstruction failure [19]. A large multicenter retrospective study by Choi et al found that implant volumes over 400 g were associated with increased rates of infection and post-mastectomy flap necrosis [20]. However, the choice of implant volume is largely dependent on mastectomy skin flap health and patient's body habitus. If the mastectomy skin flaps are thick and healthy and the patient has a larger BMI to accommodate large volume implants, the use of large breast implants is safe in prepectoral breast reconstruction (Fig. 8.4). If the mastectomy skin flaps are threatened or thin or if the patient has a low BMI, a smaller implant may be selected. There are no definitive cut-offs when determining which implant volume to use in prepectoral breast reconstruction, but mastectomy skin flap thickness and patient BMI should both be considered when choosing implant size.

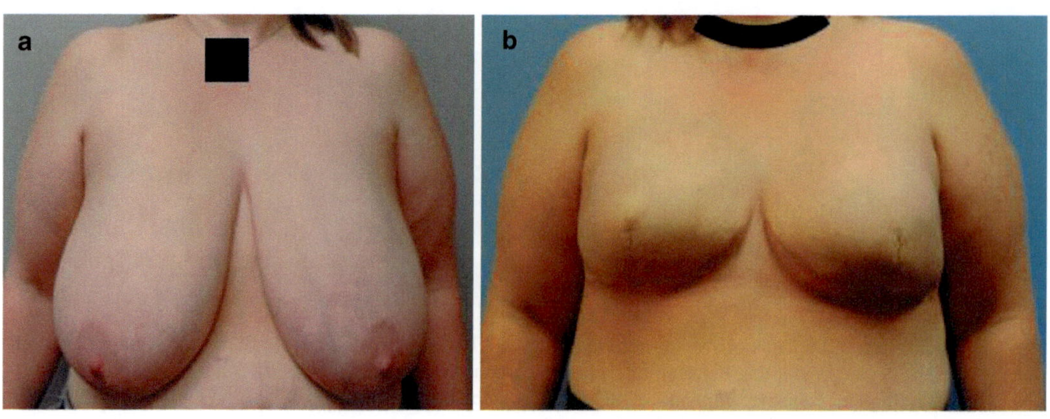

Fig. 8.4 Photograph demonstrating that patients with a large BMI can safely undergo prepectoral breast reconstruction with large breast implants. Photographs are of patient pre-operatively (**a**), and post-operatively in AP (**b**), oblique (**c**), and lateral (**d**) views. Patient was reconstructed using mentor smooth, round, extra high-profile 790 mL silicone gel implants

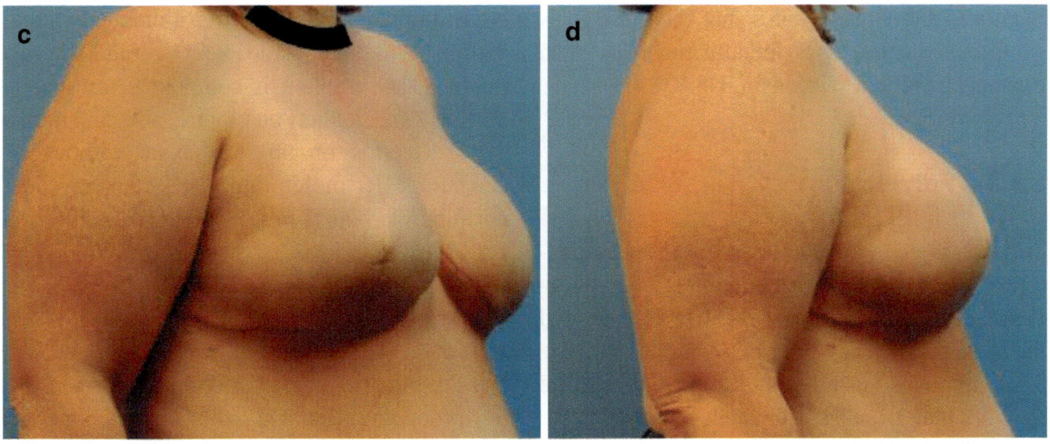

Fig. 8.4 (continued)

8.3 Implant Manufacturers

A thorough search of published literature, social media support groups, blogs, and local surgeon websites was reviewed to create the following list of implants in popular use. There are many manufacturers of breast implants globally, and this section is by no means meant to be an exclusive list. There are other breast implants that are likely available and should be considered for use even if not reviewed in this chapter.

8.3.1 Allergan

Allergan is a worldwide manufacturer of breast implants, producing both saline and silicone Natrelle implants of varying cohesivity. Formerly called McGhan and then Inamed, they are now called Allergan. Their products (NuSil silicone) are manufactured in Costa Rica. They recently removed their macro-textured breast implant from the market after its association with BI-ALCL was established. They are one of four companies currently producing breast implants for sale in America [21].

8.3.2 Sientra

Sientra is a company that supplies breast implants solely within the United States. Sientra was previously the North American distributor of Brazilian Silimed breast implants. However, Silimed's manufacturing plant in Brazil was found to be contaminated in 2014, so Sientra discontinued its association with Silimed and moved its manufacturing headquarters to the United States in Franklin, WI. Sientra provides exclusively silicone gel implants (round or anatomic, smooth or textured), with no saline implants offered [22].

8.3.3 Mentor

Mentor is an American company based out of California that supplies breast implants within the United States. They are owned by Johnson & Johnson company, and they offer both silicone and saline breast implants. Their silicone is manufactured in Costa Rica and imported to the US where the implants are handmade. They offer a special adjustable saline filled breast implant, the Spectrum implant, which allows surgeons to adjust the volume of the implant for up to 6 months postoperatively through a removable fill tube [23].

8.3.4 Silimed

Silimed is a Brazilian company that is the largest supplier of breast implants in Latin America. They offer silicone breast implants in round, anatomic, smooth, and textured options. Silimed previously manufactured the implants supplied by

Sientra in the United States, but the companies split and Sientra now manufactures its own implants locally in Wisconsin, USA [24].

8.3.5 Polytech

Polytech is one of the world's leading manufacturers of silicone breast implants, supplying breast implants throughout most of Europe and the middle east. They offer both smooth and textured implants, using polyurethane to texture their implants (a substance which is banned in the United States) [25].

8.3.6 Ideal Implant

Ideal implant is another company that sells implants solely within the United States. Their silicone is imported from Costa Rica, and the implants are manufactured in the US in Vesta, WI. The company offers saline only implants in a dual silicone shell designed to minimize rippling. The goal is to provide the feel and look of a silicone implant with the peace of mind of a saline implant (no risk of silicone rupture) [26].

8.3.7 CG Aesthetics

GC aesthetics is an aesthetic company that manufactures breast implants through two branching companies: Nagor (in Scotland and England) and Eurosilicone (in France). They supply silicone breast implants to over 70 countries worldwide but are not available for sale in the United States [27].

8.3.8 Laboratories Arion

Laboratories Arion is a company that supplies breast implants to South America, Europe, Northern Africa, areas in the middle East, and Vietnam. In addition to a Monoblock silicone breast implant line, they offer a unique biocompatible and biodegradable hydrogel breast implant. The implant is completely transparent on X-ray and deflates on rupture, allowing immediate detection on physical exam without the need for MRI monitoring. This company does not supply products in the United States [28].

8.3.9 Hans Biomed

Hans Biomed is an Asian company responsible for producing BellaGel, the first silicone gel breast implant manufactured in Asia (Oh). The implant is certified in Europe with hopes to expand sales to China and the United States [29].

8.3.10 Ceraplas

Cereplas is a company in France that offers Cereform silicone gel implants in round, anatomic, smooth, and textured options. They are predominately sold in Europe, the Middle East, and South America [30].

8.3.11 Establishment Labs

Establishment labs produce silicone Motiva breast implants for countries throughout Europe, Japan, Australia, and South Korea. They are currently undergoing clinical safety trials within the United States with hopes to start sales in North America soon. They are the only company offering smooth anatomic implants, which are secured to the chest wall with tabs [31].

8.3.12 Sebbin

Sebbin is a French company producing silicone breast implants manufactured entirely by hand with sales throughout Europe, Africa, South America, Australia, and India [32].

8.3.13 Guangzhou Wanhe

Guangzhou Wanhe Plastic Materials is a Chinese company specialized in creating silicone breast implant products.

8.3.14 CollPlant

Collplant is a company in Israel that is currently working on developing 3D bioprinted breast implants. These products are not yet commercially available [33].

8.4 Tissue Expanders

For patients undergoing mastectomy, immediate breast reconstruction is the most popular reconstructive method utilized globally. Immediate breast reconstruction can be performed as a single stage operation with direct placement of an implant, or as a staged procedure with initial placement of a tissue expander and a later expander to implant exchange. Many surgeons prefer a two-stage approach as the expander acts as an initial template and ensures that insurance will pay for the exchange during which the surgeon can fine tune the pocket and optimize the outcome. Expanders can also be indicated for planned radiation therapy, in the setting of threatened mastectomy skin flap perfusion (where the expander can be initially left empty or filled with air), or in patients who desire a larger cup size than they had pre-operatively [34, 35]. In the United States, approximately 80% of alloplastic breast reconstruction is performed in a staged manner.

Although immediate breast reconstruction is the standard of care, some patients are still reconstructed in a delayed fashion. This can be due to patient preference, planned post-mastectomy radiation therapy, or in patients with significant comorbidities preventing them from undergoing elective reconstruction at the time of mastectomy. In the case of delayed reconstruction, placement of a tissue expander is a necessity.

Zenn described a staged immediate breast reconstruction technique in 2015, which addresses the risk factors of skin and nipple necrosis seen in immediate breast reconstruction while also avoiding the issue of nipple malpositioning seen in staged reconstruction with tissue expansion [35]. His team delays reconstruction 2 weeks following mastectomy in high-risk patients or those with thin mastectomy flaps, allowing skin flap perfusion to improve without placing tissue expanders and thus avoiding nipple malposition seen secondary to expansion (Fig. 8.5).

When selecting a tissue expander for prepectoral breast reconstruction, the surgeon must remember that the tissue expander chosen must create a well-controlled pocket that will tightly accommodate a future implant. If the pocket is over-expanded, the implant will not sit tightly within the pocket and will be at risk of rippling, migrating, and flipping. The tissue expander should be underfilled so that the final implant will sit snuggly within the pocket without excess skin laxity. This is an important distinction between prepectoral and submuscular reconstructions. Short to medium height expanders are typically chosen for round implants, and full height expanders are typically chosen for anatomic implants [4]. Tissues expanders with a base width 0.5–1.0 cm narrower than the desired final implant are typically chosen to ensure the pocket is not over-expanded [18]. Choice of height depends on several factors considered together including patient body habitus, measurement-based planning, patient wishes, and surgeon preference. The goal of the first stage of surgery is to create a breast footprint with a well-defined pocket that will require minimal alterations at the second stage.

Tissue expanders, like breast implants, are available in both textured and smooth options. With the discovery of BI-ALCL's association with textured implants, textured devices are used less commonly and with more caution than in prior years. Mentor, Allergan, and Sientra all offer smooth tissue expanders within the United States. Mentor's Artoura tissue expander is designed with dynamic control technology,

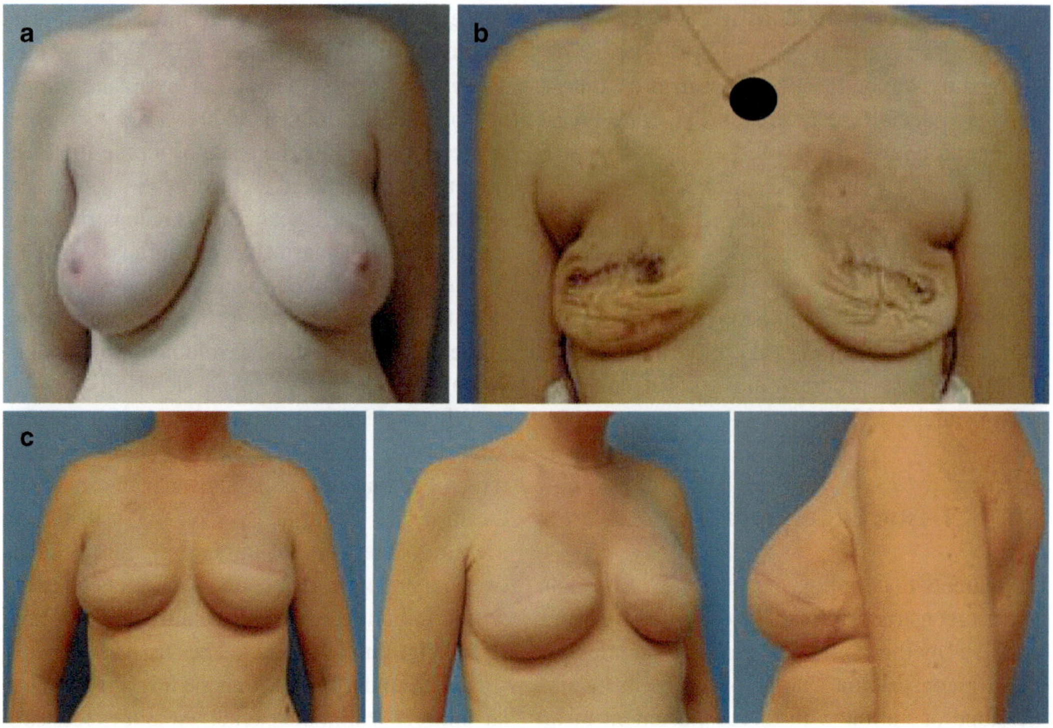

Fig. 8.5 Photograph of a patient reconstructed using a direct-to-implant reconstruction in a staged immediate technique. Images include pre-operative breasts (**a**), 1 week following mastectomy, showing recovering mastectomy skin flaps (**b**), 3 months following a direct-to-implant reconstruction using mentor smooth high-profile Xtra MemoryGel round 700 mL implants bilaterally. Reconstruction was performed 2 weeks after the mastectomy, allowing the mastectomy skin flaps to heal (**c**)

which has an internal architecture that allows only the lower pole of the expander to expand, delivering precisely controlled pocket expansion [36]. Sientra recently released their dual port smooth tissue expander which has two ports: one for injecting fluid to fill the expander and one to drain serous fluid surrounding the implant, theoretically negating the need for surgical drains [37]. This is especially helpful in prepectoral breast reconstruction given that seroma rates are higher with prepectoral implant placement compared to submuscular implant placement. PMT Corporation and CG Aesthetics offer smooth tissue expanders in Europe, although many of the implant manufacturing companies overseas only offer textured breast tissue expanders.

8.5 Mesh Selection

The advancements in mesh in recent years have allowed prepectoral breast reconstruction to increase in both success and popularity. The added layer of coverage improves rippling, helps secure implant positioning on the chest wall, minimizes migration and malrotation, defines and reinforces the inframammary fold, may potentially minimize the inflammatory response, and reduces pressure points on mastectomy skin flaps [38, 39]. Meshes have revolutionized prepectoral breast reconstruction and are paramount to its success.

Acellular dermal matrix (ADM) was first introduced in 2006, and its use in breast reconstruction surgery was quickly realized [3]. ADM was initially used in subpectoral reconstructive surgery to supplement muscle coverage along the inferior border of the pectoralis muscle in patients who were expected to receive post-operative radiation therapy [40]. With improvements in capsular contracture and pocket control, ADM use was then expanded to prepectoral breast reconstruction. Studies have shown that ADM results in less implant rippling, allows immediate breast reconstruction in the setting of thin mastectomy skin flaps that would otherwise require delayed reconstruction, and allows for the use of larger implants and larger initial tissue expander fill volumes compared to reconstructions that do not use ADM [4–6]. Since the advent of ADM, the market of biologic and synthetic meshes has expanded, allowing a concomitant expansion of the indications for prepectoral breast reconstruction.

When using biologic and synthetic meshes intraoperatively, the mesh can be used to cover the implant and reinforce areas where the skin is thin, or the mesh can be used to circumferentially wrap the implant. Wrapping an implant in ADM is considered an off-label use in the United States. Biologic meshes should additionally have optimal contact with tissue to promote integration when they are placed in the body.

8.6 Biologic Meshes

Biologic meshes include acellular dermal matrices composed of fetal bovine, porcine, and human cadaver skin components. The downside of biologic meshes is that they are expensive and come with a risk of seroma and possibly higher rates of infection. They average 20–30$/cm^2, costing anywhere from 5,000 to 20,000$ per breast [39, 41]. A study by Chun comparing submuscular implant-based breast reconstruction with ADM to reconstruction without ADM demonstrated that infection and seroma rates were significantly higher in the ADM group [42]. Although her research was on submuscular breast reconstruction, it can be extrapolated that this difference would be even more relevant in prepectoral breast reconstruction, where larger pieces of mesh are used. A systematic review by Ho et al reviewed 16 articles comparing ADM-assisted breast reconstruction to breast reconstruction without ADM [43]. They found that ADM-assisted breast reconstruction was nearly 4 times as likely to be complicated by seroma, nearly 3 times as likely to be complicated by infection, and nearly 3 times as likely to result in reconstructive failure compared to breast reconstruction performed without ADM. These numbers seem to be corroborated by Marks et al in a survey of members of the American Society of Plastic Surgeons [8]. However, Ho et al. also found that ADM allowed for larger intra-operative expander fill volumes and served a protective role in preventing capsular contracture.

There are several different manufacturers of human cadaveric dermal matrices including Alloderm, Cortiva, Dermamatrix, FlexHD, and Dermacell.

8.6.1 Alloderm

Alloderm is a human cadaveric STSG that has been aseptically processed and freeze dried. It requires refrigeration (with a shelf life of 2 years) and rehydration, and must be used within 4 h of rehydration. It must be placed with the correct side down, as the basement membrane side repels blood and should be oriented to the implant and the dermal side absorbs blood and integrates into tissues. It comes in various thicknesses (0.23–3.30 mm) and sheet sizes [44].

8.6.2 Cortiva

Cortiva was previously known as AlloMax/NeoForm and is the only terminally sterilized human dermal graft. It does not have an orientation in the human body and comes in one thickness sheets (0.8–1.8 mm) of various sizes [45].

8.6.3 Dermamatrix

Dermamatrix is an acellular human dermis, with the epidermis chemically removed during processing. It does not require refrigeration (3 year shelf life) and does require rehydration. It comes in variable thicknesses (0.2–4 mm, 0.4–0.8 mm, 0.8–1.7 mm, and 1.71 mm) and sheet sizes and has a required orientation in the body. It is not recommended for use in patients with autoimmune connective tissue disorders [46].

8.6.4 FlexHD

FlexHD is decellularized human allograft stored in ethanol with no rehydration required. It comes in three thicknesses (thin 0.4–0.8 mm, thick 0.8–1.7 mm, and ultrathick 1.8 mm) and multiple sheet sizes. Like Dermamatrix, is not recommended for use in patients with autoimmune connective tissue disorders [47].

8.6.5 Dermacell

Dermacell is an acellular dermal matrix that is processed with the antibiotics vancomycin and gentamycin. It is stored at room temperature with no rehydration needed and comes in three thicknesses (0.2–1.0 mm, 0.75–1.5 mm, and 1.25–2.0 mm) and variable sizes [48].

In addition to human cadaveric biologic matrices, biologic meshes can also be produced from animal products. Bovine and porcine-based meshes are the two most commonly produced animal matrices.

8.6.6 SurgiMend

SurgiMend is the only fetal bovine dermal collagen matrix, which claims to contain three times more collagen than other skin substitutes. It is produced in Boston and is available in the US, UK, and parts of England. It is a pre-fenestrated flat sheet that has no required orientation, with a range of 1.0–4.0 mm thicknesses available. It is stored at room temperature and requires rehydration [41, 49].

8.6.7 Strattice

Strattice is one of two predominately porcine dermal matrices produced. It is manufactured produced in New Jersey and available in the US, UK, and some parts of Europe. It is a terminally sterilized porcine dermis with stabilizers to reduce tissue adhesions [19]. It was designed to reduce tissue adhesions in hernia repair, but could theoretically reduce rates of capsular contracture in breast reconstruction. It comes in both pliable and firm options and requires rehydration. It comes in a single thickness sheet (1.5–2.0 mm thick) in various sizes [50].

8.6.8 Braxon

Braxon is the other predominately porcine dermal matrix available. It is the only pre-shaped ADM available and is produced in Italy and predominately used throughout Europe. It is designed to completely wrap around an implant up to 500 cc in size and comes in one thickness (0.6 mm). It is the thinnest biologic porcine mesh available, which the company claims was intentionally done to promote faster integration. It is stored dry and requires rehydration [19, 51].

Other biologic meshes aside from dermal matrices are also available. Meso Biomatrix is a porcine peritoneum matrix that comes in 0.3 mm sheets of variable sizes [52]. Biodesign (previously known as Surgisis) is a matrix designed from bovine small intestine submucosa [53]. Tutopatch and Veritas are bovine pericardium matrices available [54]. Although less commonly used, all of these matrices have been reported in the literature as being used in breast reconstruction.

8.7 Synthetic Meshes

Synthetic meshes are a less expensive alternative to biologic meshes. The challenge with synthetic meshes is finding a way to increase strength without losing elasticity or causing excessive inflammation [55, 56]. They typically come in knitted and woven options and can be both absorbable and non-absorbable. Knitted meshes are typically more porous and flexible than woven meshes, which are usually stronger [56]. Absorbable meshes are designed to act similarly to biologic meshes in that they incorporate into the tissues slowly over time, although they do not allow the degree of tissue ingrowth and neovascularization that a biologic mesh offers. The downside to absorbable synthetic meshes is that they still increase the risk of infection and seroma (although not to the same extent as biologic meshes), and it is doubtful that they add additional support in the long term [57–59]. Permanent meshes do not resorb and remain in the body indefinitely. This must be considered, as a permanent mesh utilized in prepectoral breast reconstruction underneath the skin can remain palpable for life and will make future revisions extremely challenging.

8.7.1 Absorbable Mesh

Common absorbable meshes include TIGR matrix, SERI surgical scaffold, and Galatea scaffold.

8.7.2 Galatea Scaffold

Galatea scaffold is a polymer that is metabolized by the Krebs cycle and fully resorbed by 18–24 months (Levy). It retains 50% of its strength by 16 weeks and also allows tissue ingrowth and neovascularization as it is replaced [60].

8.7.3 TIGR Matrix

TIGR matrix is a long lasting resorbable mesh. It has a combination of both fast resorbing fibers (6 months) and slow resorbing fibers (3 years) [61].

8.7.4 SERI Surgical Scaffold

SERI surgical scaffold is similarly designed to resorb slowly to preserve strength during the resorption process. On microscopic examination, substantial resorption is seen at 12 months, with only traces of the fibers visible on inspection at 24 months [62].

8.7.5 Permanent Mesh

Non-absorbable meshes do not resorb over time. Polypropylene meshes are the only non-absorbable meshes utilized in breast reconstruction, with examples including TriLoop Bra, ULTRAPRO, and SERAGYN BR.

8.7.6 TriLoop Bra

TriLoop Bra is a monofilament polypropylene mesh exposed to gaseous titanium to reduce the inflammatory response. It is designed to wrap around the breast implant in prepectoral breast reconstruction, and it carries a possible risk of granuloma formation [63].

8.7.7 ULTRAPRO

ULTRAPRO is comprised of equal parts of absorbable poliglecaprone monofilaments and non-absorbable polypropylene monofilaments. The absorbable component is designed to resorb within 84 days [64].

8.7.8 SERAGYN

SERAGYN is a partially resorbable mesh that is more firm than TriLoop Bra, with the absorbable component designed to resorb within 90–120 days [65].

Although meshes have helped to revolutionize prepectoral breast reconstruction, they are not always necessary. Becker et al presented a retrospective review of 25 suboptimal patients who underwent single-stage direct-to-implant breast reconstruction using a Mentor Spectrum implant without the use of ADM or mesh [66]. His patients represented a group of patients who would otherwise not be deemed candidates for prepectoral breast reconstruction because of obesity, chest wall radiation, significant breast ptosis, and breast hypertrophy. He utilized the concept of a spacer for these high-risk patients, filling the implant with air for a period of time before exchanging the air for saline in an off-label use of Spectrum implants. One patient with radiation history suffered from implant extrusion requiring explantation, and five patients had mastectomy flap skin edge necrosis requiring debridement with no further intervention needed. This study demonstrated that high-risk patients can safely be reconstructed in a single-stage operation without the use of ADM, thus saving costs, shortening operative times, and reducing overall complication rates.

Similarly, Manrique studied complication rates and aesthetic outcomes in patients who underwent prepectoral breast reconstruction with ADM versus without ADM. He found no difference in complication rates (including seroma and hematoma) or in aesthetic outcomes between the two groups, again showing that prepectoral breast reconstruction without the use of ADM can be successful [67].

8.8 Surgical Tips

In spite of the growing body of evidence on this topic, there is no specific recommendation that we can provide that will fit every patient and every surgeon. Unfortunately, there is a learning curve associated with the use of the different implants and meshes in prepectoral reconstruction, and each surgeon will have to determine what works best for his or her locale.

We do believe that a successful reconstruction with ADM is usually going to be superior to one without mesh or with a synthetic mesh, as the ADM might provide long-term support and additional thickness to the mastectomy skin flap and will possibly decrease the risk of capsular contracture. However, this has to be considered in light of the increased risk of complications (namely seroma, infection and implant loss) and the exuberant cost of the product. If the reconstructive surgeon has the luxury of thick, well-vascularized mastectomy skin flaps and his practice has a low incidence of infection, then an ADM might be his best option. However, this is often not the case and alternatives might need to be considered. This also largely depends on the thickness of the mastectomy skin flap. If the flaps are thick, then we prefer to not use any mesh and place an expander to allow a capsule to form before placing the implant. If the flaps are thin, then an absorbable mesh is our first choice. ADM can be added later if needed although that is rarely the case.

Choosing the appropriate size of the expander is a more important choice than the brand. There are a few things to consider when placing the expander that are different from submuscular reconstructions. First, it is extremely important that the most superior tab (the 12 o'clock tab) is sutured to the chest wall. In a submuscular reconstruction, the pectoralis muscle will support the superior edge of the expander against the chest wall, and suturing this tab is less important. However, in a prepectroal reconstruction, the superior edge of the expander might migrate anteriorly if the superior tab is not sutured, and in severe cases the expander might assume a horizontal lie; a condition that will necessitate a return to the OR. Second, the expander should be fixed securely at multiple points using a permanent suture that includes a good thickness of the chest wall. If this is not done, then the chance of expander rotation or migration is high. Third, choosing the appropriate width and height of the expander is more important than in submuscular reconstruction. A properly sized expander will a) make the expander to implant exchange extremely easy and even doable under local anesthesia with sedation and b) decrease the need for capsulotomy and allow the surgeon to fat graft the entire anterior envelope. Fourth, we have had mixed results when the expander is overinflated. In some cases, this can lead to loss of the anatomic shape of the pocket and downgrade the aesthetic result.

Finally, implant choice can also make a difference in outcome. Rippling continues to be a significant downside to prepectoral reconstruction [8]. One should not expect that fat grafting will treat symptomatic rippling. However, choosing an implant with a higher cohesivity will make a difference in rippling and this continues to be our preference for all prepectoral reconstructions. We also believe that the ratio of implant size to the patient's BMI is a more important factor than absolute implant volume. We continue to use the largest implants available in patients with high BMI, but are more conservative in thinner patients.

While prepectoral breast reconstruction is now considered standard in many institutions, we expect that there will continue to be significant improvements in materials available as well as techniques used. Hopefully one day we can identify the meshes and implants that will suit a large majority of patients, have an acceptable complication rate, and come at an acceptable cost.

References

1. Schlenker JD, Bueno RA, Ricketson G, Lynch JB. Loss of silicone implants after subcutaneous mastectomy and reconstruction. Plast Reconstr Surg. 1978;62(6):853–61.
2. Gruber RP, Kahn RA, Lash H, Maser MR, Apfelberg DB, Laub DR. Breast reconstruction following mastectomy: a comparison of submuscular and subcutaneous techniques. Plast Reconstr Surg. 1981;67(3):312–7.
3. Salzberg CA. Nonexpansive immediate breast reconstruction using human acellular tissue matrix graft (AlloDerm). Ann Plast Surg. 2006;57(1):1–5.
4. Kim SE. Prepectoral breast reconstruction. Yeungnam Univ J Med. 2019;36(3):201–7.
5. Jones G, Antony AK. Single stage, direct to implant pre-pectoral breast reconstruction. Gland Surg. 2019;8(1):53–60.
6. Preminger BA, McCarthy CM, Hu QY, Mehrara BJ, Disa JJ. The influence of AlloDerm on expander dynamics and complications in the setting of immediate tissue expander/implant reconstruction: a matched-cohort study. Ann Plast Surg. 2008;60(5):510–3.
7. Nguyen J, Carey J, Wong A. Use of human acellular dermal matrix in implant- based breast reconstruction: evaluating the evidence. J Plast Reconstr Aesthet Surg. 2011;64(12):1553–61.
8. Marks JM, Farmer RL, Afifi AM. Current trends in prepectoral breast reconstruction: a survey of american society of plastic surgeons members. Plast Reconstr Surg Glob Open. 2020;8(8):e3060.
9. Surgeons ASoP. Plastic Surgery Statistics Report. 2019. Available from: https://www.plasticsurgery.org/documents/News/Statistics/2019/reconstructive-breast-procedures-age-2019.pdf.
10. Heidekrueger PI, Sinno S, Hidalgo DA, Colombo M, Broer PN. Current trends in breast augmentation: an international analysis. Aesthet Surg J. 2018;38(2):133–48.
11. Van Slyke AC, Carr M, Carr NJ. Not all breast implants are equal: a 13-year review of implant longevity and reasons for explantation. Plast Reconstr Surg. 2018;142(3):281e–9e.
12. Spies RJ, Robert J. SPIES, MD, FACS BOARD CERTIFIED IN PLASTIC AND RECONSTRUCTIVE SURGERY [updated May 16, 2012]. Available from: https://www.azplasticsurgerycenter.com/blog/which-breast-implant-weighs-more-silicone-or-saline/#:~:text=A%20400cc%20saline%20implant%20weighs,%2F20%20of%20a%20pound).&text=Silicone%20implants%20are%20more%20similar,breast%20tissue%20than%20saline%20impla.
13. Maxwell GP, Scheflan M, Spear S, Nava MB, Heden P. Benefits and limitations of macrotextured breast implants and consensus recommendations for optimizing their effectiveness. Aesthet Surg J. 2014;34(6):876–81.
14. Webb LH, Aime VL, Do A, Mossman K, Mahabir RC. Textured breast implants: a closer look at the surface debris under the microscope. Plast Surg (Oakv). 2017;25(3):179–83.
15. Castel N, Soon-Sutton T, Deptula P, Flaherty A, Parsa FD. Polyurethane-coated breast implants revisited: a 30-year follow-up. Arch Plast Surg. 2015;42(2):186–93.
16. Labs, Establishment: Motiva; [updated 2019]. Available from: https://motiva.health/patients/implants/anatomical-truefixation-breast-implant/?rtid=3b79abf43c0e4ff0a9cf11dd03296f960e29699e53e54bf0808467c32fca3285.

17. Boschert M. American Society of Plastic Surgeons 2020 [updated March 2020]. Available from: https://www1.plasticsurgery.org/members/discussions/Topic.aspx?id=3531.
18. Gabriel A, Maxwell GP. Implant selection in the setting of prepectoral breast reconstruction. Gland Surg. 2019;8(1):36–42.
19. Vidya R, Berna G, Sbitany H, Nahabedian M, Becker H, Reitsamer R, et al. Prepectoral implant-based breast reconstruction: a joint consensus guide from UK, European and USA breast and plastic reconstructive surgeons. Ecancermedicalscience. 2019;13:927.
20. Choi M, Frey JD, Alperovich M, Levine JP, Karp NS. "Breast in a Day": examining single-stage immediate, permanent implant reconstruction in nipple-sparing mastectomy. Plast Reconstr Surg. 2016;138(2):184e–91e.
21. Natrelle: Allergan; [updated 2020]. Available from: https://www.natrellesurgeon.com/.
22. Sientra 2020 [updated 2020]. Available from: https://sientra.com/for-us-surgeons/.
23. Breast Implants by Mentor [updated 2020]. Available from: https://www.breastimplantsbymentor.com/Products/MENTOR-breast-implants.
24. Silimed [updated 2020]. Available from: http://silimed.com/.
25. Polytech [updated 2020]. Available from: https://polytech-health-aesthetics.com/en/products/breast-implants/.
26. Ideal Implant [updated 2020]. Available from: https://idealimplant.com/overview.
27. GC Aesthetics. Available from: https://www.gcaesthetics.com/products/surgery/breast/.
28. Laboratories Arion [updated 2020]. Available from: https://www.laboratoires-arion.fr/en/.
29. Hans Biomed [updated 2020]. Available from: https://www.hansbiomed.com/en/.
30. Cereplas [updated 2020]. Available from: https://www.cereplas.com/en/produits/implants-mammaires/rondes.html.
31. Establishment Labs [updated 2020]. Available from: https://establishmentlabs.com/our-products/.
32. Sebbin [updated 2020]. Available from: https://www.sebbin.com/en/category/mammary-implants/.
33. Collplant [updated 2020]. Available from: https://collplant.com/products/breast-implants/.
34. Becker H, Zhadan O. Filling the spectrum expander with air-a new alternative. Plast Reconstr Surg Glob Open. 2017;5(10):e1541.
35. Zenn MR. Staged immediate breast reconstruction. Plast Reconstr Surg. 2015;135(4):976–9.
36. Mentor [updated 2020]. Available from: https://www.jnjmedicaldevices.com/en-US/product/mentor-artoura-breast-tissue-expanders.
37. Sientra [updated 2020]. Available from: https://sientra.com/for-us-surgeons/breast-tissue-expanders/.
38. Rebowe RE, Allred LJ, Nahabedian MY. The evolution from subcutaneous to prepectoral prosthetic breast reconstruction. Plast Reconstr Surg Glob Open. 2018;6(6):e1797.
39. Ter Louw RP, Nahabedian MY. Prepectoral breast reconstruction. Plast Reconstr Surg. 2017;140(5S Advances in Breast Reconstruction):51S–9S.
40. Breuing KH, Warren SM. Immediate bilateral breast reconstruction with implants and inferolateral AlloDerm slings. Ann Plast Surg. 2005;55(3):232–9.
41. Cheng A, Saint-Cyr M. Comparison of different ADM materials in breast surgery. Clin Plast Surg. 2012;39(2):167–75.
42. Chun YS, Verma K, Rosen H, Lipsitz S, Morris D, Kenney P, et al. Implant-based breast reconstruction using acellular dermal matrix and the risk of postoperative complications. Plast Reconstr Surg. 2010;125(2):429–36.
43. Ho G, Nguyen TJ, Shahabi A, Hwang BH, Chan LS, Wong AK. A systematic review and meta-analysis of complications associated with acellular dermal matrix-assisted breast reconstruction. Ann Plast Surg. 2012;68(4):346–56.
44. Allergan [Available from: https://media.allergan.com/actavis/actavis/media/allergan-pdf-documents/labeling/alleoderm_rtm_ifu.pdf.
45. RTI Surgical Implants [updated 2020]. Available from: https://www.rtix.com/en_us/implants/cortiva-1mm-allograft-dermis.
46. Synthes [Available from: http://synthes.vo.llnwd.net/o16/Mobile/Synthes%20North%20America/Product%20Support%20Materials/Brochures/CMF/MXBRODermaMatrixAcellular-J7237D.pdf.
47. MTF Biologics [updated 2020]. Available from: https://www.mtfbiologics.org/our-products/detail/flexhd-structural.
48. Stryker [updated 2020]. Available from: https://www.stryker.com/us/en/endoscopy/products/dermacell.html.
49. Surgimend. Available from: https://www.surgimend.com/products/by-brand/surgimend.
50. Strattice [updated 2020]. Available from: http://hcp.stratticetissuematrix.com/en/products.
51. Raise Healthcare [updated 2020]. Available from: https://www.raisehealthcare.co.uk/products/breast-reconstruction/braxon/.
52. MTF Biologics [updated 2020]. Available from: https://www.mtfbiologics.org/our-products/detail/mesobiomatrix.
53. Cook Medical [updated 2020]. Available from: https://www.cookmedical.com/surgery/the-path-from-surgisis-to-biodesign.
54. rti Surgical [updated 2020]. Available from: https://www.rtix.com/en_us/implants/tutopatch-bovine-pericardium%2D%2Dtutomesh-fenestrated-bovine-pericardium.
55. Breast Cancer and Breast Reconstruction. In: Luis Tejedor SGM, Lachezar Manchev, Arli Aditya Parikesit editor. London: IntechOpen; 2020.
56. FitzGerald JF, Kumar AS. Biologic versus synthetic mesh reinforcement: what are the pros and cons? Clin Colon Rectal Surg. 2014;27(4):140–8.
57. Potter S, Conroy EJ, Cutress RI, Williamson PR, Whisker L, Thrush S, et al. Short-term safety out-

comes of mastectomy and immediate implant-based breast reconstruction with and without mesh (iBRA): a multicentre, prospective cohort study. Lancet Oncol. 2019;20(2):254–66.
58. Dieterich M, Angres J, Stachs A, Glass A, Reimer T, Gerber B, et al. Patient-report satisfaction and health-related quality of life in TiLOOP(R) bra-assisted or implant-based breast reconstruction alone. Aesthetic Plast Surg. 2015;39(4):523–33.
59. Hallberg H, Rafnsdottir S, Selvaggi G, Strandell A, Samuelsson O, Stadig I, et al. Benefits and risks with acellular dermal matrix (ADM) and mesh support in immediate breast reconstruction: a systematic review and meta-analysis. J Plast Surg Hand Surg. 2018;52(3):130–47.
60. Galatea Surgical [updated 2020]. Available from: https://www.galateasurgical.com/surgical-scaffolds/what-is-p4hb/.
61. Novus Scientific [updated 2020]. Available from: https://novusscientific.com/row/products/tigr-matrix/.
62. Seri Surgical Scaffold [updated 2020]. Available from: https://seri.com/about/product-characteristics.html.
63. PFM Medical [updated 2020]. Available from: https://www.pfmmedical.com/productcatalogue/mesh_implants_breast_surgery/tiloopr_bra/index.html.
64. Ethicon [updated 2020]. Available from: https://www.jnjmedicaldevices.com/en-US/product/ultrapro-mesh-ethicon.
65. Serag Wiessner [updated 2020]. Available from: https://www.serag-wiessner.de/en/products/textile-implants/seragyn-br/.
66. Becker H, Mathew PJ. Immediate prepectoral breast reconstruction in suboptimal patients using an air-filled spacer. Plast Reconstr Surg Glob Open. 2019;7(10):e2470.
67. Manrique OJ, Huang TC, Martinez-Jorge J, Ciudad P, Forte AJ, Bustos SS, et al. Prepectoral two-stage implant-based breast reconstruction with and without acellular dermal matrix: do we see a difference? Plast Reconstr Surg. 2020;145(2):263e–72e.

9 Prepectoral Implant-Based Breast Reconstruction: Complete Cover with Preshaped Mesh

Raghavan Vidya and Simon Cawthorn

Approximately, one million new cases of breast cancer are diagnosed globally per year. In the United Kingdom (UK), about 50, 000 new cases of breast cancer are diagnosed each year with four in ten women undergoing mastectomy as their primary therapeutic procedure [1]. Implant-based breast reconstructions account for 40–60% of all breast reconstructions performed in the UK and about 75% in the United States [2, 3].

Over the last decade, innovations and advances in meshes and implants have revolutionized implant-based breast reconstruction. The classical submuscular implant-based breast reconstruction is based on the principle of lower lateral pole coverage using a mesh after pectoralis muscle detachment. However, this caused animation deformity and impairment of shoulder function due to detachment of the muscle [4]. This led surgeons to introduce and adopt prepectoral or muscle sparing technique in their practice. The advantages of this technique over traditional submuscular implant-based breast reconstruction was preservation of normal chest wall anatomy with restoration of body image with minimal morbidity [5].

R. Vidya (✉)
The Royal Wolverhampton NHS Trust, Wolverhampton, UK
e-mail: Raghavan.Vidya@nhs.net

S. Cawthorn
The Breast Unit, Southmead Hospital, Bristol, UK

Implant-based reconstruction is the most common method of immediate breast reconstruction with majority of them being carried out as a single-stage procedure in the UK and Europe or as a two-staged process in the US: the first stage involving a tissue expander and a second stage where the expander is exchanged for a prosthetic breast implant [6, 7].

9.1 Selection of Patients

Prepectoral implant reconstruction can be considered in anyone who would normally be considered suitable for an implant based reconstruction. Preoperatively, the patient should undergo normal counselling including discussion of diagnosis, potential treatments and the associated risks & benefits [8]. Patient choice and selection are important particularly balancing the increased risk of perioperative complications in the presence of elevated BMI (>35), poorly controlled diabetes mellitus, immunosuppression, and previous radiation damage - these conditions can be considered as relative contraindications [9]. Oncologically, the procedure should be avoided in locally advanced tumors, involvement of skin or chest wall muscle, and in inflammatory breast cancers [9, 10]. Preoperative assessment of breast morphology including its footprint, breast size,

© The Author(s), under exclusive license to Springer Nature Switzerland AG 2023
R. Vidya, H. Becker (eds.), *Prepectoral Breast Reconstruction*,
https://doi.org/10.1007/978-3-031-15590-1_9

and ptosis is essential. Preoperative estimation of skin thickness with a pinch test is useful to assess prepectoral implant placement. Techniques such as digital mammography or magnetic resonance imaging (MRI) to predict skin thickness have also been described [11, 12]. Based on the footprint and the breast morphology, a detailed discussion takes place preoperatively about the suitability of the implants, viz. round vs anatomical. The patients are offered a choice between textured and smooth implants, and the benefits and risks are discussed in detail based on the current evidence. In the UK, single-stage implant-based breast reconstruction is commonly carried out. However, two -stage breast reconstruction using tissue expanders is considered in patients with compromised mastectomy flap perfusion, smokers, and anticipated breast weight replacement greater than 550 cc.

9.2 Indications

Although prepectoral breast reconstruction is mainly carried out as primary procedure (Fig. 9.1) following breast cancer surgery, its role has extended to risk reducing and revision surgery [13].

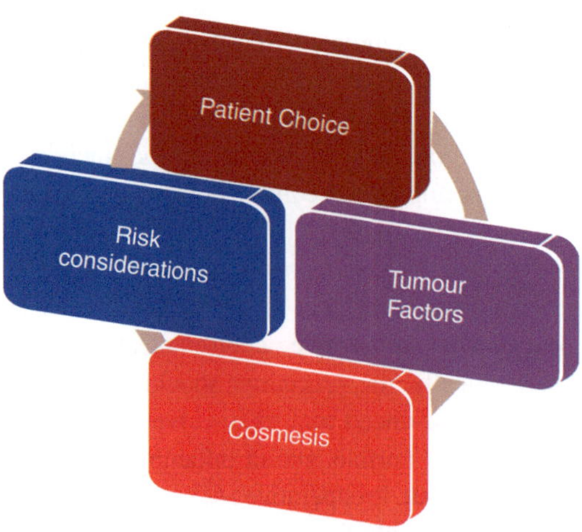

Fig. 9.1 Factors influencing the need for mastectomy

9.3 Planning

It is essential to the plan the type of incision depending on the site of tumor, breast morphology, need for axillary staging, patient and surgeon's preference. In general, incisions should be planned to minimize interruption of subcutaneous vasculature. The common incisions for nipple sparing or skin sparing mastectomy [14] include inframammary, vertical, lateral lazy S shaped approach; non-nipple sparing includes the standard elliptical approach. The option that can be used when the nipple needs to be removed is areola-sparing mastectomy where the nipple can later be reconstructed from the areola. Preoperatively the footprint of the breast including the takeoff, inframammary fold, lateral and medial extent should be marked to guide accurate surgical dissection.

9.4 Technique

Prepectoral space is the potential space that arises following the removal of the breast [15]. The volume of the space depends on the dimensions of the chest wall, along with the elasticity and quality of the skin, which dictates the degree to which it can safely accommodate the implant/mesh coverage.

In one-stage mastectomy, success is largely dependent on the quality of the mastectomy flap. The patients should be kept warm throughout the procedure, and alcohol-based skin preparations are used. A single dose of intravenous antibiotic depending on the local hospital policy should be used.

Preservation of the subcutaneous layer of the mastectomy flaps and the perforators that vascularize them is the key to success of this surgery [15]. The mastectomy is carried out in the normal breast oncological plane [16] using monopolar electrocautery in low settings in order to maintain a well-perfused skin envelope and reduce the risks of thermal injury. It is essential to ensure as much as possible that all breast tissue is removed, but the limits of the plane need to be respected. Intraoperatively, preservation of good skin flap vascularity is the key to the success of this surgery. Most authors clinically assess flap vascularity based on color, absence of dermal exposure, and flap damage from diathermy [15, 17]. If devices were available, to assess skin flap vascularity, the authors would advise to use it, particularly in situations when there is uncertainty about flap viability [17, 18]. If skin flap vascularity is compromised, other methods of reconstruction must be considered. The authors recommend an excision of the wound edges before wound closure to improve the blood flow at the flaps suture line. This visible increase in the bleeding at the flap extremity following excision on the 2 mm strip of skin traumatized by the retraction required to perform the flap dissection is very reassuring to witness. The mastectomy cavity should be washed with plenty of warm saline until clear, and 1 or 2 closed suction drains placed within the prepectoral pocket.

Braxon® is a preshaped (Decomed S.r.l., Venezia, Italy), 0.6 mm thick, porcine, non-cross-linked acellular dermal matrix (ADM). It needs to be hydrated in saline for a minimum of 10 minutes. The mesh is manufactured in a single size of 30 × 20 cm and can accommodate implants up to 500 cc and if meshed can accommodate up to 560 cc. The mesh has an anterior flap with a central slit, which when sutured gives the shape. The posterior flap with 2 windows prevents seroma fluid collecting around the implant. The anterior slit and the 2 wings are closed using 2-0 vicryl continuous suture [19]. Figure 9.2a–i demonstrates the procedure of creating a mesh implant wrap.

The type of implants used can be fixed volume silicone or saline, anatomical or round depending on the need to match symmetry. If there is concern following dissection of the skin flap viability, an adjustable expander implant can be used. The implant is placed underfilled, causing no increased pressure on to the flaps and expanded at a later date once viability of the flaps is confirmed [20].

The desired implant is placed inside the ADM. A marking pen is used to define the exact size of the matrix that is required to form a wrap around the implant so that the ADM snugs the implant and there is no redundant space inside. It is also useful to leave a 2–5 mm rim around the edges, which will enable easy anchorage to the chest wall. The anterior and posterior edges of the ADM are sutured together using 2-0 vicryl to form a pocket for the implant. The inferior aspect of Braxon® provides the required ptosis and does not require any anchorage. The lateral space should be closed to improve the shape and reduce any dead space. The new reconstructed ADM implant unit is placed in the prepectoral space and anchored to the muscle using cardinal sutures at 3, 9, and 12-clock positions using 2-0 vicryl sutures (Fig. 9.2). Other sutures can be placed especially laterally and anteriorly between the matrix and subcutaneous layer before the closure of the skin. Preservation of pectoralis fascia enables easy fixation of implant wrap. It is desirable to close the lateral wall from the axilla and reduce dead space inside the chest wall by quilting.

We usually use absorbable 2-0 vicryl for subcutaneous and 3-0 monocryl for subcuticular skin closure. Usually one to two closed suction drains are used and well tunnelled away from the implant pocket (6–8 cm away). If simultaneous axillary clearance is performed, a separate drain is placed in the axilla. Meticulous care of drain exit sites is necessary, and drains are left in place until the drainage is below 20 cc over two consecutive days (48 h) prior to drain removal. Perioperative antibiotics (oral) are administered, and the duration of administration can be stratified based on the risk factors [21, 22].

A well-supporting sports bra is fitted (Fig. 9.3a) before discharge from hospital which may be the same day as surgery since post-operative pain is not a significant problem allowing patients to be safely be cared for in their own homes. The author uses negative pressure dressing prophylactically in patients who are anticipated to develop post-operative wound problems [23] (Fig. 9.3b). This group includes patients with high BMI 35, comorbidities such as diabetes, undergone neoadjuvant chemotherapy,

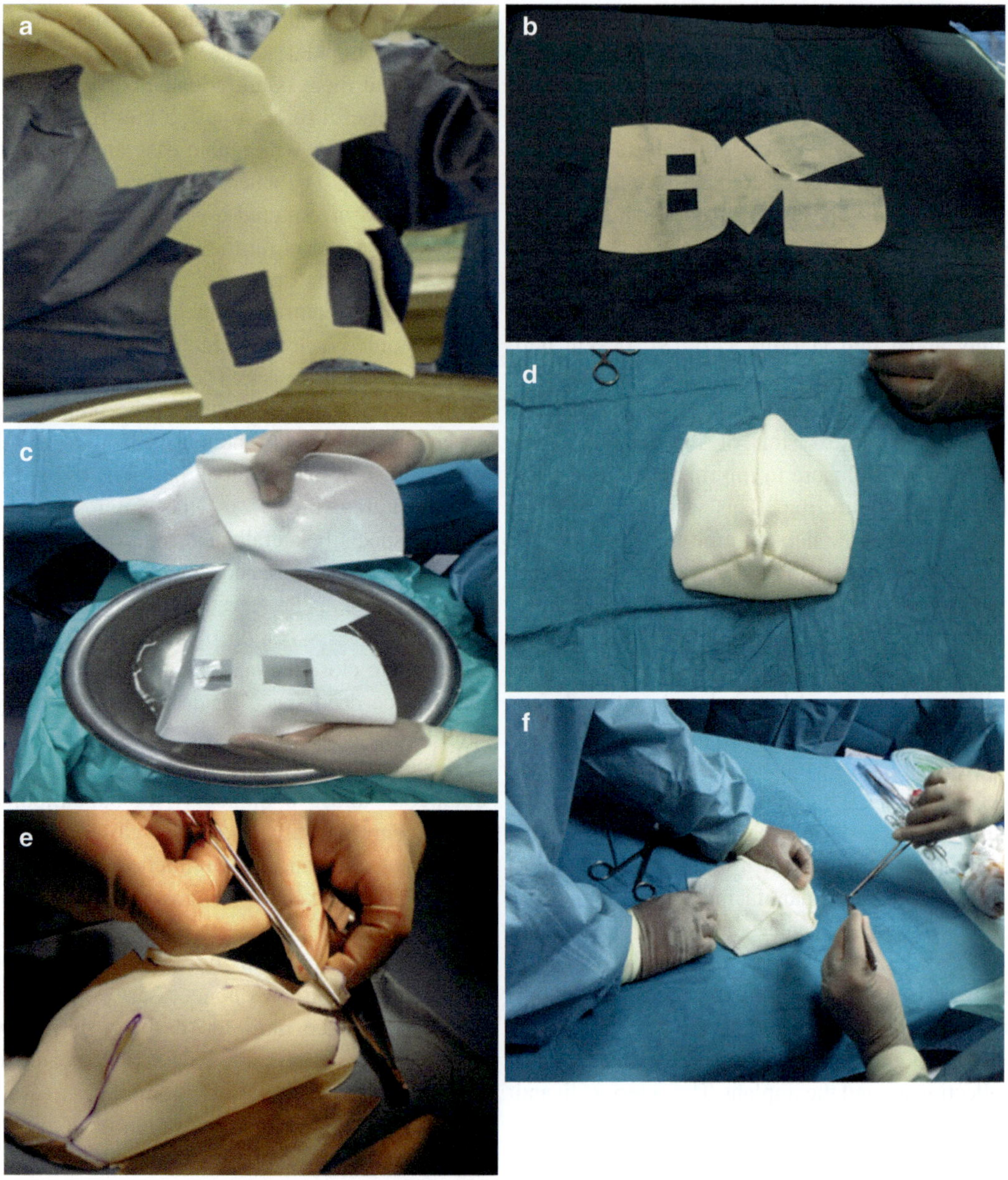

Fig. 9.2 The technique of preparing the breast implant wrap using the preshaped Braxon® mesh. (**a, b**) Braxon is a porcine acellular dermal matrix (ADM), 0.6 mm thick, without preservatives and dry. The windowed part of the matrix (posterior wrap) is design to form the rear portion of the implant wrap, preventing seroma formation. (**c**) The mesh is rinsed in cold or saline at room temperature for a minimum of 5–10 minutes and it becomes soft and well hydrated. (**c**) Suture of the anterior shell of the dermal implant pocket with absorbable suture (Vicryl 2/0). (**d**) Suturing of the frontal and posterior part of Braxon®. (**e**) Trimming of the excess matrix after marking with a pen and leaving a 2 mm rim to enable fixation to the chest wall. (**f**) Suture of the anterior and posterior shell to form a snug mesh implant wrap using absorbable suture (Vicryl 2/0). (**g**) Posterior part of Braxon with windows to prevent fluid accumulation. This part of the wrapped implant will be placed over the pectoralis muscle and sutured to the chest wall. (**h**) The picture shows the frontal part of the wrapped implant. (**i**) The mesh implant wrap is placed over the pectoralis muscle and secured to the chest wall

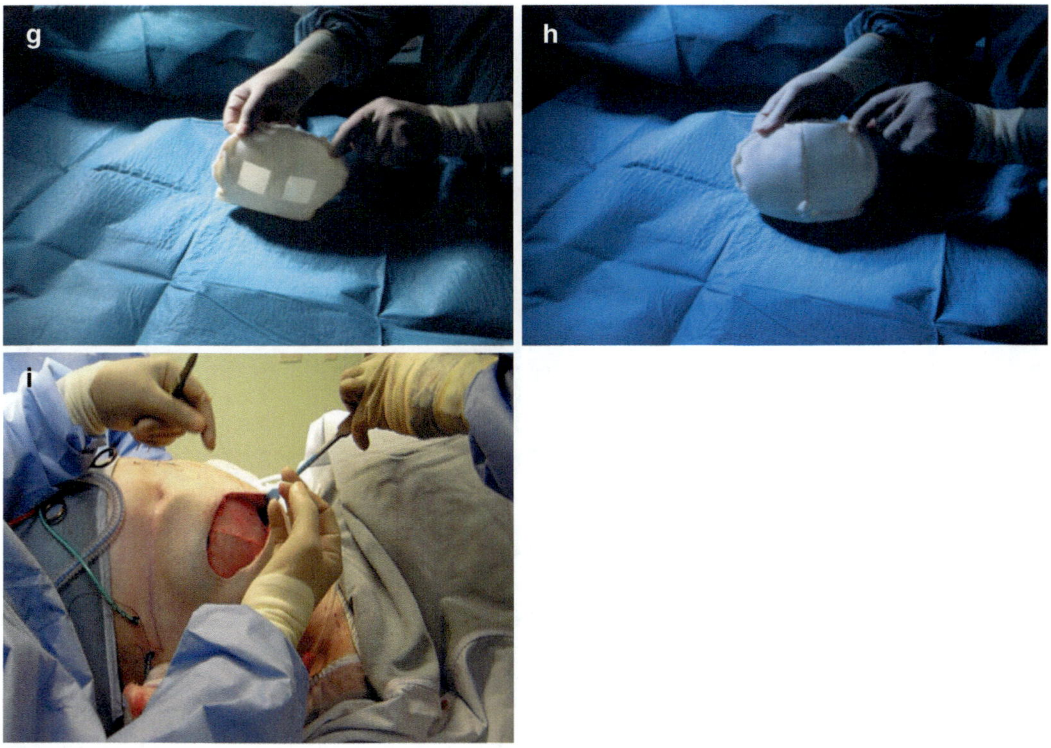

Fig. 9.2 (continued)

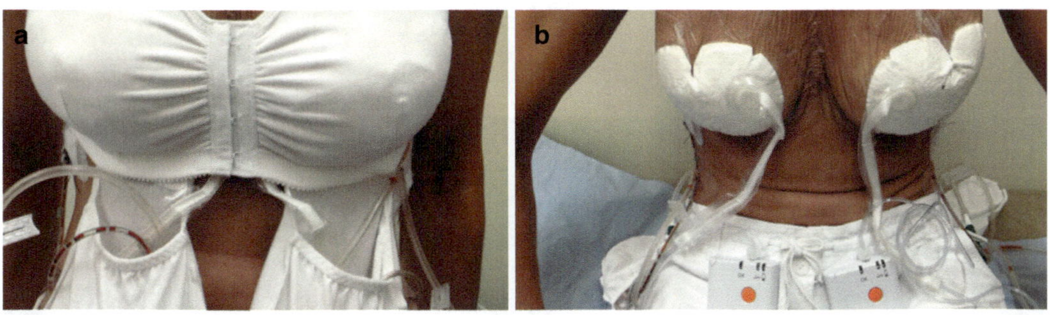

Fig. 9.3 (**a**) Simple dressing and immediate post op bra applied. (**b**) Special dressing such as negative pressure dressing used prophylactically in high-risk patients

needing concurrent axillary clearance with mastectomy and previous radiotherapy. We observed good integration of the matrix both on ultrasound imaging and histologically [24]. The histological and ultrasound follow-up has been described in detail by Marucci et al. [25] in the next chapter. Figures 9.4a–f and 9.5a–f demonstrates the pre and post operative photographs using this technique.

Patients undergoing Prepectoral implant based reconstruction reported less discomfort, less post-operative pain, no shoulder dysfunction or animation, and early recovery. Patients had high rates of overall satisfaction including psychosocial and sexual well-being [26, 27]. Results on cosmetic and patient-reported outcomes are also promising, though further long-term studies are needed.

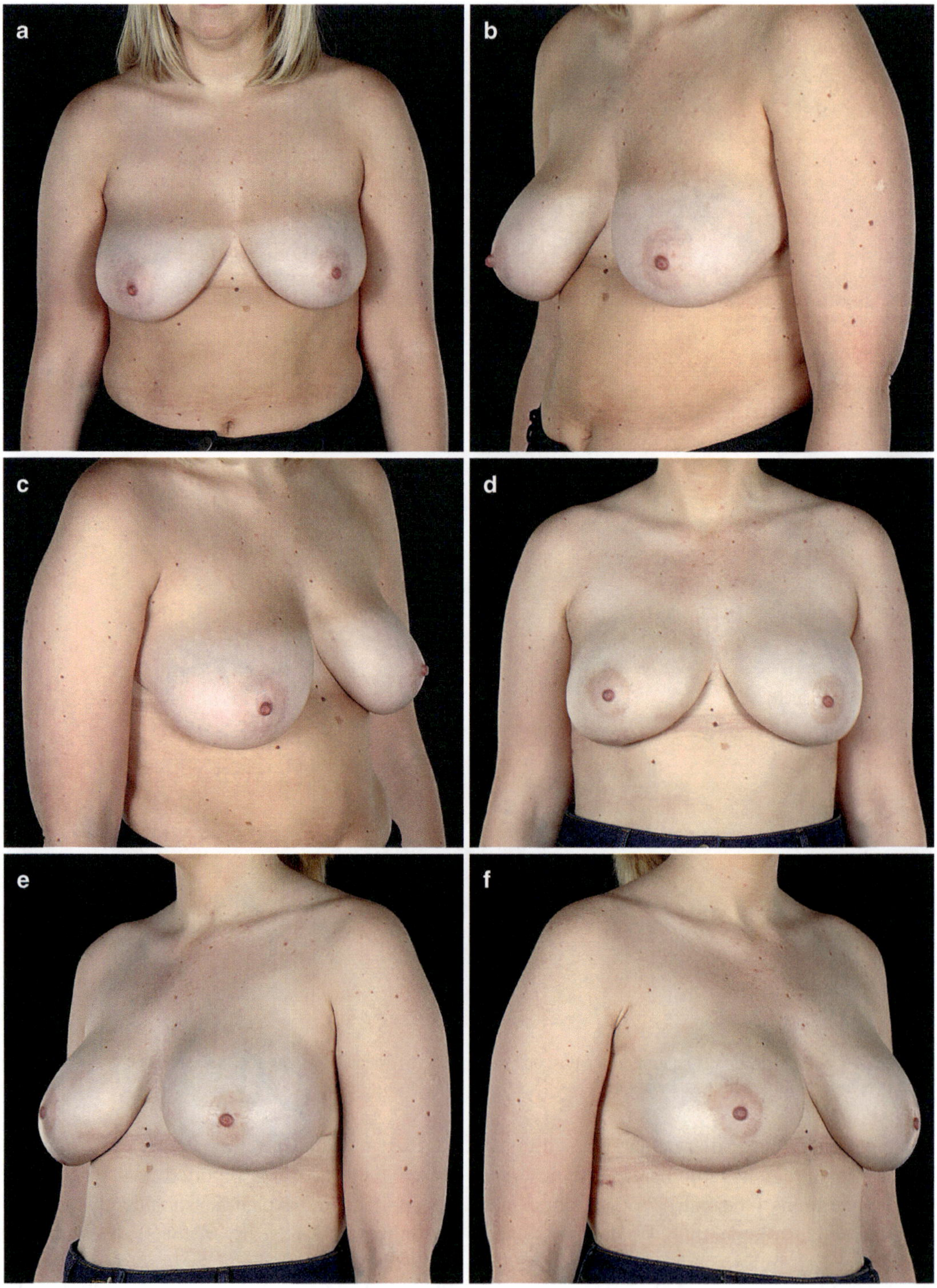

Fig. 9.4 (**a–f**) 40 year-old woman with a diagnosis of positive BRCA gene undergoing bilateral skin nipple sparing mastectomy and prepectoral breast reconstruction. Preoperative (up) and post-operative views (below) at 1 year follow up. Anatomical silicone breast implants (560cc) and Braxon® ADM has been used

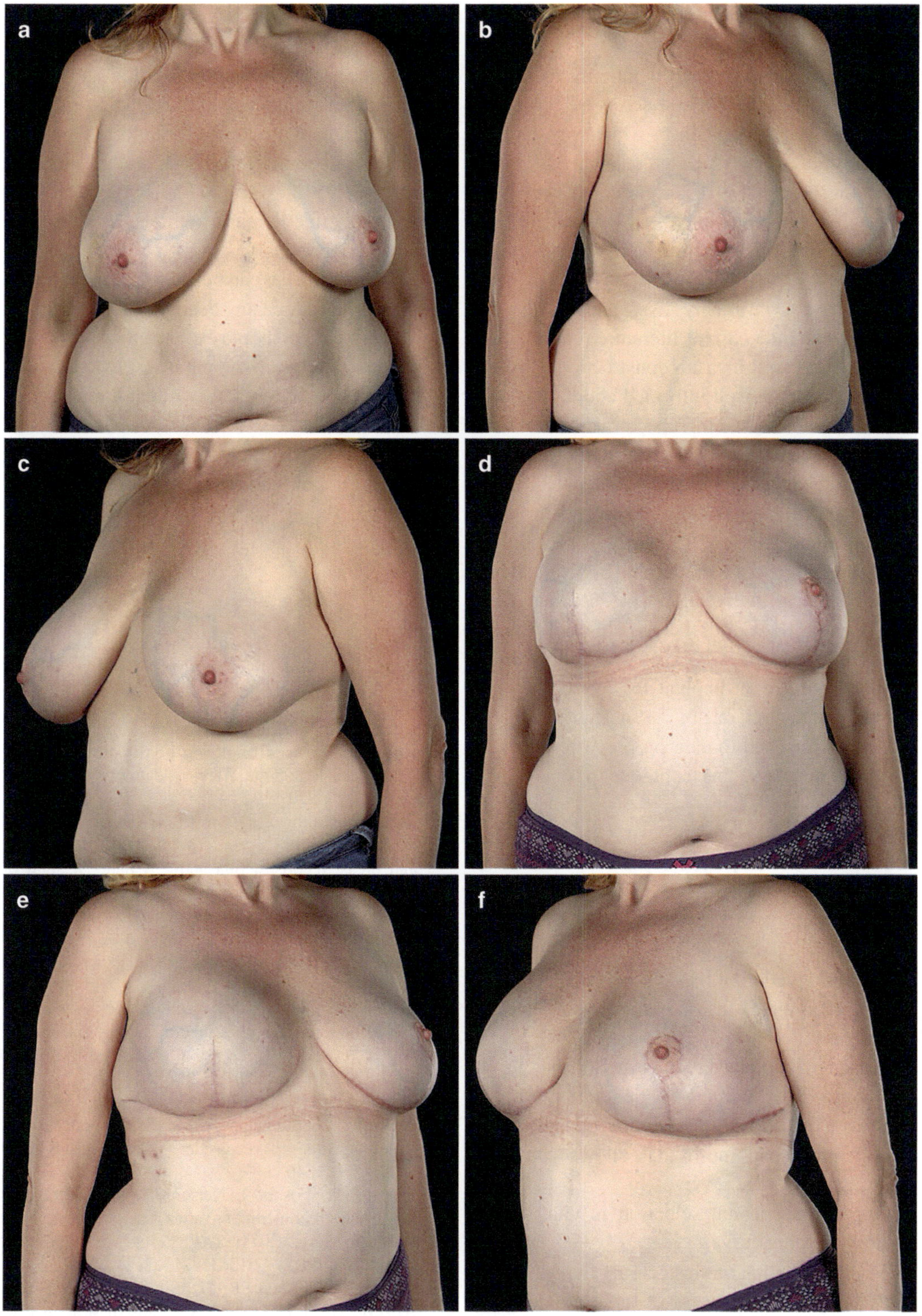

Fig. 9.5 (**a–f**) 48 year-old woman diagnosed with invasive ductal carcinoma of the right breast undergoing right skin sparing non nipple sparing mastectomy with axillary clearance with prepectoral implant based breast reconstruction (550cc) with dermal sling with axillary clearance and contra lateral left breast matching reduction. Preoperative views (up) and post-operative views (below) at 6 months follow up

9.5 Review of Literature

The technique was described initially by Berna et al. in 2014 [28]. The first series of 100 cases were reported by the author, which was carried out in a cohort of high selected patients with minimal comorbidities [29]. The outcome was good with a low complication rate, which could be accounted by the selection bias and surgical expertise.

Rippling is invariably associated with this technique, and the current literature reports up to 35% in prepectoral breast reconstruction [30]. All patients should be well informed about this complication associated with prepectoral breast reconstruction. Techniques to minimize rippling include uniform subcutaneous layer, good volume of implant to skin ratio, and use of silicone implants. Lipomodelling is a useful adjunct to correct rippling and in our own series about 10% of patients needed surgical intervention [31]. Recently, the largest audit IBAG has been published involving 1450 procedures with a 6- year follow-up. It has demonstrated an implant loss of 6.1% and a capsular contracture rate of 2.1%. This is the largest series published to date on prepectoral breast reconstruction using this technique [32].

9.6 Summary and Tips

9.6.1 Preshaped Mesh

- The introduction of meshes has enabled adoption of minimal invasive surgery in surgical practice.
- Prepectoral implant reconstruction has minimal morbidity and good patient outcomes.
- Braxon® is the only ADM currently available as a preshaped mesh that allows complete implant coverage ex-vivo.
- Appropriate patient selection is vital in the early learning curve.
- The preservation of mastectomy flap vascularity is the key to success of this surgical technique. The preservation of pectoralis fascia enables anchorage of the mesh.
- The dissection can be carried using preferred technique but it is important to minimize traction and thermal injury to the skin flaps.
- The mesh implant must be snug to promote integration and reduce seroma formation.
- The mastectomy cavity should be washed with plenty of warm saline until clear. This reduces infection and removes free-floating fat and debris.
- The lateral space can be closed to improve the shape and reduce any dead space.
- Theater traffic should be kept to a minimum, as should duration of operative procedure. For bilateral procedures, a two-team approach is beneficial.
- Seroma is detrimental to prepectoral breast reconstruction, and every effort should be made to reduce it. Seroma should be drained immediately as it can lead to wound dehiscence.

References

1. Cancer Research UK. Breast Cancer Statistics. http://www.cancerresearchuk.org/health-professional/cancer-statistics/statistics-by-cancer-type/breast-cancer. 04/13/2016.
2. Jeevan R, Cromwell D, Browne J, Van Der Meulen J, Pereira J, Caddy C, et al. The National Mastectomy and breast reconstruction audit. A national audit of provision and outcomes of mastectomy and breast reconstruction surgery for women in England. Second Annu Rep; 2009.
3. ASoP surgeons. Plastic surgery statistics report. Am Soc Plast Surg Arlingt Height; 2012.
4. Sbitany H, Serletti JM. Acellular dermis–assisted prosthetic breast reconstruction: a systematic and critical review of efficacy and associated morbidity. Plast Reconstr Surg. 2011;128(6):1162–9.
5. Tasoulis MK, Iqbal FM, Cawthorn S, MacNeill F, Vidya R. Subcutaneous implant breast reconstruction: time to reconsider? Eur J Surg Oncol. 2017;43(9):1646–3.
6. Serletti JM, Fosnot J, Nelson JA, Disa JJ, Bucky LP. Breast reconstruction after breast cancer. Plast Reconstr Surg. 2011;127(6):124e–35e. https://doi.org/10.1097/PRS.0b013e318213a2e6.
7. Albornoz CR, Bach PB, Mehrara BJ, Disa JJ, Pusic AL, McCarthy CM, et al. A paradigm shift in U.S. breast reconstruction: increasing implant rates. Plast Reconstr Surg. 2013;131(1):15–23.

8. Vidya R, Berna G, Sbitany H, Nahabedian M, Becker H, Reitsamer R, Rancati A, Macmillan D, Cawthorn S. Prepectoral implant-based breast reconstruction: a joint consensus guide from UK, European and USA breast and plastic reconstructive surgeons. Ecancermedicalscience. 2019;13:927.
9. Sbitany H. Important considerations for performing Prepectoral breast reconstruction. Plast Reconstr Surg. 2017;140(6S):7S–13S.
10. Abbate O, Rosado N, Sobti N, Vieira BL, Liao EC. Meta-analysis of prepectoral implant-based breast reconstruction: guide to patient selection and current outcomes. Breast Cancer Res Treat. 2020;182(3):543–54.
11. Rancati AO, Angrigiani CH, Hammond DC, et al. Direct to implant reconstruction in nipple sparing mastectomy: patient selection by preoperative digital mammogram. Plast Reconstr Surg Glob Open. 2017;5(6):e1369. https://doi.org/10.1097/GOX.0000000000001369.
12. Frey JD, Salibian AA, Choi M, Karp NS. Mastectomy flap thickness and complications in nipple-sparing mastectomy: objective evaluation using magnetic resonance imaging. Plast Reconstr Surg Glob Open. 2017;5(8):e1439.
13. Vidya R, Iqbal FM. A guide to prepectoral breast reconstruction: a new dimension to implant-based breast reconstruction. Clin Breast Cancer. 2017;17(4):266–71.
14. Frey JD, Salibian AA, Levine JP, Karp NS, Choi M. Incision choices in nipple-sparing mastectomy: a comparative analysis of outcomes and evolution of a clinical algorithm. Plast Reconstr Surg. 2018;142:826e–35e.
15. Vidya R, Iqbal FM. Breast anatomy: time to classify the subpectoral and prepectoral spaces. Clin Anat. 2017;30(4):434–5.
16. Rehnke RD, Groening RM, Buskirk ERV, Clarke JM. Anatomy of the superficial fascia system of the breast. Plast Reconstr Surg. 2018;142(5):1135–44. https://doi.org/10.1097/prs.0000000000004948.
17. Phillips BT, Lanier ST, Conkling N, et al. Intraoperative perfusion techniques can accurately predict mastectomy skin flap necrosis in breast reconstruction: results of a prospective trial. Plast Reconstr Surg. 2012;129:778e–88e.
18. Mattison GL, Lewis PG, Gupta SC, et al. SPY imaging use in postmastectomy breast reconstruction patients: preventative or overly conservative? Plast Reconstr Surg. 2016;138:15e–21e.
19. Vidya R. Prepectoral breast reconstruction or muscle-sparing technique with the Braxon porcine acellular dermal matrix. Plast Reconstr Surg Glob Open. 2017;5(6):e1364.
20. Becker H, Zhadan O. Filling the spectrum expander with air-a new alternative. Plast Reconstr Surg Glob Open. 2017;5(10):e1541. https://doi.org/10.1097/GOX.0000000000001541.
21. Vidya R. Risk assessment and antibiotic administration model. Plast Reconstr Surg. 2017;139(5):1206e–7e.
22. Barr SP, Topps AR, Barnes NL, Henderson J, Hignett S, Teasdale RL, McKenna A, Harvey JR, Kirwan CC, Northwest Breast Surgical Research Collaborative. Infection prevention in breast implant surgery - A review of the surgical evidence, guidelines and a checklist. Eur J Surg Oncol. 2016;42(5):591–603.
23. Irwin GW, Boundouki G, Fakim B, Johnson R, Highton L, Myers D, Searle R, Murphy JA. Negative pressure wound therapy reduces wound breakdown and implant loss in prepectoral breast reconstruction. Plast Reconstr Surg Glob Open. 2020;8(2):e2667. https://doi.org/10.1097/GOX.0000000000002667.
24. Iqbal FM, Bhatnagar A, Vidya R. Host integration of an acellular dermal matrix: Braxon mesh in breast reconstruction. Clin Breast Cancer. 2016;16(6):e209–11. https://doi.org/10.1016/j.clbc.2016.06.009.
25. Onesti MG, Maruccia M, Di Taranto G, et al. Clinical, histological, and ultrasound follow-up of breast reconstruction with one-stage muscle-sparing "wrap" technique: a single-center experience. J Plast Reconstr Aesthet Surg. 2017;70(11):1527–36.
26. Walia GS, Aston J, Bello R, Mackert GA, Pedreira RA, Cho BH, et al. Prepectoral versus subpectoral tissue expander placement: a clinical and quality of life outcomes study. Plast Reconstr Surg Glob Open. 2018;6(4):e1731.
27. Vidya R, Green M. Minimal pain with prepectoral implant based breast reconstruction. Plast Reconstr Surg. 2019;143(1):236e. https://doi.org/10.1097/PRS.0000000000005135.
28. Berna G, Cawthorn SJ, Papaccio G, Balestrieri N. Evaluation of a novel breast reconstruction technique using the Braxon® acellular dermal matrix: a new muscle-sparing breast reconstruction. ANZ J Surg. 2017;87(6):493–8. Epub 2014 Sep 29
29. Vidya R, Masià J, Cawthorn S, et al. Evaluation of the effectiveness of the prepectoral breast reconstruction with Braxon dermal matrix: first multicenter European report on 100 cases. Breast J. 2017;23(6):670–6.
30. Downs RK, Hedges K. An alternative technique for immediate direct-to-implant breast reconstruction-a case series. Plast Reconstr Surg Glob Open. 2016;4:e821. https://doi.org/10.1097/GOX.0000000000000839.
31. Vidya R, Iqbal FM, Becker H, Zhadan O. Rippling associated with pre-pectoral implant based breast reconstruction: a new grading system. World J Plast Surg. 2019;8(3):311–5. https://doi.org/10.29252/wjps.8.3.311.
32. Masià J, iBAG Working Group. The largest multicentre data collection on prepectoral breast reconstruction: The iBAG study. Surg Oncol. 2020;122(5):848–60. https://doi.org/10.1002/jso.26073.

Prepectoral Implant-Based Breast Reconstruction with Anterior Implant Coverage

10

Roland Reitsamer and Andreas Sir

10.1 Introduction

Nowadays, nipple-sparing mastectomy (NSM) is the standard mastectomy technique for patients, who require mastectomy, if the skin overlying the breast gland is not infiltrated by the tumor. The local recurrence rates after NSM are low and comparable to conventional mastectomies, and the oncologic safety of NSM was demonstrated in multiple studies [1]. The autologous or heterologous breast reconstruction is an essential component of NSM. In 80% of patients after conservative mastectomy, implant-based breast reconstruction is performed in 20% of patients autologous reconstruction. The subpectoral implant placement was standard of care for many decades. The subpectoral implant placement with complete muscle coverage using the pectoralis major muscle (PMM), parts of the serratus muscle and the fascia of the rectus muscle, performed with multiple variations, has many disadvantages compared to the prepectoral implant placement. The partial implant coverage with the PMM for the upper pole and partial coverage with acellular dermal matrix (ADM) for the lower pole results in better cosmesis, but still has the disadvantages of the PMM disruption. The consideration of the insertion of an ADM was to cover the lower pole of the implant, to stabilize the dissected PMM, and to serve as a hammock for the implant. This theory was questioned very soon. If the implant is located in a pocket like a hammock, that means a very loose ADM is covering the lower pole of the implant, the PMM contracts anyway, because there is no stabilization for the PMM. If the ADM is very tight around the lower pole of the implant, the PMM may be stabilized, but if the PMM contracts, the ADM and the implant will be retracted and pulled upwards, resulting in a bad cosmesis and asymmetry of the breasts. Due to the variance of the origin of the PMM, the percentage of coverage with the PMM can vary significantly from two-thirds of the implant to only on third of the implant [2, 3], which means up to two-thirds of the implant have to be covered by a matrix or mesh. The disadvantages of the subpectoral implant placement as the reduced muscle strength, the increased postoperative pain, the prolonged recovery time, and the breast animation deformity, persist. The prepectoral implant placement without any detachment of the PMM has many advantages and may equalize the disadvantages of the subpectoral implant placement, but requires a full implant coverage of the surface of the implant and an implant fixation. The implant fixation can be performed with various ADMs, various meshes, or autologous deepithelialized dermal flaps.

R. Reitsamer (✉) · A. Sir
Department of Senology, Breast Center Salzburg, Paracelsus Medical University Salzburg, Salzburg, Austria
e-mail: r.reitsamer@salk.at; a.sir@salk.at

© The Author(s), under exclusive license to Springer Nature Switzerland AG 2023
R. Vidya, H. Becker (eds.), *Prepectoral Breast Reconstruction*,
https://doi.org/10.1007/978-3-031-15590-1_10

10.2 Single-Stage Direct-to-Implant (DTI) or Two-Stage Reconstruction

The question of single-stage direct-to-implant (DTI) or two-stage breast reconstruction has been discussed repeatedly and there are arguments for both types of surgery. The decision depends on various factors as skin thickness and skin quality, viability of the flaps, prior and adjuvant therapy and radiotherapy as well as patient's desires.

Advantages of single-stage direct-to-implant (DTI) breast reconstruction:

Mastectomy and breast reconstruction can be performed in one single surgery. Primarily, there are psychologic considerations as the patients awakes with a breast after surgery, and secondary the avoidance of a second surgery reduces costs. A DTI breast reconstruction can be performed in patients who desire an identical breast size, or slightly larger breast, but can also be performed in patients with large and ptotic breasts as a reduction mastectomy.

The two-stage reconstruction offers the advantage for a correction in the second step. Results of the final pathological report are available, adjuvant therapy planning can be included in the consideration. The skin viability can be assessed, and patients with desire for larger breast can have the expander inflated.

Disadvantages of DTI are the risk of problems with the skin or nipple viability. The final pathological report can necessitate a second procedure in rare cases.

Many publications on prepectoral implant placement report on two-stage expander-to-implant breast reconstructions [4–6]. Recently, increasing numbers of papers report on DTI prepectoral implant breast reconstruction [7–20].

10.3 Advantages and Disadvantages of Prepectoral Implant Placement

The main advantage of prepectoral implant placement is the integrity of the PMM, compared to subpectoral implant placement. The dissection or elevation of the PMM is not performed, and a muscular deficit cannot be generated. Particularly, sportive activities and work out or heavy physical labor can be compromised by the dissection of the PMM. Postoperative pain is less if the PMM is not dissected and the breast animation deformity, the so-called jumping breast, does not occur. Additional advantages are shorter operation time, better cosmetic result, less capsular fibrosis, particularly after radiotherapy.

10.3.1 Disadvantages of Prepectoral Implant Placement

Problems of prepectoral implant placement are the visibility and palpability of the implants in slim patients. When the patients bend forward the rippling is becoming more prominent. In some patients after radiotherapy, the skin tightens over the implant and aggravates the visibility of the implant and the rippling.

These disadvantages of the prepectoral implant placement can be improved by fat grafting and lipofilling. This simple procedure is a perfect adjunct, and rippling or small tissue defects in the cleavage zone can be adjusted.

10.4 How to Cover the Implant

Since the beginning of the NSM and implant-based breast reconstruction, the question how to cover the implant is subject of discussion. Various techniques are described as the partial coverage with matrix or mesh and partially subpectoral implant placement, or the prepectoral implant placement with anterior coverage, complete coverage, or no coverage at all in selected patients. In our experience, the application of a matrix or mesh is helpful to fix the implant, and to have a regeneration plane between the implant and the skin. We propose and prefer the anterior coverage of the implant with partial coverage of the backside of the implant with the excess matrix or mesh.

10.5 Technique of the Anterior Coverage of the Implant

After selection of the implant, the ADM or the synthetic mesh was prepared for the coverage of the implant. We used either the porcine ADMs Strattice™ or Artia™ reconstructive tissue matrices (LifeCell™ Corporation, Bridgewater, NJ, USA). Since ADMs in the desired size were not available in Europe, two sheets of Strattice™ 8x16 cm or Artia™ 8x16 cm were sutured together with interrupted Vicryl® 3/0 sutures after washing of the ADMs in saline thoroughly. The enlarged 16 × 16 cm ADM was incised twice on each longitudinal edge and was meshed to make it more pliable. This type of incision allowed to create four straight flaps, which were fixed by sutures, and four angular flaps at the corners which were wrapped around the implant (Fig. 10.1), and created an anterior implant pocket. The superior straight flap of the ADM was fixed to the tight connective tissue between the fascia of the PMM and the superficial thoracic fascia with three interrupted sutures. In the next step, the medial straight flap of the ADM was sutured to the fascia with three sutures. Then the implant with the appropriate size was placed prepectorally beneath this ADM envelope. The angular ADM flaps were wrapped around the implant medial-cranially and medial-caudally as well as lateral-cranially and lateral-caudally, in a way that a complete ADM-covered implant pocket could be achieved. Then three sutures fixed the lateral straight flap, and in the final step, three interrupted sutures were used to fix the caudal straight flap to the fascia. One suction drain was inserted, and a double layer wound closure was performed. The drain was removed when less than 20 ml of wound fluid within 24 h was produced.

If the synthetic matrix TIGR™ (Novus Scientific AB, Uppsala, Sweden, 10 × 15 cm or 20 × 30 cm) was used, the mesh was trimmed and incised in a similar way, but the mesh was fixed with 3 sutures at the superior edge of the mesh only (Fig. 10.1b). The mesh was wrapped around the implant, covering the surface and partially the backside with the excess mesh and the wrapped

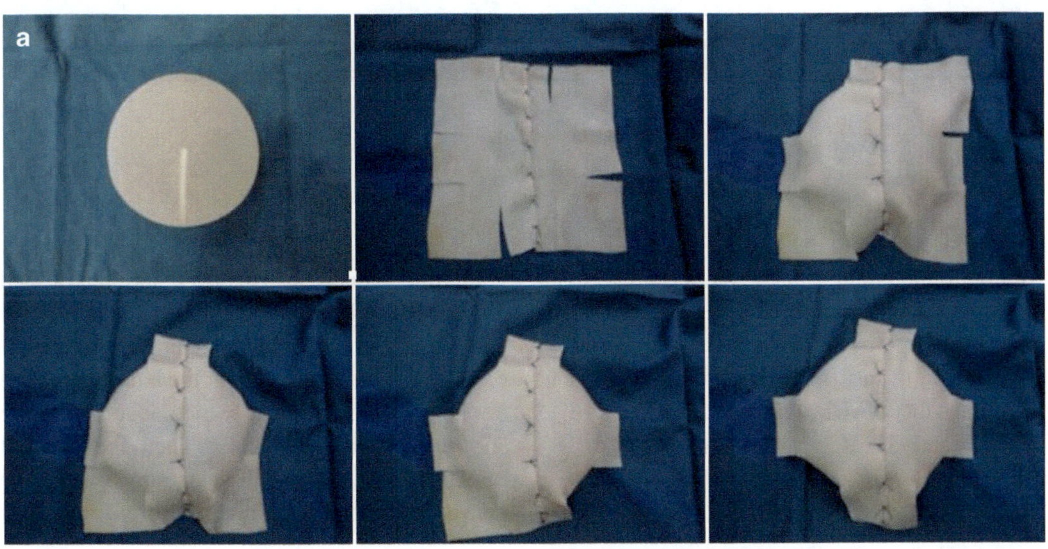

Fig. 10.1 (**a**) Implant wrapping with porcine ADM Strattice®. (**b**) Implant wrapping with synthetic mesh TIGR®. (**c**) Implant wrapping with bovine ADM Surgimend® meshed

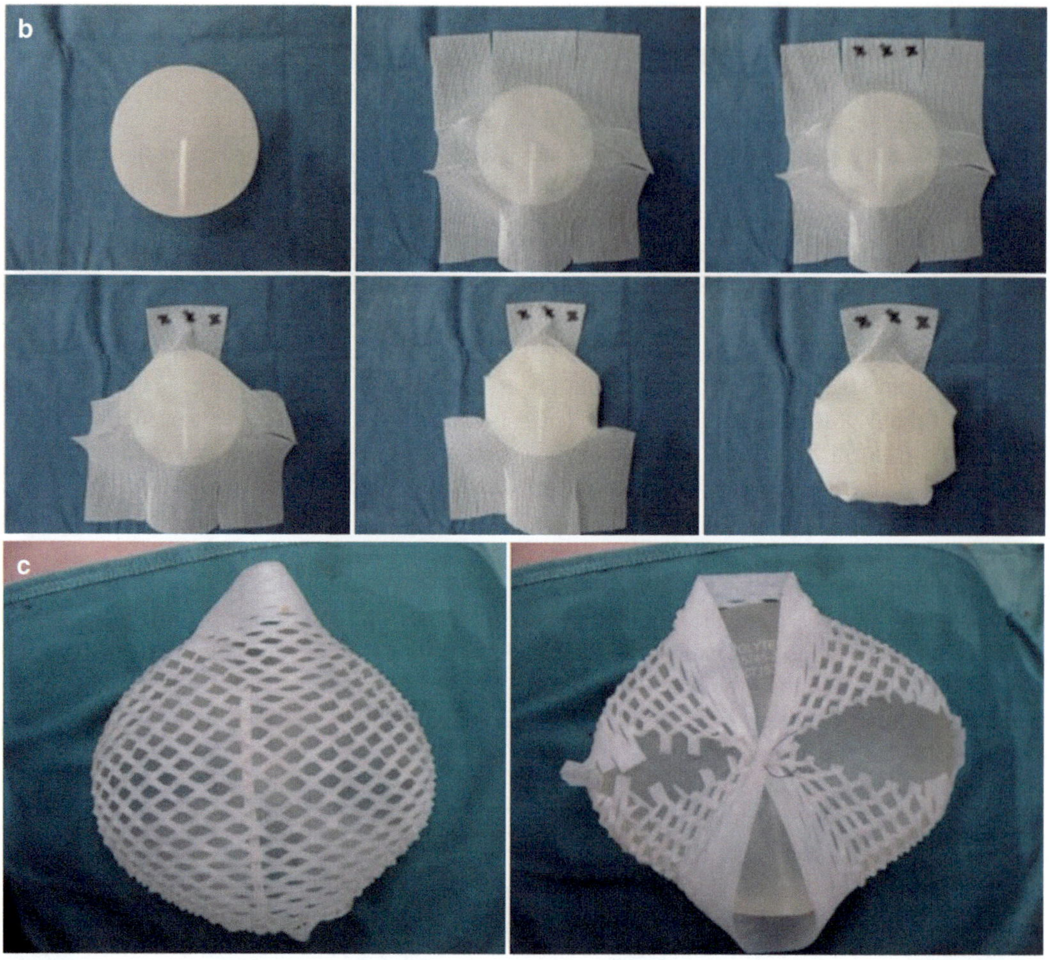

Fig. 10.1 (continued)

implant was put into the mastectomy pocket and fixed with three laid sutures. TIGR™ matrix is a long-term resorbable, synthetic surgical mesh with dual-stage degradation and full resorption, containing of fast resorbing fibers and slow resorbing fibers. ADM was used in 113 (56.5%) breasts, and TIGR™ matrix was used in 87 (43.5%) breasts.

10.6 Advancements in Technique and Materials

We replaced the porcine matrices Strattice® and Artia®, by Surgimend® meshed (Fig. 10.1c), a bovine ADM (Integra LifeSciences Corporation, Boston, MA, USA) for handling reasons and surgery time reduction. This soft and fenestrated ADM can easily be stretched over the surface of the implant without any folds, and the excess of the ADM can be sutured over the back side of the implant within minutes, which is comfortable and surgery time reducing. Then the covered implant can be fixed with few sutures within the pocket to avoid implant malposition.

10.7 The Seroma Discussion

There is an ongoing discussion on seroma formation after NSM and implant-based breast reconstruction. ADMs and meshes are considered to be in charge of seroma formation. The comparison between various ADMs or meshes in the literature is impossible, as there are no standards for the evaluation of seroma rates. Even in a review of 12 studies performing exclusively prepectoral implant-based breast reconstruction using one specific ADM, a huge variation of seroma formation was reported by Glenda Caputo [21]. The seroma rate ranged from 1.4% to 23.4%. The authors found interestingly that the ADM is not causative of the seroma formation, but a surgery-related origin is discussed. Nevertheless, this conclusion is not surprising at all. We always suggested that seroma formation is due to surgery with a large inner wound surface of the skin flaps. Every surgeon is aware of the occurrence of seroma after simple or modified radical mastectomy without any breast reconstruction. This is an unavoidable reaction of the tissue, according to the size of the inner wound and the type and technique of surgery, and a consequence of the interrupted lymphatic flow, but not a complication using the one or the other matrix, as mentioned in most reports.

10.8 Prepectoral DTI Breast Reconstruction

We performed and published [22] a series of 200 consecutive NSMs and direct-to-implant breast reconstructions with prepectoral implant placement and complete anterior implant coverage either with the porcine ADMs, Strattice™ or Artia™, or with the synthetic surgical mesh, TIGR® Matrix.

Shortly we present the key facts of the study: In 134 patients and 200 breasts, NSM and single-stage DTI breast reconstruction with prepectoral implant placement was performed. Sixty-six of 134 (49.3%) patients were treated with bilateral mastectomy, and 68/134 (50.7%) patients were treated with unilateral mastectomy. Fifty-eight of 200 (29.0%) breasts received some form of radiotherapy, 32/200 (16.0%) breasts had radiotherapy after NSM and DTI reconstruction. Twenty-six of 200 (13.0%) breasts had a history of radiotherapy and recurrent invasive breast cancer or recurrent DCIS and were treated with NSM and DTI. The mean volume of the removed breasts was 342 ml (range 59–1092 ml), and the mean implant weight was 340 g (range 110–735 g). Nipple-sparing mastectomy was performed in all patients. In the majority of operations (79.5%), inframammary fold incision was chosen.

10.9 Results

In this series, 200 breasts were reconstructed. Postoperative complications included minor complications with minimal nipple necrosis in 14 breasts (7.0%), and major complications including implant loss in 7 breasts (3.5%) and hematoma with revision surgery and evacuation in 8 breasts (4.0%). Mean duration of drainage was 5 days (range 3–12 days).

After a mean follow-up of 36 months (range 3–68 months), cosmetic results were excellent for 117 breasts (58.5%), good for 63 breasts (31.5%), sufficient for 13 breasts (6.5%), and insufficient for 7 breasts (3.5%). Implant displacement occurred in none of the patients, while implant rotation could be observed in 5 patients (2.5%). The implant rims were visible and palpable in the upper poles of the breasts in 3 very skinny patients, and rippling could be observed in 2 other very skinny patients.

Thirty-two (16.0%) patients received postoperative radiotherapy to one breast. Thirty-one patients did not have severe radiotherapy-induced side effects (Fig. 10.2). In one patient, the implant had to be removed 4 weeks after radiotherapy due to massive swelling, edema, and infection (Fig. 10.3). Capsular contractures grade III or IV could not be observed, and cosmetic results were excellent at the short-term follow-up. Twenty-six (13.0%) patients had prior radiotherapy to one breast. Six (23.0%) of those 26 breasts developed some kind of complication, 4/26 (15.3%) developed major complications. One patient suffered implant loss, three patients developed hematoma with revision surgery, and 2/26 (7.7%) showed minimal nipple necrosis. There were no differences in complication rates nor in cosmetic results according to the utilization of ADMs or synthetic meshes.

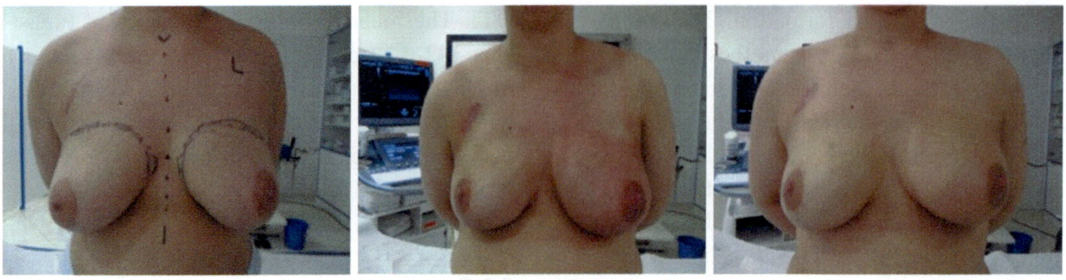

Fig. 10.2 Cosmetic result, bilateral NSM and postoperative radiotherapy to the left breast after radiotherapy and after 1 year

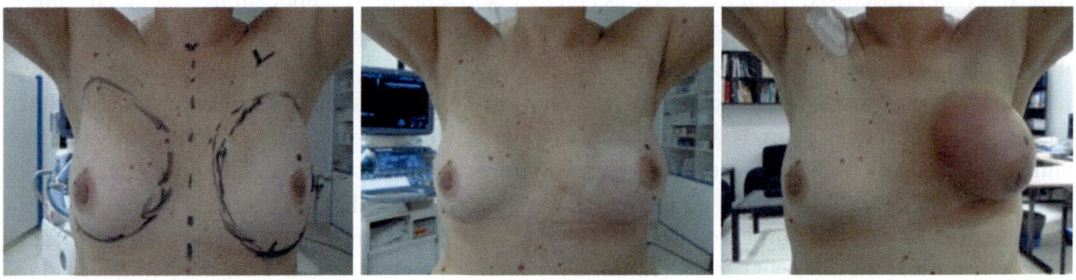

Fig. 10.3 Cosmetic result, NSM left side after surgery and after radiotherapy

The updated dataset comprises 350 reconstructed breasts, and the total results do not vary to the previous publication. Minor complications comprised minimal nipple necrosis in 23/350 breasts (6.6%), major complications comprised implant loss due to skin flap necrosis or infection in 14/350 breasts (4.0%), and hematoma with revision surgery in 10/350 breasts (2.9%).

10.10 Prepectoral DTI in Large and Ptotic Breasts

Direct-to-implant breast reconstruction in a single-stage procedure is an excellent option for many patients with small- and medium-sized breasts. For patients with large and ptotic breasts, usually a two-stage procedure or even a three-stage procedure (breast reduction mastopexy followed by nipple-sparing mastectomy and expander reconstruction, followed by expander-to-implant exchange) was suggested. Skin reduction nipple-sparing mastectomy (SR-NSM) is an option to reduce the excessive skin envelope, to use the deepithelialized autoderm as an implant coverage and to facilitate implant-based prepectoral breast reconstruction. The large and ptotic breast offers a perfect option for the substitution of ADMs or meshes with autoderm to cover the implant. A single-stage SR-NSM and direct-to-implant breast reconstruction with prepectoral implant placement and complete or partial coverage with deepithelialized autoderm are the further development for breast reconstruction for large and ptotic breasts after complete removal of the entire breast gland [23–25]. We performed a series of 20 breasts in 12 patients with large and ptotic breasts. The median age of the patients was 42 years, the median weight was 73 kg, and the median BMI was 25. The median sternal-notch-to-nipple distance was 27 cm. Wise incision was performed in all patients, the excessive skin was completely deepithelialized. An inferior and superior pedicled nipple–areola complex was designed, and the resection of the complete breast gland was easily performed by a dual access from medially and laterally of the pedicled NAC. SLNs were identified and removed from the same incision for patients with breast cancer. The chosen implant was inserted prepectorally and completely covered and fixed by the autoderm. If the autoderm did not cover the implant completely, a small piece or sling of ADM or synthetic mesh was shaped and sutured to the autoderm and to the thoracic superficial fascia. The skin was closed over the implant and the autoderm in a usual way, and the position of the NAC was excised and the NAC sutured in the correct position. The median weight of the removed breasts was 663 g (max 1092, min 500), and the median volume of the implants was 393 ml (max 495, min 255). Minor complications comprised superficial nipple necrosis without further intervention and complete healing in 4 breasts (20%), and major complications with hematoma and revision surgery in 2 breasts (10%) and full nipple necrosis in one breast (5%). In 13 breasts (65%), no complication occurred. SR-NSM and single-stage DTI breast reconstruction is a reasonable option for patients with large and ptotic breasts scheduled for mastectomy for breast cancer or risk-reducing purposes.

10.11 Conclusion

NSM and breast reconstruction is the new standard of care for conventional mastectomies in most cases. Yet in the seventies, the question of subcutaneous or subpectoral prosthesis positioning and single-stage breast reconstruction was discussed [26, 27]. The superiority of subpectoral implant placement is being questioned due to improvements in implant technology, ADMs, and surgical techniques. Pain and discomfort after detachment of the PMM are well-known postoperative complaints. Animation deformities while PMM contraction are common side effects. The substantial strength loss of the PMM and the muscular deficit in women with subpectoral prosthetic breast reconstruction are adequately described [28]. There is no data supporting subpectoral implant placement to be superior to prepectoral implant placement for breast reconstruction. For prepectoral implant placement, the ADM serves as soft tissue support, by acting as a tissue regeneration interlayer between the skin and the implant. The ADM prevents breast implant displacement. The development of form-stable silicone gel-filled breast implants and the advent of various acellular dermal matrices enable the prepectoral implant placement with complete wrapping of the implant and therefore the reconstruction of a natural looking soft breast without detaching the PMM. Capsular fibrosis is a well-known problem of implant-based breast reconstruction, and there are some reports that the additional use of ADM could further reduce the capsular contracture rate [29–33]. Furthermore, there are reports on reduced capsule formation in patients with ADM envelope and postoperative radiotherapy [34, 35]. ADM may slow the progression of capsule formation, fibrosis, and contraction via a decreased radiation-related inflammation [31, 32]. Recent publications on prepectoral implant placement and postmastectomy radiotherapy show promising results [6, 35]. Most publications on prepectoral placement are reports on two-stage breast reconstruction [4–6, 35]. There are only few reports on prepectoral implant placement in a one-stage procedure [7–17], with different approaches to cover the implant. Coverage techniques with various ADMs or with titanized polypropylene meshes or with synthetic absorbable meshes are described [10–18].

Complication rates of prepectoral implant placement are reasonable and comparable to subpectoral implant placement. The cosmetic results are appealing, one of the most displeasing side effect is rippling, especially in a bent forward position. This rippling can be improved by fat grafting easily. However, rippling is not only observed in prepectoral implant placement, but also in subpectoral implant placement, as the PMM atrophies over time. In our experience, most women preferred an identical breast size after NSM. In those women or women with a desire for slight augmentation, DTI reconstruction easily can be performed in a one-stage procedure. However, in women with desire for breast reduction after NSM, the DTI procedure can be performed either [23–25].

Prepectoral direct-to-implant breast reconstruction after NSM is a promising and feasible method which allows the reconstruction of a soft, appealing, and good-looking breast in most women. Advantages are intact thoracic musculature, less postoperative pain, no breast animation deformity, and in most cases one single surgical procedure. Prospective randomized multicentric trials comparing pre- versus subpectoral implant placement are ongoing (OPBC-2/PREPEC), and results are awaited eagerly [36].

References

1. Headon HL, Kasem A, Mokbel K. The oncologic safety of nipple-sparing mastectomy: a systematic review of the literature with a pooled analysis of 12,358 procedures. Arch Plast Surg. 2016;43(4):328–38.
2. Madsen RJ Jr, Chim J, Ang B, Fisher O, Hansen J. Variance in the origin of the pectoralis major muscle: implications for implant-based breast reconstruction. Ann Plast Surg. 2015;74(1):111–3.
3. Wy B, Byun IH, Seok Kim Y, Jung BK, Yun IS, Roh TS. Variance of the pectoralis major in relation to the inframammary fold and the pectoralis minor and its application to breast surgery. Clin Anat. 2017;30(3):357–61.
4. Sbitany H, Piper M, Lentz R. Prepectoral breast reconstruction: a safe alternative to submuscular prosthetic reconstruction following nipple-sparing mastectomy. Plast Reconstr Surg. 2017;140(3):432–43.
5. Salibian AH, Harness JK, Mowlds DS. Staged suprapectoral expander/implant reconstruction without acellular dermal matrix following nipple-sparing mastectomy. Plast Reconstr Surg. 2017;139(1):30–9.
6. Sigalove S, Maxwell GP, Sigalove NM, et al. Prepectoral implant-based breast reconstruction: rationale, indications, and preliminary results. Plast Reconstr Surg. 2017;139(2):287–94.
7. Colwell AS, Damjanovic B, Zahedi B, Medford-Davis L, Hertl C, Austen WG Jr. Retrospective review of 331 consecutive immediate single-stage implant reconstructions with acellular dermal matrix: indications, complications, trends, and costs. Plast Reconstr Surg. 2011;128(6):1170–8.
8. Reitsamer R, Peintinger F. Prepectoral implant placement and complete coverage with porcine acellular dermal matrix: a new technique for direct-to-implant breast reconstruction after nipple-sparing mastectomy. J Plast Reconstr Aesthet Surg. 2015;68(2):162–7.
9. Berna G, Cawthorn SJ, Papaccio G, Balestrieri N. Evaluation of a novel breast reconstruction technique using the Braxon® acellular dermal matrix: a new muscle-sparing breast reconstruction. ANZ J Surg. 2017;87(6):493–8.
10. Casella D, Bernini M, Bencini L, et al. TiLoop®bra mesh used for immediate breast reconstruction: comparison of retropectoral and subcutaneous implant placement in a prospective single-institution series. Eur J Plast Surg. 2014;37(11):599–604.
11. Casella D, Di Taranto G, Marcasciano M, et al. Evaluation of prepectoral implant placement and complete coverage with TiLoop®Bra mesh for breast reconstruction: a prospective study on long-term and patient reported BREAST-Q outcomes. Plast Reconstr Surg. 2019;142(1):1e–9e.
12. Vidya R, Masià J, Cawthorn S, et al. Evaluation of the effectiveness of the prepectoral breast reconstruction with Braxon dermal matrix: first multicenter European report on 100 cases. Breast J. 2017;23(6):670–6.
13. Onesti MG, Maruccia M, Di Taranto G, et al. Clinical, histological, and ultrasound follow-up of breast reconstruction with one-stage muscle-sparing "wrap" technique: a single-center experience. J Plast Reconstr Aesthet Surg. 2017;70(11):1527–36.
14. Bernini M, Calabrese C, Cecconi L, et al. Subcutaneous direct-to-implant breast reconstruction: surgical, functional, and aesthetic results after long-term follow-up. Plast Reconstr Surg Glob Open. 2016;3(12):e574. https://doi.org/10.1097/GOX.0000000000000533.
15. Downs RK, Hedges K. An alternative technique for immediate direct-to-implant breast reconstruction – a case series. Plast Reconstr Surg Glob Open. 2016;4(7):e821. https://doi.org/10.1097/GOX.0000000000000839.
16. Highton L, Johnson R, Kirwan C, Murphy J. Prepectoral implant-based breast reconstruction. Plast Reconstr Surg Glob Open. 2017;5(9):e1488. https://doi.org/10.1097/GOX.0000000000001488.
17. Jones G, Yoo A, King V, et al. Prepectoral immediate direct-to-implant breast reconstruction with anterior AlloDerm coverage. Plast Reconstr Surg. 2017;140(6S Prepectoral Breast Reconstruction):31S–8S. https://doi.org/10.1097/PRS.0000000000004048.
18. Hallberg H, Lewin R, Elander A, Hansson E. TIGR® matrix surgical mesh – a two-year follow-up study and complication analysis in 65 immediate breast reconstructions. J Plast Surg Hand Surg. 2018;52(4):253–8.
19. Masià J, iBAG Working Group. The largest multicentre data collection on prepectoral breast reconstruction: the iBAG study. J Surg Oncol. 2020;122(5):848–60.
20. Khan A, Tasoulis MK, Teoh V, Tanska A, Edmonds R, Gui G. Pre-pectoral one-stage breast reconstruction with anterior biological acellular dermal matrix coverage. Gland Surg. 2021;10(3):1002–9.
21. Caputo GG, Mura S, Albanese R, Zingaretti N, Parodi PC. Seroma formation in pre-pectoral implant-based ADM assisted breast reconstruction: a comprehensive review of current literature. Chirurgia. 2021;116:16–23.
22. Reitsamer R, Peintinger F, Klaassen-Federspiel F, Sir A. Prepectoral direct-to-implant breast reconstruction with complete ADM or synthetic mesh coverage – 36-months follow-up in 200 reconstructed breasts. Breast. 2019;48:32–7.
23. Nava MB, Ottolenghi J, Pennati A, et al. Skin/nipple sparing mastectomies and implant-based breast

reconstruction in patients with large and ptotic breast: oncological and reconstructive results. Breast. 2012;21(3):267–71.
24. Caputo GG, Marchetti A, Dalla Pozza E, et al. Skin-reduction breast reconstruction with prepectoral implant. Plast Reconstr Surg. 2016;137(6):1702–5.
25. Onesti MG, Di Taranto G, Ribuffo D, Scuderi N. ADM-assisted prepectoral breast reconstruction and skin reduction mastectomy: expanding the indications for subcutaneous reconstruction. J Plast Reconstr Aesthetic Surg. 2019 Nov 28. pii:S1748-6815(19)30492-9.
26. Hüter J, Clemens H, Ogbukagu A. Subcutaneous or subpectoral prosthesis positioning? Arch Gynecol. 1979;228(1–4):290.
27. Apfelberg DM, Laub DR, Maser MR, Lash H. Submuscular breast reconstruction – indications and techniques. Ann Plast Surg. 1981;7(3):213–21.
28. De Haan A, Toor A, Hage JJ, Veeger HE, Woerdeman LA. Function of the pectoralis major muscle after combined skin-sparing mastectomy and immediate reconstruction by subpectoral implantation of a prosthesis. Ann Plast Surg. 2007;59(6):605–10.
29. Stump A, Holton LH III, Connor J, Harper JR, Slezak S, Silverman RP. The use of acellular dermal matrix to prevent capsule formation around implants in a primate model. Plast Reconstr Surg. 2009;124:82–91.
30. Komorowska-Timek E, Oberg KC, Timek TA, Gridley DS, Miles DA. The effect of Alloderm envelopes on periprosthetic capsule formation with and without radiation. Plast Reconstr Surg. 2009;123:807–16.
31. Schmitz M, Bertram M, Kneser U, Keller AK, Horch RE. Experimental total wrapping of breast implants with acellular dermal matrix: a preventive tool against capsular contracture in breast surgery? J Plast Reconstr Aesthet Surg. 2013;66(10):1382–9.
32. Cheng A, Lakhiani C, Saint-Cyr M. Treatment of capsular contracture using complete implant coverage by acellular dermal matrix: a novel technique. Plast Reconstr Surg. 2013;132(3):519–29.
33. Salzberg CA, Ashikari AY, Berry C, Hunsicker LM. Acellular dermal matrix-assisted direct-to-implant breast reconstruction and capsular contracture: a 13-year experience. Plast Reconstr Surg. 2016;138(2):329–37.
34. Tang R, Coopey SB, Colwell AS, et al. Nipple-sparing mastectomy in irradiated breasts: selecting patients to minimize complications. Ann Surg Oncol. 2015;22(10):3331–7.
35. Elswick SM, Harless CA, Bishop SN, et al. Prepectoral implant-based breast reconstruction with Postmastectomy radiation therapy. Plast Reconstr Surg. 2018;142(1):1–12. https://doi.org/10.1097/PRS.0000000000004453.
36. Kappos EA, Schulz A, Regan MM, et al. Prepectoral versus subpectoral implant-based breast reconstruction after skin-sparing mastectomy or nipple-sparing mastectomy (OPBC-2/PREPEC): a pragmatic, multicentre, randomized, superiority trial. BMJ Open. 2021;11(9):e045239.

11 Prepectoral Anterior Coverage Breast Reconstruction

Glyn Jones

11.1 Introduction

The breast is a prepectoral structure, yet for decades surgeons have been reconstructing the breast in a sub-pectoral plane. Initially, implant-based breast reconstructions were performed in a subcutaneous plane, but the assumption that muscle coverage would provide better implant camouflage, reduce rippling, and lower capsular contracture rates resulted in the acceptance of sub-pectoral positioning [1–13]. Current evidence regarding capsular contracture points more towards bacterial contamination at the time of implant insertion causing biofilm formation as the primary culprit, rather than with implant pocket position [6, 8, 13]. Biofilm reduction techniques have resulted in a significant decrease in capsular contracture rates, thus rendering the need for sub-pectoral placement somewhat redundant [14–16].

Tissue expanders have been used routinely for two-stage breast reconstruction in order to recover domain lost after traditional mastectomy [9]. Skin sparing and nipple-sparing techniques have replaced conventional mastectomies, eliminating much of the need for expansion [17, 18]. Conceptually, total sub-muscular coverage had been conceived in part to control expander position at the time of mastectomy. This function was largely replaced by the adoption of lower pole coverage with acellular dermal matrices (ADMs) and meshes. ADMs not only provided tissue reinforcement, but also better pocket control, and shape without the compressive effects of total sub-muscular coverage [19, 20].

This tension could theoretically impede tissue perfusion and prevent tension free closure, both of which are necessary for uncomplicated wound healing. Further complicating the issue was the fact that tissue perfusion assessment was at best an inexact science during the dawn of implant-based breast reconstruction. Surgeons were reliant on clinical assessment and use of fluorescein. The advent of indocyanine green laser-induced fluorescence angiography was a turning point in mastectomy skin flap perfusion assessment, and the newer technology of multispectral imaging is making perfusion assessment even more accurate [21].

Two-stage sub-pectoral implant reconstruction gave reasonable results, but there were significant physical limitations accompanying sub-pectoral implant placement. Most patients exhibit a degree of animation deformity during activity, [12, 22–24] and patient function may be compromised. MRI studies have documented a 50% reduction in volume of the pectoral muscle at 12 months following sub-pectoral breast augmentation [25]. Additionally, there are reports of up to 15% reduction in strength amongst patients with sub-pectoral implants [22, 26–31].

G. Jones (✉)
University of Illinois College of Medicine at Peoria, Peoria, IL, USA

© The Author(s), under exclusive license to Springer Nature Switzerland AG 2023
R. Vidya, H. Becker (eds.), *Prepectoral Breast Reconstruction*,
https://doi.org/10.1007/978-3-031-15590-1_11

As a consequence of these developments, prepectoral implant-based breast reconstruction has become increasingly popular. On the positive side of the equation, prepectoral placement:

1. Eliminates the pain of muscle division.
2. Minimizes animation deformity.
3. Enables better medial implant placement with cleavage creation.
4. Has not been associated with increased incidence of skin necrosis.
5. Does not predispose the patient to increased risk of bottoming out.

On the negative side of the equation, prepectoral reconstruction poses the challenges of:

1. Loss of the "support" structure of muscle to control implant position following mastectomy.
2. Requiring the surgeon to precisely control implant position, particularly when performing direct-to-implant (DTI) reconstruction.
3. Exposing the patient to potentially higher risk of visible rippling.

In order to mitigate these risks and difficulties inherent to the procedure, pocket control with anterior coverage using biologic or synthetic meshes becomes of paramount importance. It is true to say that tabbed expanders have solved some of the issues with regard to controlling the position of expanders in the prepectoral space, allowing for reconstruction without mesh if the surgeon feels so inclined. I personally feel the many longer term benefits of ADM outweigh such arguments. However when single stage prepectoral implant insertion is proposed, the use of mesh to control placement becomes immensely important. Most breast surgeons breach the lateral breast crease during dissection of the axillary tail, thereby obliterating an important natural landmark in breast esthetics while creating a lateral space into which an unconstrained implant tends to fall. Lateral displacement of the implant not only creates a bizarre-looking breast, but also drastically limits cleavage formation. The use of anterior coverage with ADM (or synthetic mesh) allows for precise positioning of the implant, control of the lateral breast crease, and the ability to encourage inferior placement of the implant to mimic the lower pole fullness of a natural breast.

11.2 Anterior Coverage Versus Full Device Wrap?

There is much debate about the pros and cons of anterior versus full device wrapping with ADM or mesh. The author has experience with both techniques utilizing ADM.

Completely wrapping an implant or expander requires considerably more material, which is costly. Wrapping a deflated expander in 1 sheet of ADM is certainly easy, allowing the surgeon to tack the wrapped device to the chest wall using peripheral interrupted sutures either through the ADM, or if expanders are used, through the suture tabs. Proponents of full wrap suggest that creating an inferior cuff to support the device is key to preventing inferior malposition of the reconstruction. While that may sound logical, it is not strictly true. Of far greater importance is defining the inframammary fold (IMF) by suturing the ADM or mesh securely to the chest wall and not to Scarpa's fascia. If suturing is performed to the fascia, it allows the implant to slide inferiorly beneath the fascia on the muscle surface resulting in fold malposition. By suturing to the chest wall muscle at the fold, a new IMF is delineated securely and accurately and creating a trough or gutter into which the implant can lie is really unnecessary. This allows for more ADM to be applied to contouring the anterior surface of the pocket to achieve the most generous amount of ptosis for breast shaping instead of wasting valuable surface area behind the device. For these reasons I have elected to focus my surgical practice entirely on the use of anterior coverage for both implants and expanders in the prepectoral space. Prepectoral direct-to-implant reconstruction provides consistent single stage outcomes for a majority of patients (Fig. 11.1a, b).

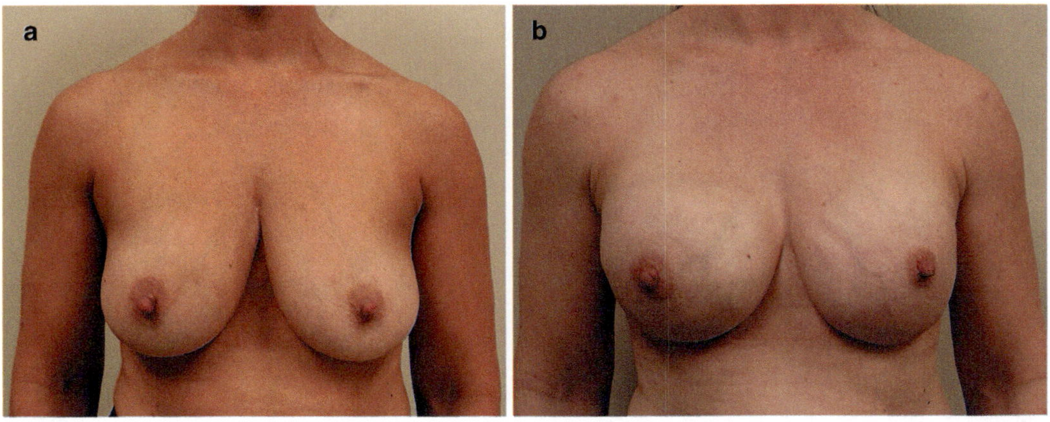

Fig. 11.1 (**a**) Pre-operative view of a 55-year-old woman with right breast carcinoma. (**b**) Postoperative view 1 year following bilateral nipple-sparing mastectomies with immediate single stage prepectoral breast reconstruction

11.3 Materials and Methods

In my current practice, 96% of patients are reconstructed using single stage prepectoral DTI. Two-stage expander reconstructions comprise only 4% of cases, again in the prepectoral plane, and are reserved for patients with questionable skin envelope perfusion (usually heavy smokers) as assessed by multispectral near-infrared imaging using the Kent Snapshot device (Kent Medical Imaging, Calgary, Alberta). This device has replaced the use of indocyanine green fluorescence imaging in our practice as the multispectral camera is inexpensive, more accurate, and non-invasive.

Mastectomy skin flap perfusion is the key determinant when deciding to proceed with single-stage reconstruction. The decision is based entirely on adequacy of mastectomy skin flap perfusion with a temporary sizer in place. In over 12 years of direct-to-implant reconstruction, the author has come to the conclusion that skin flap thickness is of little concern; *what matters is perfusion*. Thin skin flaps can always be augmented with later fat grafting if necessary. If skin perfusion is adequate with an appropriate temporary sizer in place, a decision is made to proceed. If perfusion is marginal, either an under-filled expander is inserted, or the procedure can be aborted and converted to a delayed-immediate approach within 2 weeks.

11.4 Operative Procedure

Following mastectomy, the skin is re-prepped with either chlorhexidine alcohol or betadine solution. A temporary sizer is placed, and skin perfusion is assessed using multispectral near-infrared imaging (Fig. 11.2). This modality provides rapid assessment of cutaneous flap oxygenation as a surrogate of perfusion and correlates better with clinical outcomes than the indocyanine green fluorescence imaging I used to use. Multispectral imaging is non-invasive, handheld, inexpensive and can be repeated multiple times during a given procedure. The mastectomy pocket is lavaged with saline and then full-strength betadine solution [16, 32].

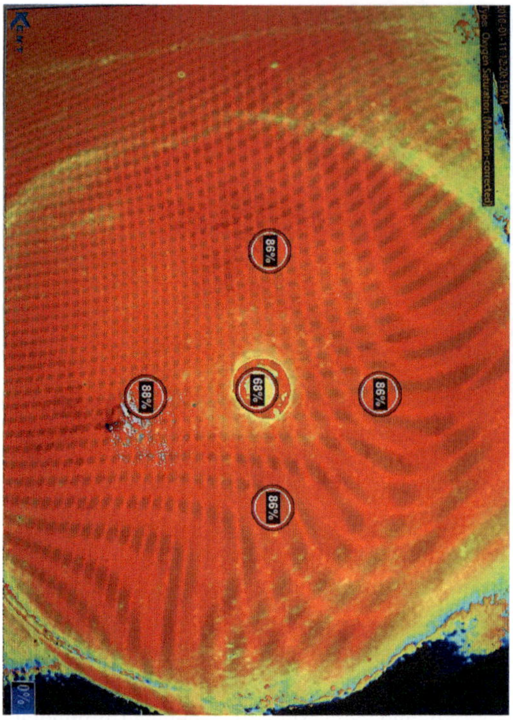

Fig. 11.2 Multispectral near-infrared perfusion imaging of mastectomy blood flow

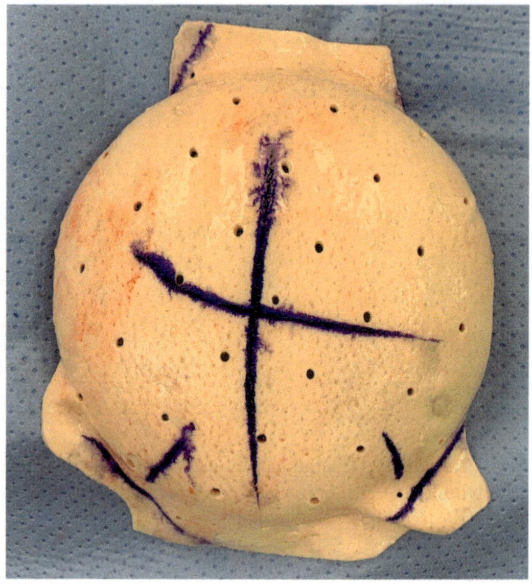

Fig. 11.3 Shaping of the ADM to the contour of the implant prior to inset

11.5 Anterior Suturing Technique

A sheet of 16x20cm thick ADM (AlloDerm, Allergan Inc) is washed according to manufacturer protocol. The material is draped over the temporary sizer and using a fresh marking pen, is marked for shaping using a central cross for orientation within the pocket. I typically remove 2 small triangles of ADM to achieve narrowing of the upper pocket so as to limit upward migration of the implant (Fig. 11.3). Suturing is performed *without* the implant in place. The ADM is draped over the anterior surface of the pectoralis major muscle, and the 12 o'clock position is determined using the ink marks for orientation. Suturing is performed to the anterior surface of pectoralis major using the anterior tenting approach [33].

Using 2–0 PDS, continuous suturing is performed from 12 o'clock to 5 o'clock and 12 to 7 o'clock leaving an inferior access window for implant insertion, assuming either an inframammary incision or central breast incision has been utilized for mastectomy. Laterally, the ADM is sutured to an elevated cuff of serratus fascia or muscle if the fascia is deficient (Fig. 11.4a). If a lateral incision was used, then suturing is performed from 12 to 10 o'clock and from 12 to 3 to 7 o'clock (in a right mastectomy), leaving a lateral access window for implant insertion. Suturing should be performed in such a way as to leave as much redundancy as possible in the ADM envelope inferiorly, so as to permit more ADM bulging over the lower pole of the implant for lower pole fullness. The prepared pocket is re-checked with a sizer in place to ensure correct shape and position of the reconstruction. The sizer is removed, and the pocket is washed again with full-strength betadine solution. The surgeon changes gloves, and the implant is inserted using a Keller funnel or equivalent to ensure no contact between the implant and the skin in an effort to minimize biofilm formation [15, 16, 34]. The ADM is then pulled taught over the dome of the implant to create a snug "hand-in-glove" fit. The inferior aspect of the ADM is then sutured to the chest wall (not Scarpa's fascia) with the remaining tails of 2–0 PDS (Fig. 11.4b). Suturing the ADM to Scarpa's fascia should never be performed as it can result in inferior displacement of

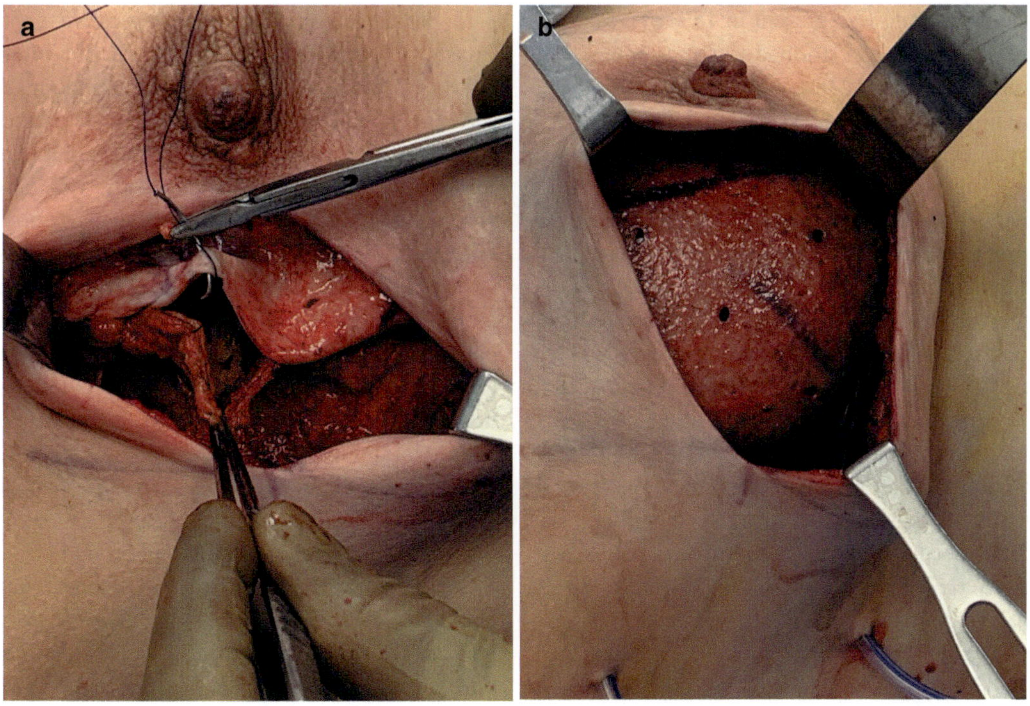

Fig. 11.4 (**a**) Suturing of the lateral edge of the ADM to serratus fascia. (**b**) The completed prepectoral construct with implant in place prior to skin closure

the implant down the chest wall under the influence of gravity resulting in abnormal lowering of the inframammary fold. Closure is performed over 2 channel drains. The entire construct is covered with a Tegaderm occlusive dressing, which is left in place for 2 weeks. The first drain is removed at 1 week postoperatively whilst the second remains in place until drainage is less than 20–25 cc per 24 h period. We have been evaluating our results regarding 1 versus 2 drains and in our practice it appears that double drain use does result in a lower rate of postoperative seromas or infections.

11.6 Results

In reviewing the first 194 breasts in 140 patients, maximum follow-up was 3.8 years. Over 500 breasts have now been operated on with similar long-term outcomes. The initial data was based on anatomic textured cohesive gel implants (Allergan Inc.) which are no longer available. For the past 2 years, the author has converted to using only smooth round moderately cohesive gel implants with either full or moderate profiles. Initial experience with highly cohesive round smooth gel implants, particularly those with extra high profiles, was associated with an unacceptably high incidence of antero-posterior flipping and was abandoned in our practice for this reason, hence the use of full profile moderately cohesive devices. There have been no cases of breast implant-associated anaplastic large cell lymphoma (BIA-ALCL) in our textured surface implant reconstructions. Successful outcome was achieved in 93.3% of cases (Fig. 11.1a, b). The most common complications were very minor contour deformities (slight implant edge visibility or hollowing) at 44.3%, benign seromas 5.2%, and cellulitis in 5.7% patients. Explantation for any reason occurred in 6.7% of cases. There were no major full thickness skin necrosis requiring debridement and closure in the operating room. Partial thickness cutaneous blistering was treated conservatively with topical therapy in 4.1%.

Minor rippling was present in 15% of cases, and fat grafting was performed to soften minor contour deformities in 38% when we were using anatomic highly cohesive gel implants, which is significantly lower than rates of fat grafting in our sub-pectoral reconstruction patients. Since converting to round smooth implants, our fat graft rates have risen dramatically to over 90% in order to backfill the upper pole contour of the chest and reduce visible rippling associated with the slightly less cohesive devices. There was 0% capsular contracture in non-radiated patients and 0% animation deformity. We attribute the consistently low capsular contracture rate to the use of biofilm reduction techniques and the use of ADM. Long-term revision for implant size change occurred in 7.2% of cases, which is significantly lower than in our sub-pectoral single stage reconstructions.

11.7 Discussion

Numerous studies have corroborated the effectiveness of prepectoral reconstruction [35–44]. Gabriel report acceptable results in 39 obese patients undergoing prepectoral breast reconstruction, with only one reconstructive failure [35]. Several studies have looked at prepectoral breast reconstruction after post-mastectomy radiation therapy (PMRT) [37, 42, 43]. Both Elswick et al. and Sigalove et al. found no statistically significant increased risk of adverse outcomes in prepectoral breast reconstructions that underwent PMRT based on short-term retrospective data in 93 and 52 breasts, respectively [37, 42]. Sinnot found that patients who underwent sub-pectoral breast reconstruction and PMRT had a greater rate of capsular contracture than patients undergoing prepectoral reconstruction [43]. This is most likely due to the effects of radiation fibrosis within the pectoralis major muscle causing tightness deformity and shoulder stiffness. Lastly, when comparing prepectoral breast reconstruction to sub-pectoral breast reconstruction, several studies since our last publication found positive results. Cattelani et al. found less postoperative pain, faster recovery from postoperative upper extremity functional morbidity, and earlier return to work in a small, prospective, nonrandomized series [44]. Walia reported significantly decreased postoperative pain in two-stage prepectoral breast reconstruction patients. Their study was also without significant differences in patient reported outcomes based on BREAST-Q analysis. However, there was a statistically significant increase in nipple ischemia amongst prepectoral patients [39]. Finally, Baker et al. reported no significant difference in pain scores, early complications, or postoperative length of stay between direct-to-implant prepectoral and sub-pectoral breast reconstruction groups. By contrast, more patients were dissatisfied with the amount of implant rippling in the prepectoral group [41].

Whilst an increasing number of studies report favorable data on direct-to-implant prepectoral breast reconstruction, a majority of surgeons still practice two-stage expander based reconstruction [36, 37, 43, 44]. This may seem incongruous given that current mastectomy techniques have resulted in the preservation of ever increasing amounts of skin, culminating in nipple-sparing mastectomy [17, 18]. The need for expansion to recruit skin has decreased exponentially as these newer mastectomy approaches have been adopted. Releasing the fascial constraints of the breast at mastectomy results in the breast skin envelope being able to accommodate a similar, or even larger, sized implant than the original breast volume. This challenges the second commonly proposed indication for expansion. By contrast, we are often able to augment breast size in one stage after reconstruction. Reimbursement is certainly higher with 2 stage expander-implant reconstruction and may affect decision-making. Single stage reconstruction offers a far more practical solution to breast reconstruction in socialized healthcare systems .

As was mentioned earlier, skin flap perfusion is the primary determinant of direct-to-implant reconstruction rather than skin flap thickness. Mastectomy skin flap thickness per se had *no* impact on outcomes, if the flaps were shown to be well perfused on perfusion assessment imaging [13, 35]. If skin perfusion is adequate with a temporary sizer in place, single-stage prepectoral direct-to-implant reconstruction is a safe, reproducible technique. While many hospitals do not have access to some of the costly ICG-based devices, the use of the handheld Kent Snapshot near-infrared multispectral device (Kent Imaging, Alberta Canada) makes perfusion assessment accurate, simple, and completely non-invasive. It's accuracy in our hands has been shown to be superior to that of ICG-based technology in a recent about-to-be published study.

The benefits of the technique in our practice can be divided into acute and long term. In the acute setting, the use of anterior coverage helps to control the mastectomy space and implant position resulting in a much more accurate, reproducible outcome. In the longer term, it is associated with much less patient discomfort, no need for postoperative expansion, reduced tissue flap edema, and virtually no subjective negative impact on upper extremity function. Animation deformity has been completely eliminated.

Whilst fat grafting was required less frequently (38%) in prepectoral patients than in our sub-pectoral patients when anatomic cohesive gel implants were in use, this changed with the use of round implants. This is a reflection of the deficiencies innate to round implant shapes.

Rippling perpendicular to the contraction of the pectoralis major muscle has been eliminated and is now a function primarily of the gel consistency used. Limited cleavage formation by the pectoralis major muscle preventing more medial implant placement is no longer an issue with prepectoral implant placement. The ADM pocket can be constructed as medially as required in order to achieve better cleavage using the anterior approach. Very precise control can be achieved. The results have been so encouraging that the authors have completely abandoned sub-pectoral implant-based breast reconstruction. The authors have also almost entirely abandoned routine two-stage reconstruction in favor of single stage prepectoral reconstruction assuming acceptable skin flap perfusion.

11.8 Conclusion

Improvements in mastectomy technique have resulted in preservation of most if not all of the mastectomy skin envelope. The use of anterior coverage of round implants with ADM or mesh allows for greater accuracy and planning of the single-stage reconstruction, incurring much less discomfort and inconvenience for the patient. Single-stage prepectoral DTI has become an excellent alternative to 2-stage expander reconstruction, facilitated by the use of anterior coverage. With 10-year follow-up available, the technique demonstrates maintenance of the integrity and quality of the reconstructions with minimal rates of capsular contracture and complete absence of animation deformity. Previously voiced concerns about late implant ptosis, erosion, or unacceptable rippling have simply not materialized.

References

1. Freeman BS. Subcutaneous mastectomy for benign breast lesions with immediate or delayed prosthetic replacement. Plast Reconstr Surg Transplant Bull. 1962;30:676–82.
2. Berens JJ, Stapley LA. Breast tumors treated by mastectomy (subcutaneous) with mammary replacement. Ariz Med. 1969;26(8):651–7.
3. Hueston J, McKenzie G. Breast reconstruction after radical mastectomy. Aust N Z J Surg. 1970;39(4):367–70.
4. Snyderman RK, Guthrie RH. Reconstruction of the female breast following radical mastectomy. Plast Reconstr Surg. 1971;47(6):565–7.
5. Guthrie RH. Breast reconstruction after radical mastectomy. Plast Reconstr Surg. 1976;57(1):14–22.
6. Schlenker JD, Bueno RA, Ricketson G, Lynch JB. Loss of silicone implants after subcutaneous mastectomy and reconstruction. Plast Reconstr Surg. 1978;62(6):853–61.
7. Blevins PK. Subcutaneous mastectomy and breast replacement: its role in the treatment of benign, premalignant, and malignant breast disease. Am Surg. 1981;47(7):281–6.
8. Gruber RP, Kahn RA, Lash H, Maser MR, Apfelberg DB, Laub DR. Breast reconstruction following mastectomy: a comparison of submuscular and subcutaneous techniques. Plast Reconstr Surg. 1981;67(3):312–7.

9. Radovan C. Breast reconstruction after mastectomy using the temporary expander. Plast Reconstr Surg. 1982;69(2):195–208.
10. Giraud B, Dauplat J, Gadonneix P, Jany M, Rodier JF, Issert B, et al. [Subcutaneous mammectomy with prosthetic inclusion. Apropos of 114 cases]. Chirurgie 1986;112(5):402–412.
11. Scarfì A, Ordemann K, Hüter J. Reconstruction of an ablated breast. Eur J Gynaecol Oncol. 1986;7(2):93–6.
12. Artz JS, Dinner MI, Sampliner J. Breast reconstruction with a subcutaneous tissue expander followed with a polyurethane-covered silicone breast implant. Ann Plast Surg. 1988;20(6):517–21.
13. Artz JS, Dinner MI, Foglietti MA, Sampliner J. Breast reconstruction utilizing subcutaneous tissue expansion followed by polyurethane-covered silicone implants: a 6-year experience. Plast Reconstr Surg. 1991;88(4):635–9. discussion640–1
14. Ajdic D, Zoghbi Y, Gerth D, Panthaki ZJ, Thaller S. The relationship of bacterial biofilms and capsular contracture in breast implants. Aesthet Surg J. 2016;36(3):297–309.
15. Deva AK, Adams WP Jr, Vickery K. The role of bacterial biofilms in device-associated infection. Plast Reconstr Surg. 2013;132(5):1319–28.
16. Jewell ML, Adams WP Jr. Betadine and breast implants. Aesthet Surg J. 2018;38(6):623–6.
17. Toth BA, Lappert P. Modified skin incisions for mastectomy: the need for plastic surgeons input. Plast Reconstr Surg. 1991;87(6):1048–53.
18. Bishop CC, Singh S, Nash AG. Mastectomy and breast reconstruction preserving the nipple. Ann R Coll Surg Engl. 1990;72(2):87–9.
19. Duncan DI. Correction of implant rippling using allograft dermis. Aesthet Surg J. 2001;21(1):81–4.
20. Baxter RA. Intracapsular allogenic dermal grafts for breast implant-related problems. Plast Reconstr Surg. 2003;112(6):1692–6.
21. Gurtner GC, Jones GE, Neligan PC, Newman MI, Phillips BT, Sacks JM, et al. Intraoperative laser angiography using the SPY system: review of the literature and recommendations for use. Ann Surg Innov Res. 2013;7(1):1–1.
22. Spear SL, Schwartz J, Dayan JH, Clemens MW. Outcome assessment of breast distortion following submuscular breast augmentation. Aesth Plast Surg. 2009;33(1):44–8.
23. Becker H, Fregosi N. The impact of animation deformity on quality of life in post-mastectomy reconstruction patients. Aesthet Surg J. 2017;37(5):531–6.
24. Nigro LC, Blanchet NP. Animation deformity in Postmastectomy implant-based reconstruction. Plast Reconstr Surg Glob Open. 2017;5(7):e1407–4.
25. Weck Roxo AC, Nahas FX, Salin R, de Castro CC, Aboudib JH, Marques RG. Volumetric evaluation of the mammary gland and pectoralis major muscle following subglandular and submuscular breast augmentation. Plast Reconstr Surg. 2016;137(1):62–9.
26. Banbury J, Yetman R, Lucas A, Papay F, Graves K, Zins JE. Prospective analysis of the outcome of subpectoral breast augmentation: sensory changes, muscle function, and body image. Plast Reconstr Surg. 2004;113(2):701–7.
27. Beals SP, Golden KA, Basten M, Kelly KM. Strength performance of the pectoralis major muscle after subpectoral breast augmentation surgery. Aesthet Surg J. 2003;23(2):92–7.
28. Becker H, Lind JG II, Hopkins EG. Immediate implant-based Prepectoral breast reconstruction using a vertical incision. Plast Reconstr Surg Glob Open. 2015;3(6):e412–9.
29. de Haan A, Toor A, Hage JJ, Veeger HEJ, Woerdeman LAE. Function of the pectoralis major muscle after combined skin-sparing mastectomy and immediate reconstruction by subpectoral implantation of a prosthesis. Ann Plast Surg. 2007;59(6):605–10.
30. Hage JJ, van der Heeden JF, Lankhorst KM, Romviel SMG, Vluttters ME, Woerdeman LAE, et al. Impact of combined skin sparing mastectomy and immediate subpectoral prosthetic reconstruction on the pectoralis major muscle function. Ann Plast Surg. 2014;72:631–7.
31. Sarbak J, Baker J. Effects of breast augmentation on pectoralis major muscle function in the athletic woman. Aesthet Surg J. 2004;24(3):224–8.
32. Campbell CA. The role of triple-antibiotic saline irrigation in breast implant surgery. Ann Plast Surg. 2018;80:S398–402.
33. Jones G, Yoo A, King V, Jao B, Wang H, Rammos C, et al. Prepectoral immediate direct-to-implant breast reconstruction with anterior AlloDerm coverage. Plast Reconstr Surg. 2017;140:31S–8S.
34. Flugstad NA, Pozner JN, Baxter RA, Creasman C, Egrari S, Martin S, et al. Does implant insertion with a funnel decrease capsular contracture? A Preliminary Report Aesthet Surg J. 2016;36(5):550–6.
35. Gabriel A, Maxwell GP. Prepectoral breast reconstruction in challenging patients. Plast Reconstr Surg. 2017;140:14S–21S.
36. Jafferbhoy S, Chandarana M, Houlihan M, Parmeshwar R, Narayanan S, Soumian S, et al. Early multicentre experience of pre-pectoral implant based immediate breast reconstruction using Braxon®. Gland Surg. 2017;6(6):682–8.
37. Sigalove S, Maxwell GP, Sigalove NM, Storm-Dickerson TL, Pope N, Rice J, et al. Prepectoral implant-based breast reconstruction and Postmastectomy radiotherapy. Plast Reconstr Surg Glob Open. 2017;5(12):e1631–7.
38. Paydar KZ, Wirth GA, Mowlds DS. Prepectoral breast reconstruction with fenestrated acellular dermal matrix. Plast Reconstr Surg Glob Open. 2018;6(4):e1712–4.

39. Walia GS, Aston J, Bello R, Mackert GA, Pedreira RA, Cho BH, et al. Prepectoral versus subpectoral tissue expander placement. Plast Reconstr Surg Glob Open. 2018;6(4):e1731–6.
40. Pittman TA, Abbate OA, Economides JM. The P1 method: Prepectoral breast reconstruction to minimize the palpable implant edge and upper pole rippling. Ann Plast Surg. 2018;80(5):487–92.
41. Baker BG, Irri R, MacCallum V, Chattopadhyay R, Murphy J, Harvey JR. A prospective comparison of short-term outcomes of subpectoral and Prepectoral Strattice-based immediate breast reconstruction. Plast Reconstr Surg. 2018;141(5):1077–84.
42. Elswick SM, Harless CA, Bishop SN, Schleck CD, Mandrekar J, Reusche RD, et al. Prepectoral implant-based breast reconstruction with Postmastectomy radiation therapy. Plast Reconstr Surg. 2018;142(1): 1–12.
43. Sinnott CJ, Persing SM, Pronovost M, Hodyl C, McConnell D, Young AO. Impact of postmastectomy radiation therapy in prepectoral versus subpectoral implant-based breast reconstruction. Ann Surg Oncol. 2018:1–10. Springer International Publishing
44. Cattelani L, Polotto S, Arcuri MF, Pedrazzi G, Linguadoca C, Bonati E. One-step Prepectoral breast reconstruction with dermal matrix-covered implant compared to submuscular implantation: functional and cost evaluation. Clin Breast Cancer. 2018;18(4):e703–11. Elsevier Inc

Further Reading

Gur E, Hanna W, Andrighetti L, Semple JL. Light and electron microscopic evaluation of the pectoralis major muscle following tissue expansion for breast reconstruction. Plast Reconstr Surg. 1998;102(4):1046–51.

Maxwell GP, Tornambe R. Management of mammary subpectoral implant distortion. Clin Plast Surg. 1988;15(4):601–11.

Hammond DC, Schmitt WP, O'Connor EA. Treatment of breast animation deformity in implant-based reconstruction with pocket change to the subcutaneous position. Plast Reconstr Surg. 2015;135(6):1540–4.

Lesavoy MA, Trussler AP, Dickinson BP. Difficulties with subpectoral augmentation Mammaplasty and its correction: the role of subglandular site change in revision aesthetic breast surgery. Plast Reconstr Surg. 2010;125(1):363–71.

Gabriel A, Sigalove S, Sigalove NM, Storm-Dickerson TL, Rice J, Pope N, et al. Prepectoral revision breast reconstruction for treatment of implant-associated animation deformity: a review of 102 reconstructions. Aesthet Surg J. 2018;38(5):519–26.

Hammond DC. Commentary on: Prepectoral revision breast reconstruction for treatment of implant-associated animation deformity: a review of 102 reconstructions. Aesthet Surg J. 2018;38(5):527–8.

12 Breast Reconstruction Using a Prepectoral Spacer

Hilton Becker

As the advantages of prepectoral breast reconstruction are recognized, the technique is gaining increasing acceptance [1–7].

Many surgeons now report that not only is prepectoral placement their procedure of choice, but some are even reluctant to use sub-pectoral implant placement at all [8].

Prepectoral placement not only avoids animation deformity, muscle discomfort chronic pain, and impairment of shoulder function, but the cosmetic results are often superior to that of sub-pectoral reconstruction [9].

However, optimal results can only be obtained when the resultant skin flaps following the mastectomy are sufficiently thick and well vascularized.

What is a surgeon to do when the flaps are sub-optimal?

The three most common options include.

Submuscular placement, delayed or immediate delayed reconstruction [10].

A promising alternative includes the placement of a "spacer," which is effectively equivalent to delayed reconstruction as it is only filled once circulation is assured. The spacer is an under filled (or empty), smooth adjustable implant that is placed in the prepectoral pocket. When there is a concern of vascular compromise, minimal mesh is used to avoid possible contamination should the incision edge need debridement.

The implant is initially partially filled with air, thus reducing pressure on the thin skin flaps, particularly inferiorly, where the implant is beneath the incision. The air is evenly dispersed in the implant compared to saline which pools inferiorly. By leaving the implant underfilled, the skin contracts, resulting in some degree of thickening and lifting of the skin flap (Figs. 12.1 and 12.2).

Should further thickening of the skin flaps be necessary, serial fat grafting or delayed mesh insertion can be performed [11].

H. Becker (✉)
Department of Surgery, Charles E. Schmidt College of Medicine, Boca Raton, FL, USA

Florida Atlantic University, Boca Raton, FL, USA
e-mail: Hilton@beckermd.com

© The Author(s), under exclusive license to Springer Nature Switzerland AG 2023

R. Vidya, H. Becker (eds.), *Prepectoral Breast Reconstruction*,
https://doi.org/10.1007/978-3-031-15590-1_12

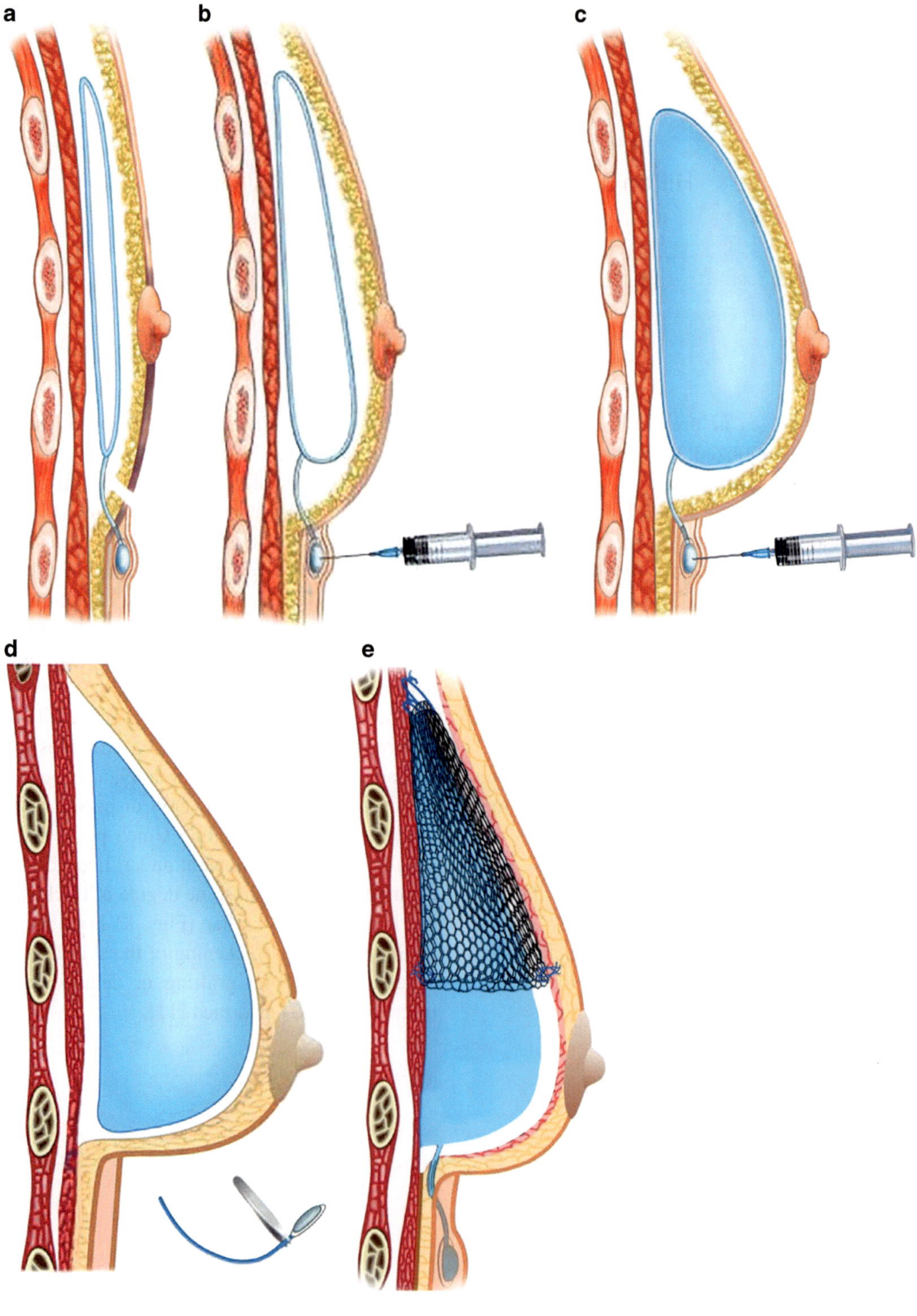

Fig. 12.1 (**a**) A Pre pectoral placement of adjustable saline implant Implant underfilled with air acts as a spacer. (**b**) Further air is added to implant once circulation is assured Flap contracts over spacer Thickens and elevates. (**c**) Air is replaced with saline. the Injection port is removed once satisfactory volume is achieved. (**d**) Fat graft to skin flap, Injection port removed, or implant replaced with silicone gel implant. (**e**) Double layer long term absorbable mesh sutured to upper pole

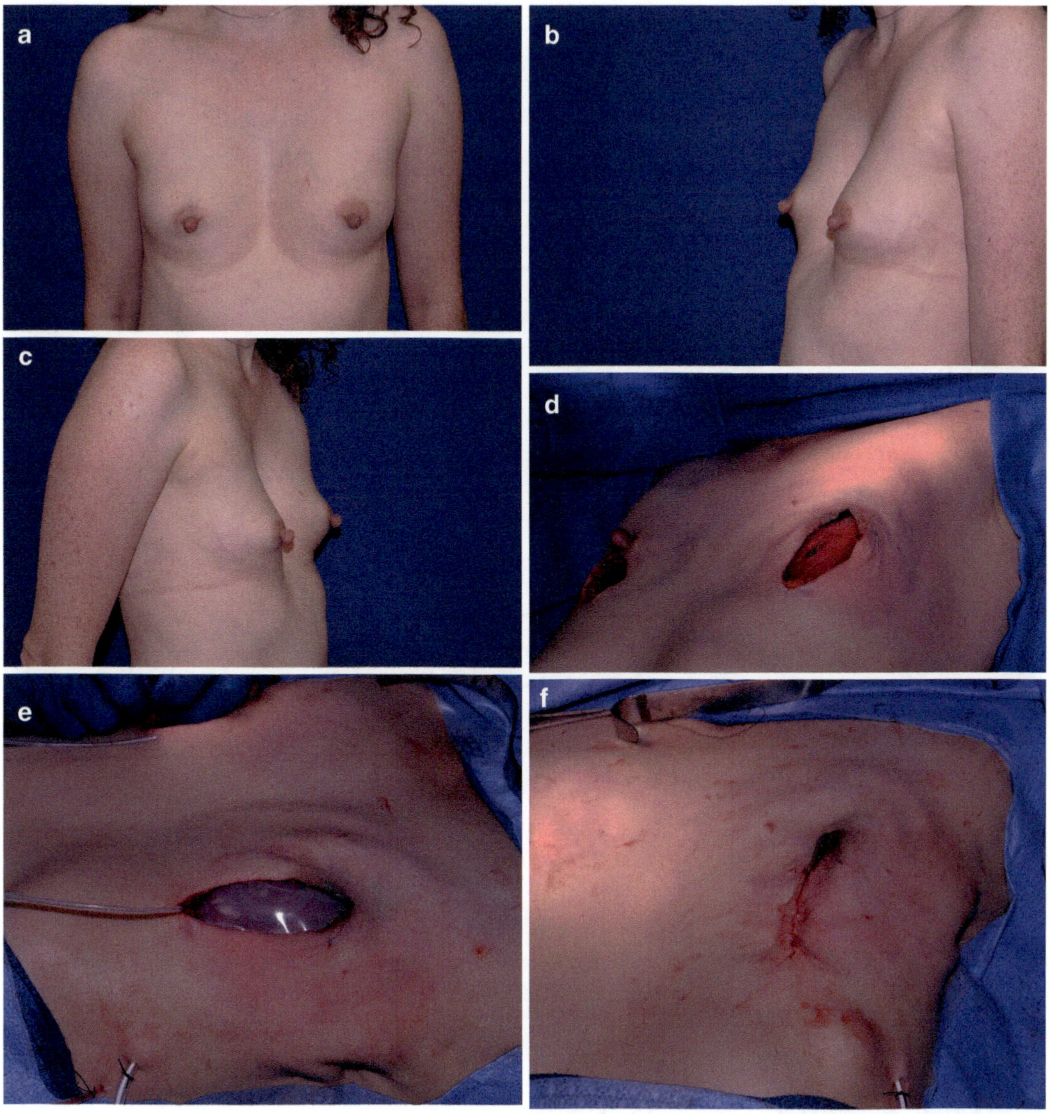

Fig. 12.2 (**a**, **b**, **c**) Patient with carcinoma of the l breast Scheduled for bilateral mastectomies. (**d**) Following L skin sparing sparing mastectomy and R nipple sparing mastectomy. (**e**) Insertion of an adjustable temporary sizer noting tightness of flaps. (**f**) Placement of a Spacer (virtually empty spectrum implant). (**g**) Early post operative result with cyanosis of L mastectomy flap. (**h**) Further air added. (**i**) Implant overfilled with air. (**j**) Air replaced with saline Nipple reconstructed with a composite graft from the R nipple. (**k**, **l**, **m**) L Adjustable saline implant replaced with smooth silicone gel implants

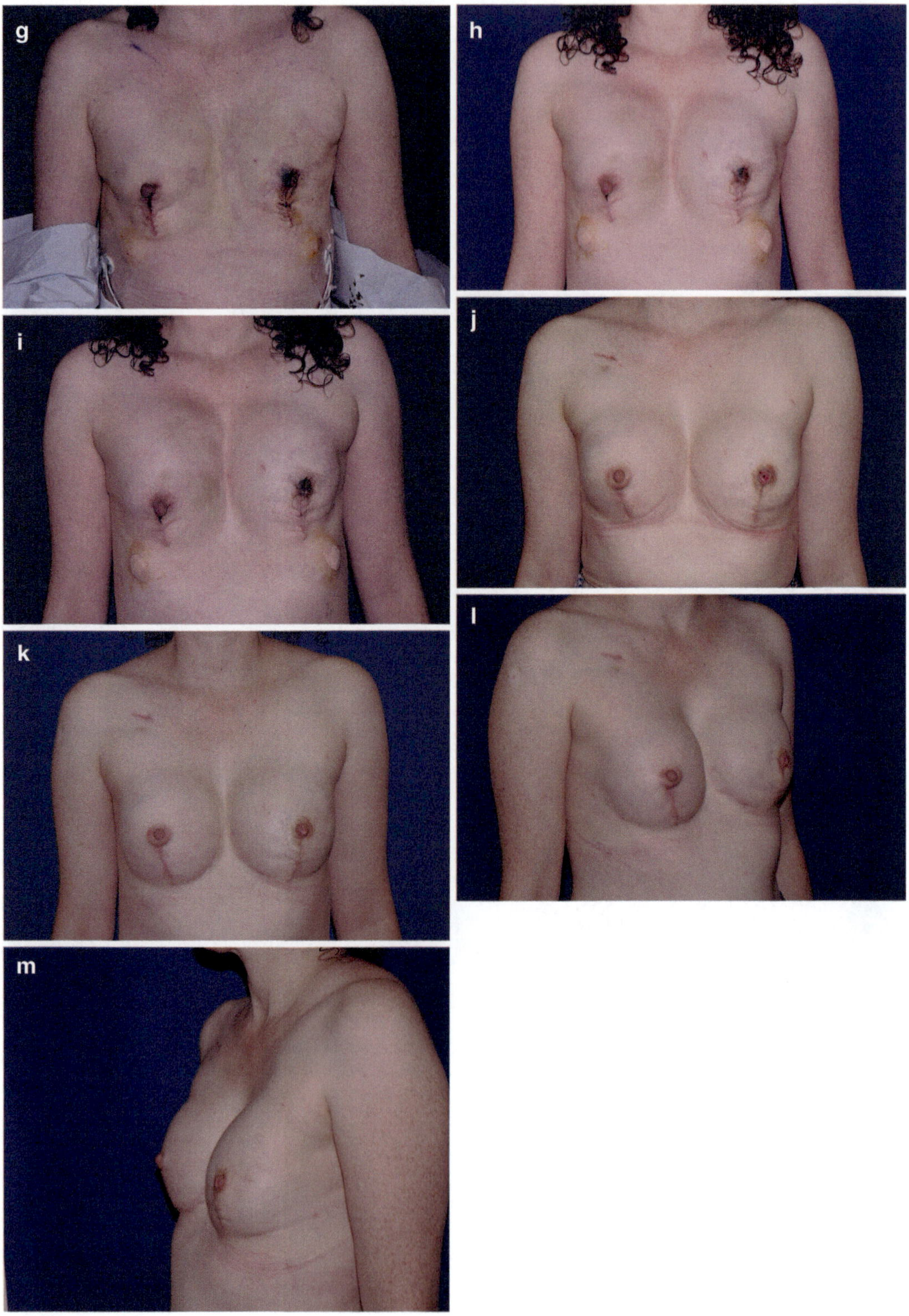

Fig. 12.2 (continued)

12.1 Procedure

All options including prepectoral reconstruction are discussed with the patients.

Once the surgeon has completed the mastectomy, the flaps are assessed. If the flaps are optimal, direct to gel implant, prepectoral reconstruction can be considered. If the flaps are sub-optimal or there is concern about the circulation, a spacer will be inserted.

SPY (Indocyanine) imaging is not used, as delaying of the skin flap provides an opportunity for circulation to the flaps to recover, thus enabling retention of a flap that may otherwise be sacrificed due to poor circulation.

The lateral pocket and entrance to the axilla are closed off with 2-0 Vicryl sutures, thus restoring the lateral breast fold.

Two drains are placed through long subcutaneous tunnels and sutured to the skin.

Hemostasis is checked, and the pocket irrigated with triple antibiotic solution.

The smooth adjustable implant is then prepared for insertion. The implant can be placed in the pocket without ADM or mesh support.

Where necessary anterior sheet of fully-resorbable, mono-filamentous mesh such as DuraSorb (SIA) is used. It has been found that a double layer of mesh results in a 3-dimensional effect matching capsule thickness otherwise achieved using ADM [12].

Recently, the double layered mesh is impregnated with PRP and fat, thus Fat SVF simulating a biological mesh (Fig. 12.3).

As the implant is pre-filled with air, the desired amount of air is removed, and the underfilled implant is then placed in the pocket. The filling tube is cut to the desired length and attached to the injection port. The mesh is sutured to the upper pole of the pectoralis muscle with Stratafix (Ethicon) sutures (Fig. 12.3e). The injection port is placed in a subcutaneous pocket lateral to the incision and secured with one or two Vicryl sutures (Fig. 12.4). The skin edges are then approximated in layers using 3/0 Vicryl to the subcutaneous layer and two rows of 4-0 Monocryl (Ethicon) to the skin.

A Biopatch (Ethicon) and Tegaderm (3 M) dressing is applied to the drain.

A large Tegaderm dressing is placed over the skin flap together with a light cotton gauze dressing.

The flap is assessed the following day, and additional air is injected/added to the implant by means of a 23 g butterfly needle inserted into the injection port. A sterile 0.2-μm syringe filter is used when air is added. When the fill is adequate for the patient, the air is replaced with saline.

Should wound edge necrosis occur, the spacer is emptied, and debridement carried out. Secondary skin closure is usually successful as tension on the skin flap is minimized (Fig. 12.3).

Once the correct size and shape of the breast have been achieved, the injection port can be removed. Port removal is usually done under local anesthesia. The original mastectomy incision is used, and dissection carried down to the port. The port is partially retrieved, and the connection on the filling tube retracted. The filling tube is grasped distal to the connector and removed from the self-sealing valve on the implant.

If the patient is scheduled for radiation, it is preferable to leave the injection port in position until radiation is complete. The implant volume can be adjusted to meet the radiation requirements. At the completion of radiation, the implant can be over expanded for a few weeks to help reduce capsular contracture.

Fat grafting is performed to thicken the flaps if needed (Fig. 12.5).

If rippling persists, the saline implant can be replaced with a smooth silicone gel implant. At this stage, mesh and/or fat grafting can also be performed.

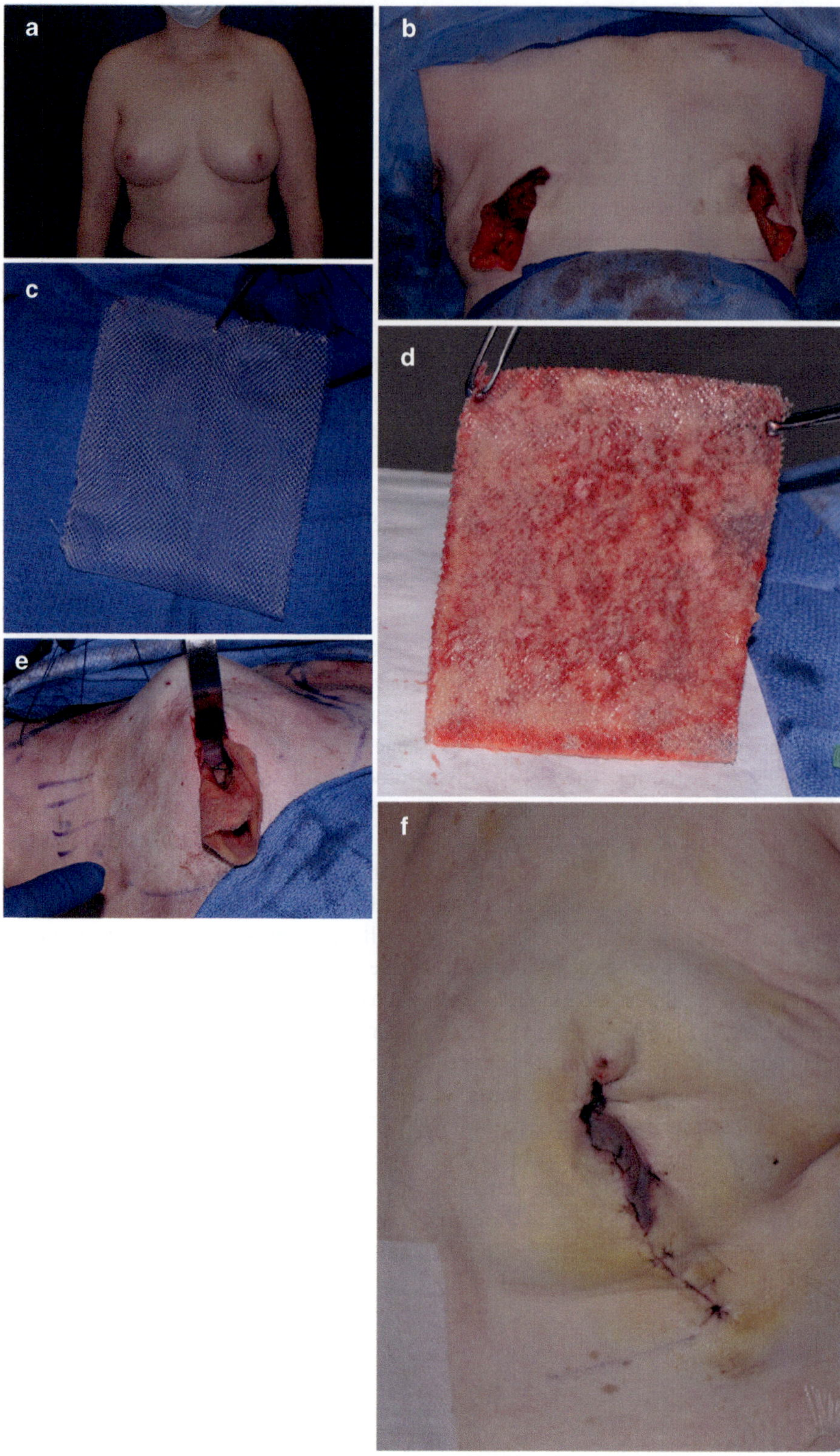

Fig. 12.3 (**a**) 33 year old patient with r Breast carcinoma and BRCA positive. JPG. (**b**) Following bilateral mastectomy. (**c**) Double layered mesh. (**d**) d (Bio-mesh) Fat/SVF and PRP). (**e**) Insertion of mesh. (**f**) Necrosis at skin edge. (**g**) Following debridement of necrotic flap and secondary closure. (**h**) Circulation improved further air added. (**i**) Air removed and replaced with saline. (**j**) Spacer replaced with gel implant nipple tattoo

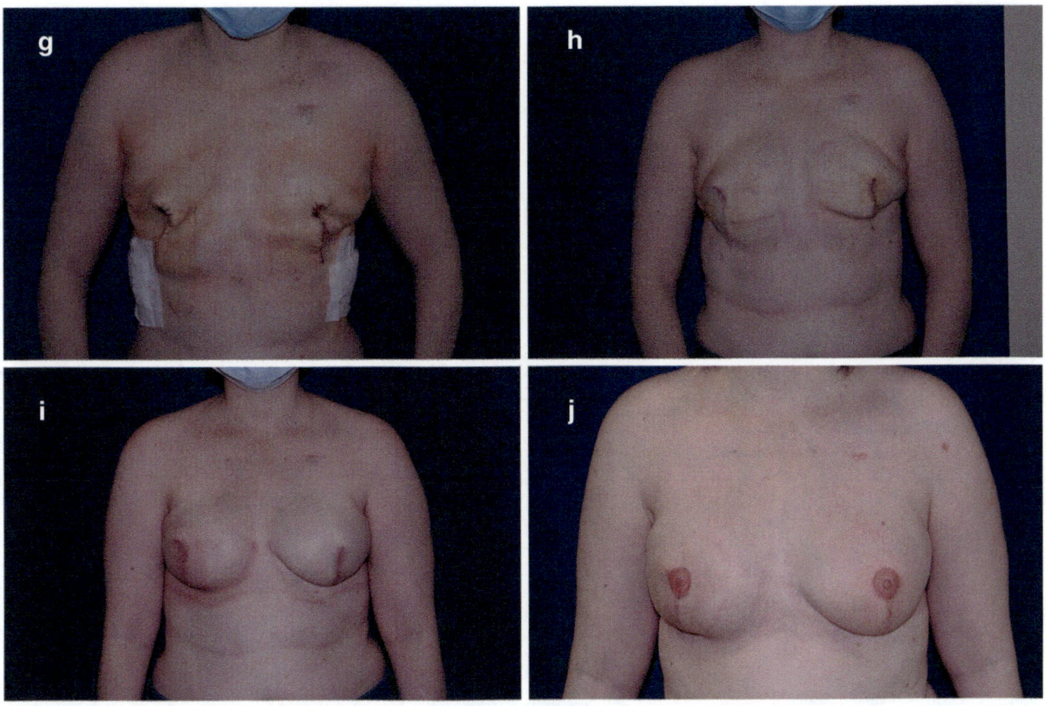

Fig. 12.3 (continued)

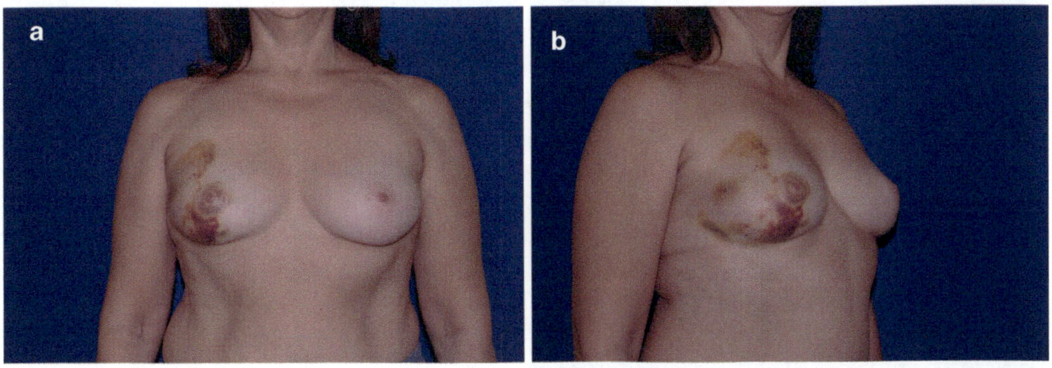

Fig. 12.4 (**a**, **b**) Patient with carcinoma of the R breast (**c**) Spacer containing air (**d**) Spacer placed beneath skin flap (**e**) injection port placed lateral to the incision (**f**) Post operative implant partially filled with air (**g**) Air replaced with saline (**h**, **i**) spacer replaced with silicone gel implant

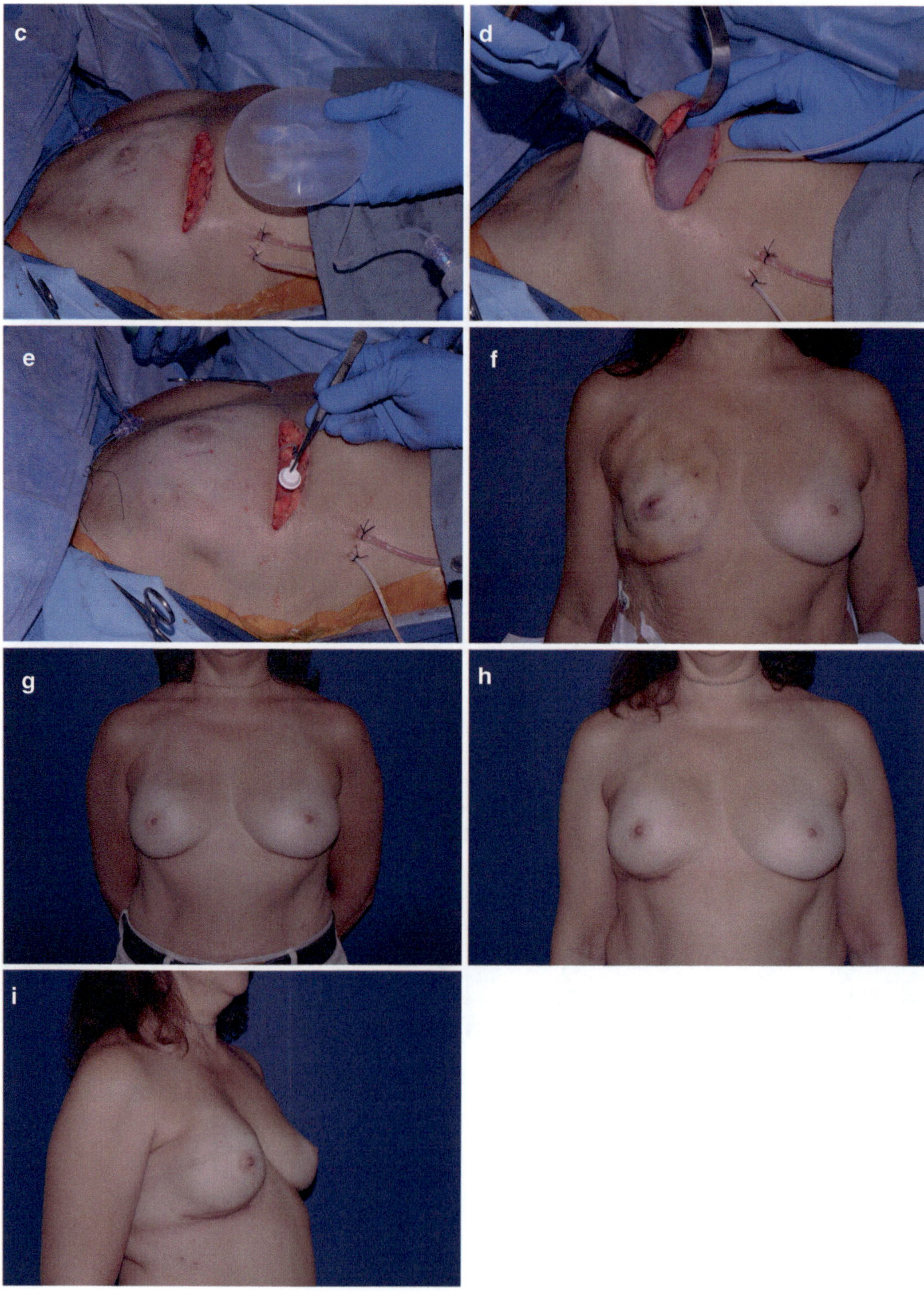

Fig. 12.4 (continued)

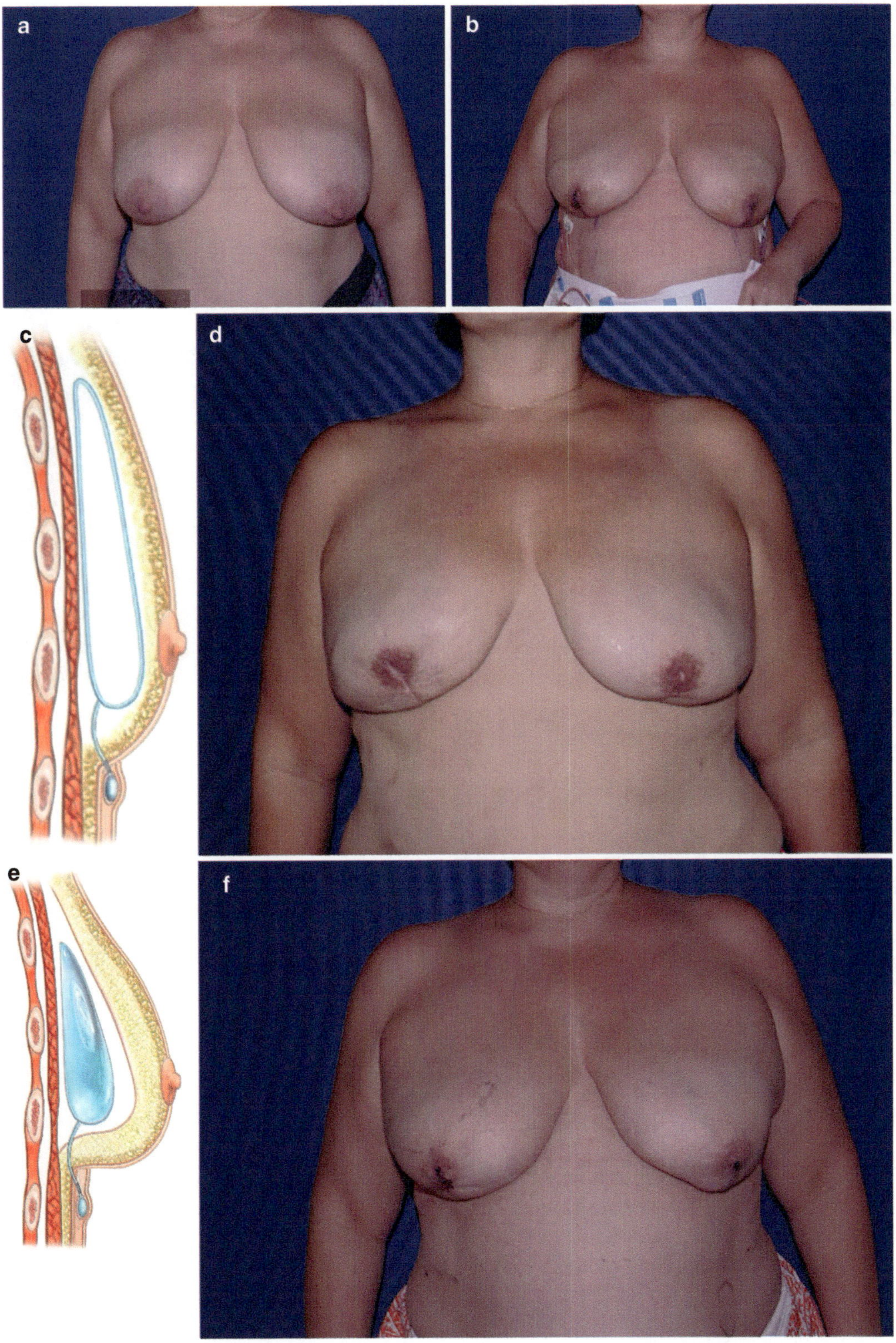

Fig. 12.5 (**a**) Patient with Ca R breast BRCA positive. (**b**, **c**) Following bilateral skin sparing mastectomy. Partially air filled spacer placed pre pectorally. (**d**, **e**) Air replaced with saline, fat graft to skin flap. (**f**, **g**, **h**) Volume of implant reduced further fat grafted. (**i**) implant removed, long term result. (**j**, **k**) Final result

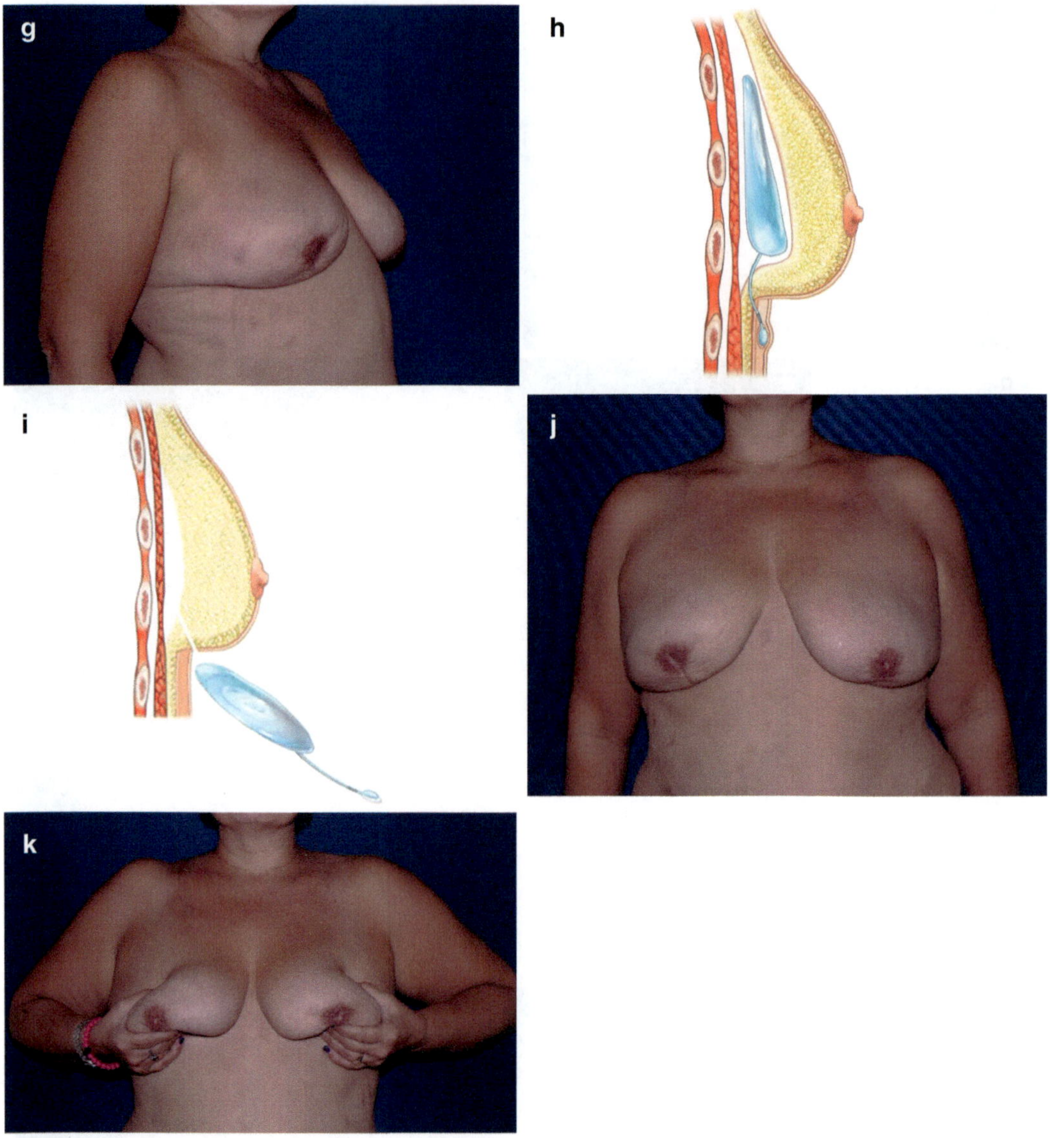

Fig. 12.5 (continued)

12.2 Discussion

Prepectoral breast reconstruction is becoming the procedure of choice in immediate breast reconstruction. When skin flaps are sub-optimal, most surgeons will assess the flaps with indocyanine imaging. If circulatory compromise is seen, the surgeon may debride the flap or place the implant in the submuscular position. Alternatively, delayed or immediate delayed reconstruction can be performed, thus allowing the circulation to recover thereby avoiding unnecessary skin excision.

In a similar fashion placement of a spacer (adjustable implant) at the time of reconstruction allows for the delay effect flap, thus giving the flap the benefit of the doubt, and allowing the circulation to recover.

Immediate breast reconstruction carries a relatively high risk. Prepectoral placement carries additional risks especially for patients with sub-optimal flaps. Therefore, all possible means of risk reduction need to be considered:

1. Minimal flap manipulation: No further skin incision on the compromised flap. The nipple–areolar complex is not elevated at the initial procedure.
2. Placement of a smooth spacer deflated: It is felt that a smooth surface has less immediate complications such as seroma or infections compared to a textured implant. The adjustable implant is partially filled with air or deflated from its packaged state. This results in a more even surface with no pooling of saline at the bottom of the implant [13, 14].
3. Further filling is done when circulation is assured.
4. Use of a fine, long-term absorbable (by 1 year), monofilament mesh has proven to be very beneficial having virtually no infections. Two layers are often used to create a 3-dimensational lattice. Which can be further enhanced with fat and or PRP.
5. Tension-free flap closure.

12.3 Poorly Vascularized Portions of the Flap Are Not Excised at the Time of the Mastectomy

The incision is closed tension-free giving the flaps the opportunity to recover. Should wound edge debridement be necessary, the implant is emptied, and secondary wound closure completed without tension on the incision.

By leaving the implant underfilled with air, the pocket contracts, resulting in elevation and thickening of the flap [15].

One of the remaining problems encountered with prepectoral implant reconstruction is loss of upper pole fullness due to the absence of the pectoral muscle. Suturing multiple layers of DuraSorb (SIA) mesh impregnated with Fat/SVF and PRP (Bio-Mesh) to the upper pectoralis major muscle extending to the upper edge of the areola helps correct the deficient upper pole (Fig. 12.3).

12.4 Conclusion

Prepectoral reconstruction usually requires robust thick flaps for optimal results. The use of a “Spacer” should be considered is cases where breast flaps are sub-optimal following mastectomy.

Additional thickening of the flap can be achieved by allowing natural skin contraction to take place, delayed fat grafting and placement of a multiple layer of long-term absorbable, monofilament mesh.

References

1. Sbitany H, Piper M, Lentz R. Prepectoral breast reconstruction: a safe alternative to submuscular prosthetic reconstruction following nipple-sparing mastectomy. Plast Reconstr Surg. 2017;140(3):432–43.
2. Vidya R, Iqbal FM. A guide to prepectoral breast reconstruction: a new dimension to implant-based breast reconstruction. Clin Breast Cancer. 2017;17(4):266–71.
3. Becker H, Lind JG 2nd, Hopkins EG. Immediate implant-based prepectoral breast reconstruction using a vertical incision. Plast Reconstr Surg Glob Open. 2015;3(6):e412.
4. Ter Louw RP, Nahabedian MY. Prepectoral breast reconstruction. Plast Reconstr Surg. 2017;140(5 Suppl):51S–9S.
5. Eskenazi LB. New options for immediate reconstruction: achieving optimal results with adjustable implants in a single stage. Plast Reconstr Surg. 2007;119:28–37.
6. Woo A, Harless C, Jacobson SR. Revisiting an old place: single-surgeon experience on post-mastectomy subcutaneous implant-based breast reconstruction. Breast J. 2017;23:545–53.
7. The aesthetic meeting 20/20 april Aesthetic Breast Reconstruction Co-Chairs: Nolan Karp, MD and John Kim, MD: Pre-Pectoral Breast Reconstruction.
8. Hilton Becker MD. Correction of animation deformity. Plastic surgery pulse news. 2017;7(1).
9. Zenn MR. Staged immediate breast reconstruction. Plast Reconstr Surg. 2015;135(4):976–9.
10. Mayer HF, editor. Breast reconstruction: modern and promising surgical techniques. Springer Nature; 2020.
11. Becker H. Breast reconstruction using an inflatable breast implant with detachable reservoir. Plast Reconstr Surg. 1984;73:678–3.

12. Becker H, Zhadan O. Filling the spectrum expander with air—a new alternative. Plast Reconstr Surg Glob Open. 2017;6:e1541.
13. Becker H, Carlisle H, Kay J. Filling of adjustable breast implants beyond the manufacturer's recommended fill volume. Aesthetic Plast Surg. 2008;32(3):432–41.
14. 15 Tissue Contraction—A New Paradigm in Breast Reconstruction Hilton Becker, MD, FACS*†‡ Olga Zhadan, MD, MS §PRS Global Open • 2018.
15. Becker H, Maraist F. Immediate breast reconstruction after mastectomy using a permanent tissue expander. South Med J. 1987;80(2):154–60.

13 Synthetic Meshes in Prepectoral Breast Reconstruction

D. Casella, J. Kaciulyte, V. Restaino, F. Lo Torto, and M. Marcasciano

13.1 Introduction

Prepectoral immediate breast reconstruction (IBR) was introduced in 1971 by Snyderman and Guthrie [1]. It was acknowledged as a great advancement in prosthetic breast reconstruction, as it allowed shorter recovery period and major patients' satisfaction, when compared to traditional submuscular reconstruction [2]. Despite the expected benefits, subcutaneous heterologous reconstructions have been soon associated with elevated incidences of capsular contracture, implant visibility, palpability, rippling, high risk of mastectomy skin flap necrosis, and implant extrusion. The introduction of synthetic meshes (SM) and acellular dermal matrixes (ADM) progressively affirmed the concept of complete prosthesis wrapping, thus opening new horizons in implant-based procedures and in particular, prepectoral breast reconstruction.

D. Casella (✉) · V. Restaino
Department of Breast Cancer Surgery, UOC Chirurgia Oncologica Della Mammella, Azienda Ospedaliero-Universitaria Senese, University Hospital of Siena, Siena, Italy

J. Kaciulyte · F. L. Torto
Department of Surgery "P.Valdoni", Unit of Plastic and Reconstructive Surgery, Sapienza University of Rome, Policlinico Umberto I, Roma, Italy

M. Marcasciano
Experimental and Clinical Medicine Department, Division of Plastic and Reconstructive Surgery, "Magna Graecia" University of Catanzaro Germaneto, Catanzaro, Italy

In 2013, Cheng et al. [3] reported for the first time the treatment of capsular contracture following retro-muscular breast reconstructions with the introduction of a novel surgical technique using acellular dermal matrix to completely cover anteriorly a new breast implant.

In 2014, as far as we know, for the first time breast implants completely wrapped by a titanium-coated polypropylene mesh (TCPM) have been placed in a subcutaneous pocket, in a series of patients diagnosed with breast cancer and undergoing skin- or nipple-sparing mastectomy [4].

Either ADM or synthetic meshes are considered safe devices and show good aesthetic and functional outcomes in prepectoral IBR [5]. Subcutaneous breast reconstruction reduces morbidity and preserves breast natural anatomy, by sparing muscles. The support of wrapping devices allows a complete coverage of the implant, thus avoiding its direct contact with the mastectomy flaps.

If compared to the traditional submuscular procedures, prepectoral approach significantly reduces postoperative pain and surgical time. Moreover, literature registers mainly excellent cosmetic outcomes and complication rates that appear to be similar nowadays [6].

To date, as a matter of fact, a gold standard procedure suitable for every patients does not exist. Indeed, either subpectoral or prepectoral breast reconstruction can lead to good results. Nevertheless, a thorough understanding of the benefits and drawbacks of every single technique is necessary, in order to offer every single patient

© The Author(s), under exclusive license to Springer Nature Switzerland AG 2023
R. Vidya, H. Becker (eds.), *Prepectoral Breast Reconstruction*,
https://doi.org/10.1007/978-3-031-15590-1_13

the best reconstructive approach, tailored on physiological and anamnestic characteristics.

Prepectoral breast reconstruction as any other procedure presents limitations: valid skin flaps' vascular support and consistent subcutaneous thickness are primary conditions for a comprehensive success. A major risk of implant exposure and reconstructive failure is described for patients with poor soft tissue quality, as a consequence of compromised skin flaps or microvascular circulation [7].

Accurate preoperative planning and proper patient selection are always critical to achieve surgical success; they become mandatory when dealing with prepectoral breast reconstruction [8].

Since the introduction of the Halstead radical mastectomy in 1882, more conservative breast oncologic surgeries have been developed, aiming to spare the skin and the nipple–areola complex. Umberto Veronesi introduced an important shift towards less invasive surgeries, "from maximum tolerable treatment to minimum effective treatment." [9] The recent concepts of the "*aesthetic cancer cure*" and "*oncoplastic surgery*" followed as natural consequence of this trend, showing a dynamic way of patient's care, with efficacious cancer surgery together with preservation or improvement of the breast aesthetic [10].

Prepectoral breast reconstruction technique goes along with this modern approach. Lately advances in implant material and surgical devices such as SM made this technique reliable, safe, and aesthetically feasible, with low and acceptable overall complication rates [11].

13.2 Patients' Selection

Accurate patient selection is mandatory, along with a tight screening of the multiple pre and intraoperative variables. Surgical risks should be assessed with a precise and personalized method and, in this regard, literature offers several reports that should help surgeons in the decision-making process and on the feasibility of prepectoral breast reconstruction. In 2017, Rancati et al. [12] proposed an algorithm that focuses on preoperative flap thickness evaluation through the use of digital mammograms, to orient the surgical planning. Similarly, Mlodinow et al. [13] introduced the Breast Reconstruction Risk Assessment (BRA) Score, to estimate the postoperative complication risk in both autologous and implant-based IBR procedures. In 2019, Vidya et al. [14] proposed an international consensus signed by European and USA breast and plastic reconstructive surgeons, that may act as a guide guide to prepectoral breast reconstruction, with particular emphasis on patient selection, technique, and postoperative outcomes. Despite these useful tools, there is still no consensus on the definitive criteria to be used for the identification of patients suitable for subcutaneous breast reconstruction and eventually, to accurately foresee the best candidate for direct-to-implant (DTI), or two-stage reconstruction with tissue expander. Numerous variables are to be considered before going Prepec, in order to eventually predict the risk of mastectomy flaps ischemic stress or necrosis. Patients global health evaluation including full personal history and general clinical exams is mandatory. Elderly as well as patients with non-regular BMI, active smokers or suffering for diabetes mellitus will present a potentially compromised microvascular circulation, with an increased risk of skin flap necrosis and extrusion or infection of the implant [15–17]. Alike, evidence of breast ptosis requiring skin-reducing mastectomy is associated with an increased risk of implant exposure at the inframammary fold [18].

Patient's medical history has to be scrupulous, as previous breast surgeries and previous radiotherapies are associated with high risk of wound dehiscence and infection [19]. Intraoperative evaluation of mastectomy skin flap thickness and potential viability is also crucial: reasonable thickness with moderate and vascularized subcutaneous fat is favorable as they are associated with more successful outcomes [20]. Recently, indocyanine green fluorescence angiography has been proposed as a reliable, objective assessment method for postmastectomy skin flaps viability evaluation. Nevertheless, it is claimed to be a quite expensive procedure and not everywhere at disposal for the breast surgeons. Moreover, there is still a lack of high-quality evidence proving its superiority to an accurate clinical intraoperative exam, and larger studies are required to impulse the spreading of this innovative technique [21].

13.3 Synthetic Meshes

The recent shift of the reconstructive trends from submuscular to the prepectoral approach has occurred mainly as a consequence of the development of new technologies and improvement of synthetic and biological devices, together with the advances in autologous fat grafting techniques [22]. Synthetic meshes were introduced in breast surgery almost 20 years ago [23]. If compared to ADMs, they offer good strength and pliability, at lower price, nevertheless it has been stated that surgeons present a significant learning curve in performing breast reconstruction with meshes [24]. SM provide a complete implant envelope and act like an additional layer between the prosthesis and the subcutaneous tissue, stimulating the formation of a sort of "neo-fascia" [25].

SM are flexible absorbable, partially absorbable or non-absorbable sheets providing tensile support to the implant. There is a compromise between strength and elasticity, as with strength increase, elastic properties lower and inflammatory response may rise [26]. Mesh incorporation capacity into the surrounding tissues derives from its pore sizes. Ingrowth and fibrous tissue formation appear to be directly associated with pores' diameter [26]. Strength and flexibility properties derive from SM creation process, consisting in knitting or weaving. Stronger meshes are generally woven, for high density of fibers. On the other side, knitted meshes are characterized by porosity and flexibility [27].

Table 13.1 resumes the specific characteristics of the main SM used in breast reconstruction field [28–33].

Absorbable meshes present various absorption timing, from few months (Copolymer of glycolide and lactide - Vicryl) [34] to 2 or 3 years (Seri Surgical Scaffold, TIGR Matrix) [35, 36]. The rational for long-term absorption is the dual presence of fast degrading fiber to give extra support during the wound healing phase, while the slow absorbing fibers support the implant for years [37]. Seri Surgical Scaffold is made of silk and behaves more like an ADM since its incorporation is followed by new tissue formation, to which its strength is transferred [38, 39].

Among the non-absorbable meshes, only those made of polypropylene (PP) are used for breast reconstruction (TiLOOP Bra and Pocket, TiO2Mesh BRA) [40, 41]. Finally, some meshes are made of hybrid material and they are partially absorbable (ULTRAPRO pro, SERAGYN BR)

Table 13.1 Synthetic meshes for breast reconstruction

Absorbable polymers		Material source	Absorption time	Final tensile strenght (Newton or Newton/cm)	Literature reference in breast reconstruction
	Vicryl mesh	Copolymer of glycolide and lactide	3 months	–	Faulkner et al. [29]
	Seargyn BR (partially absorbable)	Polyglycol acid-caprolacton and polypropylene	3–4 months	41 N/cm	Machleidt et al. [31]
	ULTRAPRO (partially absorbable)	Poliglecaprone-25 monofilament and nonabsorbable polypropylene	3–4 months	–	József et al. [32]
	Seri Surgical Scaffold	Silk	2 years	99.7 N	van Turnhout et al. [28]
	TIGR Matrix	Copolymer of lactide, glycolide and trimethylene carbonate	3 years	86.6 N/cm	Hallberg et al. [33]
Non-absorbable titanium-coated polymers					
	TiLOOP Bra	Titanium-coated polypropylene	–	37 N/cm	Casella et al. [30]
	TiO_2 Mesh Bra	Monofilament polypropylene with titanium oxide surface	–	–	–

[31, 42]. Recently, Eichler et al. [43] carried out a comparative study between the non-absorbable TiLOOP mesh and the partially absorbable Seragyn. According to their findings, there was no significant difference in complication rates between the two devices. Moreover, they showed comparable overall implant loss rates to the considerably more expensive ADMs based reconstructions.

Many years ago, our group somehow pioneered the use of TiLoop® Bra meshes (TiLoop® Bra, pfm medical, Cologne, Germany) in prepectoral breast reconstruction, sharing the experience in several papers [44–47]. This ready-to-use mesh does not require any rehydration, is made of non-resorbable titanized type 1a polypropylene and it has been introduced and approved for surgical use. Recently, it has been introduced an upgrade version of the mesh, as a pre-shaped pocket with the aim to ease the device positioning over the implant and to achieve intraoperative time shortening. As all synthetic meshes with titanized surface, it helps to achieve good cell growth and it decreases scarring, shrinkage, inflammation, and capsular contracture rate [48–50].

13.4 Surgical Technique

Breast unit surgical team is usually composed by general and plastic surgeons, who provide independent skills. However, it has been pointed out that a single surgeon, dual-trained in breast oncology and plastic surgery could handle the entire surgical treatment. This thorough figure benefits from a comprehensive understanding of the breast cancer treatment, leading to wider offer of surgical options and higher rates of successful outcomes [51]. In our experience, all prepectoral breast reconstructions either with definitive or temporary implants are always performed by a dual-trained surgeon, taking care of the oncological and the reconstructive step at once [52].

Preoperative full patient evaluation is mandatory. Prepectoral reconstruction is scheduled if viable and reliable mastectomy skin flaps are foreseen, still keeping in mind the possibility to switch into submuscular plane, after intraoperative evaluation. Markings are drawn with the patient in an upright position and including the middle and parasternal lines, inframammary folds, and the incision site. Depending on oncological features, tumor location, patients, and breast characteristics, surgeons may choose among inframammary fold, inverted T, "Italic S," or peri-areolar access for mastectomy. Skin flaps are raised in the subdermal plane. Dissection is performed through the suspensory ligaments of Cooper, and margins bleeding and flap viability are carefully evaluated before placing a prepectoral definitive prosthesis. In case of thin or questionable skin flaps, two step reconstruction with temporary expanders represents the first choice.

In fact, when skin coverage after nipple-sparing mastectomy appears too feeble to support a definitive prosthesis, a tissue expander is inserted as a temporary spacer.

The 30% of subcutaneous pocket is filled, to avoid stress over skin flaps while complete tissue healing is reached. Tissue expanders have a slightly different role if placed after skin-sparing mastectomies. They are progressively filled in order to create an adequate cutaneous coverage for the definitive implant. In either DTI or two-stage reconstructions, SM is folded onto the implants and is sutured to the pectoralis major fascia with apical, medial, and lateral stitches. Moderate compression is applied with wound dressing immediately after surgery and it is substituted with post-surgical bra for about 60 days. When indicated, especially after skin-reducing mastectomies or procedures performed in patients with higher risk of developing postoperative complications, negative pressure wound dressings (e.g., PICO, Smith & Nephew, London, UK) may be applied in order to prevent wound complications, reduce cicatrization time, and minimize the number of postoperative accesses [53].

In cases of a two-stage reconstruction, the first postoperative expansion is usually scheduled 3 weeks following discharge.

13.5 Autologous Adipose Tissue Grafting

Since 2007, when Rigotti et al. [54] first showed the beneficial effects of fat grafting, the procedure gained importance in breast reconstructive surgery and nowadays, it became an integral part of the prepectoral reconstructive path. Autologous adipose tissue contains stem/progenitor cells (ASC) in the stromal vascular fraction and may be easily harvested from multiple donor sites. Once injected, ASC organize and differentiate, thus promoting the secretion of soluble factors that enhance angiogenesis, decrease apoptosis, and/or modulate the immune response [55]. These characteristics are exploited to manage or prevent postoperative complications such as rippling, capsular contracture, infection, ulceration, and implant exposure, that are eventually associated with breast reconstructive surgery or radiotherapy as well [56]. In this regard, specific protocols with autologous fat grafting have been developed either for prepectoral and submuscular breast reconstructions, as ASC have proven being oncologically safe and not increasing the likelihood of oncologic recurrence [57].

The timing of fat grafting in the setting of expander/implant-based breast reconstruction is debated, and several protocols have been proposed [58, 59].

Nevertheless there is still a lack of info regarding fat grafting protocols following prepectoral breast surgery. In our experience, when a tissue expander wrapped in a synthetic mesh is placed subcutaneously, a session of lipofilling may be performed during the second reconstructive step, and only eventually repeated. In this way, three surgical procedures (two plus one) are shrinked into the classic two steps. The quality of the mastectomy flaps that will cover the definitive implant is enhanced, while implant superficialization, capsular contracture, rippling, and wrinkling may be prevented, resulting in better aesthetic and functional outcomes. In patients who underwent postoperative radiotherapy, fat grafting is particularly beneficial, as it is related to lower rates of local infection/ulceration, extrusion of the implant and capsular contracture, achieving comparable results to those of reconstructed patients who did not receive radiotherapy [60].

13.6 Complications

Prepectoral approach is safe, fast, and easy to perform and well tolerated by patients. Nevertheless it is not without drawbacks. According to a recent systematic review, capsular contracture is the most common complication following prepectoral breast reconstruction, with an incidence up to 8.8% [61]. Capsular contracture physiopathology is considered a multifactorial process, resulting from human body reaction, biofilm activation, bacteremic seeding, or silicone exposure. It frequently follows breast radiation therapy, leading to breast distortion, pain, and unsatisfactory aesthetic appearance [56]. As already mentioned, fat grafting may help preventing or managing early capsular contracture stages, nevertheless reoperation with capsulotomy or capsulectomy and implant exchange may be required [62, 63]. According to Sinnott et al., prepectoral breast reconstructions show three times lower incidence of capsular contracture following radiation therapy, if compared to submuscular ones (16.1% versus 52.2%) [64].

This difference in post-radiotherapy contracture rates may be the consequence of a particularly fibrotic, radiated muscle, applying additional force to the implant and resulting in displacement and capsular contracture [65].

On the other hand, missing the muscular cover, another concern is represented by the risk of visible implant rippling as a consequence of thin or inconsistent mastectomy flaps, especially at the upper and medial poles. Rippling and edge visibility are observed in 12.9–19.4% of cases, depending on follow-up length [66]. Fat grafting may mitigate this condition, especially in the upper-medial and lateral quadrants. Keeping in mind that DTI reconstructions are frequently followed by revision procedures as lipofilling, it is important to counsel patients by explaining them that they may need ulterior procedures to reduce rippling and implant visibility.

Other complications such as seroma (5.1%), hematoma (2.4%), and mastectomy flap or NAC necrosis with consequent implant loss (3.3%) are less common but dreadful events [61].

Meticulous hemostasis and thoughtful drain placement may prevent these complications. Seroma may lead to pain, discomfort, or more impacting issues such as infection and mastectomy flap necrosis. Therefore, it should be properly handled and always aspired when necessary. Needle aspiration can be performed under ultrasound guidance or even freehand in case of temporary expanders, by exploiting the safe area around the injection port to drain serum located between the prosthesis and surrounding tissues and simultaneously perform tissue expansion, while preventing accidental ruptures [67].

Mastectomy flap or NAC necrosis is a consequence of vascular impairment due to the oncologic surgical step and eventually, to the excessive pressure applied by the implant on excessively thin and stressed mastectomy flaps. Loss of this overlying soft tissue coverage can be devastating and may result in reconstruction failure. This complication might be prevented or at least decreased with an accurate preoperative patient selection and intraoperative evaluation of mastectomy skin flap viability, (indocyanine green tissue perfusion assessment). As stated before, in cases of questionable skin flaps' reliability, we suggest to defer DTI and switch to a two-stage reconstruction with tissue expanders. Peri-prosthetic infection rates range from 1.1–2.5% to 35%, depending on the implant insertion site and reason [68].

Although infection incidence is similar in submuscular and prepectoral breast reconstructions [69], in the last case there is very little information published in literature and no consensus on its management protocols. Traditional strategies consist in antibiotic administration and revision surgery with partial or complete capsulectomy and implant discharge, in order to remove colonized tissues [70]. When revising a prepectoral pocket, capsule's proximity to the skin brings the risk of excessive tissue thinning and compromise of skin flaps vitality. In this regard, pulse lavage appears to be a useful tool, thanks to its ability to alternatively eject and aspirate a flow of sterile saline solution, thus performing a hydrodynamic cleansing [71–73]. When dealing with prepectoral implant infection, we apply pulse lavage during the breast expander removal. Accurate debridement and bonification of the subcutaneous pocket are carried out. Accordingly, the definitive implant is placed in a new clean setup, thus sparing further surgical steps. Finally, Red Breast Syndrome is an idiopathic temporary postoperative erythema that has been described only after breast reconstructions with ADMs, with an incidence being reported as high as 7.6%. The condition may mimic cellulitis, with possible presence of pruritus and pain, associated with absence of clinical findings of infection [74]. To date, there is only one report that describes a single case of Red Breast Syndrome that followed an immediate IBR with synthetic polyglycolic acid mesh, and resolved spontaneously [75].

Prepectoral implant-based breast reconstruction with SM can provide excellent results; however, a comprehensive identification of its inclusion criteria and a thorough acquaintance with possible complications and their management is crucial to achieve successful outcomes.

13.7 Review of Short Literature to Date

Breast reconstruction presents a variety of options, from autologous tissues to prosthetic devices. Since the introduction of silicone gel breast implants in 1960s, IBR became the most common, being performed in 70% of cases, nowadays [76]. Along with reconstructive techniques, breast oncologic surgery developed and conservative approaches are favored nowadays, thus withdrawing the olden demolitive Halstead approach of the nineteenth century [77].

Breast oncologic and reconstructive surgeries have evolved together over time, along with innovative implants and covering devices, technologies to assess flap perfusion and combination with well-known techniques as fat grafting allowed to improve surgical outcomes. In particular, implant-covering devices (ADMs and SM) were introduced in 2006 and played a significant role in giving new perspectives to prepectoral breast reconstruction [78].

Prepectoral breast reconstruction implies implant positioning in its anatomical plane, with minimized morbidity and good cosmesis. As its resurgence is relatively recent, literature dealing with prepectoral breast reconstruction with SM shows narrow follow-up and limited long-term outcomes [79]. The first report on the use of a synthetic mesh in breast reconstruction was published in 1997, by Rietjens et al. [80] Nevertheless, it describes a series of subpectoral implant-based reconstructions, alike the majority of the articles at disposal in literature, in which SM are placed to reinforce the lateral-inferior pole of the submuscular prosthesis.

Concerning the SM use in prepectoral breast reconstruction, Reitsamer et al. [81] described successful outcomes in their 200 cases of IBR with either ADM or absorbable TIGR SM, with a mean follow-up of 36 months. Similarly, Casella et al. [30] reported satisfactory patient-related and aesthetic results with TiLoop SM, with low-complication rates, in an even longer mean follow-up period (38.5 months).

Investigations have been conducted to compare complications' incidence between prepectoral and submuscular breast reconstructions, showing similar infection, skin necrosis, and seroma rates [82]. Other reports aimed to widen prepectoral reconstruction application. Caputo et al. [83] described successful results in patients requiring significant skin reduction, and Marcasciano et al. [84] reported similar results in skin-reduction breast reconstructions with prepectoral implant covered by a combination of lower dermal flap and synthetic mesh.

Innovation and continuous evolution characterize modern oncologic breast surgery. Salibian et al. [85] reported that viable and well represented mastectomy skin flaps and strict preservation of the native inframammary fold may obviate the need for implant-covering devices.

As the quality of breast reconstructive result raises and gains importance, modern breast surgeons have to face the importance of continuous update and interspecialty collaboration, as innovation and improvement do not come from isolated work, rather from cooperation and sharing of ideas and knowledge. According to recent literature, a shift in healthcare culture is taking place, with increased patient's participation and attention to reconstructive outcomes and their impact on patient's quality of life [86]. Even in hazardous times as the actual Covid-19 pandemic, research, and sharing knowledge must not stop and breast surgeons may find modern ways to connect, update, and improve, in order to keep providing the best treatment options for their patients [87]. Indeed, prepectoral breast reconstruction revival is the example of how scientific research that may advance not only with new inventions, but also by revisiting old places and refining historical techniques.

13.8 Summary with Tips

- Implant-based breast reconstruction represents the most common approach following mastectomy.
- Traditionally, submuscular breast reconstruction was considered the gold standard technique.
- The introduction of ADMs and SM progressively affirmed the concept of complete prosthesis wrapping, opening new horizons in implant-based procedures, and giving new revival to prepectoral breast reconstruction.
- Subcutaneous breast reconstruction with SM spares muscles, therefore postoperative pain and surgical time are reduced. Cosmetic outcomes are improved while complication rates appear to be similar to submuscular reconstructions.
- The necessity of valid skin vascular support and consistent mastectomy flaps may represent a limitation to prepectoral breast reconstruction. Thus, accurate preoperative planning and proper patient selection are crucial.
- Autologous fat grafting should be considered an integral part of the prepectoral reconstructive path. It is proven to reduce postoperative complications such as rippling, capsular contracture, infection, ulceration, and risk of implant exposure.

References

1. Snyderman RK, Guthrie RH. Reconstruction of the female breast following radical mastectomy. Plast Reconstr Surg. 1971;47:565–7.
2. Kobraei EM, Cauley R, Gadd M, Austen WG Jr, Liao EC. Avoiding breast animation deformity with

pectoralis-sparing subcutaneous direct-to-implant breast reconstruction. Plast Reconstr Surg Glob Open. 2016;4:e708.
3. Cheng A, Lakhiani C, Saint-Cyr M. Treatment of capsular contracture using complete implant coverage by acellular dermal matrix: a novel technique. Plast Reconstr Surg. 2013;132:519–29.
4. Casella D, Bernini M, Benci ni L, Roselli J, Lacaria MT, Martellucci J, Banfi R, Calabrese C, Orzalesi L. TiLoop® bra mesh used for immediate breast reconstruction: comparison of retropectoral and subcutaneous implant placement in a prospective single institution series. Eur J Plast Surg. 2014;37:599–604.
5. Lo Torto F, Cigna E, Kaciulyte J, Casella D, Marcasciano M, Ribuffo D. National breast reconstruction utilization in the setting of postmastectomy radiotherapy: two-stage implant-based breast reconstruction. J Reconstr Microsurg. 2017;33:e3.
6. Jafferbhoy S, Chandarana M, Houlihan M, Parmeshwar R, Narayanan S, Soumian S, Harries S, Jones L, Clarke D. Early multicentre experience of pre-pectoral implant based immediate breast reconstruction using Braxon®. Gland Surg. 2017;6:682–8.
7. Cattelani L, Polotto S, Arcuri MF, Pedrazzi G, Linguadoca C, Bonati E. One-step prepectoral breast reconstruction with dermal matrix-covered implant compared to submuscular implantation: functional and cost evaluation. Clin Breast Cancer. 2018;18:e703–11.
8. Sbitany H. Important considerations for performing Prepectoral breast reconstruction. Plast Reconstr Surg. 2017;140:7S–13S.
9. Zurrida S, Veronesi U. Milestones in breast cancer treatment. Breast J. 2015;21:3–12.
10. Kaufman CS. Increasing role of oncoplastic surgery for breast cancer. Curr Oncol Rep. 2019;21:111.
11. Maxwell GP, Gabriel A. Bioengineered breast: concept, technique, and preliminary results. Plast Reconstr Surg. 2016;137:415–21.
12. Rancati AO, Angrigiani CH, Hammond DC, Nava MB, Gonzalez EG, Dorr JC, Gercovich GF, Rocco N, Rostagno RL. Direct to implant reconstruction in nipple sparing mastectomy: patient selection by preoperative digital mammogram. Plast Reconstr Surg Glob Open. 2017;5:e1369.
13. Mlodinow AS, Lanier ST, Galiano RD, Kim JYS. Using the breast reconstruction risk assessment (BRA) score: an individualized risk calculator to assist expectation management and reconstructive decision making in the mastectomy patient. In: Harness J, Willey S, editors. Operative approaches to nipple-sparing mastectomy. Springer: Cham; 2017. p. 117–26.
14. Vidya R, Berna G, Sbitany H, Nahabedian M, Becker H, Reitsamer R, Rancati A, Macmillan D, Cawthorn S. Prepectoral implant-based breast reconstruction: a joint consensus guide from UK, European and USA breast and plastic reconstructive surgeons. Ecancermedicalscience. 2019;13:927.
15. Srinivasa DR, Holland M, Sbitany H. Optimizing perioperative strategies to maximize success with prepectoral breast reconstruction. Gland Surg. 2019;8:19–26.
16. Gabriel A, Maxwell GP. Prepectoral breast reconstruction in challenging patients. Plast Reconstr Surg. 2017;140:14S–21S.
17. Casella D, Di Taranto G, Lo Torto F, Marcasciano M, Kaciulyte J, Greco M, Onesti MG, Ribuffo D. Body mass index can predict outcomes in DTI prepectoral breast reconstruction. Plast Reconstr Surg. 2020;145:867e–8e.
18. Komorowska-Timek E, Merrifield B, Turfe Z, Davis AT. Subcutaneous prosthetic breast reconstructions following skin reduction mastectomy. Plast Reconstr Surg Glob Open. 2019;7:e2078.
19. Spear SL, Boehmler JH, Bogue DP, Mafi AA. Options in reconstructing the irradiated breast. Plast Reconstr Surg. 2008;122:379–88.
20. Khavanin N, Qiu C, Darrach H, Kraenzlin F, Kokosis G, Han T, Sacks JM. Intraoperative perfusion assessment in mastectomy skin flaps: how close are we to preventing complications? J Reconstr Microsurg. 2019;35:471–8.
21. Pruimboom T, Schols RM, Van Kuijk SM, Van der Hulst RR, Qiu SS. Indocyanine green angiography for preventing postoperative mastectomy skin flap necrosis in immediate breast reconstruction. Cochrane Database Syst Rev. 2020;4:CD013280.
22. Lo Torto F, Relucenti M, Familiari G, Vaia N, Casella D, Matassa R, Miglietta S, Marinozzi F, Bini F, Fratoddi I, Sciubba F, Cassese R, Tombolini V, Ribuffo D. The effect of postmastectomy radiation therapy on breast implants: material analysis on silicone and polyurethane prosthesis. Ann Plast Surg. 2018;81:228–34.
23. Jacobs JM, Salzberg CA. Implant-based breast reconstruction with meshes and matrices: biological vs synthetic. Br J Hosp Med (Lond). 2015;76:211–6.
24. Rolph R, Farhadi J. The use of meshes and matrices in breast reconstruction. Br J Hosp Med (Lond). 2018;79:454–9.
25. Sigalove S, Maxwell GP, Sigalove NM, Storm-Dickerson TL, Pope N, Rice J, Gabriel A. Prepectoral implant- based breast reconstruction: rationale, indications, and preliminary results. Plast Reconstr Surg. 2017;139:287–94.
26. Gómez-Modet S, Tejedor L. Synthetic mesh in immediate breast reconstruction. Breast cancer and breast reconstruction. IntechOpen. 2020. https://doi.org/10.5772/intechopen.90884.
27. Fitzgerald JF, Kumar AS. Biologic versus synthetic mesh reinforcement: what are the pros and cons? Clin Colon Rectal Surg. 2014;27(4):140–8.
28. Van Turnhout AAWM, Franke CJJ, Vriens-Nieuwenhuis EJC, Van der Sluis WB. The use of SERI™ surgical scaffolds in direct-to-implant reconstruction after skin-sparing mastectomy: a retrospective study on surgical outcomes and a systematic

review of current literature. J Plast Reconstr Aesthet Surg. 2018;71:644–50.
29. Faulkner HR, Shikowitz-Behr L, McLeod M, Wright E, Hulsen J, Austen WG Jr. The use of absorbable mesh in implant-based breast reconstruction: a 7-year review. Plast Reconstr Surg. 2020;146:731e–6e.
30. Casella D, Di Taranto G, Marcasciano M, Sordi S, Kothari A, Kovacs T, Lo Torto F, Cigna E, Calabrese C, Ribuffo D. Evaluation of prepectoral implant placement and complete coverage with TiLoop Bra mesh for breast reconstruction: a prospective study on long-term and patient-reported BREAST-Q outcomes. Plast Reconstr Surg. 2019;143:1e–9e.
31. Machleidt A, Schmidt-Feuerheerd N, Blohmer JU, Ohlinger R, Kueper J, von Waldenfels G, Dittmer S, Paepke S, Klein E. Reconstructive breast surgery with partially absorbable bi-component Seragyn® BR soft mesh: an outcome analysis. Arch Gynecol Obstet. 2018;298:755–61.
32. József Z, Újhelyi M, Ping O, Domján S, Fülöp R, Ivády G, Ráchel T, Rubovszky G, Mészáros N, Kenessey I, Mátrai Z. Long-term dynamic changes in cosmetic outcomes and patient satisfaction after implant-based postmastectomy breast reconstruction and contralateral mastopexy with or without an ultrapro mesh sling used for the inner bra technique. A retrospective correlational study. Cancers (Basel). 2020;13:E73.
33. Hallberg H, Lewin R, Elander A, Hansson E. TIGR® matrix surgical mesh - a two-year follow-up study and complication analysis in 65 immediate breast reconstructions. J Plast Surg Hand Surg. 2018;52:253–8.
34. Tessler O, Reish RG, Maman DY, Smith BL, Austen WG Jr. beyond biologics: absorbable mesh as a low-cost, low-complication sling for implant-based breast reconstruction. Plast Reconstr Surg. 2014;133:90–9.
35. Cuffolo G, Holford NC, Contractor K, Tenovici A. TIGR matrix for implant-based breast reconstruction - a long-term resorbable mesh. Expert Rev Med Dev. 2018;15:689–91.
36. Pompei S, Evangelidou D, Arelli F, Ferrante G. The use of TIGR matrix in breast aesthetic and reconstructive surgery: is a resorbable synthetic mesh a viable alternative to acellular dermal matrices? Clin Plast Surg. 2018;45(1):65–73.
37. Becker H, Lind JG. The use of synthetic mesh in reconstructive, revision, and cosmetic breast surgery. Aesthet Plast Surg. 2013;37:914–21.
38. Fine NA, Lehfeldt M, Gross JE, Downey S, Kind GM, Duda G, Kulber D, Horan R, Ippolito J, Jewell M. SERI surgical scaffold, prospective clinical trial of a silk-derived biological scaffold in two-stage breast reconstruction: 1-year data. Plast Reconstr Surg. 2015;135:339–51.
39. De Vita R, Buccheri EM, Pozzi M, Zoccali G. Direct to implant breast reconstruction by using SERI, preliminary report. J Exp Clin Cancer Res. 2014;33:78.
40. Dieterich M, Reimer T, Dieterich H, Stubert J, Gerber B. A short-term follow-up of implant based breast reconstruction using a titanium-coated polypropylene mesh (TiLoop(®) Bra). Eur J Surg Oncol. 2012;38:1225–30.
41. TiO2Mesh™ – Surgical Mesh Implant. Available at: http://www.biosermedikal.com/en/tio2mesh-surgical-mesh-implant. Accessed on January 2021
42. Pukancsik D, Kelemen P, Gulyás G, Újhelyi M, Kovács E, Éles K, Mészáros N, Kenessey I, Pálházi P, Kovács T, Kásler M, Mátrai Z. Clinical experiences with the use of ULTRAPRO® mesh in single-stage direct-to-implant immediate postmastectomy breast reconstruction in 102 patients: a retrospective cohort study. Eur J Surg Oncol. 2017;43:1244–51.
43. Eichler C, Schulz C, Thangarajah F, Malter W, Warm M, Brunnert K. A retrospective head-to-head comparison between TiLoop Bra/TiMesh® and Seragyn® in 320 cases of reconstructive breast surgery. Anticancer Res. 2019;39:2599–605.
44. Bernini M, Calabrese C, Cecconi L, Santi C, Gjondedaj U, Roselli J, Nori J, Fausto A, Orzalesi L, Casella D. Subcutaneous direct-to-implant breast reconstruction: surgical, functional, and aesthetic results after long-term follow-up. Plast Reconstr Surg Glob Open. 2016;3:e574.
45. Casella D, Calabrese C, Bianchi S, Meattini I, Bernini M. Subcutaneous tissue expander placement with synthetic titanium-coated mesh in breast reconstruction: long-term results. Plast Reconstr Surg Glob Open. 2016;3:e577.
46. Lo Torto F, Marcasciano M, Kaciulyte J, Redi U, Barellini L, De Luca A, Perra A, Frattaroli JM, Cavalieri E, Di Taranto G, Greco M, Casella D. Prepectoral breast reconstruction with TiLoop® bra pocket: a single center prospective study. Eur Rev Med Pharmacol Sci. 2020;24:991–9.
47. Casella D, Di Taranto G, Marcasciano M, Sordi S, Kothari A, Kovacs T, Lo Torto F, Cigna E, Ribuffo D, Calabrese C. Nipple-sparing bilateral prophylactic mastectomy and immediate reconstruction with TiLoop® Bra Mesh in BRCA1/2 mutation carriers: a prospective study of long-term and patient reported outcomes using the BREAST-Q. Breast. 2018;39:8–13.
48. PFM Medical. TiLoop ® Bra Pocket. Available at: https://www.pfmmedical.com/en/productcatalogue/mesh_implants_breast_surgery/tiloopR_bra_pocket. Accessed: December 2020
49. Mowlds DS, Salibian AA, Scholz T, Paydar KZ, Wirth GA. Capsular contracture in implant-based breast reconstruction: examining the role of acellular dermal matrix fenestrations. Plast Reconstr Surg. 2015;136:629–35.
50. Dessy LA, Corrias F, Marchetti F, Marcasciano M, Armenti AF, Mazzocchi M, Carlesimo B. Implant infection after augmentation mammaplasty: a review of the literature and report of a multidrug-resistant candida albicans infection. Aesthet Plast Surg. 2012;36:153–9.
51. Shaterian A, Saba SC, Yee B, Tokin C, Mailey B, Dobke MK, Wallace AM. Single dual-trained surgeon

for breast care leads to higher reconstruction rates after mastectomy. World J Surg. 2013;37:2600–6.
52. Casella D, Di Taranto G, Marcasciano M, Lo Torto F, Barellini L, Sordi S, Gaggelli I, Roncella M, Calabrese C, Ribuffo D. Subcutaneous expanders and synthetic mesh for breast reconstruction: long-term and patient-reported BREAST-Q outcomes of a single-center prospective study. J Plast Reconstr Aesthet Surg. 2019;72:805–12.
53. Casella D, Fusario D, Cassetti D, Miccoli S, Pesce AL, Bernini A, Marcasciano M, Lo Torto F, Neri A. The patient's pathway for breast cancer in the COVID-19 era: an italian single-center experience. Breast J. 2020;26:1589–92.
54. Rigotti G, Marchi A, Galiè M, Baroni G, Benati D, Krampera M, Pasini A, Sbarbati A. Clinical treatment of radiotherapy tissue damage by lipoaspirate transplant: a healing process mediated by adipose-derived adult stem cells. Plast Reconstr Surg. 2007;119:1409–22.
55. Cigna E, Ribuffo D, Sorvillo V, Atzeni M, Piperno A, Calò PG, Scuderi N. Secondary lipofilling after breast reconstruction with implants. Eur Rev Med Pharmacol Sci. 2012 Nov;16(12):1729–34.
56. Ribuffo D, Lo Torto F, Atzeni M, Serratore F. The effects of postmastectomy adjuvant radiotherapy on immediate two-stage prosthetic breast reconstruction: a systematic review. Plast Reconstr Surg. 2015;135:445e.
57. Calabrese C, Kothari A, Badylak S, Di Taranto G, Marcasciano M, Sordi S, Barellini L, Lo Torto F, Tarallo M, Gaggelli I, D'Ermo G, Fausto A, Casella D, Ribuffo D. Oncological safety of stromal vascular fraction enriched fat grafting in two-stage breast reconstruction after nipple sparing mastectomy: long-term results of a prospective study. Eur Rev Med Pharmacol Sci. 2018;22:4768–77.
58. Ribuffo D, Atzeni M, Guerra M, Bucher S, Politi C, Deidda M, Atzori F, Dessi M, Madeddu C, Lay G. Treatment of irradiated expanders: protective lipofilling allows immediate prosthetic breast reconstruction in the setting of postoperative radiotherapy. Aesthet Plast Surg. 2013;37:1146–52.
59. Vaia N, Lo Torto F, Marcasciano M, Casella D, Cacace C, De Masi C, Ricci F, Ribuffo D. From the "Fat Capsule" to the "Fat Belt": limiting protective lipofilling on irradiated expanders for breast reconstruction to selective key areas. Aesthet Plast Surg. 2018;42:986–94.
60. Vyas KS, DeCoster RC, Burns JC, Rodgers LT, Shrout MA, Mercer JP, Coquillard C, Dugan AJ, Baratta MD, Rinker BD, Vasconez HC. Autologous fat grafting does not increase risk of oncologic recurrence in the reconstructed breast. Ann Plast Surg. 2020;84:S405–10.
61. Wagner RD, Braun TL, Zhu H, Winocour S. A systematic review of complications in prepectoral breast reconstruction. J Plast Reconstr Aesthet Surg. 2019;72:1051–9.
62. Chopra K, Gowda AU, Kwon E, Eagan M, Grant SW. Techniques to repair implant malposition after breast augmentation: a review. Aesthet Surg J. 2016;36:660–71.
63. Harris R, Raphael P, Harris SW. Thermal capsulorrhaphy: a modified technique for breast pocket revision. Aesthet Surg J. 2014;34:1041–9.
64. Sinnott CJ, Persing SM, Pronovost M, Hodyl C, McConnell D, Ott YA. Impact of postmastectomy radiation therapy in prepectoral versus subpectoral implant-based breast reconstruction. Ann Surg Oncol. 2018;25:2899–908.
65. Casella D, Di Taranto G, Onesti MG, Greco M, Ribuffo D. A retrospective comparative analysis of risk factors and outcomes in direct-to-implant and two-stages prepectoral breast reconstruction: bmi and radiotherapy as new selection criteria of patients. Eur J Surg Oncol. 2019;45:1357–63.
66. Nahabedian MY. What are the long-term aesthetic issues in prepectoral breast reconstruction? Aesthet Surg J. 2020;40:S29–37.
67. Marcasciano M, Kaciulyte J, Marcasciano F, Lo Torto F, Ribuffo D, Casella D. "No drain, no gain": simultaneous seroma drainage and tissue expansion in pre-pectoral tissue expander-based breast reconstruction. Aesthet Plast Surg. 2019;43:1118–9.
68. Washer LL, Gutowski K. Breast implant infections. Infect Dis Clin North Am. 2012;26:111–25.
69. Avila A, Bartholomew AJ, Sosin M, Deldar R, Griffith KF, Willey SC, Song DH, Fan KL, Tousimis EA. Acute postoperative complications in prepectoral versus subpectoral reconstruction following nipple-sparing mastectomy. Plast Reconstr Surg. 2020;146:715e–20e.
70. Spear SL, Howard MA, Boehmler JH, Ducic I, Low M, Abbruzzesse MR. The infected or exposed breast implant: management and treatment strategies. Plast Reconstr Surg. 2004;113:1634–44.
71. Prince MD, Suber JS, Aya-Ay ML, Cone JD Jr, Greene JN, Smith DJ Jr, Smith PD. Prosthesis salvage in breast reconstruction patients with periprosthetic infection and exposure. Plast Reconstr Surg. 2012;129:42–8.
72. De Lorenzi C. Successful treatment of acute periprosthetic breast infection with curettage, pulse lavage, and immediate device exchange. Aesthet Plast Surg. 2005;29:400–3.
73. Antoniazzi E, Villani R, Fabbri E, Vietti Michelina V, D'Angelo G, Summo V, Cipriani R, Morselli PG, Fasano D. Management of the exposed and/or infected breast prosthesis: a proposal for a standardized approach. Plast Reconstr Surg Glob Open. 2016;4:e658.
74. Ganske I, Hoyler M, Fox SE, Morris DJ, Lin SJ, Slavin SA. Delayed hypersensitivity reaction to acellular dermal matrix in breast reconstruction: the red breast syndrome? Ann Plast Surg. 2014;73:S139–43.
75. Mayer HF, Perez Colman M, Stoppani I. Red breast syndrome (RBS) associated to the use of polyglycolic

mesh in breast reconstruction: a case report. Acta Chir Plast. 2020;62:50–2.
76. Vidya R, Iqbal FM. A guide to prepectoral breast reconstruction: a new dimension to implant-based breast reconstruction. Clin Breast Cancer. 2017;17:266–71.
77. Akram M, Siddiqui SA. Breast cancer management: past, present and evolving. Indian J Cancer. 2012;49:277–82.
78. Salzberg CA. Nonexpansive immediate breast reconstruction using human acellular tissue matrix graft (AlloDerm). Ann Plast Surg. 2006;57:1–5.
79. Ter Louw RP, Nahabedian MY. Prepectoral Breast reconstruction. Plast Reconstr Surg. 2017;140:51S–9S.
80. Rietjens M, Garusi C, Lanfrey E, Petit JY. La Suspension cutanée: Reconstruction Mammaire immédiate Avec Avancement cutané Abdominal à l'aide d'une Plaque Non résorbable. Résultats préliminaires à Propos de Vingt-Neuf Cas [Cutaneous suspension: immediate breast reconstruction with abdominal cutaneous advancement using a non-resorptive mesh. preliminary results and report of 28 cases]. Ann Chir Plast Esthet. 1997;42:177–82.
81. Reitsamer R, Peintinger F, Klaassen-Federspiel F, Sir A. Prepectoral direct-to-implant breast reconstruction with complete ADM or synthetic mesh coverage - 36-months follow-up in 200 reconstructed breasts. Breast. 2019;48:32–7.
82. Zhu L, Mohan AT, Abdelsattar JM, Wang Z, Vijayasekaran A, Hwang SM, Tran NV, Saint-Cyr M. Comparison of subcutaneous versus submuscular expander placement in the first stage of immediate breast reconstruction. J Plast Reconstr Aesthet Surg. 2016;69:e77–86.
83. Caputo GG, Marchetti A, Dalla Pozza E, Vigato E, Domenici L, Cigna E, Governa M. Skin-reduction breast reconstructions with prepectoral implant. Plast Reconstr Surg. 2016;137:1702–5.
84. Marcasciano Md M, Kaciulyte J, Gentilucci M, Barellini L, Ribuffo D, Casella D. Skin-reduction breast reconstructions with prepectoral implant covered by a combined dermal flap and titanium-coated polypropylene mesh. J Plast Reconstr Aesthet Surg. 2018;71:1123–8.
85. Salibian AH, Harness JK, Mowlds DS. Staged suprapectoral expander/implant reconstruction without acellular dermal matrix following nipple-sparing mastectomy. Plast Reconstr Surg. 2017;139:30–9.
86. Marcasciano M, Frattaroli J, Mori FLR, Lo Torto F, Fioramonti P, Cavalieri E, Kaciulyte J, Greco M, Casella D, Ribuffo D. The new trend of pre-pectoral breast reconstruction: an objective evaluation of the quality of online information for patients undergoing breast reconstruction. Aesthet Plast Surg. 2019;43:593–9.
87. Marcasciano M, Kaciulyte J, FLR M, Lo Torto F, Barellini L, Loreti A, Fanelli B, De Vita R, Redi U, Marcasciano F, Di Cesare F, dal Prà G, Conversi A, Elia L, Montemari G, Vaia N, Bernini M, Sordi S, Luridiana G, D'Ermo G, Monti M, De Luca A, Ricci F, Mazzocchi M, Gentilucci M, Greco M, Losco L, Valdatta LA, Raposio E, Giudice G, Maruccia M, Di Benedetto G, Cigna E, Casella D, Ribuffo D. Breast surgeons updating on the thresholds of COVID-19 era: results of a multicenter collaborative study evaluating the role of online videos and multimedia sources on breast surgeons education and training. Eur Rev Med Pharmacol Sci. 2020;24:7845–54.

Hybrid Prepectoral Breast Reconstruction: Combining Flaps and Implants

14

Arash Momeni and Anna Zhou

14.1 Introduction

Since the first report of implant-based breast reconstruction five decades ago, tremendous advances have been made in regard to surgical approaches to post-mastectomy reconstruction. These advances have been paralleled by a substantial improvement of clinical outcomes, thus cementing the central role of breast reconstruction in breast cancer care. The transition from submuscular approaches to prepectoral implant-based breast reconstruction, for example, illustrates how modern techniques have resulted in a reduction of surgical morbidity. Furthermore, numerous studies have documented the beneficial impact of breast reconstruction on patient-reported outcomes and health-related quality of life [1–3].

Historically, patients have been offered either implant-based or autologous reconstruction in order to achieve the goals of breast reconstruction, namely reconstruction of a breast of adequate size, shape, symmetry, softness, and sensation (i.e., "5S") [4]. While this binary approach to breast reconstruction is appropriate in the vast majority of patients, there remains a subset of patients for whom this simplistic approach is not adequate. This is particularly relevant given the increasing number of bilateral mastectomies [5], as donor-site tissue volume may be insufficient in those instances. The reconstructive challenge, therefore, is characterized by a patient who either desires or requires bilateral autologous breast reconstruction, yet, has insufficient donor-site volume. A variety of solutions have been proposed in the literature, including primary and/or secondary fat grafting following flap transfer, reconstruction with stacked flaps, and hybrid breast reconstruction, i.e., the combination of autologous tissue with prosthetic implants [6–11].

While autologous fat grafting is a short outpatient procedure that can significantly improve clinical outcomes and patient satisfaction by correcting contour deformities and volume deficiencies [12], it has several drawbacks, including a variable fat absorption rate, risk of fat necrosis, need for multiple procedures, and lack of structural support to the reconstructed breast [13]. Furthermore, it is worthwhile to consider that patients who have insufficient abdominal tissue for bilateral breast reconstruction may also lack adequate fat deposits at other anatomical sites to permit secondary fat grafting in the amount required to obtain an appealing result.

A. Momeni (✉) · A. Zhou
Division of Plastic & Reconstructive Surgery, Stanford University School of Medicine, Stanford, CA, USA
e-mail: amomeni@stanford.edu; Atzhou@stanford.edu

© The Author(s), under exclusive license to Springer Nature Switzerland AG 2023
R. Vidya, H. Becker (eds.), *Prepectoral Breast Reconstruction*,
https://doi.org/10.1007/978-3-031-15590-1_14

Reconstruction with stacked flaps, in contrast, permits single-stage transfer of a large soft tissue volume, thus permitting a totally autologous breast reconstruction. Importantly, the transferred tissue is not subject to secondary absorption. Yet, flap harvest from multiple donor sites not only increases surgical duration and complexity but also increases patient morbidity. Furthermore, while excellent results have been reported following breast reconstruction with stacked flaps, the technical expertise necessary to perform these reconstructions may not be widely available [9, 14].

Hybrid reconstruction may, therefore, represent an ideal solution to address the reconstructive challenge of patients with inadequate donor-site volume who desire autologous reconstruction.

Hybrid breast reconstruction is characterized by the combination of autologous tissue with prosthetic implants. The most common form of hybrid reconstruction is the combination of a latissimus dorsi (LD) flap with an implant [15, 16]. Disadvantages of this reconstructive modality, however, include the donor-site morbidity associated with LD muscle harvest, need for intraoperative repositioning, risk of postoperative animation deformity, difficulty in creating a natural breast ptosis, and secondary soft tissue atrophy with resultant implant visibility and rippling [6, 17, 18]. An expansion of this concept, however, namely the combination of free abdominal flap transfer with simultaneous implant placement addresses these shortcomings successfully.

Abdominal flap harvest is not only associated with placement of a scar in a more concealed location, it also allows for a greater volume of soft tissue to be transferred that is not prone to atrophy, thus minimizing the risk of implant visibility and rippling [11, 19]. Furthermore, the greater amount of abdominal flap volume permits placement of smaller implants and explains why the final breast appearance following hybrid reconstruction with free abdominal flaps is determined by the abdominal flap rather than the implant; this is in contrast to LD flap-based reconstructions. It is important to consider the different purpose an implant serves in abdominal flap- vs. LD flap-based reconstruction. In the former scenario, the implant is used to define projection and serves as a foundation over which the abdominal flap is draped. The bulk of volume is provided by the free abdominal flap, thus, defining the final breast shape, size, and suppleness. Decreasing the ratio of implant contribution to overall breast volume is, furthermore, believed to reduce long-term implant-related complications. In contrast, in LD flap-based reconstruction, the implant is the major determinant of breast volume and appearance, with the LD flap merely serving as a vascularized soft tissue cover.

14.2 Timing of Implant Placement

An important consideration is related to the timing of implant placement, with options including immediate vs. delayed insertion. Delayed implant placement has been favored by some authors who have reported greater control over the final reconstructive outcome. Reported reasons include an increased control and accuracy in creating the implant pocket and determining implant size, respectively [20]. Disadvantages of this delayed approach, however, include an increased technical difficulty with implant pocket dissection, particularly in patients who have undergone adjuvant radiotherapy [21]. Furthermore, delayed implant insertion has been associated with a greater number of revisions, with as many as six procedures being reported before the final result is achieved [22].

In contrast, immediate implant placement avoids the mandatory second procedure associated with delayed implant insertion. While early studies commented on an increased rate of implant-related complications associated with simultaneous implant placement and transverse rectus abdominis myocutaneous (TRAM) flap transfer, including infection rates as high as 19%, recent studies have not corroborated these concerns [19, 23–25]. In a retrospective analysis of

57 patients who had undergone bilateral hybrid breast reconstruction, only a single case of postoperative infection was noted [26]. Advantages of immediate implant insertion include avoidance of a mandatory second procedure; excellent control over implant position, particularly with the use of mesh products; and improved postoperative breast appearance as the discrepancy between breast skin envelope and breast volume is corrected at the index operation rather than secondarily. This is particularly relevant in patients who are scheduled to undergo adjuvant radiotherapy. Once the mastectomy skin flap has healed to a smaller free flap, re-expansion of the skin envelope to the original dimension is challenging as the free flap and mastectomy skin flap no longer move independent from one another; a phenomenon that is more pronounced following radiotherapy, subsequent to which the skin envelope is densely adherent to the smaller flap. While secondary implant placement in these instances will increase breast volume, breast shape and contour may not be ideal [26].

Despite the advantages of immediate hybrid reconstruction, implant selection can be challenging, as evidenced by an over 10% revision rate related to implant size following immediate hybrid reconstruction [10]. An elegant solution to this challenge is delayed-immediate hybrid reconstruction, whereby a staged approach is implemented characterized by immediate prepectoral tissue expander-based reconstruction (stage 1), followed by tissue expander removal with free abdominal flap transfer with simultaneous implant placement (stage 2) [27]. This approach permits a more precise determination of implant size, defined by the difference between final tissue expander volume and flap weight. An additional benefit of a delayed-immediate approach is the fact that the occurrence of mastectomy skin necrosis following stage 1 does not compromise final breast aesthetics, as the ensuing expansion process permits recruitment of lost skin prior to the critical second stage of reconstruction. Importantly, given that patients can provide input during the expansion process, it is quite easy to meet patients' expectations in regard to final breast size.

14.3 Radiation Therapy

Another important factor to consider is radiotherapy, as higher rates of mastectomy skin flap necrosis, higher rates of capsular contracture, and increased rates of fat necrosis after deep inferior epigastric perforator (DIEP) flap transfer have been reported following radiotherapy [28]. While mastectomy skin necrosis following prepectoral implant-based reconstruction jeopardizes the entire reconstruction, this is not the case following hybrid reconstruction, as the implant is separated from the area of mastectomy skin necrosis by the well-vascularized abdominal flap. Hence, surgical intervention is not mandatory for management of mastectomy skin necrosis following hybrid reconstruction. While implant-related complications occur more frequently when placed within an irradiated field, the addition of autologous tissue seems to reduce radiation-induced implant-related problems [29].

Particularly, thin patients who will require radiotherapy represent a challenging patient population, as implant-based reconstruction in this cohort is associated with high failure rates and aesthetic shortcomings [30, 31]. Certainly, prepectoral device placement has improved outcomes, secondary to avoiding the detrimental effects of radiation-induced muscle fibrosis and contracture seen with subpectoral reconstructions [32]; yet, challenges related to the tenuous soft tissue cover remain. Autologous reconstruction in thin patients is similarly challenging, however, as reconstruction of an appealing breast in regard to size and shape is difficult when faced with insufficient flap volume. Hybrid reconstruction is that patient population, thus, represents an elegant reconstructive solution.

14.4 Plane of Implant Placement

Similar to the evolution in implant-based breast reconstruction, hybrid breast reconstruction has evolved in regard to plane of implant placement and degree of muscle coverage. Early reports of combined free tissue transfer and implant placement favored total muscle coverage of the implant, with implant coverage being provided by the pectoralis major muscle and occasionally serratus anterior muscle, as well as muscle component of the TRAM flap [6, 33]. Following the report of favorable outcomes using mesh products for improved implant pocket control in the setting of simultaneous pedicled flap transfer [25, 34], this concept was expanded to include microsurgical hybrid reconstruction. Hence, the advent of mesh products resulted in the introduction of hybrid breast reconstruction in which the implant was placed in the subpectoral plane with inferolateral implant support being provided by acellular dermal matrices or polyglactin mesh [24]. This marked a major advancement, as it permitted precise implant pocket definition, a key component in achieving an optimal result. In an attempt to further minimize patient morbidity and simplify the procedure, hybrid prepectoral breast reconstruction was introduced thereafter, whereby pectoral major muscle elevation was avoided altogether [10, 26].

Not only has the plane of implant insertion changed, but also the intraoperative sequence. While early clinical studies reported implant insertion prior to flap transfer, we now perform flap transfer first and insert the implant following completion of microvascular anastomoses.

14.5 Surgical Technique

Preoperative markings are made in standard fashion and include the midline, inframammary fold, upper breast border, and abdominal flap outline (Fig. 14.1). Abdominal flap harvest is performed using established techniques. Following completion of mastectomy, the pectoralis major muscle is divided along its fibers at the level of the third costal cartilage. Thereafter, the third rib cartilage is removed, although a rib-sparing approach is occasionally used when a large intercostal space is encountered. Following dissection of the internal mammary vessels, the abdominal flap is transferred to the chest and microvascular anastomosis of the deep inferior epigastric vessels is performed to the internal mammary vessels. The abdominal flap is then inserted into the breast pocket. At this point, the decision regarding implant size is made using implant sizers. It is noteworthy, that the implant chosen has a base width that is routinely 2–3 cm less than the preoperative breast width of the patient. This facilitates flap inset and permits complete anterior coverage of the implant by the flap. Once the implant size is determined, the final implant

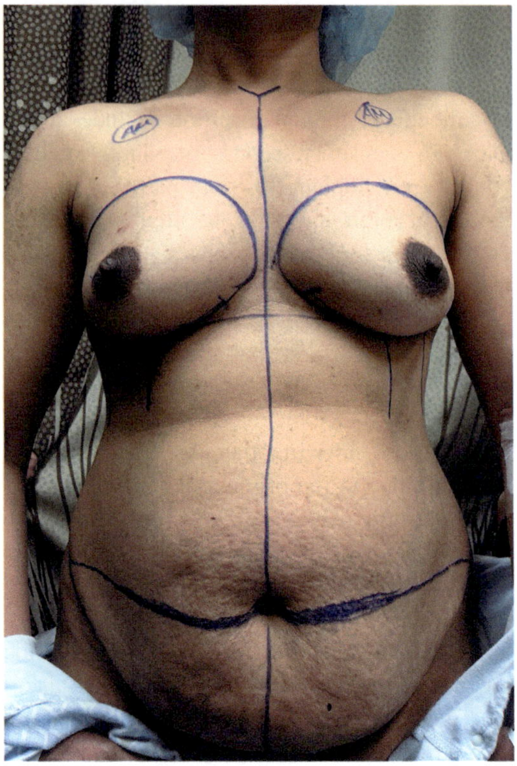

Fig. 14.1 Standard preoperative markings, including midline, inframammary fold, upper breast border, and abdominal flap outline. Note, that the upper border of the abdominal flap courses below the level of the umbilicus

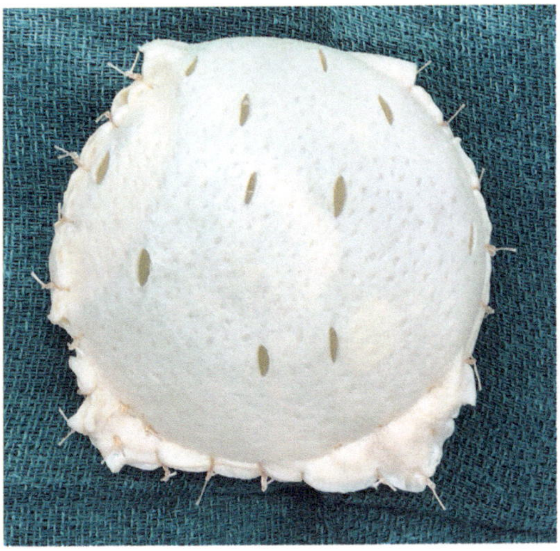

Fig. 14.2 Silicone gel implant wrapped with acellular dermal matrix

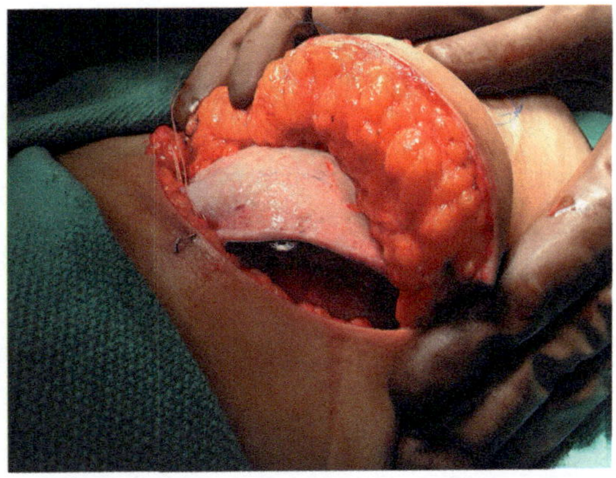

Fig. 14.3 Robust well-vascularized soft tissue coverage of the prepectoral acellular dermal matrix-implant-construct

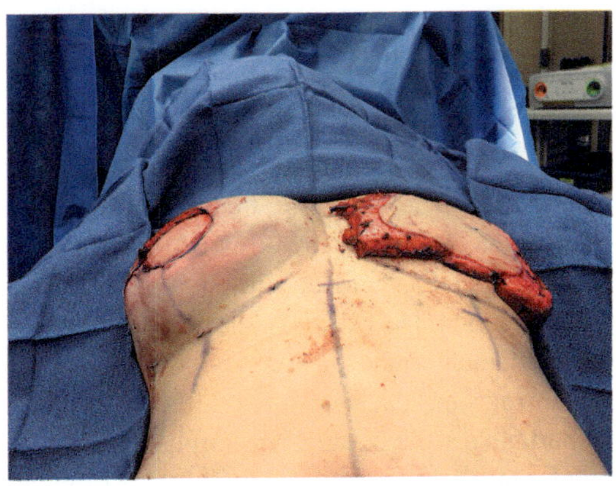

Fig. 14.4 The contribution of the implant to breast projection as seen intraoperatively

along with a sheet of ADM is brought onto the sterile field. The implant is wrapped in ADM and the wrap secured with 2-0 polyglactin sutures (Fig. 14.2). Of note, depending on the implant size, a complete wrap may not be possible. The implant-ADM construct is placed in dilute betadine solution and subsequently inserted into the breast pocket. It is pivotal during implant insertion to visualize the flap pedicle in order to avoid undue tension or kinking of the vascular pedicle. After the desired implant location has been determined, 2–0 polyglactin sutures are used to secure the ADM to the chest wall, thus securing the implant position. The abdominal flap is draped over the anterior surface of the ADM-implant construct, providing robust coverage with vascularized tissue (Fig. 14.3), and secured to the chest wall with 2–0 polyglactin sutures. While the implant size is rather small, commonly between 150 and 210 cc [10, 24], its contribution to the projection of the reconstructed breast becomes immediately evident (Fig. 14.4). Figure 14.5 demonstrates pre- and postoperative images following immediate hybrid reconstruction.

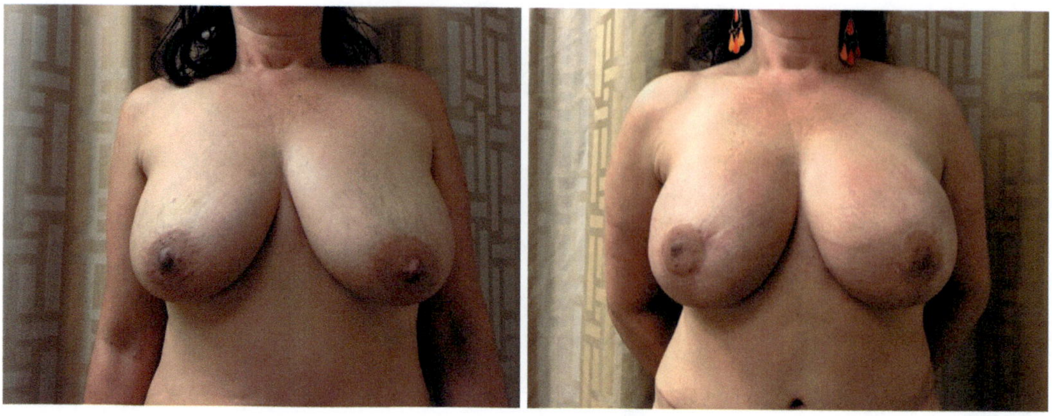

Fig. 14.5 Pre- and postoperative images of a 49-year-old patient following bilateral nipple-sparing mastectomy with immediate hybrid reconstruction with free abdominal flaps and 175 cc silicone gel implants

14.6 Advantages of Hybrid Breast Reconstruction

Hybrid breast reconstruction permits a departure from the rather simplistic binary approach to post-mastectomy breast reconstruction, which is defined by either implant-based or autologous reconstruction. Hence, it expands the reconstructive armamentarium, thus allowing a more individualized approach to breast reconstruction. Importantly, it neither replaces implant-based nor autologous reconstruction but seeks to offer an elegant reconstructive solution for select patients. These patients are characterized by the desire or need to undergo autologous reconstruction, yet, have insufficient donor-site volume. When determining whether a patient is a candidate for hybrid reconstruction, it is important to assess the degree of abdominal skin/soft tissue laxity as its presence generally confers eligibility for this reconstructive modality.

The robust vascularized soft tissue coverage following hybrid reconstruction addresses many of the challenges seen following implant-based reconstruction, notably implant visibility and rippling. Furthermore, the shift of implant-to-tissue ratio in favor of autologous tissue is believed to reduce long-term implant-related complications. Finally, abdominal flap harvest not only corrects infraumbilical soft tissue laxity, but results in a significantly lower abdominal scar when compared to conventional abdominal flap-based reconstruction [4].

14.7 Literature Review

A number of clinical studies have documented the safety of microsurgical hybrid breast reconstruction. The ability to control implant position in immediate hybrid breast reconstruction was demonstrated in series of 19 patients who underwent 38 breast reconstructions using mesh products, notably acellular dermal matrix and polyglactin. No cases of implant malposition, implant infection, or flap loss were noted. Of note, all patients in this study underwent subpectoral implant placement, with mesh being used for inferolateral support [24]. In an attempt to reduce patient morbidity while also simplifying the procedure, clinical outcomes following prepectoral hybrid breast reconstruction were studied in a cohort of 57 patients who underwent 114 breast reconstructions and confirmed the safety associated with this reconstructive modality [26]. The >10% rate of mastectomy skin necrosis, however, prompted the introduction of an alternative approach to hybrid reconstruction, namely the delayed-immediate approach, whereby hybrid reconstruction is performed in a staged manner following conventional prepectoral tissue expander-based reconstruction. Clinical outcomes following this approach were reported in a retrospective study of 31 patients who underwent 62 breast reconstructions [27]. Importantly, patients neither desired secondary implant exchange for size correction, thus demonstrating an improved ability to determine the desired implant size, nor was any case of mastectomy skin necrosis noted following the critical second reconstructive stage [27]. More recently, secondary outcome parameters following hybrid reconstruction have been investigated, such as abdominal scar location and aesthetic rating of the donor site. Comparing the abdominal appearance following conventional flap-based reconstruction, hybrid reconstruction, and cosmetic abdominoplasty, a significantly lower abdominal scar position was noted following abdominoplasty and hybrid reconstruction when compared to conventional abdominal flap-based reconstruction. Importantly, the lower scar location was also associated with a higher abdominal aesthetic rating [4].

It is noteworthy that hybrid reconstructions have also been successfully performed with flaps other than the traditional LD flap or free abdominal flap. To reduce the donor-site morbidity associated with LD muscle harvest, the thoracodorsal artery perforator flap (TDAP) has been successfully combined with the use of a tissue expander or permanent implant [35]. The value of acellular dermal matrix in providing soft tissue support and controlling implant position has, furthermore, been demonstrated in several retrospective clinical studies [25, 34].

14.8 Summary

In summary, hybrid breast reconstruction expands the reconstructive armamentarium by offering a reconstructive modality that avoids some of the limitations of traditional forms of breast reconstruction. The combination of implant placement with free abdominal tissue transfer, in particular, is associated with excellent clinical outcomes, as the generous soft tissue provided by the abdominal flap allows for stable soft tissue coverage of the implant, thereby reducing the risk of implant palpability and rippling. The implant, in return, improves projection of the reconstructed breast without negatively impacting flap-related outcome metrics. Furthermore, as the abdominal donor site is no longer the sole contributor to the volume of the reconstructed breast, a lower abdominal flap can be designed, thus resulting in a lower abdominal scar with improved abdominal aesthetics.

As with any reconstructive approach, patient selection is key. The main factor determining whether a patient is a candidate for hybrid breast reconstruction is the presence of abdominal skin/soft tissue laxity in a patient who wishes correction thereof. The intraoperative use of implant sizers is recommended to determine the ideal implant size. While several different intraoperative sequences have been described, our preference is currently prepectoral implant placement after flap transfer and completion of microvascular anastomoses, as we have found that this sequence best allows determination of the ideal implant position and is least disruptive to the flow of the procedure.

References

1. Alderman AK, Kuhn LE, Lowery JC, Wilkins EG. Does patient satisfaction with breast reconstruction change over time? Two-year results of the Michigan breast reconstruction outcomes study. J Am Coll Surg. 2007;204(1):7–12.
2. Hu ES, Pusic AL, Waljee JF, Kuhn L, Hawley ST, Wilkins E, et al. Patient-reported aesthetic satisfaction with breast reconstruction during the long-term survivorship period. Plast Reconstr Surg. 2009;124(1):1–8.
3. Nelson JA, Allen RJ Jr, Polanco T, Shamsunder M, Patel AR, McCarthy CM, et al. Long-term patient-reported outcomes following Postmastectomy breast reconstruction: an 8-year examination of 3268 patients. Ann Surg. 2019;270(3):473–83.
4. Li AY, Momeni A. Abdominal flap-based breast reconstruction versus abdominoplasty: the impact of surgical procedure on scar location. Plast Reconstr Surg Glob Open. 2020;8(9):e3112.
5. Albornoz CR, Bach PB, Mehrara BJ, Disa JJ, Pusic AL, McCarthy CM, et al. A paradigm shift in U.S. breast reconstruction: increasing implant rates. Plast Reconstr Surg. 2013;131(1):15–23.

6. Serletti JM, Moran SL. The combined use of the TRAM and expanders/implants in breast reconstruction. Ann Plast Surg. 1998;40(5):510–4.
7. Laporta R, Longo B, Sorotos M, Pagnoni M, Santanelli di Pompeo F. Breast reconstruction with delayed fat-graft-augmented DIEP flap in patients with insufficient donor-site volume. Aesthet Plast Surg. 2015;39(3):339–49.
8. Zhu L, Mohan AT, Vijayasekaran A, Hou C, Sur YJ, Morsy M, et al. Maximizing the volume of latissimus Dorsi flap in autologous breast reconstruction with simultaneous multisite fat grafting. Aesthet Surg J/ Am Soc Aesthet Plast Surg. 2016;36(2):169–78.
9. Stalder MW, Lam J, Allen RJ, Sadeghi A. Using the retrograde internal mammary system for stacked perforator flap breast reconstruction: 71 breast reconstructions in 53 consecutive patients. Plast Reconstr Surg. 2016;137(2):265e–77e.
10. Momeni A, Kanchwala S. Hybrid Prepectoral breast reconstruction: a surgical approach that combines the benefits of autologous and implant-based reconstruction. Plast Reconstr Surg. 2018;142(5):1109–15.
11. Chu MW, Samra F, Kanchwala SK, Momeni A. Treatment options for bilateral autologous breast reconstruction in patients with inadequate donor-site volume. J Reconstr Microsurg. 2017;33(5):305–11.
12. Kanchwala SK, Glatt BS, Conant EF, Bucky LP. Autologous fat grafting to the reconstructed breast: the management of acquired contour deformities. Plast Reconstr Surg. 2009;124(2):409–18.
13. Khouri RK, Rigotti G, Khouri RK Jr, Cardoso E, Marchi A, Rotemberg SC, et al. Tissue-engineered breast reconstruction with Brava-assisted fat grafting: a 7-year, 488-patient, multicenter experience. Plast Reconstr Surg. 2015;135(3):643–58.
14. Mayo JL, Allen RJ, Sadeghi A. Four-flap breast reconstruction: bilateral stacked DIEP and PAP flaps. Plast Reconstr Surg Glob Open. 2015;3(5):e383.
15. Slavin SA. Improving the latissimus dorsi myocutaneous flap with tissue expansion. Plast Reconstr Surg. 1994;93(4):811–24.
16. Biggs TM, Cronin ED. Technical aspects of the latissimus dorsi myocutaneous flap in breast reconstruction. Ann Plast Surg. 1981;6(5):381–8.
17. Figus A, Mazzocchi M, Dessy LA, Curinga G, Scuderi N. Treatment of muscular contraction deformities with botulinum toxin type a after latissimus dorsi flap and sub-pectoral implant breast reconstruction. J Plast Reconstr Aesthet Surg. 2009;62(7):869–75.
18. Button J, Scott J, Taghizadeh R, Weiler-Mithoff E, Hart AM. Shoulder function following autologous latissimus dorsi breast reconstruction. A prospective three year observational study comparing quilting and non-quilting donor site techniques. J Plast Reconstr Aesthet Surg. 2010;63(9):1505–12.
19. Roehl KR, Baumann DP, Chevray PM, Chang DW. Evaluation of outcomes in breast reconstructions combining lower abdominal free flaps and permanent implants. Plast Reconstr Surg. 2010;126(2):349–57.
20. Bach AD, Morgenstern IH, Horch RE. Secondary "hybrid reconstruction" concept with silicone implants after autologous breast reconstruction - is it safe and reasonable? Medical Sci Monit Int Med J Exp Clin Res. 2020;26:e921329.
21. Walters JA 3rd, Sato EA, Martinez CA, Hall JJ, Boutros SG. Delayed mammoplasty with silicone gel implants following DIEP flap breast reconstruction. Plast Reconstr Surg Glob Open. 2015;3(10):e540.
22. Pien IJ, Anolik R, Blau J, Hollenbeck ST. Delayed implant augmentation of breast free flaps. J Reconstr Microsurg. 2015;31(4):254–60.
23. Spear SL, Wolfe AJ. The coincidence of TRAM flaps and prostheses in the setting of breast reconstruction. Plast Reconstr Surg. 2002;110(2):478–86.
24. Momeni A, Kanchwala SK. Improved pocket control in immediate microsurgical breast reconstruction with simultaneous implant placement through the use of mesh. Microsurgery. 2018;38(5):450–7.
25. Borsen-Koch M, Gunnarsson GL, Udesen A, Arffmann S, Jacobs J, Salzberg A, et al. Direct delayed breast reconstruction with TAP flap, implant and acellular dermal matrix (TAPIA). J Plast Reconstr Aesthet Surg. 2015;68(6):815–21.
26. Kanchwala S, Momeni A. Hybrid breast reconstruction-the best of both worlds. Gland Surg. 2019;8(1):82–9.
27. Momeni A, Kanchwala S. Delayed-immediate hybrid breast reconstruction-increasing patient input and precision in breast reconstruction. Breast J. 2019;25(5):898–902.
28. Khansa I, Colakoglu S, Curtis MS, Yueh JH, Ogunleye A, Tobias AM, et al. Postmastectomy breast reconstruction after previous lumpectomy and radiation therapy: analysis of complications and satisfaction. Ann Plast Surg. 2011;66(5):444–51.
29. Chang DW, Barnea Y, Robb GL. Effects of an autologous flap combined with an implant for breast reconstruction: an evaluation of 1000 consecutive reconstructions of previously irradiated breasts. Plast Reconstr Surg. 2008;122(2):356–62.
30. Yun JH, Diaz R, Orman AG. Breast reconstruction and radiation therapy. Cancer Control. 2018;25(1):1073274818795489.
31. Zhao R, Tran BNN, Doval AF, Broadwater G, Buretta KJ, Orr JP, et al. A multicenter analysis examining patients undergoing conversion of implant-based breast reconstruction to abdominally based free tissue transfer. J Reconstr Microsurg. 2018;34(9):685–91.
32. Sinnott CJ, Persing SM, Pronovost M, Hodyl C, McConnell D, Ott YA. Impact of Postmastectomy

radiation therapy in Prepectoral versus subpectoral implant-based breast reconstruction. Ann Surg Oncol. 2018;25(10):2899–908.
33. Miller MJ, Rock CS, Robb GL. Aesthetic breast reconstruction using a combination of free transverse rectus abdominis musculocutaneous flaps and breast implants. Ann Plast Surg. 1996;37(3):258–64.
34. Gunnarsson GL, Borsen-Koch M, Nielsen HT, Salzberg A, Thomsen JB. Bilateral breast reconstruction with extended thoracodorsal artery perforator propeller flaps and implants. Plast Reconstr Surg Glob Open. 2015;3(6):e435.
35. Hamdi M, Salgarello M, Barone-Adesi L, Van Landuyt K. Use of the thoracodorsal artery perforator (TDAP) flap with implant in breast reconstruction. Ann Plast Surg. 2008;61(2):143–6.

15 Prepectoral Breast Reconstruction Without Mesh

Eduardo González and Cicero Urban

15.1 Introduction

The evolution of immediate breast reconstruction with expanders or implants in one or two stages varied according to complications and cosmetic results. One of the factors that influenced these points and caused paradigm changes was the making of the pockets where to place the prostheses, and if necessary, add other materials to improve results without increasing complications.

In the past [1–3], there have been attempts at subcutaneous reconstructions with smooth implants but with more radical mastectomy techniques in the management of the thickness of the flaps and the limits of breast resection. These techniques were abandoned due to poor results and especially due to the high rate of complications, as Schlenker [4] published, who observed 13.5% of skin necrosis, 6.7% of device extrusion, 56% of capsular contracture, and 28% of explantation and replaced by submuscular pockets that were used for many years [5].

In our experience, due to the unsatisfactory cosmetic results of the complete submuscular reconstruction and the difficulty that it produced in the expansion of the lower pole since 2004, we used the partial submuscular technique of the dual plane published by Serra-Renom [6]. This technique is satisfactory but, on some occasions, it can produce excessive expansion of the lower pole, and more frequently animated deformity and the "window-shading" effect.

For the prevention of these complications, the first experiences with the use of different types of synthetic or biological meshes in reconstructions with direct implants or expanders began to be published [7–10]. The objective was to produce an elongation of the pectoralis major muscle avoiding its retraction, to control the shape and stability of the submammary groove and the lateral border of the breast, avoiding the rotation of the implant and covering it in its entirety. Here, it is good to clarify that a mastectomy performed correctly should not alter the submammary fold and should not modify the shape of the breast envelope that, associated with a correct choice of implant, would also avoid these drawbacks.

Although many of the objectives of this technique were achieved with the conventional dual plane with or without the assistance of meshes, the postoperative pain due to the elevation of the pectoralis major, the animated deformity and the capsular contractures with breast contour deformity increased with radiotherapy, they continued to observe each other. These unresolved conflicts led to the beginning of the era of prepectoral reconstruction.

E. González (✉)
Departamento de Mastología, Instituto de Oncología Ángel H Roffo, Universidad de Buenos Aires, Buenos Aires, Argentina

C. Urban
Nossa Senhora das Graças Hospital and Centro de Doenças da Mama Curitiba (PR), Curitiba, Brazil

© The Author(s), under exclusive license to Springer Nature Switzerland AG 2023
R. Vidya, H. Becker (eds.), *Prepectoral Breast Reconstruction*,
https://doi.org/10.1007/978-3-031-15590-1_15

Prepectoral reconstruction is a faster procedure that produces less pain and discomfort and quick recovery, it maintains the function of the pectoralis major muscle, without producing animated deformity, maintaining the normal shape of the breast and its anatomical limits with careful dissection and preparation of the well-vitalized flaps. But it also generates certain doubts in relation to the possibility of presenting more rippling and visualization of the implant, more extrusions, and more incidence of capsular contractures without mesh wrapping.

At this point, we will stop for a moment to analyze the impact of the meshes in this technique. It is known that there are basically two types of meshes, the synthetic ones of various types of materials, generally slow reabsorption or non-absorbable [8–10] that have the primary function of leaving the implant well positioned and secondarily improving the trophism and thickness of the flaps. Although the latter is generally not achieved. The other possibility is the use of biological meshes derived from humans (ADM), pigs, cattle, etc. that can improve tissue vascularization, trophism, and skin-adipose flap consistency by minimizing rippling with a more natural consistency. On the other hand, and very important is its function of protecting the tissues from the effects of radiotherapy and lowering the rates of capsular contractures.

When we see the extensive publications that speak of the benefits but also the complications of the use of all types of meshes, it becomes very difficult to define their usefulness, especially due to the little evidence based on prospective studies. Only in some studies such as the meta-analysis of Ho et al. [11] describe that breast reconstructions assisted by ADM had a higher rate of seroma, infection, and reconstructive failure than breast reconstructions with prostheses that use traditional musculofascial flaps, but it highlights the benefits of ADM in relation to a lower rate of capsular contracture.

In the same way, when we do the same analysis in the use of synthetic meshes in the multicenter a, prospective cohort iBRA by Potter et al. [12] on 1357 breast reconstructions with mesh (1133 biological and 243 synthetic), in the group of synthetics observed 26% infections and 10% loss of implants. The authors conclude that the rates of all these complications are higher than those in the National Quality Standards (<5% for reoperation, re-admission, and implant loss, and <10% for infection).

When the complications of prepectoral vs subpectoral reconstruction are evaluated, it has been shown that they are comparable, Chatterjee [13] in a meta-analysis of 14 studies (all with the use of biological or synthetic meshes) corroborated the above with a correct choice of patients. If we add the radiotherapy effect, we are seeing in not very long follow-ups a better cosmetic result with prepectoral reconstruction and low rates of capsular contractures (4 times less), probably related to the negative impact and production of fibrosis of the treatment on the pectoral muscle in the submuscular pockets [13, 14]. It is valid to clarify that these publications include patients with ADM use.

Single-stage direct-to-implant prepectoral breast reconstruction is currently considered a state-of-the-art breast reconstruction technique and has been found to be safe and reproducible, being the first option in most cases of immediate post-mastectomy breast reconstruction. The question we ask ourselves, and it is the basis of this experience, is whether, in this indication, it is always necessary to associate meshes or we can reproduce the results in all scenarios without them.

Therefore, the objective of this chapter is to see what impact the surgical technique of mastectomy as, regardless of the favorable or non-favorable factors prior to surgery, in breast reconstruction with direct implants but without the addition of meshes and to evaluate whether the results can be reproduced and not increase complications in all consequent scenarios of cancer treatments such as radiotherapy. We will also analyze the factors that may incline us to dispense with synthetic or biological meshes with the prepectoral technique.

15.2 Indications and Contraindications

Safety of the prepectoral breast reconstruction requires the careful selection of patients, considering the preoperative analysis of comorbidities and the intraoperative evaluation of the post-mastectomy flap viability, as well as the radiotherapy status and oncological criteria. As in any type of surgery, patients must be well selected and oriented about technical choices, their risks, and benefits, and their limitations.

Many techniques for prepectoral implant-based breast reconstruction have been described in the literature. Prepectoral reconstruction may be indicated for patients who are candidates for nipple-sparing and skin-sparing mastectomy, with indication for 2-stage tissue expander or a single-stage direct-to-implant reconstruction if the flap is adequate. Ideal candidates for prepectoral reconstruction include patients with a body mass index less than 30 kg/m^2, patients with mild to moderate breast volume, nonsmokers, patients with minimal ptosis, patients having prophylactic mastectomy, and patients with central breast tumor [15, 16].

Patient's characteristics that should be considered as contraindications to prepectoral breast reconstruction are poorly controlled diabetes mellitus, obesity (BMI greater than 35), and active or recent smokers. All these traits will result in patients with compromised microvascular circulation and poor soft-tissue quality, thus increasing the risk of skin flap necrosis and extrusion or infection implant. Another factor that should be considered is radiation status at the time of mastectomy. It is recommended that this technique be avoided in patients with a history of prior external beam radiation to the breast at the time of mastectomy and reconstruction. Tissue expansion of previously radiated skin carries a high risk of wound dehiscence and infection [17]. In these situations, the choice may be made for performing subpectoral or prepectoral reconstruction in two stages, associating the use of acellular dermal matrices or fat grafting to improve the vascularization of the flap.

From an oncological point of view, preoperative tumor location in the breast should be assessed before mastectomy. Those patients with a tumor that invades the skin or chest wall, patients with inflammatory breast cancer, patients with stage IV breast cancer or those with aggressive axillary metastasis and bulk axillary adenopathy should be considered as contraindications for prepectoral breast reconstruction [17, 18]. Patients in these cases are among those with high risk of recurrence that could delay adjuvant treatment and make it difficult to detect possible recurrences.

Based on the experience of our institutions in 2021 we sent for publication, and it was accepted in Plastic and reconstructive Surgery, the work: "Pre-pectoral direct-to-implant immediate breast reconstruction in nipple-sparing mastectomy without placement of acellular dermal matrix or mesh." In this work, we included in a multicenter cohort study immediate direct-to-implant prepectoral breast reconstruction therapeutic or risk reduction, without any type of mesh assistance (biological or synthetic), including patients with all types of breasts, without ptosis or with moderate ptosis, with different types of adipose panicle, body mass index, smokers or not and with or without prior radiation therapy. Patients who had cutaneous involvement of the disease, previous severe actinic sequela, hypertrophy, or ptosis grade 3–4 or patients with intraoperative vascularization disorders with high possibilities of cutaneous necrosis or NAC were excluded.

15.3 Surgical Technique

If the mastectomy flap is adequate, breast reconstruction with a prepectoral implant-based can be performed regardless of the mastectomy incision (periareolar, radial, inframammary fold, among others). Symmetry between the incisions is important in the case of bilateral mastectomies. Detailed preoperative planning, with well-defined breast limits and measurement of the chest wall are essential steps to be taken for a successful reconstruction, especially when we are not going to use meshes. It is also very important to preserve adipose tissue in all regions where there is no glandular tissue, such as the upper pole (Fig. 15.1).

There are no clinical studies that have prospectively evaluated the ideal thickness of the mastectomy flap and CAP to date. The thickness of the flap depends on the constitution of the patient and the amount of subcutaneous tissue found. It must be thick enough to maintain vascularity, avoiding thick flaps that increase the risk of local recurrence and trying not to leave breast tissue, even though it has been shown that total removal of it is impossible [19]. To prevent complications, it is necessary to consider all the parameters shown in Table 15.1.

It has been shown that there are incisions that generate more complications such as periareolar and others are safer [20] In our experience, we use two variants of submammary incision, a conventional one in the fold without lateral or medial projection to preserve more perforating sensory nerves (Fig. 15.2) and another midlateral curvilinear incision 1–2 cm above and along the IMC was designed, until de anterior axillary line, with the possibility to extend upward to the midaxillary line, when the sentinel node was positive and axillary dissection was necessary [21] (Fig. 15.3).

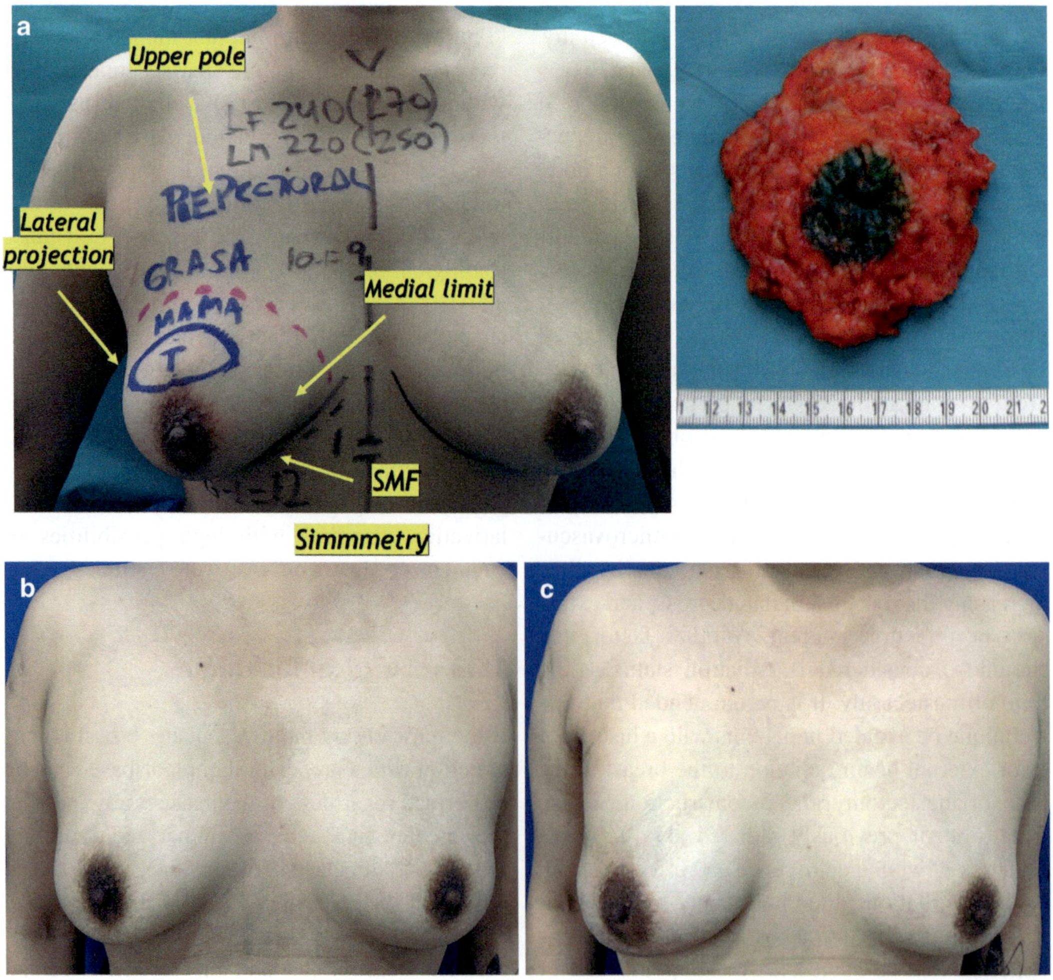

Fig. 15.1 (**a**) A good reconstruction must begin with a good mastectomy. Resect all glandular tissue without invading the anatomical limits of the breast and preserving as much adipose tissue as possible. (**b**) Pre op NSM prepectoral BR right breast. (**c**) Post op NSM prepectoral BR right breast

Table 15.1 How to prevent complications

Prepectoral Breast reconstruction—How to prevent complications	
Planning	Anatomy
	Preoperative imaging evaluation
	Previous morbidities (obesity, smoking, Radiotherapy)
	Choice of tactic (primary, surgical delay NAC, etc.)
	Choice of technique
	Incisions
Surgical technique	Flap dissection
	Limits of mastectomy
	Low temperature dissection methods
	Vitality assessment methods (Spy)
	Choice of pocket
	Choice of implant (expander/prosthesis)
	Change of conduct or intraoperative technique
	Drainage

Once the mastectomy has been performed, the flap perfusion analysis can be performed using clinical signs (color, temperature and thickness of the flap, bleeding from the dermis layer) or imaging devices such as indocyanine green angiography, allowing immediate evaluation of tissue perfusion [22, 23] (Fig. 15.4).

In the presence of signs of poor flap perfusion during the intraoperative period, prepectoral reconstruction should be discouraged. In these cases, subpectoral reconstruction or the use of temporary expanders with 2-step surgeries should be chosen.

Once the choice of the appropriate flap perfusion is contemplated, the reconstruction stage should continue [18].

Regarding the choice of the implant, it is necessary to have some clinical evaluation parameters such as the measurement of the base and height of the breast, protection of the lower pole, degree of ptosis, quantity and elasticity of the

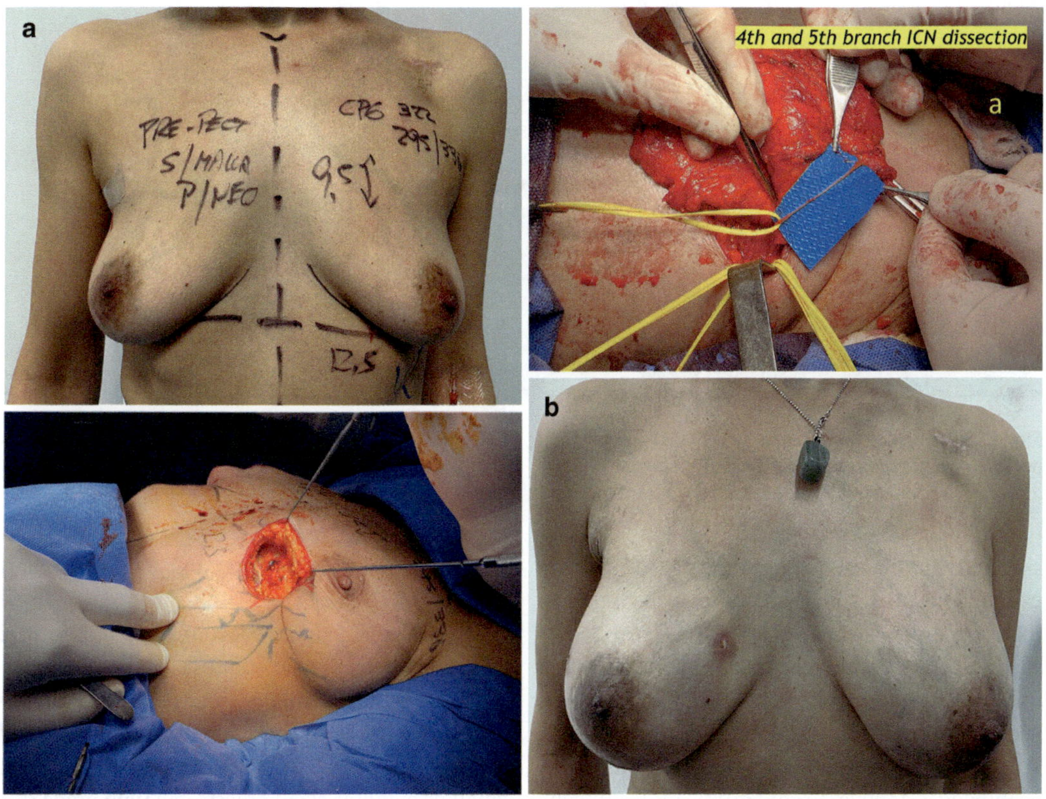

Fig. 15.2 (**a**) Bilateral Prepectoral NSM Post Neo Mutation Check 2+. Classic submammary fold incision. Preservation of sensitivity. (**b**) Post op

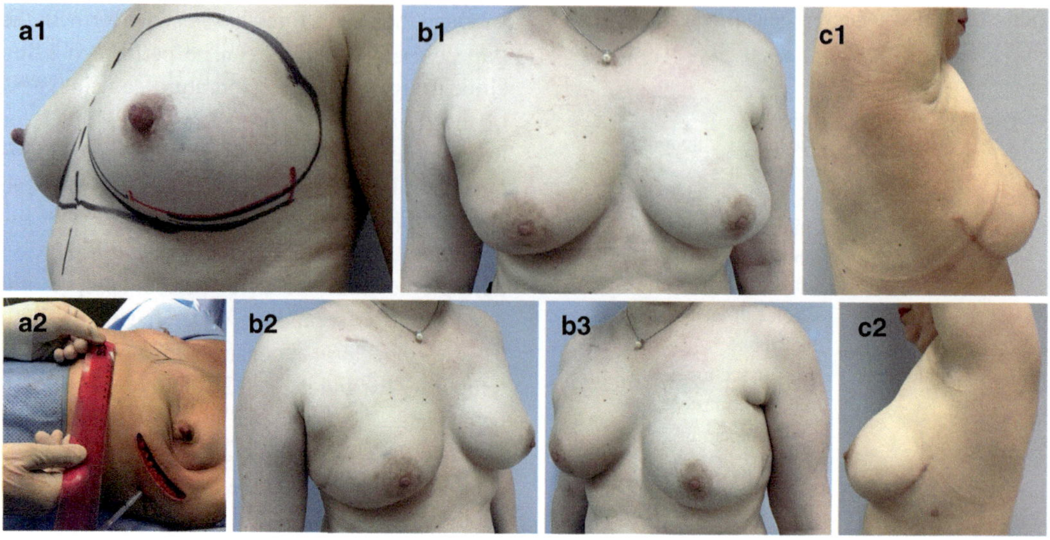

Fig. 15.3 (**a**) *Submammary* midlateral curvilinear incision 1–2 cm above and along the IMC until de anterior axillary line. (**b**) Final result. (**c**) Final result, lateral scar

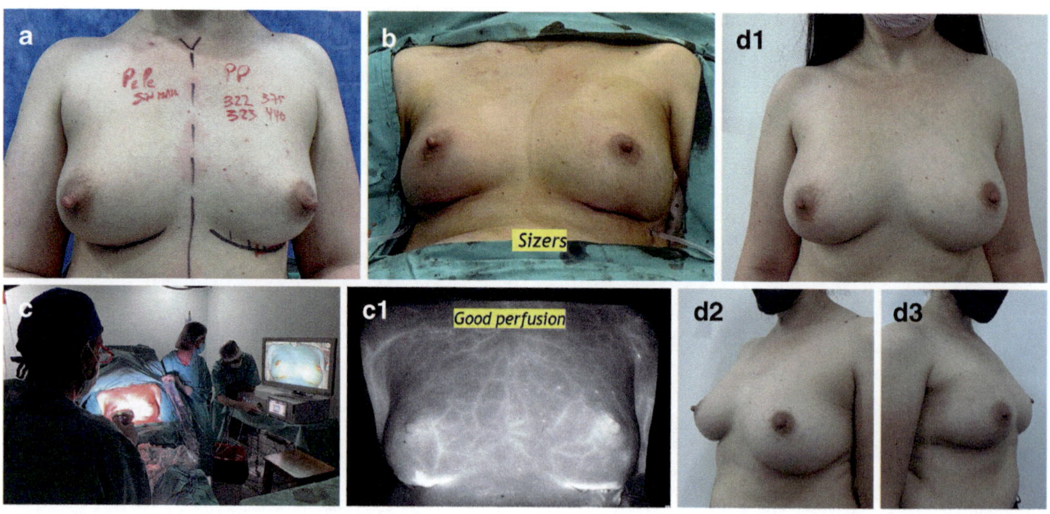

Fig. 15.4 (**a**) Bilateral risk reducing NSM—prepectoral polyurethane implants previous BCT right breast + radiotherapy. (**b**) NSM and prepectoral sizers. (**c**) Intraoperative LA-ICGA, laser-assisted indocyanine green fluorescent angiography. (**d**) Post op 2 years, no epidermolysis or necrosis

skin and thus choose the implant (Fig. 15.5). It is essential to also verify all these measurements intraoperatively and use sizers.

Different types of anatomical textured implants from the following manufactures were used such as Mentor® styles 313, 323 or 333, Allergan/Natrelle® style 410 (until their use was prohibited), Motiva Ergonomix®, or Potlytech® in the prepectoral area, chosen according to the chest wall measurements and desired breast shape.

The edges of the mastectomy are closed in 2 layers with absorbable sutures: hypodermis, subdermis, and intradermal suture. In cases of unilateral NSM, the contralateral breast was intervened in the same surgery for symmetrization in cases of small or medium-sized breasts and with grade 0–1 ptosis. In other cases, symmetrization was per-

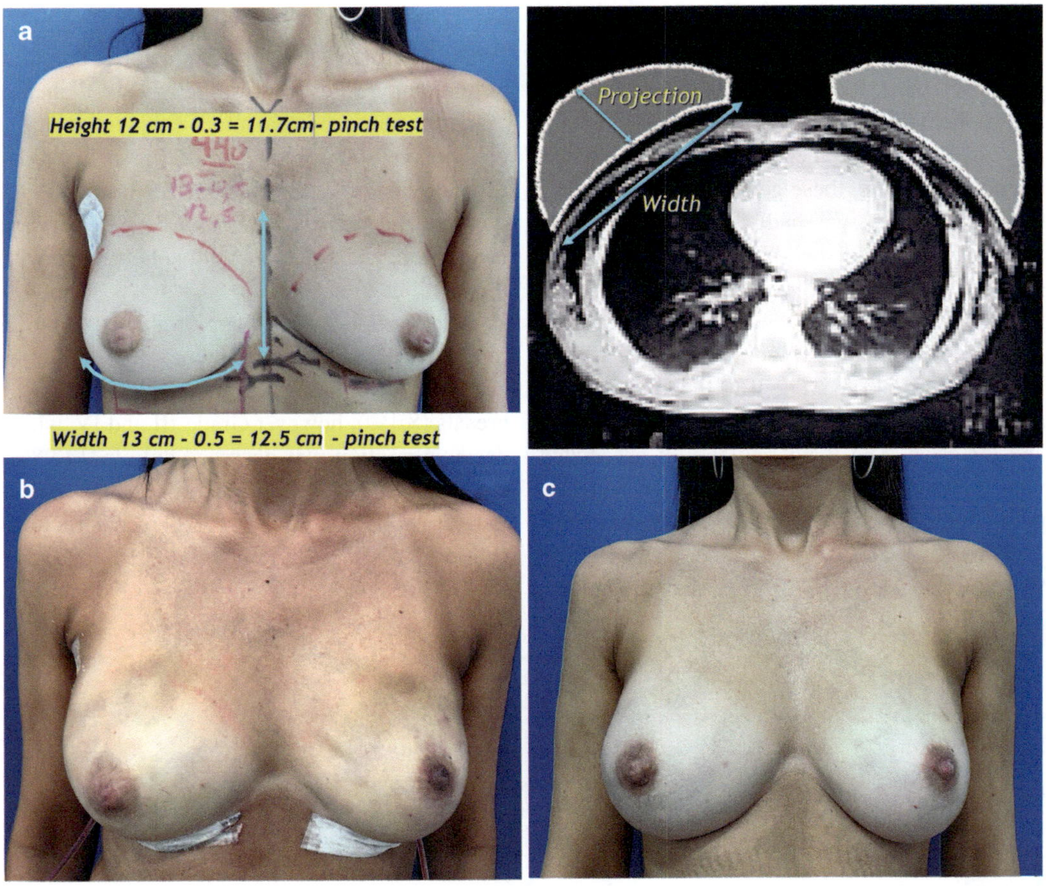

Fig. 15.5 (**a**) How to choose the implant? (**b**) Bilateral NSM and prepectoral reconstruction. 7th day post op. (**c**) Post op 1 year

formed 6 months after surgery, after the end of cancer treatment, or 6 months after the completion of radiotherapy. After the operation, all patients were followed weekly for 4 weeks, every 3 months until 6 months, 1 year after the operation and then every 4–6 months. The drains were removed when the volume was less than 30 cc in 24 h.

15.4 Clinical Outcomes

We started a multicenter cohort of patients undergoing immediate prepectoral reconstruction direct to the implant after NSM through the MFI, without adding ADM or mesh, from January 2018 to June 2020 in Curitiba (Brazil), and from June 2013 to April 2020 in Buenos Aires (Argentina). NSM was offered to all women, with all sizes and types of breasts, either for prophylactic or therapeutic purposes. Patients who underwent either unilateral or bilateral NSM were included [24].

280 immediate breast reconstructions were performed in 195 consecutive patients, using the described procedure. The mean age of the patients was 45 years, and 32.8% of them were in post menopause. Forty-two patients (15.4%) were previous or actual smokers; 92 (32.9%) had BMI over 25 (overweight or obesity) and 7 (5.4%) had diabetes. The median follow-up was 16.5 (±17.43) months. Eighty-five patients (43.6%) underwent bilateral mastectomy and IBR using this technique; 116 (41.4%) mastectomies were prophylactic and 164 (58.6%) were therapeutic.

Sixty-eight (24%) reconstructions had at least one acute complication, the most common of them being implant explantation in 26 (9.2%) breasts. Other reported complications were persistent seroma (19 cases), implant exposure (23 cases), hematoma (7 cases), and flap or NAC necrosis (4 cases). When mild or moderate epidermolysis occurs, these generally resolve spontaneously. When we had cutaneous or NAC necrosis, this established by the risk of infection or extrusion, they were intervened with different techniques according to the defect to be repaired (Fig. 15.6). Implant explantation occurred in a mid-range of 64 days (12–180 days). The most common reason for this was flap or NAC necrosis and infection. The main risk factors associated with explantation were smoking history (odds ratio [OR], 4.33; 95% confidence interval [CI], 1.81–10.37; $P = 0.0012$), BMI over 25 (OR 2.21; 95% CI, 0.98–4.99; $P = 0.077$), and chemotherapy (OR 2.23; 95%CI, 0.97–5.11; $P = 0.062$). When evaluated other risk factors, previous radiotherapy, adjuvant radiotherapy and diabetes, implant extrusion were more frequent in these patients, yet these findings did not reach statistical significance. Other factors such as axillary lymphadenectomy, previous breast surgery, breast size, and ptosis also did not correlate with this complication.

Late complications were evaluated only in reconstructions with a follow-up over 6 months ($n = 184$). Rippling grade II was identified in 15 breasts (8.1%), however Grade III and IV, which needs correction was observed only in 7 (3.8%) cases (Fig. 15.7). Capsular contracture Baker II-IV was observed in 29 (15.7%) reconstructions (Fig. 15.8), being 22 as Baker II (11.9%), 6 Baker III (3.3%), and 1 Baker IV (0.5%) No capsular

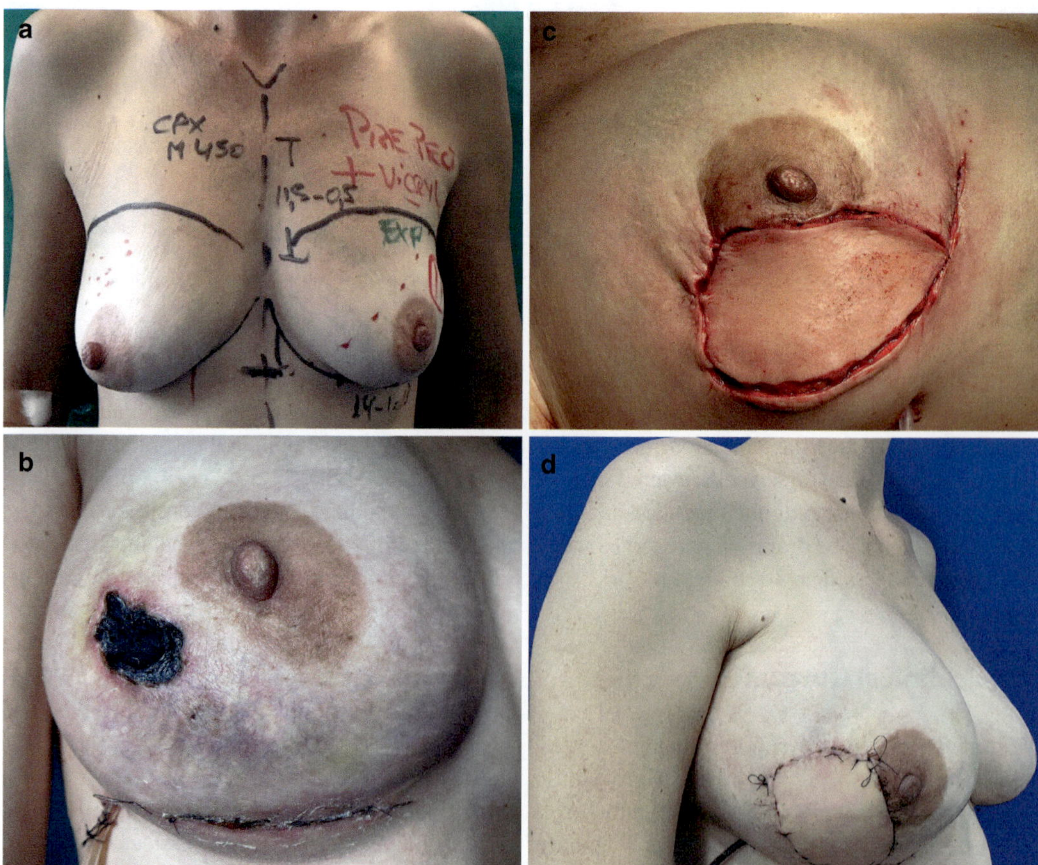

Fig. 15.6 (**a**) Bilateral NSM. Breast reconstruction DTI without mesh. (**b**) Skin necrosis right breast. (**c, d**) BR with Latissimus Dorsi Flap preserving the implant

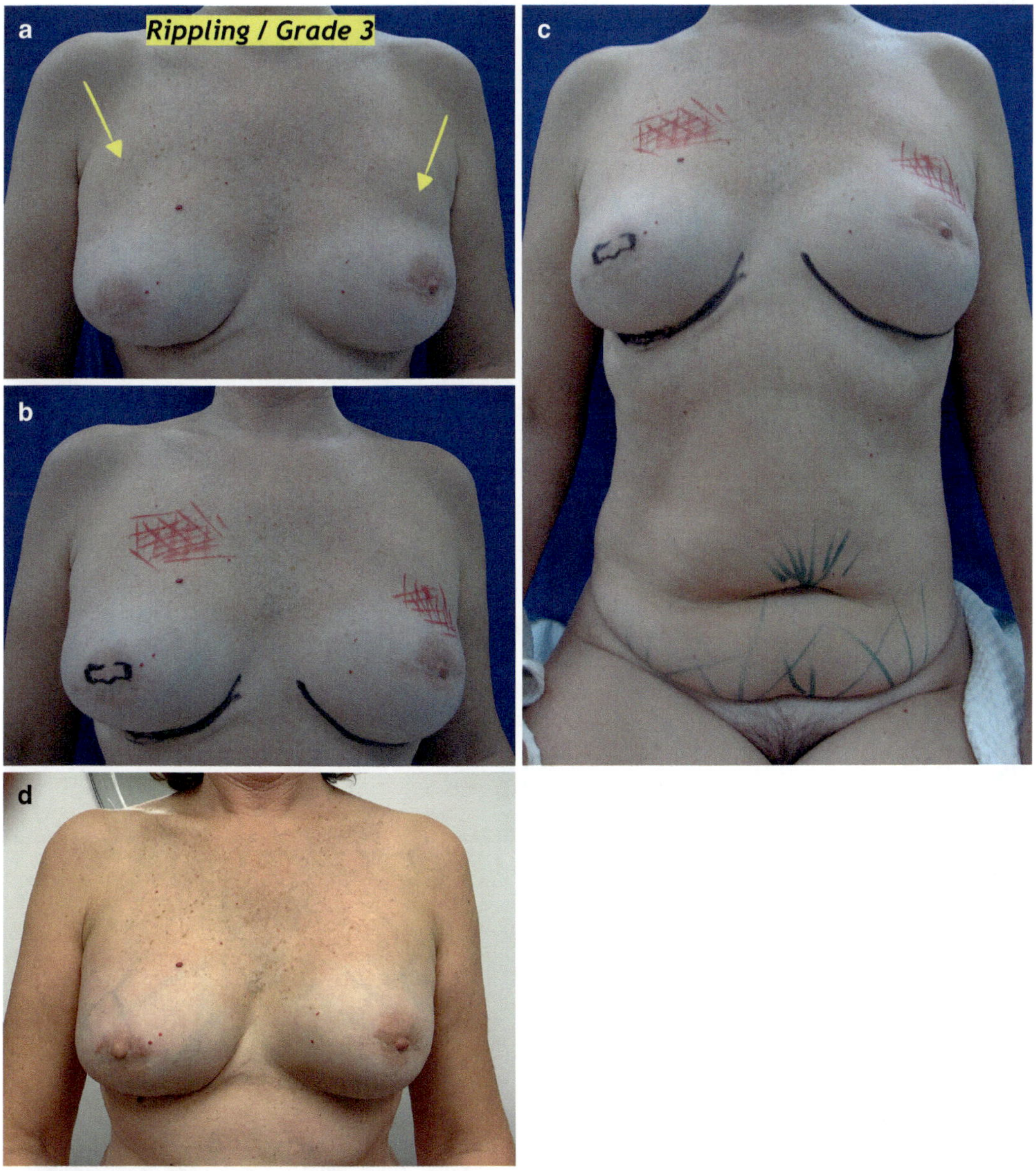

Fig. 15.7 (**a**) Bilateral NSM. Breast reconstruction DTI without mesh. Rippling, necrosis right nipple. (**b**, **c**) Planning, lipofilling, and reconstruction of the nipple. (**d**) Final result

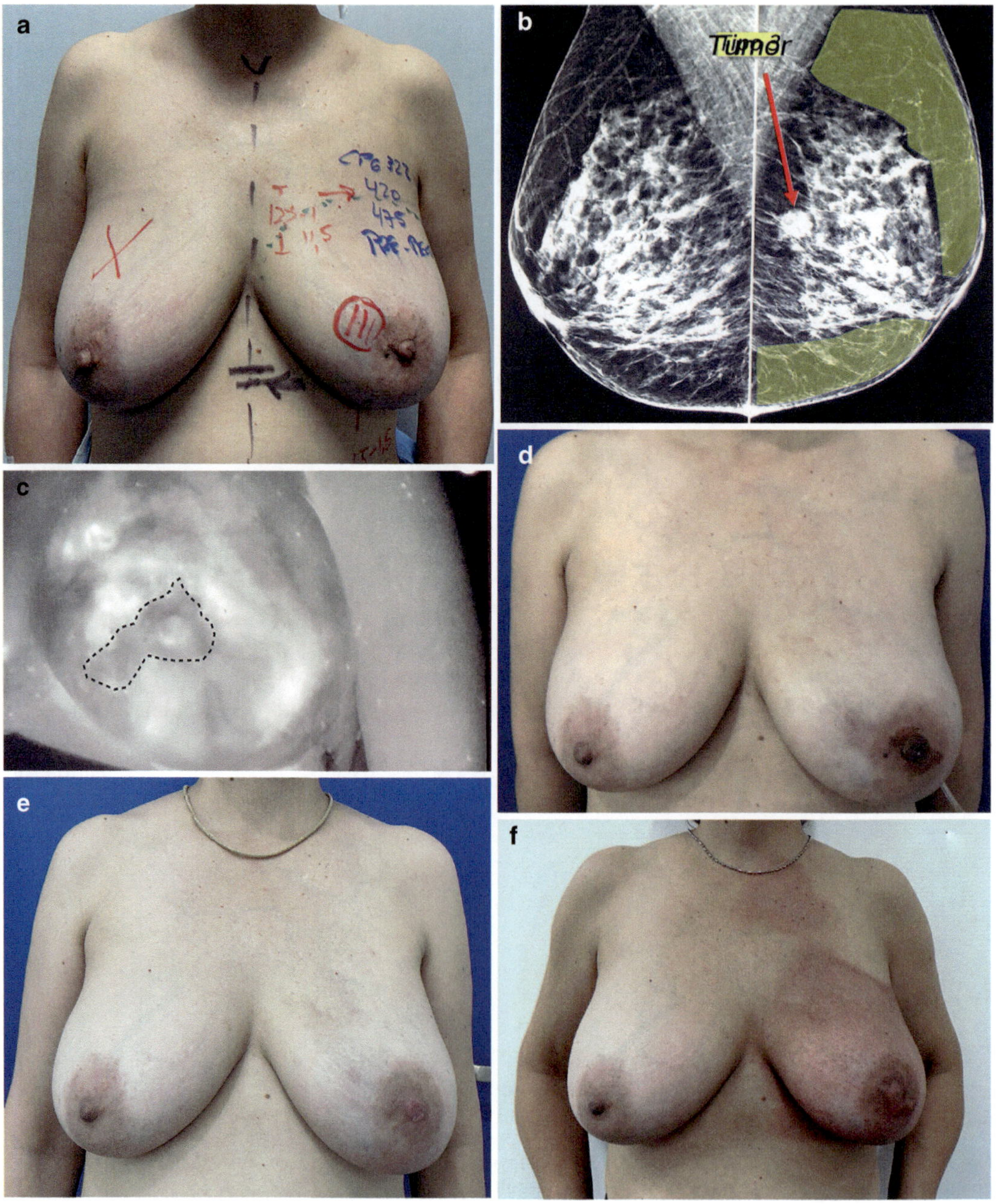

Fig. 15.8 (**a**) Left NSM post Neo. Breast reconstruction DTI prepectoral without mesh. (**b**) Mammogram with adipose panicle Type 3. (**c**) Intraoperative laser-assisted indocyanine green fluorescent angiography with moderate hypoperfusion. (**d**) Moderate necrosis of the NAC. (**e**) Total repairing. (**f**) End of radiotherapy. (**g**) 1 year post radiotherapy with mild harmonious asymmetry and capsular contracture Baker II

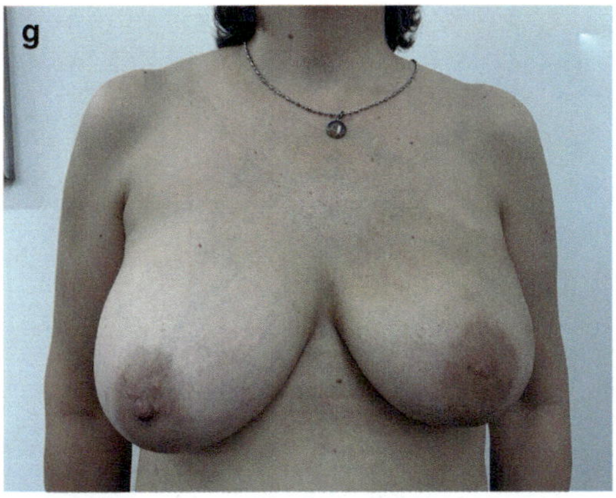

Fig. 15.8 (continued)

contracture was observed in 126 (45%) breasts (Fig. 15.9). 44 (15.7%) breasts were irradiated after surgery, loss of implant occurred in 6 (13.6%) of them, 11 (25%) were without capsular contracture (Fig. 15.10), 7 (15.9%) with Baker I, 8 (18.2%) with Baker II and 3 (6.8%) with Baker 3 (8 of them were without evaluation). One implant rotation was observed. No deformity animation was observed in this period of follow-up. Aesthetic results (evaluated with the BCCT.core software) [25] were considered satisfactory in most patients in our series, even those with large breasts. The incision in the inframammary fold was inapparent (Fig. 15.11).

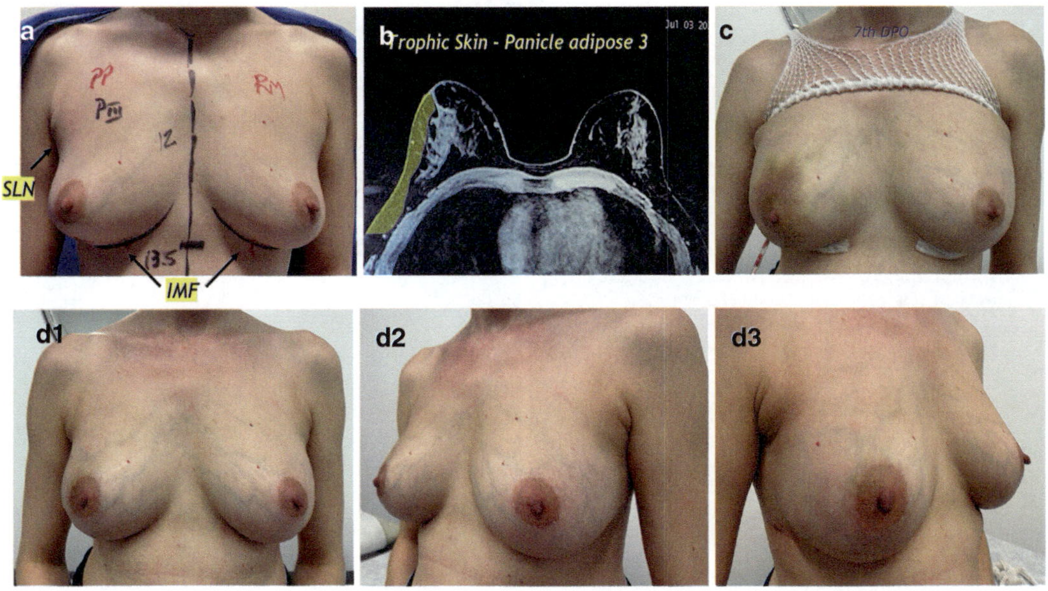

Fig. 15.9 (**a**) Right NSM. Breast reconstruction DTI prepectoral without mesh, contralateral breast augmentation. (**b**) MRIa with adipose panicle Type 3. (**c**) 7th day post op. (**d**) 1 year post op. No capsular contracture

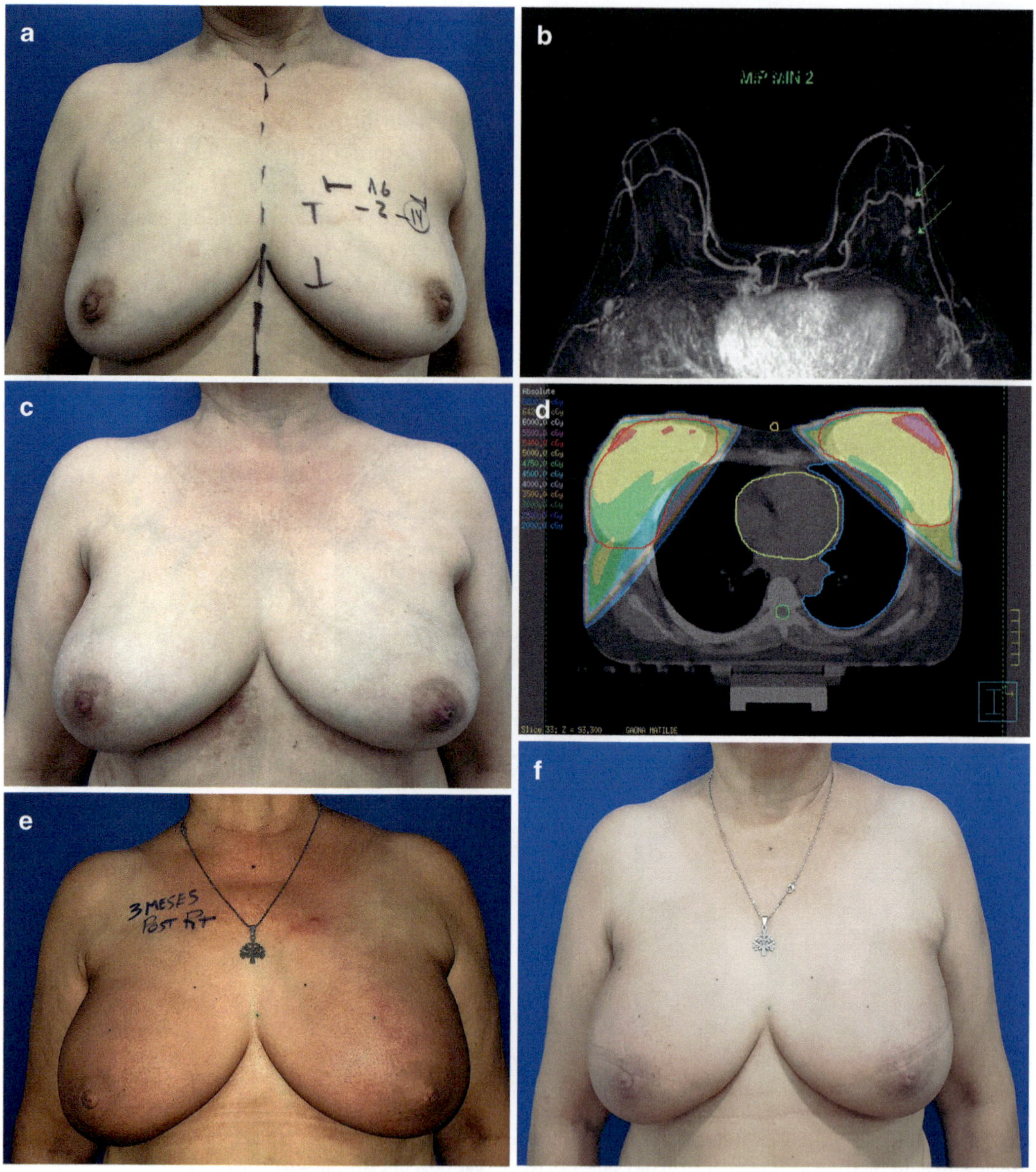

Fig. 15.10 (**a**) Bilateral NSM post Neo, triple-breast cancer. Breast reconstruction DTI prepectoral without mesh-planning. (**b**) MRI complete response in right breast and partial response in left breast. (**c**) 21 days post op. (**d**) Planning bilateral adjuvant radiotherapy. (**e**) Total repairing. (**f**) End of radiotherapy. (**e**) Immediate post radiotherapy result. (**f**) 1 year post radiotherapy without capsular contracture and good symmetry

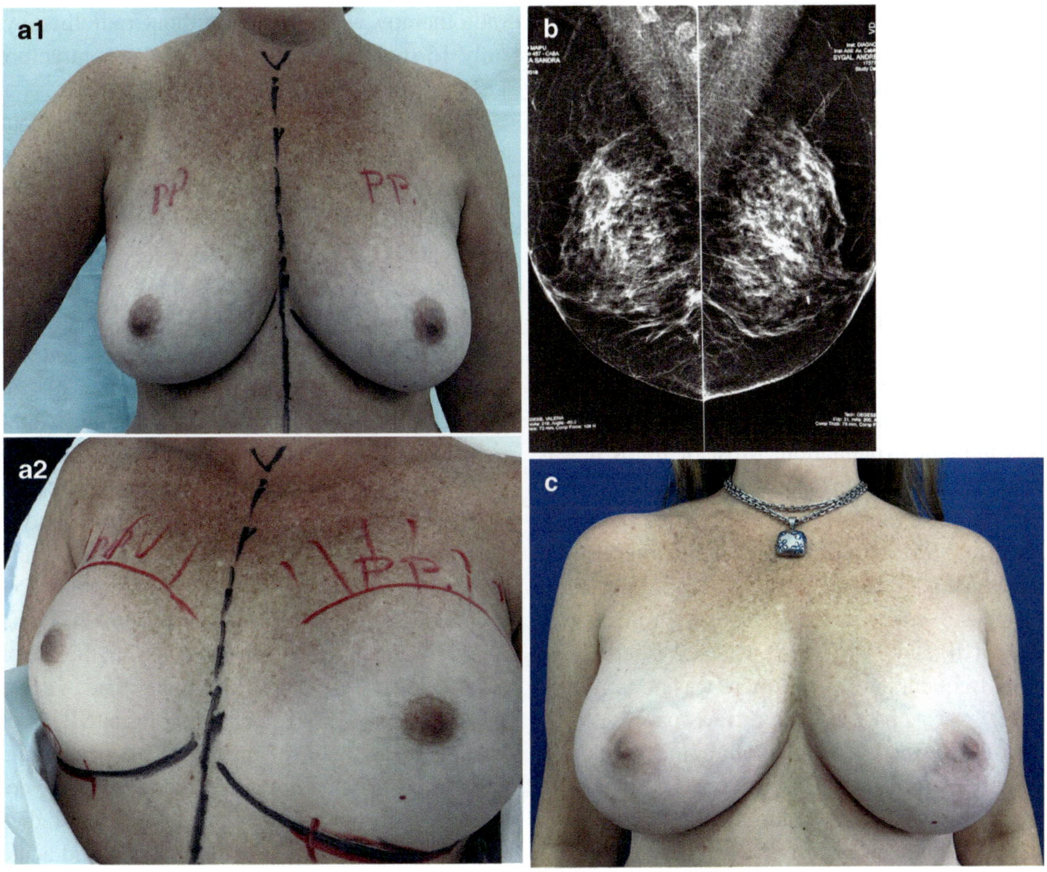

Fig. 15.11 (**a**) Bilateral NSM. BRCA 1+. Breast reconstruction DTI without mesh. (**b**) Mammogram with adipose panicle Type 3. (**c**) Final result good cosmetic result

15.5 Considerations

There are many techniques for immediate reconstruction after NSM. Patients can go to temporary expander, direct-to-implant or autologous flaps. The decision depends on the surgeon's experience, available materials on the center care, and patient's related risk factors like smoking history, diabetes, BMI, breast characteristics (size and ptosis), and the complementary cancer treatment (radiotherapy, chemotherapy, hormonotherapy, lymphadenectomy), that can add risks for bad aesthetic outcomes and increasing complications rates [26–30]. Understanding the importance of skin flap perfusion, vascular integrity and quality of the mastectomy is fundamental to the success of prepectoral technique [19–23].

The main benefits of the prepectoral approach include faster surgery, elimination of animation deformity, and less pain in the postoperatory period (decreased need for narcotics and faster recovery), as it is a less invasive procedure. Postoperative complications with the prepectoral approach have been shown to be comparable with those reported with partial muscle coverage. Although a number of studies have demonstrated advantages of prepectoral implant breast reconstruction, most studies mainly describe two-stage tissue expander approaches or direct-to-implant with the placement of ADM or mesh to support [30, 31]. Li et al., in a metanalysis with 16 comparative studies showed no statistical differences in overall complications, implant extrusion, seroma, nipple or skin flap necrosis, hematoma, reoperation, wound dehiscence, and wound-skin infection, rippling between prepectoral and subpectoral, and with a better Breast Q score and less postoperative pain [32].

Prepectoral is not suitable to all patients. Best candidates usually were the ones with small to medium size breasts, with no or low degree of ptosis. In addition, they should not have other risk factors like obesity, smoking, diabetes mellitus, and previous irradiation on the breast [8–23, 26–34] Even in these favorable cases, many surgeons opt for a 2-stage reconstruction [26–29] In our series we didn't use these criteria to select patients. The most frequent early complication was implant explantation. Most of times it was associated with flap necrosis, infection, and in smokers. The rate of 9.2% in our series is comparable to SSM, subpectoral and also prepectoral series using ADM and mesh [29–32, 34]. Rotation was observed in just one case. Significant rippling (III and IV), which was expected to be more frequent here where there was no muscular cover, was observed in a few cases (7/184 breasts). In the event of rippling and wrinkling, several factors require consideration, including the thickness flaps, the implant-to-mastectomy ratio, and implant cohesivity. Rippling and wrinkling are considerate by many surgeons as common in the setting of prepectoral reconstruction. However, there is no significant data on it and was not so frequent in our series.

Capsular contracture is a common adverse outcome following implant breast reconstruction, often associated with radiation treatment. Chu et al. in a literature review showed that also preoperative and postoperative radiation were associated with a higher rate of implant loss, with statistical significance [35]. Muscle fibrosis can be a contributor of breast reconstruction contracture after radiation. Sobti et al. found greater rates of capsular contracture in the subpectoral vs. prepectoral group ($n = 28$, 51.8% vs. $n = 12$, 30.0%, $P = 0.02$). When compared to prepectoral, DTI reconstruction in irradiated patients, subpectoral implant placement was nearly 4 times as likely to result in capsular contracture ($P < 0.01$). In addition, in our series, significant capsular contracture (Baker II to IV) was present in 29 (15.7%) cases. In 14 of them, adjuvant radiotherapy was present. Without radiotherapy, only 15 (6.3%) breasts had capsular contracture [13].

Mesh and ADM can serve as a layer of vascularized regenerative tissue between the implant and mastectomy flap and allow stabilization of reconstructed breast. [29] Though ADMs have been widely adopted by plastic surgeons, Salibian et al. have demonstrated that thick mastectomy skin flaps and strict preservation of the native inframammary fold may obviate the need for ADM. Their 10-year retrospective review of 250 prepectoral breast reconstructions without ADM reveal clinically significant capsular contracture in 7.6% of patients and implant displacement in 0.8%. Aesthetic outcomes were graded as good to very good in 85.2% of patients [31]. A systematic review and meta-analysis of complications following NSM and reconstruction with DTI and ADM by Heidemann et al. suggests that the use of ADM can be associated with a higher rate of acute complications. [36] The authors presented 4% of NAC necrosis, 12% of infection, 5% of seroma, and 1% of hematoma. All percentages were equivalent to our study, requiring further studies to prove the association between ADM and acute complications. The cost of using ADM and mesh is expensive, ranging from $1000 to more than $20,000. In our series of 280 prepectoral DTI breast reconstructions, no ADM and no mesh were used, and complication rates and outcomes were similar to ADM and mesh series. However, data on prepectoral DTI breast reconstruction without ADM and mesh are still limited.

Flap necrosis is one of the main complications and occurs in 3–7% of cases.1 A meta-analysis of Daar et al. showed a NAC necrosis rate after NSM by IMF of 6.82% [28]. In our series, NAC necrosis occurred in only 4 breasts (1.4%) and flap necrosis in 20 breasts (7.1%). Mastectomy skin flaps can vary based on thickness, dimensions, and perfusion. Therefore, skin flap assessment is a critical component and determinant of success in prepectoral reconstruction. The quality of the mastectomy, and in this way, thickness of skin flap are less important than the perfusion. Thin and young patients typically have thin mastectomy flaps, and overweight or obese and older patients tend to have thicker mastectomy skin flaps. The normal subcutaneous layer of the breast varies from person to person and ranges from 2 to 3 cm. In situations where the mastectomy skin flaps are thicker and well perfused, either a tissue expander or a permanent implant can be placed in the prepectoral space.

15.6 Conclusions

In our experience between 2013 and 2020, we included in a multicenter cohort study immediate direct-to-implant prepectoral breast reconstruction therapeutic or risk reduction, without any type of mesh assistance (biological or synthetic), including patients with all types of breasts, without ptosis or with moderate ptosis, with different types of adipose panicle, body mass index, smokers or not, and with or without prior radiation therapy.

Surgical complications with this technique did not differ substantially from the previously reported series of ADM, mesh, or subpectoral. The rates of rippling and capsular contracture were not higher here. These data demonstrated that this technique is promising, safe, and could be economically advantageous, as it is a one-stage technique without ADM or mesh. Also, there is no animated mama. However, this is only a preliminary series with short-term and long-term results. Larger and more comparative studies are required.

Key Points

- Surgical complications appear similar to series with synthetic mesh, ADM, or subpectoral reconstructions.
- Rippling rates are not higher than with other techniques.
- Capsular contracture rates not higher than with other techniques.
- Capsular contractures in patients with radiotherapy, in the follow-up to date, these present in percentages similar to the other techniques but not altering the shape of the irradiated breast, being harmonic and with a better positive impact on symmetry.
- In addition, there is no animated breast.
- This technique is promising, safe and could be economically advantageous, as it is a one-stage technique without ADM and mesh.

References

1. Freeman BS. Subcutaneous mastectomy for benign breast lesions with immediate or delayed prosthetic replacement. Plast Reconstr Surg. 1980;65(3):371–2.
2. Freeman BS. Technique of subcutaneous mastectomy with replacement; immediate and delayed. Br J Plast Surg. 1969;22(2):161–6.
3. Snyderman RK, Guthrie RH. Reconstruction of the female breast following radical mastectomy. Plast Reconstr Surg. 1971;47(6):565–7.
4. Schlenker JD, Bueno RA, Ricketson G, Lynch JB. Loss of silicone implants after subcutaneous mastectomy and reconstruction. Plast Reconstr Surg. 1978;62(6):853–61.
5. Gruber RP, Kahn RA, Lash H, Maser MR, Apfelberg DB, Laub DR. Breast reconstruction following mastectomy: a comparison of submuscular and subcutaneous techniques. Plast Reconstr Surg. 1981;67(3):312–7.
6. Serra-Renom JM, Fontdevila J, Monner J, Benito J. Mammary reconstruction using tissue expander and partial detachment of the pectoralis major muscle to expand the lower breast quadrants. Ann Plast Surg. 2004;53(4):317–21.
7. Breuing K, Warren S. Immediate bilateral breast reconstruction with implants and inferolateral AlloDerm slings. Ann Plast Surg. 2005;55(3):232–9.
8. Namnoum JD. Expander/implant reconstruction with AlloDerm: recent experience. Plast Reconstr Surg. 2009;124(2):387–94.
9. Colwell A. Direct-to-implant breast reconstruction. Gland Surg. 2012;1(3):139–41.
10. Dieterich M, Faridi A. Biological matrices and synthetic meshes used in implant-based breast reconstruction: a review of products available in germany. Geburtshilfe Frauenheilkd. 2013;73(11):1100–6.
11. Ho G, Nguyen TJ, Shahabi A, Hwang BH, Chan LS, Wong AK. A systematic review and meta-analysis of complications associated with acellular dermal matrix-assisted breast reconstruction. Ann Plast Surg. 2012;68(4):346–56.
12. Potter S, Conroy EJ, Cutress RI, Williamson PR, Whisker L, Thrush S, Skillman J, Barnes NLP, Mylvaganam S, Teasdale E, Jain A, Gardiner MD, Blazeby JM, Holcombe C, iBRA Steering Group; Breast Reconstruction Research Collaborative. Short-term safety outcomes of mastectomy and immediate implant-based breast reconstruction with and without mesh (iBRA): a multicentre, prospective cohort study. Lancet Oncol. 2019;20(2):254–66.

13. Sobti N, Weitzman RE, Nealon KP, Jimenez RB, Gfrerer L, Mattos D, Ehrlichman RJ, Gadd M, Specht M, Austen WG, Liao EC. Evaluation of capsular contracture following immediate prepectoral versus subpectoral direct-to-implant breast reconstruction. Sci Rep. 2020;10(1):1137.
14. Chatterjee A, Nahabedian MY, Gabriel A, Macarios D, Parekh M, Wang F, Griffin L, Sigalove S. Early assessment of post-surgical outcomes with prepectoral breast reconstruction: a literature review and meta-analysis. J Surg Oncol. 2018;117(6):1119–30.
15. Sigalove S, Maxwell GP, Sigalove NM, Storm-Dickerson TL, Pope N, Rice J, et al. Prepectoral implant-based breast reconstruction. Plast Reconstr Surg. 2017;139(2):287–94.
16. Sbitany H, Piper M, Lentz R. Prepectoral breast reconstruction: a safe alternative to submuscular prosthetic reconstruction following nipple-sparing mastectomy. Plast Reconstr Surg. 2017;140(3):432–43.
17. Sbitany H. Important considerations for performing prepectoral breast reconstruction. Plast Reconstr Surg. 2017;140(6S):7S–13S.
18. Nahabedian MY. Current approaches to prepectoral breast reconstruction. Plast Reconstr Surg. 2018;142(4):871–80.
19. Kaidar-Person O, Boersma LJ, Poortmans P, Sklair-Levy M, Offersen BV, Cardoso MJ, de Ruysscher D. Residual glandular breast tissue after mastectomy: a systematic review. Ann Surg Oncol. 2020;27(7):2288–96.
20. Carlson GW, Chu CK, Moyer HR, Duggal C, Losken A. Predictors of nipple ischemia after nipple sparing mastectomy. Breast J. 2014;20(1):69–73.
21. Blechman KM, Karp NS, Levovitz C, Guth AA, Axelrod DM, Shapiro RL, Choi M. The lateral inframammary fold incision for nipple-sparing mastectomy: outcomes from over 50 immediate implant-based breast reconstructions. Breast J. 2013;19(1):31–40.
22. Gurtner GC, Jones GE, Neligan PC, Newman MI, Phillips BT, Sacks JM, Zenn MR. Intraoperative laser angiography using the SPY system: review of the literature and recommendations for use. Ann Surg Innov Res. 2013;7(1):1.
23. Lauritzen E, Damsgaard TE. Use of Indocyanine Green Angiography decreases the risk of complications in autologous and implant-based breast reconstruction: A systematic review and meta-analysis. J Plast Reconstr Aesthet Surg. 2021;74(8):1703–17.
24. Urban CA, Gonzalez E, Fornazzari A, et al. Prepectoral direct-to-implant breast reconstruction without placement of acellular dermal matrix or mesh after nipple sparing mastectomy. Plast Reconstr Surg 2022;150(5):973–983. doi: https://doi.org/10.1097/PRS.0000000000009618
25. Hart A, Doyle K, Losken A, Carlson GW. Nipple malposition after bilateral nipple-sparing mastectomy with implant-based reconstruction: objective postoperative analysis utilizing BCCT.core computer software. Breast J. 2020 Jul;26(7):1270–5.
26. Weber PW, Haug M, Kurzeder C, et al. Oncoplastic Breast Consortium consensus conference on nipple-sparing mastectomy. Breast Cancer Res Treat. 2018;172:523–37.
27. Storm-Dickerson T, Sigalove N. Prepectoral breast reconstruction: the breast surgeon's perspective. Plast Reconstr Surg. 2017;140:43S.
28. Daar DA, Abdou SA, Rosario L, et al. Is there a preferred incision location for nipple-sparing mastectomy? A systematic review and meta-analysis. Plast Reconstr Surg. 2019;143:906e.
29. Storm-Dickerson T, Sigalove NM. The breast surgeons' approach to mastectomy and prepectoral breast reconstruction. Gland Surg. 2019;8(1):27–35.
30. Manrique OJ, Huang TCT, Martinez-Jorge J, et al. Prepectoral two-stage implant-based breast reconstruction with and without acellular dermal matrix: do we see a difference? Plast Reconstr Surg. 2020;145:263e.
31. Salibian AH, Harness JK, Mowlds DS. Staged suprapectoral expander/implant reconstruction without acellular dermal matrix following nipple-sparing mastectomy. Plast Reconstr Surg. 2017;139:30–9.
32. Li L, Su Y, Xiu B, et al. Comparison of prepectoral and subpectoral breast reconstruction after mastectomies: a systematic review and meta-analysis. Eur J Surg Oncol. 2019;45:1542–50.
33. Vidya R, Iqbal FM, Becker H, Zhadan O. Rippling associated with pre-pectoral implant-based breast reconstruction: a new grading system. World J Plast Surg. 2019;8:311–5.
34. Louw RPT, Nahabedian MY. Prepectoral breast reconstruction. Plast Reconstr Surg. 2017;140:51S.
35. Chu CK, Davis MJ, Winocour SJ, et al. Implant reconstruction in nipple sparing mastectomy. Semin Plast Surg. 2019;33:247–57.
36. Heidemann LN, Gunnarsson GL, Salzberg CA. Complications following nipple-sparing mastectomy and immediate acellular dermal matrix implant-based breast reconstruction—a systematic review and meta-analysis. Plast Reconstr Surg Glob Open. 2018;6:e1625.

16 Prepectoral Skin-Reducing Pattern

Glenda Giorgia Caputo and Maurizio Governa

16.1 Introduction

Skin-reduction breast reconstruction is a mastectomy/reconstruction technique involving fitting a prepectoral prosthetic implant. It is based on a technique described by Nava et al. in 2006, in which the implant was housed in a pocket comprising the pectoralis major muscle and a dermo-adipose flap created via de-epithelializing the lower pole of the breast [1]. As reported in the *PRS* in 2016 [2], we modified the technique to obviate the need to raise the pectoralis major by placing the implant in the prepectoral space in a pocket composed of a dermo-adipose flap—salvaged during the mastectomy performed according to the Wise-pattern preoperative design—below and a dermal matrix above; the dermal matrix is sutured to the pectoral fascia, thereby ensuring coverage of the upper pole of the prosthesis.

The advantages of prepectoral reconstruction are easy to see; as no muscle is raised, the surgery is less invasive, and therefore associated with a lower risk of postoperative bleeding. Furthermore, implant mobility due to contraction of the pectoralis major, a typical result of submuscular reconstruction, is absent, and, last but not least, patient comfort appears to be improved; indeed, with prepectoral reconstruction, the sensation of a bulky foreign body that is unfailingly reported with submuscular implants is not reported [3].

That being said, there are several potential complications, first and foremost being possible ischemic damage to the mastectomy flaps, which puts the patient at risk of implant exposure and therefore reconstruction failure. This chapter describes the indications, surgical technique, and most common complications of skin-reduction breast reconstruction and how to manage them, as well as several suggestions for reducing the risk that they will arise.

16.2 Indications

Achieving a good outcome of breast reconstruction must begin with accurate patient selection and impeccable surgical technique. With regard to the former, it is important to note that this particular reconstruction is indicated in focal, multifocal, or multicentric breast carcinoma patients (inflammatory breast cancer is to be excluded) with large, ptotic breasts, as ascertained with a pinch test greater than 1 cm, and no infiltration of the skin of the lower pole. It may also be used as a prophylactic mastectomy technique in cases of macromastia and breasts with a high level of ptosis, i.e., non-cancer patients in whom reduction mammoplasty or mastopexy is indicated. Indeed,

G. G. Caputo (✉)
Plastic and Reconstructive Surgery—ASUFC Udine, Udine, Italy

M. Governa
Plastic and Reconstructive Surgery—AOUI Verona, Verona, Italy

© The Author(s), under exclusive license to Springer Nature Switzerland AG 2023
R. Vidya, H. Becker (eds.), *Prepectoral Breast Reconstruction*,
https://doi.org/10.1007/978-3-031-15590-1_16

a pre- vs. post-surgical breast Q survey carried out in our OU revealed comparable scores to reduction mammoplasty patients; in other words, skin-reduction breast reconstruction patients report similar levels of postoperative well-being to those who have undergone breast reduction for macromastia.

In the beginning, when we first began to use this technique for breast reconstruction, we excluded cases in which there was a possibility of the patient receiving postoperative radiotherapy, which we viewed as an absolute contraindication. In recent years, however, we have revised this opinion due to new histological research on irradiated periprosthetic capsule tissue, which seems to be thicker and more resistant in the submuscular space with respect to the capsule that forms around subcutaneous implants covered with acellular dermal matrix (ADM) [4], and evidence that capsule contraction is reduced in ADM-assisted prosthetic breast reconstruction surgery [5, 6]. The same cannot be said of mastectomies conducted due to relapse or secondary tumor after quadrantectomy and radiotherapy QUART; in such cases, as the tissue has previously been exposed to radiation, there is the issue of vascular viability in the mastectomy flaps [7], which limits the indication of prepectoral reconstruction with inverted-T incision.

When assessing potential skin-reduction breast reconstruction surgery candidates, it is important to take a full medical history, including smoking habits, diabetes, heart disease, increased age, and high BMI, all of which expose a patient to a greater risk of postoperative complications.

16.3 Technique

16.3.1 Preoperative Drawing

Accurate preoperative drawings are to be made according to the conventional Wise-pattern method (Fig. 16.1). A vertical midline line should be marked from the sternal notch to the navel (a). From this line, along the clavicle, a distance of 7–9 cm should be measured, depending on the thoracic structure of the individual patient (b);

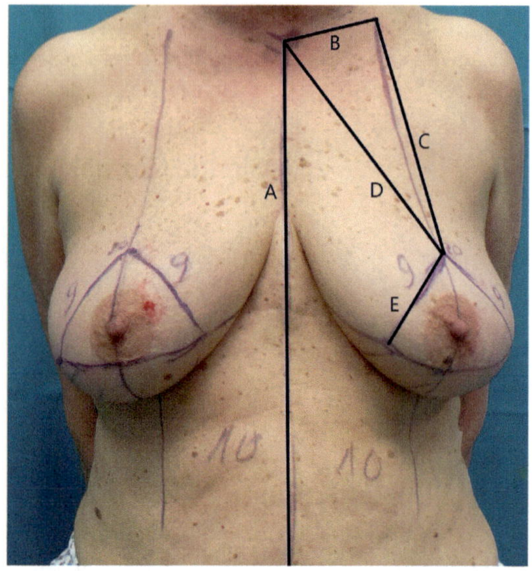

Fig. 16.1 Preoperative drawing

specifically, in patients with small thorax and narrow shoulders, the ideal distance should be 7 cm, while 9 cm is to be preferred in patients with wider chest and shoulders. From this point, a line should be traced to the nipple (c), and then continued below, to and beyond the inframammary fold, lifting the breast with the other hand, and on to the abdominal wall. The distance from this point to the midline from sternal notch to navel should be 8–11 cm, depending on the width of the thorax. Next, the point at which the nipple projection line intersects the mid-clavicle line should be marked at a variable distance from the sternal notch, from 19 to 21 cm for ptotic breasts and 21 to 24 cm in cases of macromastia (d); these measurements are indicative, because the distance between the sternal notch and nipple will depend on the desired degree of reduction or lifting of the reconstructed breast, which must be designed to be harmonious with the physical structure of the patient. In other words, the reconstructed breast should be "made to measure," bearing in mind the overall makeup of the patient's body. Hence, mammary reduction in a particularly robust patient should leave them with a relatively large breast, which in numerical terms will be reflected in the distance between the sternal notch and the nipple. Nonetheless, it is important to bear in mind that larger implants (greater than about 500 cc) expose the patient to a greater risk of complications and do not guarantee a stable long-term outcome, as the weight of the implant will gradually lead to a worsening of the ptosis (see below in the paragraph on *implant selection*).

The final phase in the preoperative marking involves moving the breast medially and then laterally in order to mark the medial and lateral arms of the vertical scar. Lines of length 8–9 cm from the point where the new nipple will be, should be measured on each line (E). This 8–9 cm is the sum of the vertical incision (6–7 cm) plus the radius of the nipple–areola complex (2 cm).

Perioperative antibiotics (cefazolin 2 g), given 30 min before the surgical incision, are, of course, routine.

16.3.2 Demolition Phase

Before beginning the skin incision according to the preoperative design, all tissue layers should be fully infiltrated with Klein solution [8] in order to obtain a bloodless field and allow hydrodissection of the cleavage planes. Specifically, infiltration should involve (1) the subcutaneous floor of the breast region, site of the mastectomy cleavage plane (Cooper's ligaments); (2) the sub-epithelial/intradermal plane of the entire area of the lower pole, which will form the periprosthetic pocket flap; and (3) the subdermal plane of the area occupied by the nipple–areola complex, which will be taken as a full-thickness skin graft, and will be grafted only if the response of the extemporaneous histological examination of the retroareolar gland sample is negative for tumor cells.

At this point, the dermo-adipose flap is de-epithelialized, which in our experience is easier with the breast still in place. In addition, it is easier to perform this operation with scissors rather than a scalpel because you can work alone, without the help of an assistant to keep the skin of the breast, which in these patients is particularly lax, under tension (which is necessary in cold scalpel de-epithelialization). Delicate surgical technique is performed aimed at reducing tissue trauma in hopes of attenuating the tissue damage [9]. The mastectomy and lymph node surgery can then be performed through the wide incision; the armpit incision should then sutured with subcutaneous stiches and isolated from the mastectomy area. Now the field is ready for the reconstruction phase.

16.3.3 Reconstruction Phase

The dermal flap of the de-epithelialized lower pole is preserved (Fig. 16.2) to be combined with a patch of ADM to create a dermal pocket (Fig. 16.3); the ADM/combined flap is used to cover the anatomical implant, over the upper pole, and held in place by resorbable sutures (Fig. 16.4). If the ADM is not fenestrated, it is then pierced with a n° 11 blade scalpel while the surgical assistant holds it tight. At this point, a test implant (if available) can be inserted and the incision temporarily closed, using metal staples, to check that the wound will close without stretching and that the breasts are volumetrically symmetrical — the contralateral breast will have undergone the same procedure in the case of bilateral mastectomy, or reduction mammoplasty in the case of monolateral mammoplasty. The size check should be performed with the patient in a sitting position (45°–60°), and at this point it

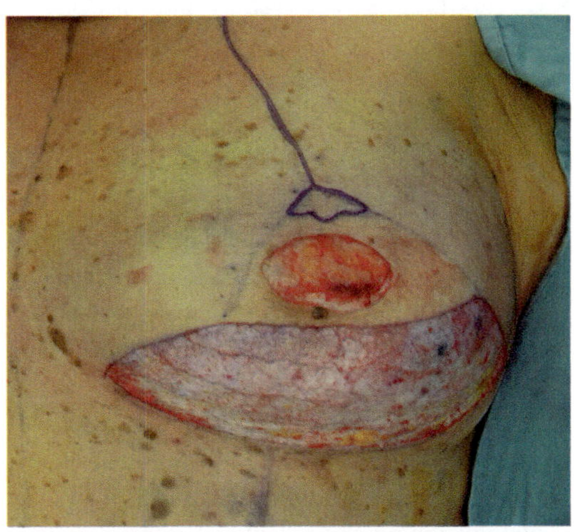

Fig. 16.2 Preservation of de-epithelialized lower pole

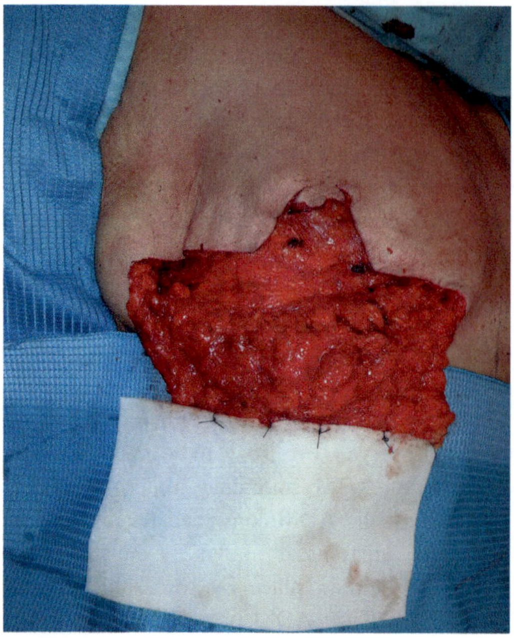

Fig. 16.3 ADM sutured to the dermal flap

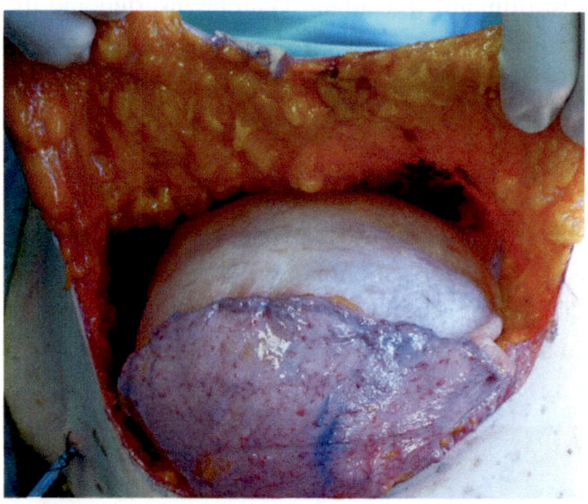

Fig. 16.4 Coverage of the implant with ADM-dermal flap

would be useful to assess the flap viability after indocyanine injection if video fluoroangiography equipment is available; any skin margins that display poor blood supply can be trimmed, and either a temporary or permanent expander or smaller, less projecting implant may be placed. If fluoroangiography is not feasible, clinical examination must determine the flap viability with a view to weighing up implant or expander options [10]. What is particularly important is that gentle handling be rigorously adhered to throughout the entire surgical procedure, beginning with the use of scissors for the mastectomy and atraumatic retractors, handled with the necessary precautions, without excessive stretching, which should, in any case, not be necessary given the large surgical field available.

Once the definitive implant or expander is in place, the pocket can be closed laterally, suturing the dermal flap to the fascia of the serratus anterior. For better inframammary fold definition, the dermal flap can be incised at its base, along the fold, up to 4 cm. The upper edge of the acellular dermal matrix should then be fixed to the anterior fascia of the pectoralis major with individual resorbable sutures. A drain should be placed in the pocket, and the skin closed in the inverted-T fashion (Fig. 16.5).

The nipple can then be reconstructed using an arrowhead flap or similar at the most protuberant point of the new breast, which corresponds to the tip of the vertical arm of the inverted T. If the fresh-frozen retroareolar biopsy results were negative, after areola marking and intraepithelial infiltration with Klein solution, the area around the new nipple can be de-epithelialized to prepare the ground for the areola graft, which should have been harvested at the beginning of the operation and preserved in a basin containing saline solution up until this point. If areolar skin is not available for graft-

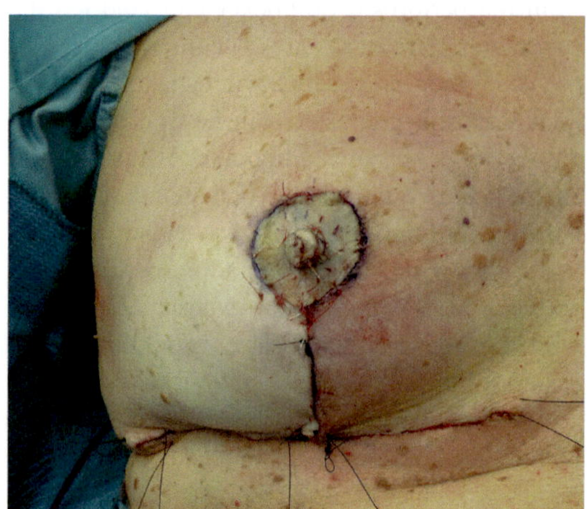

Fig. 16.5 Reconstructed breast at the end of surgery

ing, the patient can be referred for cosmetic tattooing once healing has occurred.

As regards the *implant selection*, certain considerations should be made. In particular, in our experience, textured anatomical implants result in very satisfactory outcomes, but it is important to remember that the success of implant reconstruction, especially subcutaneous, will largely depend on the viability of the mastectomy flaps as regards blood supply. Hence, it is not always possible to place a fixed-volume implant straight away in all cases. In cases in which the surgeon is not fully confident that the mastectomy flaps may be relied upon, rather than running the risk of wound dehiscence and delayed healing, it is advisable to insert an adjustable-volume implant to be later filled with saline [11], or a breast expander to be inserted with the minimum filling volume (obviously, in the latter case, a second operation will be needed to replace the expander with the permanent prosthesis). By keeping the volume of the prosthesis/expander low, the tension on the sutures will be reduced and the wound will have a better chance of healing well. Similarly, in order to reduce the tension on the central part of the inverted T, moderate or low-projection implants are to be preferred for this type of reconstruction surgery. Their transverse and vertical diameters should be carefully measured preoperatively and will vary on the basis of the anthropometric characteristics of the individual patient, seeking to remain faithful to the footprint of the natural breast.

16.4 Postoperative Care

Postoperative management of patients requires careful attention to small signs of compromised healing, which, if handled in a timely fashion, may prevent the onset of a full-blown complication necessitating implant removal. This section contains a list of things that our experience, and above all a critical behavioral assessment, dictates we look out for.

1. It is strongly recommended that a post-surgical bra be worn for the first 30 days after surgery, 24/7, and not to place a compression dressing on the upper quadrants; it is, however, advisable to make sure that the bra elastic does not excessively compress the surgical wound at the inverted T, and the submammary elastic may therefore need to be loosened.
2. The drain should be kept in place until less than 30 cc per 24 h is collected on at least 2 consecutive days, and, in any case, it should not be removed before there is evidence of viable wound margins that are healing nicely.
3. Compressive plasters, etc. should not be applied to the reconstructed nipple, but there should be some compression on the areola graft; for this purpose, we suggest cutting surgical sponges into a doughnut shape to keep the nipple free of pressure and applying some form of flat dressing over these.
4. The patient should limit movement of their upper limbs until the skin is healed in order to reduce cutaneous tension and excessive implant movement.

In such patients, rehabilitation occurs naturally, with the resumption of normal activities. In fact, as the pectoralis major has not been raised, most cases do not require special rehabilitation other than a short series of educational group meetings (5 is generally sufficient). Indeed, in a study we have conducted but not yet published at the time of writing, patients who received prepectoral direct-to-implant surgery (DTI) required less intensive rehabilitation than those who had undergone subpectoral DTI; specifically, 42% of the latter required individual rehabilitation vs. 28% in the former.

16.5 Results and Complications

Positioning an implant in the combined dermal flap-ADM pocket, created solely on the subcutaneous plane, seems to reduce the postoperative pain and discomfort that would otherwise be caused by dissection of the pectoralis major muscle. The good cosmetic outcome is maintained, without any dynamic distortion of the implant (Figs. 16.6a, b and 16.7a, b). Furthermore, the use of ADM allows custom-made coverage of the anatomical silicone implant, thereby minimizing the risk of conventional traditional techniques if needed. In addition, our patients rapidly recovered arm mobilization and were discharged in a timely manner, with quicker return to everyday life. All patients eligible for skin-reduction mastectomy with prepectoral implant reconstruction have large breasts and are stout; the upper profile of the implant is therefore hidden by a thick skin flap, but a secondary lipofilling procedure may be performed around the implant if necessary, and in occasion of this refinements surgery, if it was necessary, dog ears of the horizontal scars should be corrected (Fig. 16.8). At the end of the chapter,

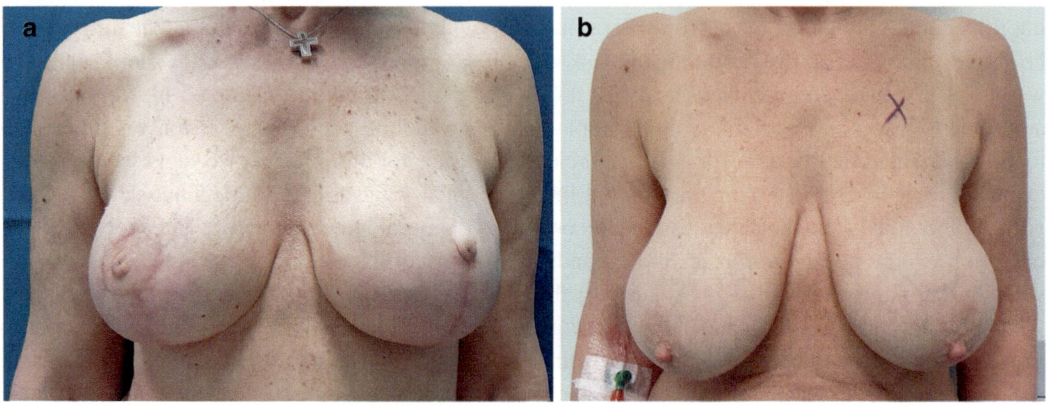

Fig. 16.6 (**a**, **b**) Nine months postoperative vs preoperative frontal view of left skin-reduction prepectoral reconstruction and right breast reduction

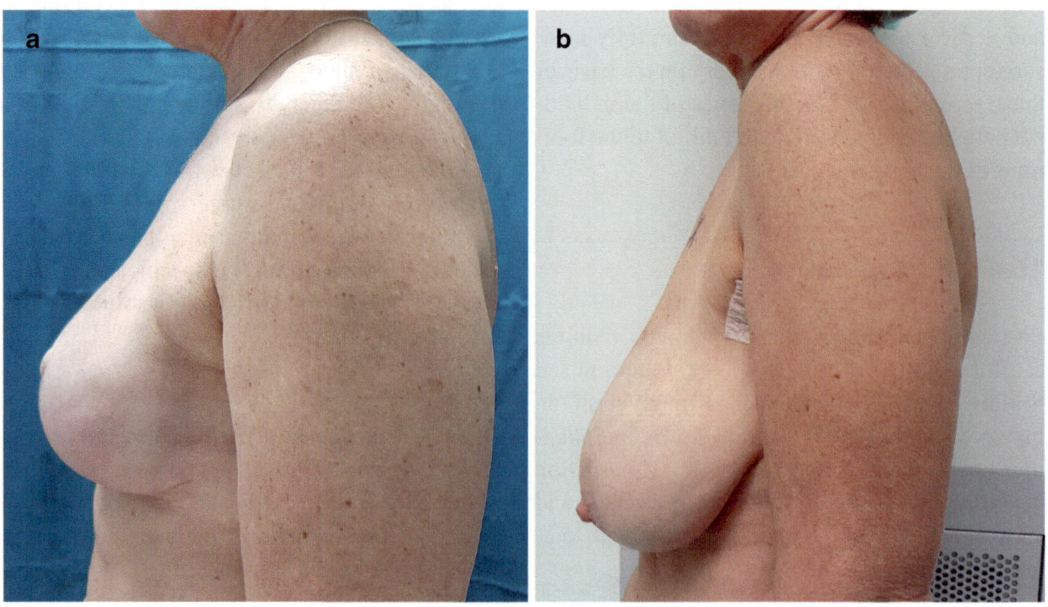

Fig. 16.7 (**a**, **b**) Nine months postoperative vs preoperative lateral view of left skin-reduction prepectoral reconstruction

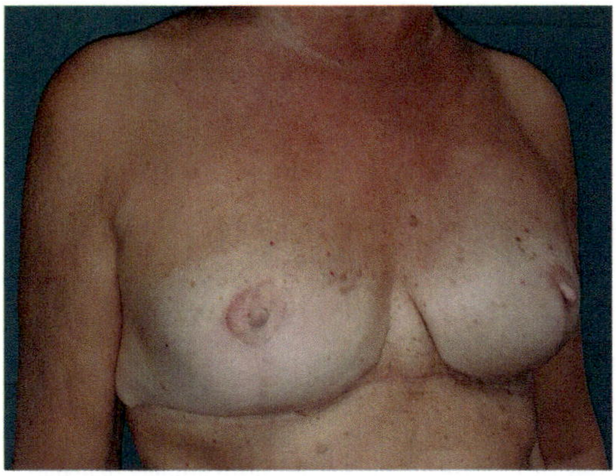

Fig. 16.8 Lateral dog ear of the horizontal scar

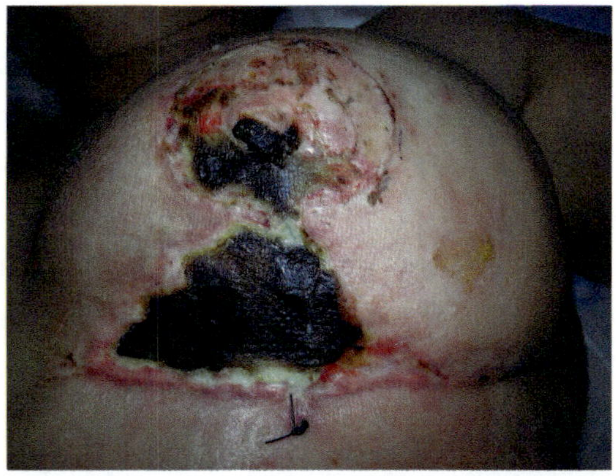

Fig. 16.9 Full-thickness necrosis of the mastectomy flap

we show our results with some pre- and postoperative pictures.

Despite very encouraging outcomes, it is important to mention the possibility that all may not always go as hoped. The most frequent complication we have encountered is *delayed healing* at the intersection of the inverted T. However, even in the first days, after the operation it is easy to identify those areas of the skin with poor blood supply and therefore at risk of de-epithelialization and eventually full-thickness necrosis; when there is an evident ischemic area, it is wise to trim the necrotic tissue until bleeding margins are exposed. Once the surgical toilette had been completed, the extent and depth of the loss of substance should be assessed in order to decide how best to proceed, as follows:

1. If the wound is small and the implant fully covered, direct cutaneous sutures and a negative pressure dressing (PICO®) [12] should be sufficient, but the implant should be deflated if possible.
2. If the wound is small but the implant exposed, it should be copiously rinsed with triple betadine [13] (50 cc of betadine, 1 g cefazolin, and 80 mg gentamicin dissolved in 500 cc of saline), closed with full-thickness sutures, the implant deflated if possible, and covered with a negative pressure dressing (PICO®).
3. If the wound is large and the implant covered (Fig. 16.9), apply a negative pressure sponge in black polyurethane with continuous suction at 75–100 mmHg. After 1 or 2 weeks of negative pressure therapy (NPWT), it can be decided whether direct suturing or grafting would be appropriate.
4. If the wound is large and the implant was only exposed under sterile conditions in the theater by the surgeon at the time of toilette, salvaging the implant/expander may be possible. The wound should therefore be copiously rinsed with triple betadine solution, the implant deflated to reduce the tension, a drain inserted, and multi-layer sutures applied. If a single-lumen implant has been fitted, however, it will be necessary to remove it and replace it with an expander or adjustable-volume implant with minimum filling in order not to generate further tension on the surgical wound.
5. If the wound is large and the implant exposed before toilette, and there is, therefore, a strong suspicion of bacterial contamination, it may be necessary to remove the prosthesis. The surgeon should decide how best to proceed, and which reconstructive solution to adopt, on a case by case basis.

Another complication, albeit rare and of late onset — it may arise even months after healing — is *scar tissue thinning* (Fig. 16.10). Linked to scar diastasis, gradual thinning may lead to breaks in the skin or a small hole (associated with decubitus of a subcutaneous point rising to the surface) and often manifests via slight serum

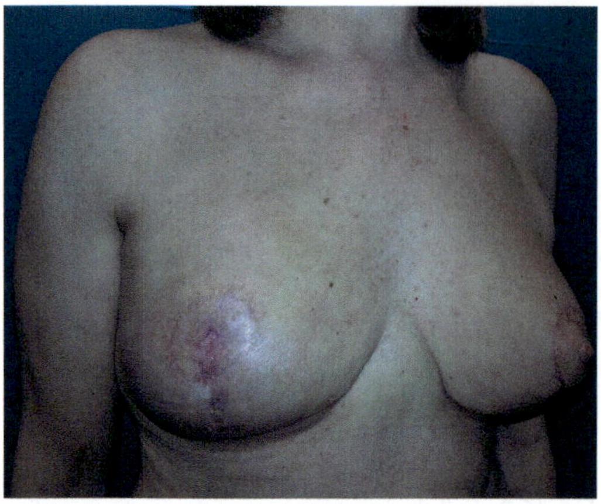

Fig. 16.10 Decubitus of a subcutaneous point at the vertical scar rising to the surface leading to serum drip through the skin of the right breast

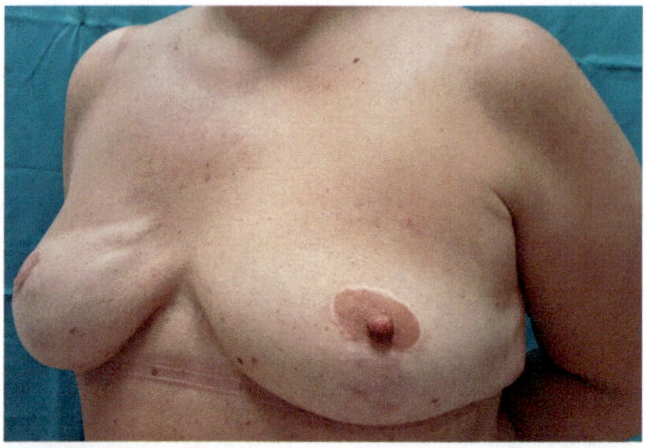

Fig. 16.11 Irregularities of the medial-upper pole due to imperfect uniformity of the mastectomy flap thicknesses (rippling) of the right breast

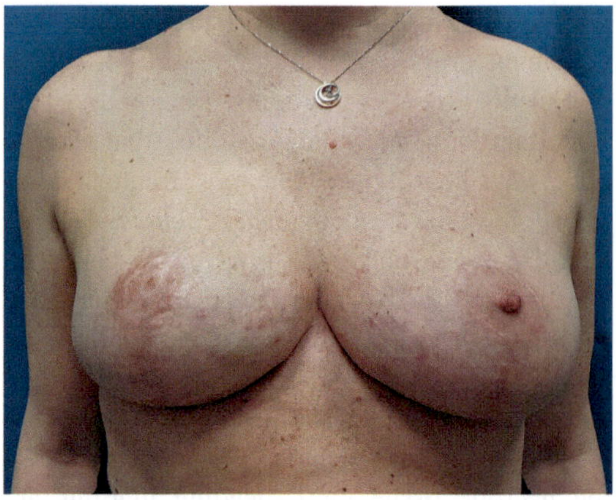

Fig. 16.12 Reconstructed nipple atrophy of the right breast

leakage. Generally speaking, the patient will contact their physician when they notice the sudden appearance of a yellow stain on their bra. In the majority of cases, timely intervention via trimming the skin margins (removing the thinning skin) and closing with full-thickness skin sutures resolves the issue. If the reason for scar diastasis is linked to the presence of a residual postoperative periprosthetic seroma, it is advisable to fit a small drainage tube, which can be removed together with the stitches (after about 14 days).

Achieving breast symmetry is one of the major goals of this type of procedure, which always requires bilateral intervention, However, a single surgery is not always sufficient to achieve perfect symmetry in terms of both shape and size. Hence, 6 months after surgery, once the outcome has stabilized, it is necessary to examine the patient to discern any discrepancy in the distribution of breast volumes. The *implant profile* may be visible, or there may be noticeable irregularities due to imperfect uniformity of the mastectomy flap thicknesses, or subsequent *subcutaneous atrophy* secondary to lipo-necrosis (Fig. 16.11). Such cases may be readily treated via fat grafting — one lipofilling session is usually sufficient to resolve the issue.

In some cases, *nipple atrophy* may occur. In general, there are likely signs of this immediately after surgery as the cause is inadequate blood supply (Fig.16.12). To resolve the issue, the nipple can be reconstructed at a later date, but often patients feel that this type of surgical correction is not indispensable, and instead prefer to turn to an expert tattoo artist who is able to simulate a three-dimensional nipple via the clever application of colors.

As a consequence of either careless execution of the reconstruction technique or the collapse of several subcutaneous sutures, the *scar may rise above the submammary fold.* This problem arises when the horizontal arm of the scar does not coincide with the submammary fold (Fig. 16.13). Going over the surgical phases of the reconstruction, it becomes clear how important it is to identify the submammary fold, with the patient in a sitting position, tracing from the outermost side of the dermo-adipose flap and placing between

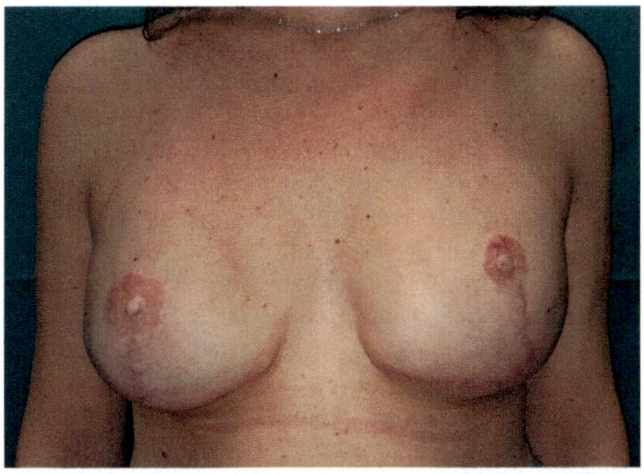

Fig. 16.13 Malpositioning of the horizontal scar which lay above the submammary fold in a bilateral prepectoral implant-based skin-reducing mastectomy

this and the serratus anterior single Vicryl 2/0 sutures, after having cut roughly 4 cm along the base of the flap. If this operation is not sufficient to obtain the desired definition, sequential sutures can be stitched along the entire submammary fold.

16.6 Review of Short Literature to Date

Over the last 10 years, post-mastectomy direct-to-implant (DTI) breast reconstruction has become common, largely due to the progress in acellular dermal matrix (ADM) technology and other coatings specifically designed for the lining of breast implants [14, 15]. Indeed, the advent of these innovations has changed the paradigm of reconstructive breast surgery, allowing a significant increase in immediate DTI reconstructions in cases of conservative mastectomies [16]; it has a growing range of indications in breast surgery and is well accepted by patients [17]. The new frontiers of DTI reconstruction with ADM began with the positioning of the implant in the submuscular plane; to complete the pocket, the lower pole of the prosthesis was covered by the matrix, in continuity with the pectoralis major muscle [18]. In the last years, we assisted to a transition to muscle-sparing techniques in which the prosthesis, completely or partially covered by ADM, is housed subcutaneously leading to much more natural looking results without animation deformities [19, 20]. For large and ptotic breasts, the traditional skin-reducing mastectomy, where the implant was placed in a submuscular plane [21], has been replaced by the prepectoral approach [22, 23].

Tips

- Preoperative drawing must be accurate (the vertical line of the inverted T no longer than 9 cm).
- The surgical field should be well infiltrated with Klein solution before cold-blade mastectomy. (scissors).
- The tissue should always be handled gently.
- If the ends of the T show signs of ischemia, trim the corner, rounding it; obviously, this must correspond to a non-de-epithelialized triangle or semicircle at the base of the dermo-adipose flap.
- Choose an implant that does not exceed a volume of 500 cc—if the implant is too heavy, it will pull on the mastectomy flaps.
- If flap viability is uncertain, insert an adjustable implant (Becker implant) or expander which can be filled with either saline or ambient air. Should you decide to use ambient air, make sure to use a sterile 0.2-micron syringe filter to minimize the risk of bacterial contamination.
- Only remove the drains when you are sure that the surgical wounds are healing well.
- If the wound margins show no signs of healing, do not delay in trimming them and deflating the implant in order to reduce the tension on the wound — second-intention healing can be very long, and exposure of the derma may, over time, lead to exposure of the implant. If a single-lumen implant has been inserted, i.e., whose volume cannot be reduced, assess whether to replace it with one that allows direct closure, or after trimming, if the implant is not exposed and the dermo-adipose tissue is healthy, apply NPT at a continuous negative pressure of 75–100 mmHg; this will allow you to keep the wound clean, promoting healing, and bring the margins together, as without

vac-therapy these would tend to pull farther apart owing to the weight of the implant.

- Make the patient wear a post-surgery bra 24/7 for 1 month, beginning immediately after surgery.

References

1. Nava MB, Cortinovis U, Ottolenghi J, et al. Skin-reducing mastectomy. Plast Reconstr Surg. 2006;118:603–10. discussion 611
2. Caputo GG, Marchetti A, Dalla Pozza E, et al. Skin-reduction breast reconstructions with Prepectoral implant. Plast Reconstr Surg. 2016;137(6):1702–5.
3. Nahabedian MY. Current approaches to prepectoral breast reconstruction. Plast Reconstr Surg. 2018;142(4):871–80.
4. Kim IK, Park SO, Chang H, Jin US. Inhibition mechanism of acellular dermal matrix on capsule formation in expander-implant breast reconstruction after Postmastectomy radiotherapy. Ann Surg Oncol. 2018;25(8):2279–87.
5. Salzberg CA, Ashikari AY, Berry C, Hunsicker LM. Acellular dermal matrix-assisted direct-to-implant breast reconstruction and capsular contracture: a 13-year experience. Plast Reconstr Surg. 2016;138(2):329–37.
6. Elswick SM, Harless CA, Bishop SN, et al. Prepectoral implant-based breast reconstruction with Postmastectomy radiation therapy. Plast Reconstr Surg. 2018;142(1):1–12.
7. Shukla L, Morrison WA, Shayan R. Adipose-derived stem cells in radiotherapy injury: a new frontier. Front Surg. 2015;2:1. Published 2015 Jan 28
8. Klein JA. The tumescent technique. Anesthesia and modified liposuction technique. Dermatol Clin. 1990;8(3):425–37.
9. Caputo GG, Franchini Z, Maritan M, et al. Daily serum collection after acellular dermal matrix-assisted breast reconstruction. Arch Plast Surg. 2015;42(3):321–6.
10. Jeon FHK, Varghese J, Griffin M, Butler PE, Ghosh D, Mosahebi A. Systematic review of methodologies used to assess mastectomy flap viability. BJS Open. 2018;2(4):175–84. Published 2018 May 28
11. Kedar D, Inbal A, Arad E, Gur E, Barnea Y. Immediate breast reconstruction in high-risk cases using an anatomically shaped permanent expandable implant. J Plast Reconstr Aesthet Surg. 2019;72(3):401–9.
12. Galiano RD, Hudson D, Shin J, et al. Incisional negative pressure wound therapy for prevention of wound healing complications following reduction mammaplasty [published correction appears in Plast Reconstr Surg Glob Open. 2018 Mar 23;6(2):e1720]. Plast Reconstr Surg Glob Open 2018;6(1):e1560. Published 2018 Jan.
13. Culbertson EJ, Felder-Scott C, Deva AK, Greenberg DE, Adams WP. Optimizing breast pocket irrigation: the breast implant-associated anaplastic large cell lymphoma (BIA-ALCL) era. Aesthet Surg J. 2020;40(6):619–25.
14. Salzberg CA. Direct-to-implant breast reconstruction. Clin Plast Surg. 2012;39(2):119–26.
15. Dieterich M, Paepke S, Zwiefel K, et al. Implant-based breast reconstruction using a titanium-coated polypropylene mesh (TiLOOP bra): a multicenter study of 231 cases. Plast Reconstr Surg. 2013;132(1):8e–19e.
16. Vidya R, Masiá J, Cawthorn S, et al. Evaluation of the effectiveness of the prepectoral breast reconstruction with Braxon dermal matrix: first multicenter European report on 100 cases. Breast J. 2017;23(6):670–6.
17. Vidya R, Green M. Minimal pain with prepectoral implant based breast reconstruction. Plast Reconstr Surg. 2019;143(1):236e.
18. Breuing KH, Colwell AS. Inferolateral AlloDerm hammock for implant coverage in breast reconstruction. Ann Plast Surg. 2007;59:250255.
19. Antony AK, Poirier J, Madrigrano A, Kopkash KA, Robinson EC. Evolution of the surgical technique for "breast in a day" direct-to-implant breast reconstruction: transitioning from dual-plane to Prepectoral implant placement. Plast Reconstr Surg. 2019;143(6):1547–56.
20. Mirhaidari SJ, Azouz V, Wagner DS. Prepectoral versus subpectoral direct to implant immediate breast reconstruction. Ann Plast Surg. 2020;84(3):263–70.
21. della Rovere GQ, Nava M, Bonomi R, Catanuto G, Benson JR. Skin-reducing mastectomy with breast reconstruction and sub-pectoral implants. J Plast Reconstr Aesthet Surg. 2008;61:1303–8.
22. Thuman J, Freitas AM, Schaeffer C, Campbell CA. Prepectoral wise-pattern staged implant-based breast reconstruction for obese or ptotic patients. Ann Plast Surg. 2019;82(6S Suppl 5):S404–9.
23. Maruccia M, Elia R, Gurrado A, et al. Skin-reducing mastectomy and pre-pectoral breast reconstruction in large Ptotic breasts. Aesthet Plast Surg. 2020;44(3):664–72.

Complications: How to Reduce and Manage

17

Jaume Masià and Cristhian D. Pomata

17.1 Introduction

The use of alloplastic materials for breast reconstruction in women undergoing mastectomy began in the second half of the 1960s [1]. Since its introduction, this technique has been accompanied by the drawbacks associated with placement of the breast implant under very thin skin. Consequently, the pre-pectoral approach was gradually abandoned due to high rates of complications and reconstruction failure [2–4].

Over the decades, the desire to reconstruct better breasts using prosthetic devices has led, first, to the refinement of mastectomy techniques that enhance the preservation of skin and subcutaneous tissue flaps, and second, to considerable technological advances in implant design including a higher performance shell, more cohesive gels, micro/nano textured surface, and a wider range of implant profiles and even shapes that can adapt to vertical and horizontal movements. However, the advent of biomaterials such as acellular dermal matrix (ADM) in the early 2000s [5] and the incorporation of fat transfer procedures have revolutionized implant-based reconstruction techniques, contributing to the resurgence of the pre-pectoral approach as a viable surgical technique after skin- or nipple-sparing mastectomy [6, 7].

Although the safety and high success rate of the pre-pectoral approach have been widely demonstrated, [6, 8] complications can still occur [9, 10]. Many of the factors associated with adverse events in pre-pectoral implant breast reconstruction (PPIBR) have been identified; therefore, the surgeon must adopt prevention strategies to reduce the risk of complications and be able to effectively manage them if they do occur, to avoid reconstruction failure.

J. Masià
Department of Plastic Surgery, Santa Creu i Sant Pau Hospital - Universitat Autonòma de Barcelona, Barcelona, Spain

Unit of Advanced Breast Reconstruction and Lymphedema Treatment, Clínica Planas, Barcelona, Spain
e-mail: jmasia@santpau.cat

C. D. Pomata (✉)
Unit of Advanced Breast Reconstruction, Clínica Planas, Barcelona, Spain
e-mail: cpomata@clinicaplanas.com

© The Author(s), under exclusive license to Springer Nature Switzerland AG 2023
R. Vidya, H. Becker (eds.), *Prepectoral Breast Reconstruction*,
https://doi.org/10.1007/978-3-031-15590-1_17

17.2 Type of Complications

Complications in PPIBR are mostly the same as with those first attempts half a century ago but with some changes in the incidence. In general, the adverse events in PPIBR can be classified as early or late. Early complications are predominantly those related to the surgery and include seroma, hematoma, nipple/skin ischemia/necrosis, infection, wound dehiscence, and implant extrusion. More recently, an inflammatory condition related to the use of dermal meshes—*red breast syndrome*—has also been described as an early complication. Late complications are those related to the interaction between the implant and the mastectomy flap. These comprise adverse effects that have repercussions on the esthetic results, such as capsular contracture, rippling/wrinkling, and implant malposition, visibility, or palpability. Reports on complication rates are variable because they can be influenced by patient-related comorbidities, inappropriate surgical technique, the use of additional materials, and the delivery of radiotherapy, among other factors [6–9]. Table 17.1 shows the complication rates in PPIBR reported in the systematic reviews published by Salibian et al. in 2017 [11] and Wagner et al. in 2019, [7] as well as in the largest multicenter collection of data on PPIBR with ADM, published by Masia et al. in 2020 [6].

Table 17.1 Complication rates in pre-pectoral implant breast reconstruction (PPIBR)

	Salibian et al. 2016 [8]			Wagner et al. [7]				Masia et al. [6]		
	General PPIBR	PPIBR – ADM	PPIBR - Mesh	General PPIBR	PPIBR - none	PPIBR - ADM	PPIBR - ADM/Mesh	PPIBR - ADM	PIBR - ADM nonirradiated	PIBR - ADM irradiated
Seroma	2.9%	8.9%	0.0%	5.1%	6.9%	5.9%	4.1%	7.7%	7.0%	11.1%
Infection	–	–	–	2.6%	1.8%	3.8%	3.5%	4.8%	3.1%	5.1%
Minor infection (antibiotic)	2.3%	0.0%	6.3%	–	–	–	–	–	–	–
Major infection (surgery)	1.2%	2.2%	0.0%	–	–	–	–	–	–	–
Wound healing problems	2.3%	4.4%	1.6%	–	–	–	–	–	–	–
Dehiscence	–	–	–	–	–	–	–	4.6%	4.5%	4.0%
Red breast syndrome	–	–	–	–	–	–	–	3.3%	3.5%	2.0%
Necrosis	–	–	–	–	–	–	–	3.2%	3.1%	4.0%
Full NAC necrosis	1.1%	2.5%	0.0%	2.7%	–	–	–	–	–	–
Partial NAC necrosis	4.5%	5.0%	4.2%	–	–	–	–	–	–	–
Major flap necrosis	1.8%	0.0%	1.6%	5.4%	4.2%	7.4%	5.6%	–	–	–
Hematoma	2.3%	2.2%	3.1%	2.4%	4.5%	2.5%	2.7%	2.1%	2.2%	2.0%
Implant loss	4.1%	6.7%	3.1%	3.3%	3.0%	7.2%	5.9%	6.5%	5.6%	11.1%
Rippling	4.7%	–	–	–	–	–		2.8%	3.1%	0.5%
Capsular contracture	1.2%	0.0%	0.0%	8.8%	12.4%	2.3%	2.4%	2.1%	1.7%	5.1%
Implant migration/rotation	0.0%	–	–	–	–	–	–	0.2%	0.2%	0.0%
Visible implant	4.3%	–	–	–	–	–	–	–	–	–
Palpable implant	8.5%	–	–	–	–	–	–	–	–	–

ADM: acellular dermal matrix; *NAC*: nipple–areola complex

17.3 Risk Factors for COMPLICACTION

Preoperative risk factors for complications in PPIBR include advanced patient age, active tobacco use, poorly controlled diabetes mellitus, use of immunosuppressive drugs, morbid obesity, and very large or ptotic breasts [6, 12–16]. Previous breast surgery and chemotherapy have also been reported to be associated with a high complication rate [6, 9]. These risk factors are mainly correlated with early complications. The combination of PPIBR and radiotherapy is another highly debated topic. Prior breast irradiation is associated with increased risk of ischemic complications, and postmastectomy radiotherapy also appears to be a statistically significant risk factor for late complications [6, 12, 17]. However, the crucial factor that exponentially increases the probability of complications in PPIBR is the surgeon's lack of experience in performing mastectomy and in handling implants or biomaterials correctly.

17.4 Early Complications

Most of the early complications in PPIBR occur immediately after surgery but they can arise over the following 2–3 months. In general, these can be divided into minor complications, which can be managed without surgical intervention, and major complications, which require readmission to hospital or unplanned return to the operating room. Such events are critical because if they are not managed properly, they can result in loss of the reconstruction. Therefore, it is essential to take all necessary precautions to reduce the risk of early adverse events. The most frequent early complications, as well as how to prevent and manage them, are described individually below.

17.4.1 Seroma

The accumulation of serous fluid is one of the most frequent postoperative complications after PPIBR surgery. The cause of seroma is not fully understood; however, the serous fluid seems to be a mixture of lymph and inflammatory exudate. Several factors are involved in its formation, including tissue inflammation generated by the surgery, together with that produced by the insertion of a foreign body (implant and ADM) and the dead space from the mastectomy and axillary dissection that facilitates serous fluid accumulation. Moreover, patients with large breasts and/or obesity tend to have larger mastectomy flaps and/or excess lateral volume, both of which can increase dead space and serous exudate. A history of cosmetic breast surgery or immunosuppressive drugs is also associated with increased risk of seroma [18].

17.4.1.1 Prevention

The accumulation of serous fluid is usually considered an expected adverse event, and various strategies have been used over the decades to decrease its incidence. The classic approach to prevention includes the use of suction drainage and avoidance of active shoulder mobilization. In addition, meticulous surgical technique with a suitable surgical cutting device can attenuate the postoperative inflammatory response, and identifying the lymphatic channels when performing axillary dissection can reduce their potential damage and consequent postoperative lymph accumulation. Likewise, techniques for obliterating dead space, such as the use of tissue sealants and quilting, or external compression, can also help reduce the risk of seroma.

Suction Drainage

The most commonly used technique to prevent serous fluid accumulation is closed suction drainage. The drains are usually placed along the inframammary crease and in the axilla, maintaining a high pressure gradient. There is a lack of consensus regarding the timing of drain removal. In general, they are kept in place until volumes are less than 20–25 ml for 24–48 h. However, one problem with leaving drains in situ for a prolonged period is their tendency to stimulate an inflammatory exudate that leads to seroma formation. In addition, they can be uncomfortable and are associated with increased risk of infection. Therefore, it is recommended to remove the drains after a maximum period of 7 days and to use prophylactic antibiotics until they are removed.

Quilting Suture

Fixation of the mastectomy flap to reduce dead space after a mastectomy is not a new technique. It can be performed in different places to form a snug pocket: the axilla, the lateral wall, or through the inframammary fold to include the surgical incision. There is a wide variety of quilting techniques that have shown a significant decrease in seroma formation. Barbed suture is currently the best option for quilting, since it allows self-anchoring, thus avoiding multiple knots. Temporary pits in the skin may develop after quilting, which usually resolve spontaneously [19].

Tissue Sealants

Fibrin sealants have been used in surgery since the 1940s [20]. Considering multiple small blood and lymphatic vessels are divided during resection of the mammary gland and axillary lymph nodes, fibrin sealants may theoretically contribute to hemostasis and tissue adherence, which may reduce postoperative serosanguinous fluid accumulation [21]. Although several studies in animal mastectomy models suggest that fibrin sealant could help prevent seroma formation, [22, 23] its application in human breast cancer surgery remains controversial [24–26]. Nevertheless, fibrin glue seems to afford additional but nonsignificant benefits in the prevention of seroma formation [27]. A more recent prospective randomized clinical trial demonstrated that cyanoacrylate adhesive can contribute to a reduction in seroma formation after mastectomy and subsequently decrease the duration of postoperative drainage and the frequency of seroma aspiration [28].

Surgical Cutting Devices

The characteristics of the cutting instrument used during mastectomy surgery have also been shown to influence the production of serous fluid. Electrocautery is the most common cutting tool; however, it has been associated with greater tissue injury and acute inflammatory response, and hence a significantly higher rate of seroma compared to scalpel dissection [29, 30]. The introduction of the PEAK Plasma Blade has revolutionized the electrosurgical device [31]. This surgical instrument uses a pulsed radiofrequency to generate a plasma-mediated discharge along the exposed rim of an insulated blade. This provides a more atraumatic cut, similar to a scalpel, with a blade temperature that remains close to body temperature, resulting in a reduction in serous fluid production and, hence, reduced drainage period and shorter hospital stay [32, 33].

Axillary Dissection Technique

When planning axillary lymph node dissection, identification of the lymphatic channels is essential not only to avoid lymph accumulation, but also to reduce the risk of limb lymphedema by performing immediate surgical repair of any damaged lymphatic channels. The use of indocyanine green lymphography and blue patent V dye are very useful for intraoperative identification of the lymphatic channels. In cases where axillary lymph node dissection is not performed, care must still be taken when dissecting the axillary tail of the mammary gland, identifying the largest lymphatic channels and clipping or coagulating them with bipolar to avoid postoperative lymph accumulation in the dead space.

Avoidance of Active Shoulder Mobilization

Active mobilization of the shoulder can cause friction between the implant, mastectomy flap, and the pectoralis major, which can further stimulate the foreign body response and prolong inflammation. It is recommended to avoid early active shoulder movements and postpone physical therapy until at least a week after surgery [19].

External Soft Compression

Soft compression bandages or a surgical bra may be helpful to prevent movement of the implant within the mastectomy pocket, which could stimulate an inflammatory response. If axillary lymph node dissection is performed, the application of an external compression dressing helps reduce dead space [19, 34].

17.4.1.2 Management

Despite efforts to prevent the accumulation of serous fluid, seroma formation after drain removal can occur and is characterized by fluctuation or increased tension in the surgical incision, which can contribute to wound dehiscence and implant exposure. Persistent seroma also interferes with ADM/mesh integration. If left untreated, fluid accumulation within the hypovascular environment of a recent mastectomy is prone to infection. For clinically significant seromas, current treatment methods consist of percutaneous needle aspiration, together with prophylactic antibiotics [18]. In case of refractory seroma, repeated aspirations can also produce infection. In this persistent situation, sclerotherapy can be a useful salvage method, utilizing a chemical agent such as doxycycline, erythromycin, ethanol, or povidone-iodine, among others [35, 36].

17.4.2 Hematoma

The risk of postoperative bleeding is inherent in any surgical intervention. It is characterized by breast enlargement, cutaneous ecchymoses, increased blood drainage, and significant pain. Hematoma frequently manifests within 24 h after the operation but can also occur during the first week after surgery or later.

In general, some drugs like platelet inhibitors, inhibitors of the coagulation cascade, and androgen hormones represent a risk for bleeding. Likewise, high blood pressure may predispose to postoperative bleeding. Regarding intraoperative circumstances, the tumescent mastectomy technique potentially reduces intraoperative blood loss and perioperative pain, but in turn can increase hematoma rates as its vasoconstrictor effects decrease postoperatively. Also, the routine participation of two different surgical teams—one to perform the mastectomy and another for the reconstruction—can be a risk factor.

17.4.2.1 Prevention

The inability to predict hematoma formation has several implications, reinforcing the need for meticulous hemostasis during mastectomy [37]. The use of intravenous tranexamic acid appears to reduce the risk of postoperative hematoma [38].

17.4.2.2 Management

When a progressive increase in blood drainage is noted, or breast size increases drastically, immediate surgical exploration should be carried out for control of bleeding and hematoma drainage. This requires a return to the operating room, usually under general anesthesia. In most cases, no distinct sites of hemorrhage are found, but if a bleeding vessel is identified, it should be carefully cauterized or clipped, especially if it is a large artery such as an internal mammary perforator. Then, the pre-pectoral pocket should be washed copiously with antibiotic solution to eliminate blood detritus, followed by placement of drains.

17.4.3 Skin/Nipple-Areola Complex Necrosis

Mastectomy flap necrosis is a potentially catastrophic complication in PPIBR. Although the incidence is not very high, it represents a significant challenge for reconstructive surgeons. As there is no vascularized tissue between the skin and the underlying implant/ADM, this complication tends to cause imminent failure of the reconstruction. Generally, most flap necroses occur within the first month after surgery. Many factors can contribute to mastectomy flap necrosis. Excessive removal of subcutaneous tissue alters the perfusion and leads to relative ischemia of the mastectomy flap. When reconstruction is performed with implants that are too large, excessive pressure increases the insult to the mastectomy flap. Smoking and cardiovascular, respiratory, or peripheral vascular disease also affect tissue oxygenation and vascular adaptation of the flap. Obesity, diabetes, hypertension, radiotherapy, and steroid administration are associated with higher rates of skin necrosis. Large breast size is also an important factor, as longer skin flaps are at higher risk of distal ischemia. Similarly, a history of prior surgery can increase the risk of complications because existing scars can compromise the blood supply to the nipple–areola complex.

17.4.3.1 Prevention

The most decisive factor for the success of PPIBR is good quality of the mastectomy flaps. This implies adequate perfusion of the mastectomy flap. The first strategy is to normalize any preexisting conditions that may affect flap perfusion. Patients who smoke should stop for at least 3 weeks prior to surgery. The second key prevention strategy is the adequate preservation of the entire skin envelope of the breast, skin, and subcutaneous tissue, as postmastectomy skin flaps receive blood supply exclusively from the subdermal plexus. The dissection must always be performed between the anterior lamella of the superficial fascia and the subcutaneous tissue, in the plane described by Bisenberger, maintaining a subcutaneous layer of at least 1 cm thick. Hydrodissection can help to improve visualization of this dissection plane. The use of diathermy to dissect skin flaps is discouraged due to the risk of thermal damage to the delicate subcutaneous vessels and the overlying skin envelope. Currently, the peak plasma blade is the best soft tissue dissection instrument for mastectomy [31, 32, 39]. Furthermore, when using retractors, care must be taken to limit the amount of traction on the skin flaps and the duration of retraction that could interrupt the blood supply, allowing sufficient time for the skin to recover between retraction periods.

Once mammary gland resection is complete, the breast skin envelope must be thoroughly evaluated for feasibility and quality. This involves examining the mastectomy flaps for signs of adequate perfusion such as skin color, capillary filling, temperature, turgor, and dermal bleeding. It is important to note that a thick mastectomy flap does not always mean good perfusion. Therefore, the use of indocyanine green with laser angiography plays a critical role in guiding intraoperative decision-making regarding the viability of the mastectomy skin flap. When assessing tissue perfusion, it may be helpful to use an implant sizer to recreate the tension that will be exerted on the flap postoperatively. It should be borne in mind that the validity of this perfusion assessment may be compromised if a solution containing epinephrine is used to facilitate subcutaneous dissection during mastectomy. If skin perfusion is compromised, it is best to organize a staged reconstruction, first inserting a tissue expander in the pre-pectoral plane to allow time for the skin flaps to develop robust perfusion through vascular adaptation, which can take 2 to 3 weeks. Another important factor is the tension on the flaps at the incision sites, especially if large amounts of skin have been resected, as excess tension can predispose to ischemia at the flap edges. Very high pressure dressings should also be avoided after surgery to maintain adequate perfusion of the mastectomy flap.

17.4.3.2 Management

Depending on the severity and the extent of the affected tissue, skin necrosis can be treated surgically or nonsurgically. Once skin flap or nipple ischemia is identified postoperatively, certain nonsurgical techniques can improve tissue perfusion. Nitroglycerin ointments can increase local blood flow to the skin by relaxing the smooth muscle walls of the subcutaneous arteries and veins [40]. Hyperbaric oxygen therapy can also contribute to tissue recovery [41].

In cases of superficial necrosis, the same nonsurgical therapies can also be helpful in combination with preparations that reduce the bacterial load, such as silver alginate dressings [42]. Usually, the healing process of this superficial necrosis involves detachment of the necrotic tissue and subsequent secondary wound healing. The use of wound management devices, such as vacuum dressings, can also facilitate wound healing, particularly when larger areas of necrosis are encountered [43–45].

Necrosis affecting most of the mastectomy flap thickness requires surgical debridement and removal of the implant. In this situation, there are then several options to treat the tissue loss. The therapeutic strategy is usually decided on a case-by-case basis, according to the experience of each surgeon (Figs. 17.1 and 17.2). Concomitant antibiotic therapy is always recommended.

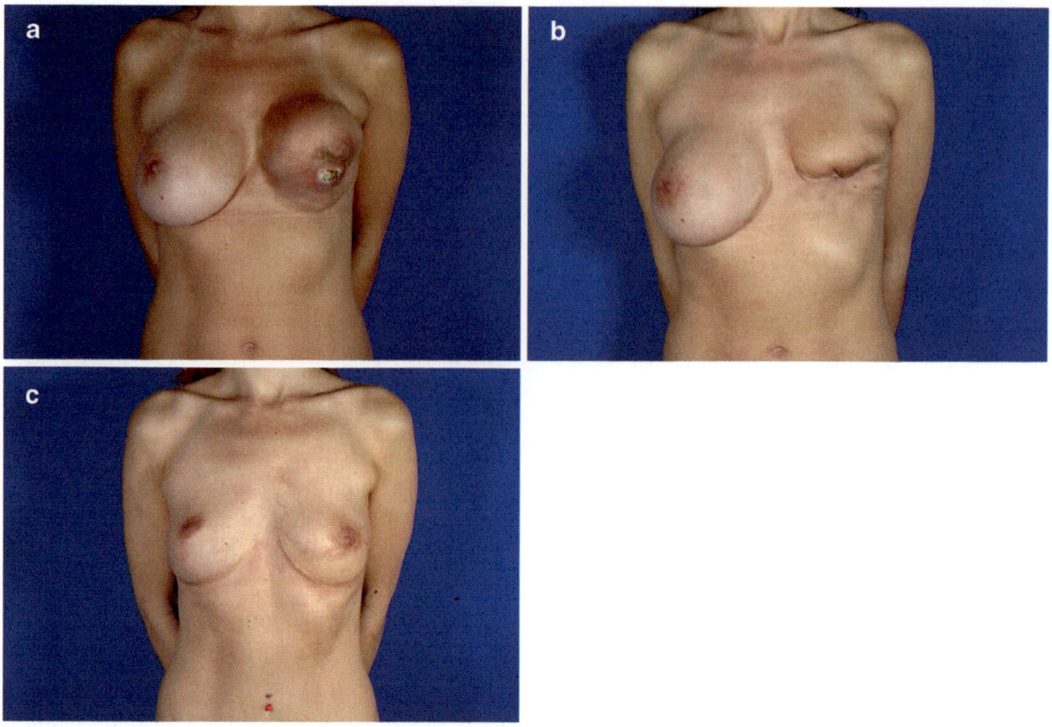

Fig. 17.1 A 34-year-old patient with a history of left nipple-sparing mastectomy and direct-to-implant reconstruction performed at another hospital. The patient underwent postmastectomy radiotherapy, and at the end of the treatment, she came to our hospital with skin necrosis and severe capsular contracture (**a**). Initially, the implant was removed (**b**). Due to insufficient tissue in the lower pole to give an adequate shape, in the second stage, breast reconstruction was performed with a deep inferior epigastric artery perforator flap, along with a contralateral breast reduction mammoplasty (**c**)

17.4.4 Infection

Infection in PPIBR is a potentially devastating complication as it tends to require additional surgery to remove the implant. According to the site, infection can be classified into superficial, involving only the skin and superficial subcutaneous tissue, and deep, involving the soft tissues and structures in contact with the implants/ ADM. This complication occurs mostly between 6 days and 6 weeks after surgery.

17.4.4.1 Prevention

In addition to confirming the absence of ongoing local or general infection, the prevention strategy in the preoperative phase includes decolonization of the skin by means of an adequate presurgical shower, preferably with antiseptic, and antibiotic prophylaxis. Intraoperative preventive measures include the following: adequate antisepsis of the skin; covering the nipple-–areola complex with an adhesive film dressing to prevent perioperative expression of bacteria from nipple ducts contaminating the operative field; change of surgical gloves every 60 min and before handling implants; washing of the pre-pectoral pocket with antiseptic and antibiotic solution; injection of antibiotic solution with a needle directly through the paper cover of the breast implant sterile package to avoid electrostatic contamination when the implants are removed; profuse washing of the ADM with antibiotic solution; minimizing the open time of the implant and ADM to reduce contamination; use of a minimal-contact technique whenever possible; drain externalization sites distant from the surgical incision, tunneling from the inside of the pre-pectoral pocket to the outside (not from outside to inside)

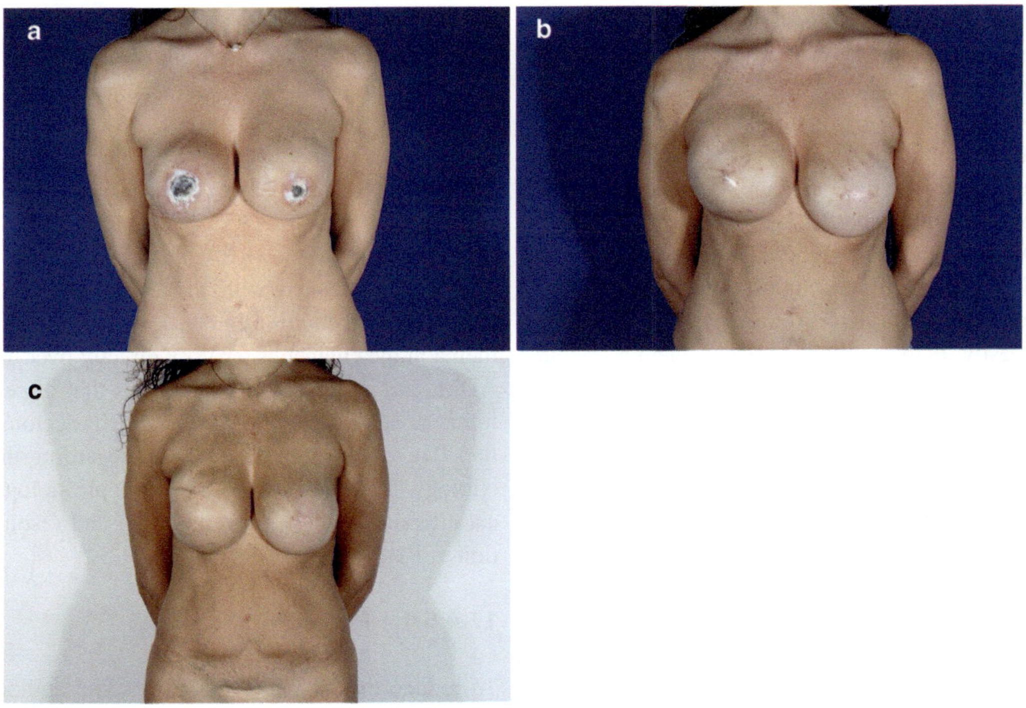

Fig. 17.2 A 53-year-old patient with a history of bilateral nipple-sparing mastectomy and direct-to-implant reconstruction performed at another hospital, who came to our clinic with necrosis of the areolas (**a**). Initially, the implants were removed, the necrosis was resected, and the defects were closed. In a second stage, tissue expanders were placed (**b**), and in a third stage, they were exchanged for implants with lipofilling (**c**)

to avoid the possible introduction of bacterial flora from the skin to the mastectomy pocket; and a suitable laminar flow ventilation system. Postoperative care is based on good daily wound care, in addition to prevention methods for seroma, hematoma, and skin necrosis [46, 47].

17.4.4.2 Management

Superficial surgical site infections limited to mild cellulitis without an exudate and without signs of systemic infection can be treated with intravenous antibiotics until the swelling and redness resolve. Then, oral antibiotic therapy must be continued for another 7 to 10 days along with close monitoring, without implant removal. In case of superficial skin necrosis infection, simultaneous local treatment includes the use of a silver-hydrofiber dressing and negative pressure therapy.

For deep subcutaneous infection, profuse washing with antibiotic solution, debridement when necessary, and implant removal are required to achieve cure. Although some surgeons will try to prevent implant removal by reopening and only washing the pocket, this may not be effective. Moreover, leaving the implant in an infected environment exposes the patient to additional risks for systemic infection. After implant removal, the breast must heal and soften before the expander/implant can be replaced, which often takes 4 to 6 months or more after completion of antibiotic therapy.

17.4.5 Wound Dehiscence

Wound dehiscence is also a frequent early complication in PPIBR. It is defined as partial or complete separation of the layers of the surgical incision. It is typically a consequence of inadequate closure or excessive tension on the incision due to the placement of very large implants.

Seroma and hematoma can also significantly increase tension on the surgical incision. A thin mastectomy skin flap in the lower part of the breast, where the pressure is higher due to gravity, is another situation that predisposes to wound dehiscence. Cutaneous trauma or ulceration, skin necrosis, and superficial infection of the surgical incision are also significant causes of wound dehiscence. Patient comorbidities have a great impact on surgical wound healing. Smoking, obesity, diabetes, hypertension, anemia, malnutrition or hypoalbuminemia, and radiotherapy represent risk factors for delayed surgical wound healing. Age over 65 years and the use of steroid medications are also associated with slow wound healing.

17.4.5.1 Prevention

The first strategy in preventing surgical incision dehiscence is avoiding wound tension. For this, care must be taken not to insert excessively large implants, especially in patients with small breasts and tight mastectomy skin flaps. Secondly, the surgical incision should always be closed in three layers, anchoring the breast tissue and Scarpa's fascia to the chest wall, followed by a subcutaneous layer of absorbable sutures and then an intradermal suture. Third, an overlay of cyanoacrylate glue can help to seal the incision, and application of an adhesive tape can be used to reinforce skin closure. It is also helpful to avoid active movement of the shoulders in the first 7 days after surgery, to prevent tension on the incision. In addition, appropriate preventive measures for seroma, hematoma, skin necrosis, and infection should also be carried out to avoid tension on the surgical incision.

17.4.5.2 Management

Minor or superficial wound dehiscence should be managed immediately. Treatment of wound dehiscence is mainly based on eliminating the factor that produces the tension. In the case of a very large implant, use of a smaller-volume implant should be considered. When a two-stage reconstruction has been carried out, partial deflation of the expander relieves tension on the surgical incision. If wound dehiscence is associated with seroma, hematoma, or skin necrosis, successful treatment of these will simultaneously lead to healing of the surgical incision.

17.4.6 Red Breast Syndrome

Red breast syndrome (RBS) is an inflammatory condition associated with the use of ADM in PPIBR. This condition is characterized by erythema in the cutaneous territory directly over the ADM, and its appearance resembles that of cellulitis or superficial infection of the mastectomy flap. There are several hypotheses regarding the etiology, but none has addressed the physiological alterations that lead to the onset and resolution of RBS [48].

17.4.6.1 Prevention and Management

To reduce the incidence of RBS, some authors suggest routine rinsing of the ADM with sterile saline followed by immersion in antibiotic solution before insertion into the mastectomy pocket [49]. An important point in the management is to differentiate RBS from infection. Although they have clearly different pathophysiology, both can occur within the same timeframe and have similar clinical characteristics. In the case of RBS, patients typically do not complain of pain and the breast is not hot to touch, differentiating it from cellulitis. Antibiotic therapy is recommended in all types of erythema in PPIBR. After 7 days, if no changes are observed and the patient remains afebrile, the erythema is probably due to RBS. Therefore, antibiotics could be discontinued because the erythema of RBS resolves spontaneously within a few weeks to a few months [48]. Use of corticosteroids may curtail the duration. Successful treatment of RBS has also been reported with montelukast [49].

17.4.7 Implant Extrusion

Implant extrusion and loss of reconstruction are closely associated, and they are a consequence of the other early complications described above.

Implant exposure can be associated with wound dehiscence, severe skin necrosis, or surgical site infection. Therefore, prevention and proper management of all the possible adverse effects described above (seroma, hematoma, infection, skin necrosis, wound dehiscence, and RBS) are the key to successful PPIBR.

17.5 Late Complications

Late complications are usually adverse effects that manifest several weeks after surgery (from around 3 months). In most cases, they are the consequence of a combination of suboptimal mastectomy technique and early adverse events. They are mainly associated with the esthetic aspect of the reconstruction; thus, most will require surgical corrective procedures. The most frequent late complications, together with their prevention measures and management, are described individually below.

17.5.1 Capsular Contracture

Capsular contracture is one of the most common late complications in PPIBR. It can be defined as a physical distortion and elevation of the reconstructed breast [50]. Signs of capsular contracture include increasing firmness or tightness in the breast and can be accompanied by chronic pain. Clinical evaluation is the simplest and most effective way to assess the presence and degree of capsular contracture. The most widespread classification is the modified Baker classification (Table 17.2) [51]. Although there are several hypotheses about the potential etiologies of capsular contracture, it is likely caused by any factor that produces inflammation within the peri-prosthetic pocket or near the developing capsule, leading to abnormal collagen and myofibroblast deposition [52, 53]. Thus, seroma, hematoma, infection, and radiotherapy are potential risk factors for capsular contracture. Some authors have also reported an increased probability of capsular contracture associated with the use of a smooth implant [54].

Table 17.2 Classification of capsular contracture after prosthetic breast reconstruction [50]

Class IA	Absolutely natural, cannot tell breast was reconstructed
Class IB	Soft, but the implant is detectable by physical examination or inspection because of mastectomy
Class II	Mildly firm reconstructed breast with an implant that may be visible and detectable by physical examination
Class III	Moderately firm reconstructed breast. The implant is readily detectable, but the result may still be acceptable
Class IV	Severe capsular contracture with an unacceptable aesthetic outcome and/or significant patient symptoms requiring surgical intervention

17.5.1.1 Prevention

The first and most important point to prevent capsular contracture is to perform the mastectomy with a reliable, meticulous technique, preserving an adequate thickness of subcutaneous tissue. Then, considering the multifactorial etiology of capsular contracture, the prevention strategies are based on taking appropriate precautions to reduce the risk of seroma, hematoma, and infection. Regarding the surface of the implants, most authors report that implants covered with polyurethane foam are associated with a lower risk of capsular contracture than smooth or textured implants [55]. Moreover, the use of ADM in PPIBR has been shown to be associated with consistently low capsular contracture rates [7]. The mechanism is not well understood but some studies have hypothesized that the presence of ADM results in a significant reduction in myofibroblast concentration in the peri-prosthetic tissue [56].

17.5.1.2 Management

In the case of mild capsular contractures, the preferred management tends to be nonsurgical. There are a variety of techniques that include mechanical displacement of the implant, external ultrasound, and certain drugs (antibiotics, vitamin E, steroids, nonsteroidal anti-inflammatory drugs, chemotherapeutics, and leukotriene inhibitors); however, no encouraging results have been reported. For severe capsular contractures (Baker III – IV) associated with chronic pain and/or significant changes in the position or shape of the breast, the treatment is surgery. This involves relaxing the capsular tissue through radial incisions (capsulotomy) or directly removing all the capsular tissue (capsulectomy). It is also advisable to replace the implant with a new one, completely covered with ADM whenever possible, and always following the prevention strategies for early complications.

17.5.2 Implant Displacement

Another late complication in PPIBR is displacement of the breast implant over time, thus losing its proper position in the breast. In general, the implant can be displaced in any direction (superiorly, inferiorly, laterally, and medially) or can even be flipped (smooth implants). Causes of this include mastectomy pockets much larger than the implant volume, ischemic or necrotic damage to the mastectomy flap that generates retraction, or the effects of radiotherapy on the reconstructed breast tissues, which is closely associated with capsular contracture.

17.5.2.1 Prevention

Prevention strategies are based initially on adjustment of the mastectomy pocket to the implant volume, anchoring the ADM that envelops the implant in the appropriate position in the chest wall, and on preventive measures for mastectomy skin flap necrosis in the postoperative period. A soft compression bra is usually applied to provide stability and maintain the implant in the preferred position. Vigorous physical activity should be avoided for the first 2–3 weeks.

17.5.2.2 Management

Treatment of breast implant displacement requires repositioning surgery. In some cases, it may be necessary to perform relaxation capsulotomies combined with contralateral capsuloplasty to delimit and narrow the mastectomy pocket and achieve the desired position.

17.5.3 Rippling

Implant rippling is a very frequent late complication following PPIBR and results in significant patient dissatisfaction. Rippling refers to contour irregularities in the breast surface, transmitted from the surface of the implant, that become clinically apparent. It is usually most evident in the upper medial or lower lateral portions of the breast. In the early stages, it is only palpable, and the edge of the implant can be felt by gently running a finger across the surface of the breast. In more advanced cases, the wrinkles or folds become visible. Risk factors for rippling include patients with a low body mass index (<20) or with thin breast skin and subcutaneous tissue (pinch test <2 cm) [57]. Saline implants or those with less cohesive silicone gel are associated with the highest risk of rippling because they are more susceptible to shape and contour change. The risk of rippling is also higher with the use of textured implants because adherence of the textured implant surface to the breast tissue and capsule can result in traction rippling. Another risk factor for rippling is when the mastectomy pocket is larger than the implant [58].

17.5.3.1 Prevention

The first step to prevent rippling is to preserve an adequate thickness of the mastectomy flap by performing subcutaneous dissection in the correct plane. The second step is to choose the new generation of highly cohesive implants. The polyurethane implant surface also appears to have the lowest risk of rippling. The third step is to use ADM to provide implant support and coverage, which may create a more favorable interface between the implant and the skin flaps, camouflaging the rippling effect. Another important point is to choose the right implant in proportion with the mastectomy pocket to avoid excess skin that can develop rippling. It is also recommended to tighten the mastectomy pocket when closing the inframammary incision [57, 58].

17.5.3.2 Management

According to the grading system described by Vidya et al. (Table 17.3), [57] grade II–III rippling can be effectively corrected by lipomodeling, which allows restoration of the thickness of the mastectomy skin flaps and camouflage of the surface defect (Fig. 17.3). In grade IV rippling, lipomodeling alone may not be enough to correct the defects. Therefore, it is usually combined with capsulotomy or partial capsulectomy. An alternative technique consists of dissecting a pocket between the posterior surface of the capsule and the underlying pectoral muscle to place the implant, thereby providing two layers of covering capsule [57, 58]. A soft breast compression with a transparent film dressing can be used to evenly distribute pressure on the skin flap.

Table 17.3 Grading system for rippling in implant-based breast reconstruction [56]

Grade 1	No evidence of rippling seen both at rest and with movement
Grade 2	Mild rippling is felt but not visualized both at rest and with movement
Grade 3	Moderate rippling visualized with movement and at rest
Grade 4	Severe - persistent rippling causing gross deformity both at rest and with movement

17.5.4 Visible Implant Edge

A visible upper medial or lateral edge of the implant is another common complication in PPIBR. It is especially frequent in slim patients with thin subcutaneous tissue. The most efficient treatment for the management of this problem is lipomodeling to regularize the transition between the chest wall and the reconstructed breast (Fig. 17.3).

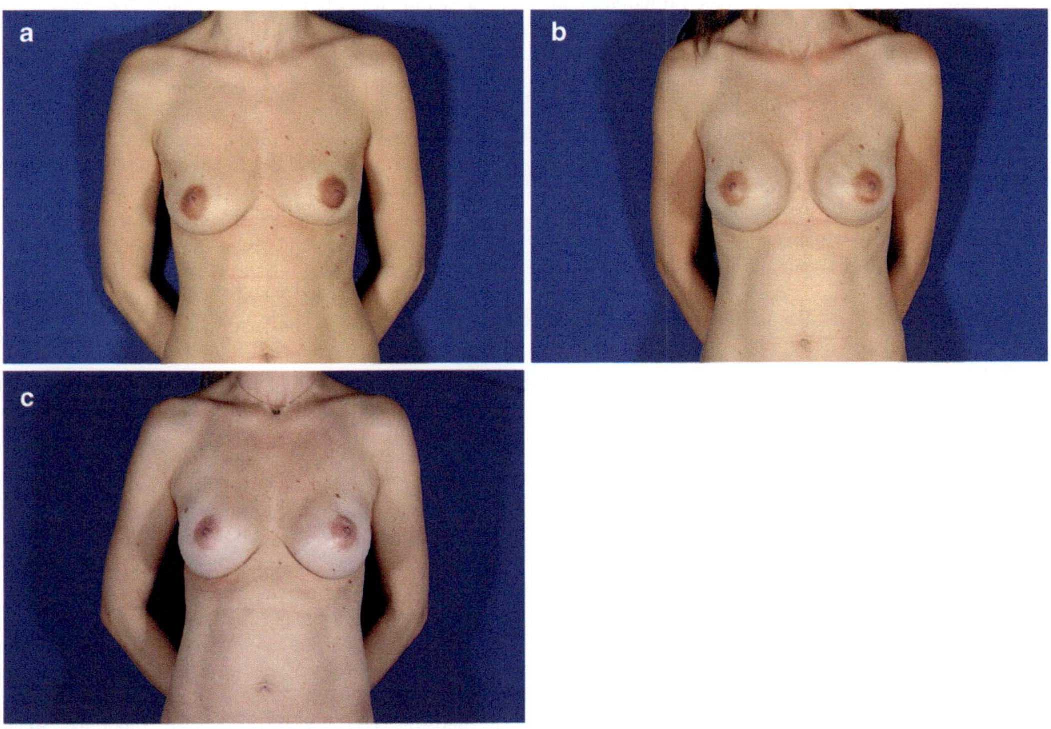

Fig. 17.3 A 36-year-old patient with a history of bilateral nipple-sparing mastectomy and direct-to-implant reconstruction. Preoperative image (**a**). After 8 months, the patient presented with visible rippling and implant edges (**b**), for which lipofilling of both breasts was carried out (**c**)

17.6 Conclusion

Comprehensive breast cancer treatment encompasses not only good oncological outcomes but also esthetic results. An effective prevention strategy for early complications is essential to avoid loss of the reconstruction and reduce the risk of late adverse events that may affect the esthetics of the reconstruction. Successful PPIBR requires appropriate patient selection, suitable preoperative planning, meticulous surgical technique, and precise intraoperative decision-making guided by the recommendations presented in this chapter, followed by proper postoperative care.

References

1. Snyderman RK, Guthrie RH. Reconstruction of the female breast following radical mastectomy. Plast Reconstr Surg. 1971;47(6):565–7.
2. Schlenker JD, Bueno RA, Ricketson G, Lynch JB. Loss of silicone implants after subcutaneous mastectomy and reconstruction. Plast Reconstr Surg. 1978;62(6):853–61.
3. Gruber RP, Kahn RA, Lash H, Maser MR, Apfelberg DB, Laub DR. Breast reconstruction following mastectomy: a comparison of submuscular and subcutaneous techniques. Plast Reconstr Surg. 1981;67(3):312–7.
4. Ward DC, Edwards MH. Early results of subcutaneous mastectomy with immediate silicone prosthetic implant for carcinoma of the breast. Br J Surg. 1983;70(11):651–3.
5. Salzberg CA. Nonexpansive immediate breast reconstruction using human acellular tissue matrix graft (AlloDerm). Ann Plast Surg. 2006;57(1):1–5.
6. Masià J, iBAG Working Group. The largest multicentre data collection on prepectoral breast reconstruction: the iBAG study. J Surg Oncol. 2020;122(5):848–60.
7. Wagner RD, Braun TL, Zhu H, Winocour S. A systematic review of complications in prepectoral breast reconstruction. J Plast Reconstr Aesthet Surg. 2019;72(7):1051–9.
8. Dave RV, Vucicevic A, Barrett E, Highton L, Johnson R, Kirwan CC, et al. Risk factors for complications and implant loss after prepectoral implant-based immediate breast reconstruction: medium-term outcomes in a prospective cohort. Br J Surg. 2021;108(5):534–41.
9. Chatterjee A, Nahabedian MY, Gabriel A, Macarios D, Parekh M, Wang F, et al. Early assessment of post-surgical outcomes with pre-pectoral breast reconstruction: a literature review and meta-analysis. J Surg Oncol. 2018;117(6):1119–30.
10. Salibian AA, Frey JD, Karp NS. Strategies and considerations in selecting between subpectoral and prepectoral breast reconstruction. Gland Surg. 2019;8(1):11–8.
11. Salibian AA, Frey JD, Choi M, Karp NS. Subcutaneous Implant-based Breast Reconstruction with Acellular Dermal Matrix/Mesh: A Systematic Review. Plast Reconstr Surg Glob Open. 2016;4(11):e1139
12. Colwell AS, Tessler O, Lin AM, Liao E, Winograd J, Cetrulo CL, et al. Breast reconstruction following nipple-sparing mastectomy: predictors of complications, reconstruction outcomes, and 5-year trends. Plast Reconstr Surg. 2014;133(3):496–506.
13. Munhoz AM, Aldrighi CM, Montag E, Arruda EG, Aldrighi JM, Gemperli R, et al. Clinical outcomes following nipple-areola-sparing mastectomy with immediate implant-based breast reconstruction: a 12-year experience with an analysis of patient and breast-related factors for complications. Breast Cancer Res Treat. 2013;140(3):545–55.
14. Hart A, Funderburk CD, Chu CK, Pinell-White X, Halgopian T, Manning-Geist B, et al. The impact of diabetes mellitus on wound healing in breast reconstruction. Ann Plast Surg. 2017;78(3):260–3.
15. Vidya R, Berna G, Sbitany H, Nahabedian M, Becker H, Reitsamer R, et al. Prepectoral implant-based breast reconstruction: a joint consensus guide from UK, European and USA breast and plastic reconstructive surgeons. Ecancermedicalscience. 2019;13:927.
16. Rifkin WJ, Kantar RS, Cammarata MJ, Wilson SC, Diaz-Siso JR, Golas AR, et al. Impact of diabetes on 30-day complications in mastectomy and implant-based breast reconstruction. J Surg Res. 2019;235:148–59.
17. Spear SL, Hannan CM, Willey SC, Cocilovo C. Nipple-sparing mastectomy. Plast Reconstr Surg. 2009;123(6):1665–73.
18. Jordan SW, Khavanin N, Kim JYS. Seroma in prosthetic breast reconstruction. Plast Reconstr Surg. 2016;137(4):1104–16.
19. van Bemmel AJM, van de Velde CJH, Schmitz RF, Liefers GJ. Prevention of seroma formation after axillary dissection in breast cancer: a systematic review. Eur J Surg Oncol. 2011;37(10):829–35.
20. Sierra DH. Fibrin sealant adhesive systems: a review of their chemistry, material properties and clinical applications. J Biomater Appl. 1993;7(4):309–52.
21. Moore MM, Freeman MG. Fibrin sealant in breast surgery. J Long-Term Eff Med Implants. 1998;8(2):133–42.
22. Lindsey WH, Masterson TM, Spotnitz WD, Wilhelm MC, Morgan RF. Seroma prevention using fibrin glue in a rat mastectomy model. Arch Surg. 1990;125(3):305–7.
23. Eroğlu E, Oral S, Unal E, Kalayci M, Oksüz O, Tilmaz M. Reducing seroma formation with fibrin glue in an animal mastectomy model. Eur J Surg Oncol. 1996;22(2):137–9.

24. Gioffrè Florio MA, Mezzasalma F, Manganaro T, Pakravanan H, Cogliandolo A. [The use of fibrin glue in the surgery of breast carcinoma]. G Chir. 1993;14(4–5):239–241.
25. Moore MM, Nguyen DH, Spotnitz WD. Fibrin sealant reduces serous drainage and allows for earlier drain removal after axillary dissection: a randomized prospective trial. Am Surg. 1997;63(1):97–102.
26. Gilly FN, François Y, Sayag-Beaujard AC, Glehen O, Brachet A, Vignal J. Prevention of lymphorrhea by means of fibrin glue after axillary lymphadenectomy in breast cancer: prospective randomized trial. Eur Surg Res. 1998;30(6):439–43.
27. Miri Bonjar MR, Maghsoudi H, Samnia R, Saleh P, Parsafar F. Efficacy of fibrin glue on seroma formation after breast surgery. Int J Breast Cancer. 2012;2012:643132.
28. Vasileiadou K, Kosmidis C, Anthimidis G, Miliaras S, Kostopoulos I, Fahantidis E. Cyanoacrylate adhesive reduces seroma production after modified radical mastectomy or Quadrantectomy with lymph node dissection-a prospective randomized clinical trial. Clin Breast Cancer. 2017;17(8):595–600.
29. Srivastava V, Basu S, Shukla VK. Seroma formation after breast cancer surgery: what we have learned in the last two decades. J Breast Cancer. 2012;15(4):373–80.
30. Keogh GW, Doughty JC, McArdle CSM, Cooke TG. Seroma formation related to electrocautery in breast surgery: a prospective randomized trial. Breast. 1998;7(1):39–41.
31. Loh SA, Carlson GA, Chang EI, Huang E, Palanker D, Gurtner GC. Comparative healing of surgical incisions created by the PEAK PlasmaBlade, conventional electrosurgery, and a scalpel. Plast Reconstr Surg. 2009;124(6):1849–59.
32. Dogan L, Gulcelik MA, Yuksel M, Uyar O, Erdogan O, Reis E. The effect of plasmakinetic cautery on wound healing and complications in mastectomy. J Breast Cancer. 2013;16(2):198–201.
33. Sowa Y, Inafuku N, Kodama T, Morita D, Numajiri T. Preventive effect on seroma of use of PEAK PlasmaBlade after latissimus Dorsi breast reconstruction. Plast Reconstr Surg Glob Open. 2018;6(12):e2035.
34. O'Hea BJ, Ho MN, Petrek JA. External compression dressing versus standard dressing after axillary lymphadenectomy. Am J Surg. 1999;177(6):450–3.
35. Sood A, Kotamarti VS, Therattil PJ, Lee ES. Sclerotherapy for the management of seromas: a systematic review. Eplasty. 2017;17:e25.
36. Throckmorton AD, Askegard-Giesmann J, Hoskin TL, Bjarnason H, Donohue JH, Boughey JC, et al. Sclerotherapy for the treatment of postmastectomy seroma. Am J Surg. 2008;196(4):541–4.
37. Seth A, Hirsch E, Kim J, Dumanian G, Mustoe T, Galiano R, et al. Hematoma after mastectomy with immediate reconstruction an analysis of risk factors in 883 patients. Ann Plast Surg. 2012;71:20–3.
38. Banuelos J, Weissler JM, Harless CA, Jacobson SR, Van Tran N, Nguyen M-DT, et al. Intravenous tranexamic acid in implant-based breast reconstruction safely reduces hematoma without thromboembolic events. Plast Reconstr Surg Glob Open. 2019;7(8 Suppl):87.
39. Ruidiaz ME, Messmer D, Atmodjo DY, Vose JG, Huang EJ, Kummel AC, et al. Comparative healing of human cutaneous surgical incisions created by the PEAK PlasmaBlade, conventional electrosurgery, and a standard scalpel. Plast Reconstr Surg. 2011;128(1):104–11.
40. Gdalevitch P, Van Laeken N, Bahng S, Ho A, Bovill E, Lennox P, et al. Effects of nitroglycerin ointment on mastectomy flap necrosis in immediate breast reconstruction: a randomized controlled trial. Plast Reconstr Surg. 2015;135(6):1530–9.
41. Fredman R, Wise I, Friedman T, Heller L, Karni T. Skin-sparing mastectomy flap ischemia salvage using urgent hyperbaric chamber oxygen therapy: a case report. Undersea Hyperb Med. 2014;41(2):145–7.
42. Robertson SA, Jeevaratnam JA, Agrawal A, Cutress RI. Mastectomy skin flap necrosis: challenges and solutions. Breast Cancer Targets Ther. 2017;9:141–52.
43. Matusiak D, Wichtowski M, Pieszko K, Kobylarek D, Murawa D. Is negative-pressure wound therapy beneficial in modern-day breast surgery? Contemp Oncol. 2019;23(2):69–73.
44. Kim JH, Kim YS, Kim YW, Kim YJ, Chun YS, Park HK, et al. A single-use negative-pressure wound therapy device can reduce mastectomy skin flap necrosis in direct-to-implant breast reconstruction. Arch Aesthet Plast Surg. 2020;26(1):12–9.
45. Irwin GW, Boundouki G, Fakim B, Johnson R, Highton L, Myers D, et al. Negative pressure wound therapy reduces wound breakdown and implant loss in Prepectoral breast reconstruction. Plast Reconstr Surg Glob Open. 2020;8(2):e2667.
46. Holland M, Lentz R, Sbitany H. Utility of postoperative prophylactic antibiotics in Prepectoral breast reconstruction: a single-surgeon experience. Ann Plast Surg. 2021;86(1):24–8.
47. Papa G, Frasca A, Renzi N, Stocco C, Pizzolato G, Ramella V, et al. Protocol for prevention and monitoring of surgical site infections in implant-based breast reconstruction: preliminary results. Med Kaunas Lith. 2021;57(2):151.
48. Nahabedian MY. Prosthetic breast reconstruction and red breast syndrome: demystification and a review of the literature. Plast Reconstr Surg Glob Open. 2019;7(5):e2108.
49. Wu PS, Winocour S, Jacobson SR. Red breast syndrome: a review of available literature. Aesthet Plast Surg. 2015;39(2):227–30.
50. Nealon KP, Weitzman RE, Sobti N, Gadd M, Specht M, Jimenez RB, et al. Prepectoral direct-to-implant breast reconstruction: safety outcome endpoints and delineation of risk factors. Plast Reconstr Surg. 2020;145(5):898e–908e.
51. Spear SL, Baker JL. Classification of capsular contracture after prosthetic breast reconstruction. Plast Reconstr Surg. 1995;96(5):1119–23. discussion 1124

52. Siggelkow W, Faridi A, Spiritus K, Klinge U, Rath W, Klosterhalfen B. Histological analysis of silicone breast implant capsules and correlation with capsular contracture. Biomaterials. 2003;24(6):1101–9.
53. Poeppl N, Schreml S, Lichtenegger F, Lenich A, Eisenmann-Klein M, Prantl L. Does the surface structure of implants have an impact on the formation of a capsular contracture? Aesthet Plast Surg. 2007;31(2):133–9.
54. Stevens WG, Nahabedian MY, Calobrace MB, Harrington JL, Capizzi PJ, Cohen R, et al. Risk factor analysis for capsular contracture: a 5-year Sientra study analysis using round, smooth, and textured implants for breast augmentation. Plast Reconstr Surg. 2013;132(5):1115–23.
55. Handel N, Silverstein MJ, Jensen JA, Collins A, Zierk K. Comparative experience with smooth and polyurethane breast implants using the Kaplan-Meier method of survival analysis. Plast Reconstr Surg. 1991;88(3):475–81.
56. Tevlin R, Borrelli MR, Irizarry D, Nguyen D, Wan DC, Momeni A. Acellular dermal matrix reduces Myofibroblast presence in the breast capsule. Plast Reconstr Surg Glob Open. 2019;7(5):e2213.
57. Vidya R, Iqbal FM, Becker H, Zhadan O. Rippling associated with pre-pectoral implant based breast reconstruction: a new grading system. World J Plast Surg. 2019;8(3):311–5.
58. Pantelides NM, Srinivasan JR. Rippling following breast augmentation or reconstruction: Aetiology, emerging treatment options and a novel classification of severity. Aesthet Plast Surg. 2018;42(4):980–5.

18 Clinical, Histological, and Ultrasound Follow-Up of Breast Reconstruction with One-Stage Prepectoral Breast Reconstruction

Maruccia Michele, Giudice Giuseppe, Gurrado Angela, Cazzato Gerardo, and Elia Rossella

18.1 Introduction

Prosthetic breast reconstruction is the most common form of reconstruction for women who undergo mastectomy and immediate reconstruction. Refinements in breast cancer treatment, mastectomy techniques, and reconstructive protocols have de facto further broadened the indications for implant-based breast reconstruction [1].

The placement of the prosthesis in a prepectoral position is currently spreading as a simpler, alternative approach to the submuscular approach. The prepectoral implant placement emerged to overcome some disadvantages related to the submuscular implant placement: (1) the reduction of muscle strength, (2) the postoperative pain, (3) a longer recovery period, (4) the breast animation deformity during contraction of the pectoralis major muscle (PPM).

Conversely, the prepectoral implant placement without any detachment of the PMM requires an implant coverage and an implant fixation with tissue support. This can be performed with acellular dermal matrices, meshes, or autologous dermofat flaps. Acellular Dermal Matrices (ADMs) and various meshes became available and together facilitated superior aesthetic outcomes with the prepectoral implant placement [2].

Furthermore, currently, an increasing number of prophylactic mastectomies and immediate breast reconstruction are being performed in younger patients at high risk for familiar cancer [3]. In these cases, patients may prefer to avoid the morbidity of pectoral disinsertion, and the prepectoral technique may ensure a rapid return to a normal lifestyle.

Insertion in a prepectoral plane of a definitive implant in one stage is predicated on adequate skin perfusion to maintain tissue viability. The eligibility of a patient for prepectoral reconstruction is based on skin perfusion, rather than flap thickness, and objective assessment with a tissue perfusion system is of critical importance to achieving suc-

M. Michele (✉) · G. Giuseppe · E. Rossella
Division of Plastic and Reconstructive Surgery, Department of Emergency and Organ Transplantation, University of Bari Aldo Moro, Bari, Italy

G. Angela
Unit of Endocrine, Digestive, and Emergency Surgery, Department of Biomedical Sciences and Human Oncology, University Medical School "Aldo Moro" of Bari, Bari, Italy

C. Gerardo
Section of Pathology, University of Bari 'Aldo Moro', Bari, Italy

© The Author(s), under exclusive license to Springer Nature Switzerland AG 2023
R. Vidya, H. Becker (eds.), *Prepectoral Breast Reconstruction*,
https://doi.org/10.1007/978-3-031-15590-1_18

cessful outcomes [4–6]. Relative contraindications include patients with comorbidities such as uncontrolled diabetes, morbid obesity, recent or current tobacco use, as well as those with a history of preoperative radiation [7, 8].

As with any form of breast reconstruction, oncologic consideration is mandatory. Prepectoral reconstruction is generally contraindicated in cases of late cancer stage or any patients deemed at high risk of recurrence [9].

18.2 Main Manuscript

The clinical, radiological, and histological follow-up of patients undergoing breast reconstruction with a one-stage prepectoral implant-based breast reconstruction (PPBR) is of significant importance to determine the safety profile of a relatively new technique. The objective is to highlight the rate of complications and the functional and aesthetic outcome of the procedure, especially in comparison to the more traditional subpectoral technique.

18.3 Clinical Follow-Up

Patients undergoing PPBR report less discomfort, no need for post-operative expansion, less tissue flap edema, and virtually no subjective negative impact on upper extremity function. Additionally, animation deformity has been completely eliminated (Fig. 18.1).

Results on cosmetic and patient-reported outcomes are also promising, though further long-term studies are needed. In several case series, patients report high rates in all the questionnaire matrices of overall satisfaction with outcome, overall satisfaction with breasts, psychosocial well-being, and sexual well-being, scoring a significant increase in these domains from the pre-operative to the postoperative periods [10, 11].

One of the main reasons why reconstructive surgeons preferred the submuscular approach to the prepectoral was the concern about capsular contracture rate (CC). In recent reports, the use of the new devices showed acceptable CC rate, similar to total submuscular reconstruction, attributing the low CC to a diminished inflammatory response [12, 13]. The ADM seemed to act like a sieve layer between the prosthesis and the subcutaneous tissue, reducing inflammatory response along with the likelihood of CC [14, 15].

With regard to further surgical complications, initially, prepectoral breast reconstruction was reported in small series that employed both immediate implant and two-stage expander reconstructions using a variety of ADMs and meshes with low complications rates [2, 11, 16–19]. These outcomes have been confirmed in a larger multicenter study [13].

Recently, a multicenter retrospective audit, promoted by the Barcelona Hospital, collected the experience of 30 centers on prepectoral breast reconstruction with Braxon ADM [20]. A total of 1450 procedures were retrospectively collected in a year period with the aim of obtaining the largest evidence on prepectoral breast reconstruction performed with a complete Braxon ADM wrapping to acquire concrete statement about outcomes and therefore improve patients' selection. Patients had a mean follow-up period of 22.7 months (range 3–75.7).

The authors reported that diabetes, smoke, and immunosuppression had an influence on complications occurrence, as well as implant weight. Capsular contracture was associated with postoperative radiotherapy, but the overall rate was low (2.1%). Complications led to implant loss in 6.5% of the cases. Besides, the multivariate analysis of the risk factors contributing to complication onset underlined an increased risk of seroma formation in patients using immunosuppressive drugs (RR = 4.56; *P*-value = .017) as well as those who had had a previous esthetic breast surgery (RR = 2.54; *P*-value = .030) or an axillary dissection during the PPBR (RR = 1.67; *P*-value = .039); also the type of tumor seemed to increase seroma onset (*P*-value = .029). Infection instead was more likely to occur in diabetics (RR = 4.026; *P*-value = .003) and ex/active smokers (value = .016) with RR = 2.15 ex. for smokers and 2.08 for active smokers. Axillary dissection

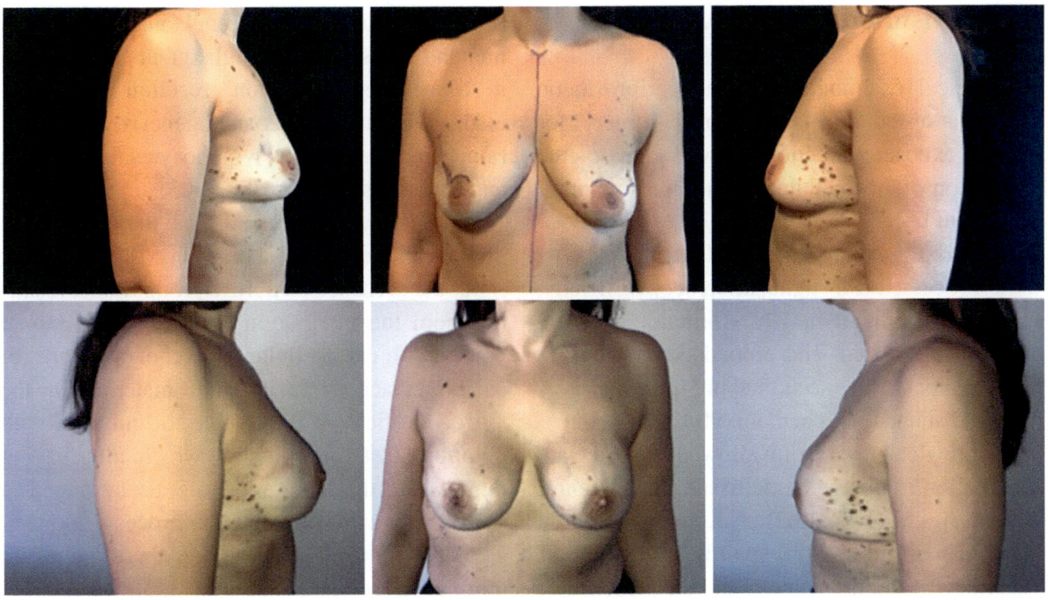

Fig. 18.1 A 45-year-old woman affected by right invasive lobular carcinoma of the breast and multiple microcalcification of the left breast, undergoing bilateral skin nipple sparing mastectomy and prepectoral breast reconstruction. Preoperative (up) and postoperative views (below) at 1 year follow-up. Round silicone breast implants (300 cc) and Braxon® ADM have been chosen

also influenced infection onset (RR = 2.17; *P*-value = .009) and an increasing implant volume showed, both in univariate and multivariate analysis, a higher risk of infection development, with an infected breast mean volume of 409.3 g compared to those of noninfected cases of 346.2 g (*P*-value = .001). Briefly, data analysis highlighted lasting results with low complication rates and defined, at the same time, the risk factors involved in the onset of postoperative complications.

If clinical outcome data are easily obtained from the several published case series on PPBR, on the contrary limited studies comparing prepectoral and subpectoral breast direct-to-implant breast reconstruction have been published so far. The PPBR has been associated with less postoperative pain, faster recovery from postoperative upper extremity functional morbidity, higher aesthetic BREAST-Q scores as well as economic advantages compared to the subpectoral procedure [21].

The outcomes of a prepectoral breast reconstruction after postmastectomy radiation therapy (PMRT) has also been investigated. PMRT is a well-known risk factor for complications after breast reconstruction, particularly capsular contracture and reconstructive failure [22]. PMRT after implant-based breast reconstruction is also associated with a higher rate of revisional surgery and worse cosmetic outcome as well as lower patient satisfaction [23].

Both Sigalove et al. and Elswick et al. found no statistically significant increased risk of adverse outcomes in prepectoral breast reconstructions that underwent PMRT based on short-term, retrospective data in 93 and 52 breasts, respectively [9, 24].

Additionally, the results of the study published by Sinnot and colleagues demonstrated that patients who underwent subpectoral breast reconstruction and receive PMRT actually had a greater rate of capsular contracture than patients that underwent prepectoral reconstruction [25].

18.4 Histological Follow-Up

Histological examination of the periprosthetic tissue harvested during revisional surgery for implant exposure/infection showed signs of the integration of the acellular dermal matrix within the patient tissue.

Biopsies of explanted ADM from the patients were processed for light microscopy. Briefly, samples were fixed in 10% formalin solution, dehydrated, cleared, and embedded in paraffin. Paraffin blocks were sectioned in 5-μm-thick sections and stained with hematoxylin and eosin.

Histological observation allowed to appreciate the creation of fibrosclerotic tissue (in the center and top right of Fig. 18.2) with modest chronic inflammatory infiltration, mainly consisting of lymphocytes and monocytes, and the presence of hemorrhagic suffusion phenomena (bottom right of Fig. 18.2) with the formation of new blood vessels, typical of any foreign body reaction.

At higher magnification (10×), it is possible to describe the presence of chronic epithelioid-granulomatous gigantocellular inflammatory infiltration that envelops up to incorporate the acellular dermal matrix, allowing integration of the material within the host tissue. In particular, we can appreciate some giant cells that are arranged "in a wheel" around a material (see the center of the field in Fig. 18.3), and some of these are in the act of "engulfing" the amorphous matrix. This represents, from the histological point of view, the primum movens for the correct disposition of the "foreign" material within human tissues. All around the giant cell focusing a "tissue-like granulation" reaction is appreciated, consisting of neoangiogenesis, extravasation of red blood cells, lymphocytes, monocytes, and focal plasma cells (Fig. 18.3).

Two different moments of the integration phase can be appreciated (Fig. 18.4). On the right, the presence of fibrosclerotic tissue, resulting from the integration of the foreign dermal matrix with extracellular matrix, of which residual proteinaceous eosinophilic material. On the left of the field, it is possible to find cells with myofibroblastic morphology which, after having migrated to the integration site, are arranged in such a way as to optimize the process, allowing greater stability, elasticity, and therefore better morpho-functional result of the graft.

These findings are consistent with the ones already published in literature [16], confirming the major peculiarity of the acellular dermal matrix compared to synthetic meshes that have been evaluated as cheaper alternatives to biological matrices in subcutaneous breast reconstruction but implanting a nonabsorbable device still represents a concern for many surgeons [26]. A biological mesh, by definition, regardless of its origin is a scaffold that is stripped of its antigenic cells through specialized processing, allowing rapid host revascularization and cell repopulation arguably facilitating a good surgical outcome.

Additional studies of the histological changes ADM use [14, 27] support the hypothesis that

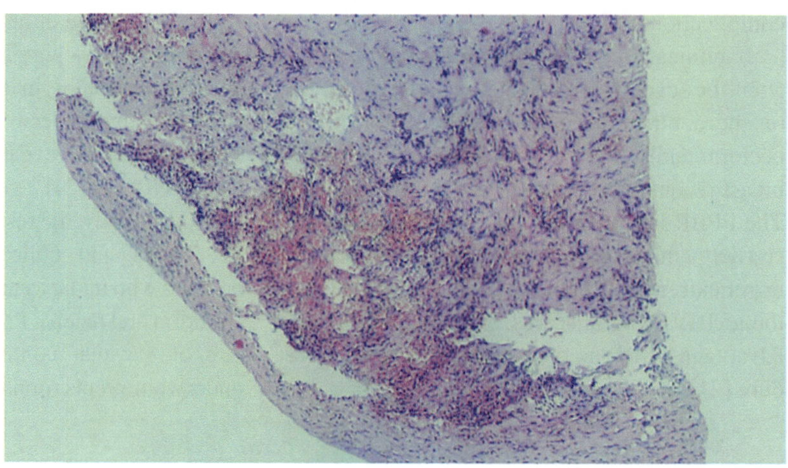

Fig. 18.2 Periprosthetic tissue biopsy. Hematoxylin-Eosin stain, Original Magnification 4×

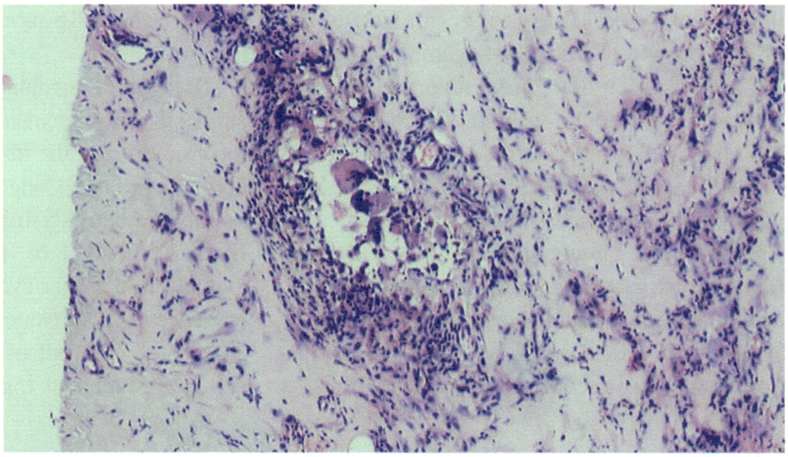

Fig. 18.3 Periprosthetic tissue biopsy. Hematoxylin-Eosin stain, Original Magnification 10×

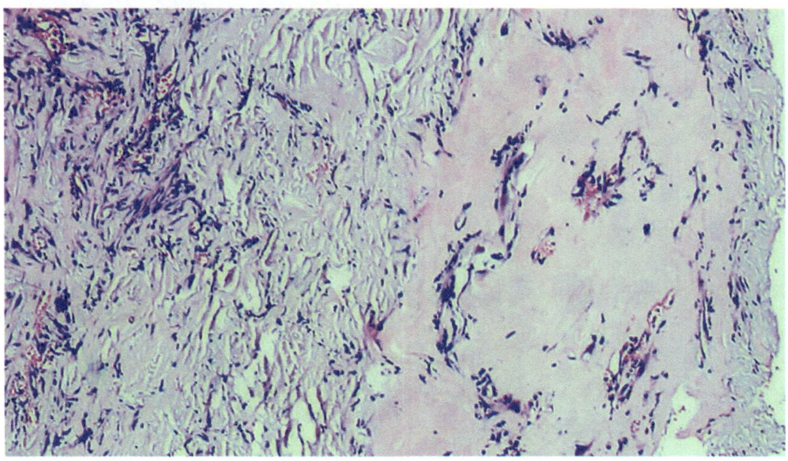

Fig. 18.4 Periprosthetic tissue biopsy. Hematoxylin-Eosin stain, Original Magnification 10×

ADMs—due to their lack of antigenic epitopes—provide a barrier to the host immune response against a foreign body (the expander/implant) and reduce capsular formation and contracture risk [28]. Komorowska-Timek et al. [27] studied the effect of an ADM on capsule formation with and without radiation and concluded that ADM reduces radiation-related inflammation and pseudoepithelium formation, resulting in slower progression of capsular formation and contraction. The incidence of capsular contracture in human subjects where ADM has been used also shows significantly reduced contracture problems, histologically and clinically [29].

18.5 Ultrasound Follow-Up

The ultrasound evaluation (US) of patients who underwent PPBR aims to highlight the signs of the ADM integration into the host tissue, including visibility and thickness of the biological membrane, the implant morphology, the implant margins, and the presence of mediolateral membrane folds.

Further, US may detect the occurrence of surgical local complications in course of follow-up, such as the presence of periprosthetic fluid, inhomogeneities of soft tissues, liponecrosis, hematoma, seroma, infection, lymphoceles, and findings of suspected disease recurrence and be of assistance to operative procedures.

Parvini et al. [30] first reported contrast-enhanced ultrasound evaluation (CEUS) to describe the vascularization of ADM after implant-based breast reconstruction. Besides, ultrasonographic contrast media that enhance the signal from the circulating blood have the potential to investigate these properties more sensitive and more reproducible. They proved the "in vivo" evaluation of vascular ingrowth and tissue formation after breast reconstruction with ADM after follow-up of 1–18 months postoperatively in 16 patients.

The early US evaluation in case of PPBR often shows the biological membrane stretched along the convexity of the implant while relaxed at the medial and lateral side of the implant, where the membrane partially fold and make some curves (Figs. 18.5 and 18.6). This feature is well appreciable in the earlier evaluations probably for the presence of periprosthetic fluid, sometimes a corpuscolated one, but over time, membrane folds can merge and stick together (Fig. 18.7).

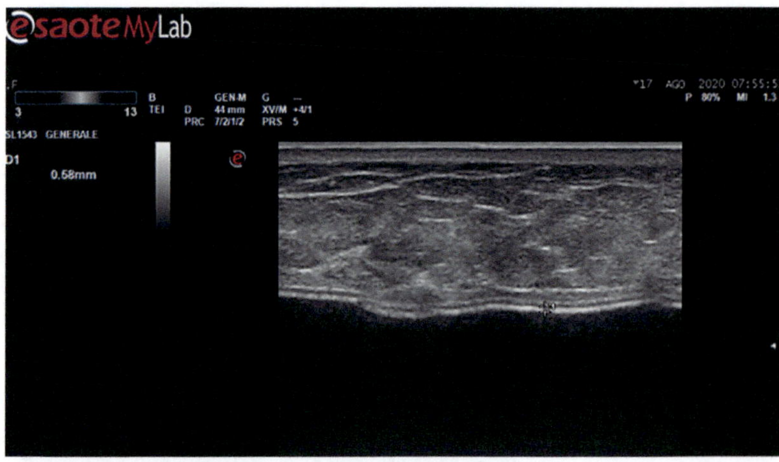

Fig. 18.5 Biological membrane presenting as a hypoechoic periprosthetic layer in the early postoperative evaluation (7 days post-op)

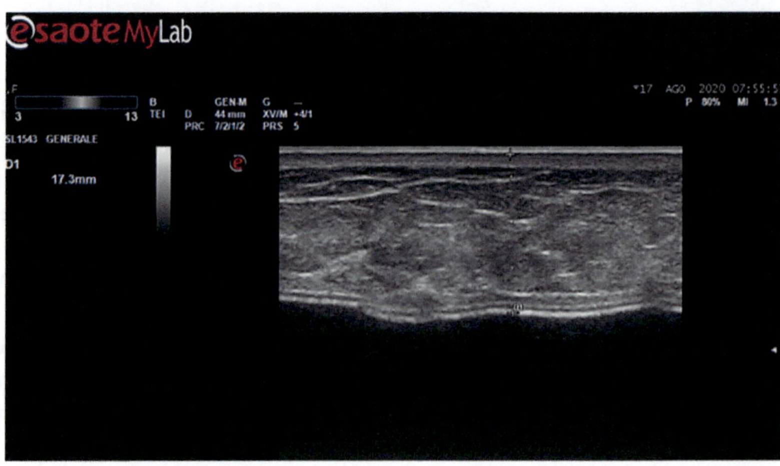

Fig. 18.6 Slight inhomogeneity and thickening of the subcutaneous adipose tissue in the early postoperative evaluation (7 days post-op)

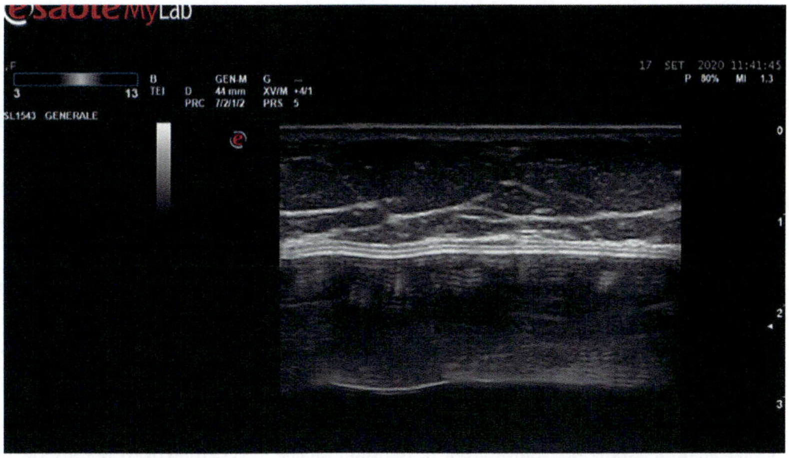

Fig. 18.7 Biological membrane is no more visible as hypoechoic periprosthetic layer, confirming the ADM's integration into the host tissue (18 months post-op)

18.6 Review of Short Literature to Date

A new method for breast reconstruction preserving the pectoralis major has been described in 2014 by Berna et al. The breast implant was placed in a subcutaneous plane, totally wrapped with a 0.6 mm-thick preshaped porcine ADM (Braxon; MBP Biologics, Neustadt-Glewe, Germany, licence holder Decomed, Marcon, Venezia, Italy) [31]. The innovative technique aimed to avoid any postoperative complication related to the detachment of the pectoralis such as muscular pain and shoulder or arm weakness and to improve the esthetic outcomes with a more physiological positioning of the breast implant.

To date, this device represents the most widely used one for PPBR in European and UK breast centers and the only ADM with a specific patented design that allows a standardized wrapping technique, reducing the number of variables so that data can be more easily compared among different centers [13] (Figs. 18.8 and 18.9).

There have been two national audits from the UK describing breast reconstruction outcomes [32]. The first audit covered breast reconstructions performed from January 2008 to March 2009 with an implant-based reconstruction cohort of more than 3000 patients. The overall complication rate in this group was 14·7%, with a return-to-theater rate of 4·6% and an implant loss rate of 9%, although all were placed in a subpectoral position. The more recent implant-based breast reconstruction evaluation (iBRA) study [20] included 2108 patients operated on for implant-based reconstruction between February 2014 and June 2016, but only 42 (2·0%) who had a prepectoral reconstruction. Overall readmission and return-to-theater rates were about 18%, and the 3-month implant loss rate was 9%. Outcomes in the prepectoral subgroup were analyzed separately and considered comparable to the overall results.

Further, the combination between a skin reducing mastectomy (SRM) through a Wise-pattern incision and ADM-implant reconstruction has been recently proposed to offer prepectoral breast reconstruction also in patients with large ptotic breasts. Wise-pattern skin-reducing mastectomies and immediate breast reconstruction for large breast volumes are inherently associated with the risk of mastectomy skin flap necrosis and "T" junction breakdown, besides the fact that larger breasted individuals requiring skin reduction may carry other contributory patient risk factors, such as an elevated BMI [33].

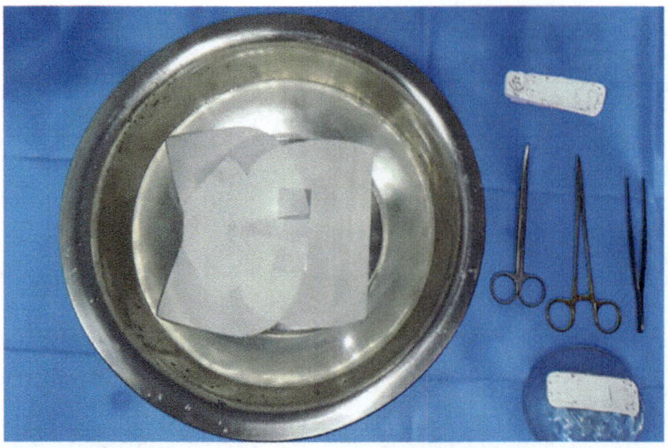

Fig. 18.8 Surgical kit for the Braxon® implantation technique. In order to allow the ADM to be incorporated into the tissue without an amplified inflammatory response, the production entails the sublimation in the final phase. This process makes the product dry so that it requires a quick rehydration for 5–10 min before use. A basic surgical kit and 2-0 Vicryl suture are used to create the pocket around the silicone sizer first and the silicone prosthesis definitively

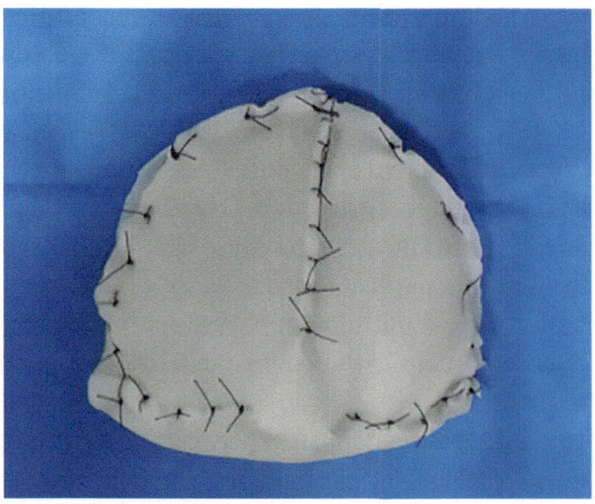

Fig. 18.9 Standardized wrapping technique of Braxon® ADM around the implant. Braxon® must be sutured to the pectoralis major and to the overlying mastectomy flaps with single stitches in order to ensure primary stability of the matrix which requires intimate contact with vascularized tissue

Caputo et al. [34] suggested to create a complete prepectoral pocket with a dermal flap along with an ADM for lower and upper pole coverage, respectively. Thuman et al. [35] demonstrated that a prepectoral, two-stages breast reconstruction with Wise-pattern skin reduction can be a suitable option in patients who have a high BMI.

A Wise-pattern SRM with prepectoral implant and complete ADM coverage with Braxon® as a single stage procedure in patients with large ptotic breasts has been described [36]. No major implant related complication was observed, and no unplanned return to operating room or readmission was required. The only two cases of wound dehiscence were managed conservatively, and no implant loss was observed. The Wise-pattern skin reducing mastectomy and prepectoral breast reconstruction can be offered to large and ptotic breasts, thereby broadening the suitable population for prepectoral implant-based reconstructions and widening patient choices. Harvesting an inferior dermal sling could act as a protector, adding little time to the overall procedure. The mastectomy flaps' perfusion still remains the key to optimize the operative procedure.

ADM-assisted one-stage prepectoral reconstruction has been proven to be the ideal approach also in cases of bilateral prophylactic surgeries. Women bearing a high risk of developing breast cancer are considered high-demanding patients because their desire for oncological safety is associated with the expectation of good aesthetic results and no functional damage. Patients with small, medium size breasts, and with large and ptotic breasts underwent a nipple-sparing mastectomy or a Wise-pattern skin reducing mastectomy as described above [36] and received Braxon® covered implants. On a total number of 46 reconstructions, no major complications were observed, as well as implant loss. Patients reported satisfaction with the outcome according to the BREAST-Q questionnaire administered postoperatively, indicating that such surgical reconstructive procedure successfully meets patients' clinical necessities and expectations [37].

18.7 New Generation ADMs: Three-Dimensional Matrices

Most of the biological matrices available for prepectoral breast reconstruction are in a flat conformation and must be tailored to fit the silhouette of the breast prosthesis. Among these matrices, Braxon® is the only one that has a pre-shaped design studied to easily adapt to the implant with minimal adjustments. Since 2021, a new version of Braxon® matrix has become available: Braxon®Fast is a biological matrix with the same characteristics as Braxon® but implemented with a three-dimensional shape. Thanks to Volumatrix® technology, Braxon®Fast is the only biological matrix presenting a dome-shape collagen sheet that is perfectly compliant to the implant's convexity on the anterior part. Complete implant coverage is maintained by means of a flat collagen sheet, connected to the dome, which allows for the formation of a closed system (Fig. 18.10). Such innovative, three-dimensional conformation is retained even after matrix hydration (Figs. 18.11 and 18.12) and speeds up the preparation of the implant wrap: after the prosthesis positioning inside the matrix and its snug coverage, only two flaps are to be stitched together (compared to the four of Braxon®) with single stitches (Fig. 18.13). Matrix excess can be removed if needed (Fig. 18.14). Implantation of the Braxon®Fast-wrapped implant follows the same procedures and rules as Braxon®-wrapped implant: parachuting stitches for placement and fixation to the pectoralis major muscle on sites distal from the incision (Fig. 18.15), stitches between the matrix and the subcutaneous tissue to ensure mechanical stillness, intimate contact of the matrix to a viable, well vascularized tissue.

The pre-curved shape of Braxon®Fast also bears advantages at the aesthetic level: by eliminating ribs and folds on the matrix surface, natural reconstructive results are easily achieved (Fig. 18.16a, b).

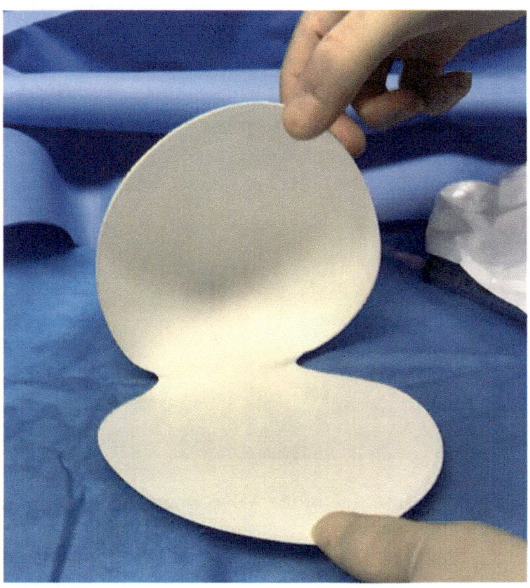

Fig. 18.10 Braxon®Fast ADM in its dry conformation, with the pre-curved dome and the flat base

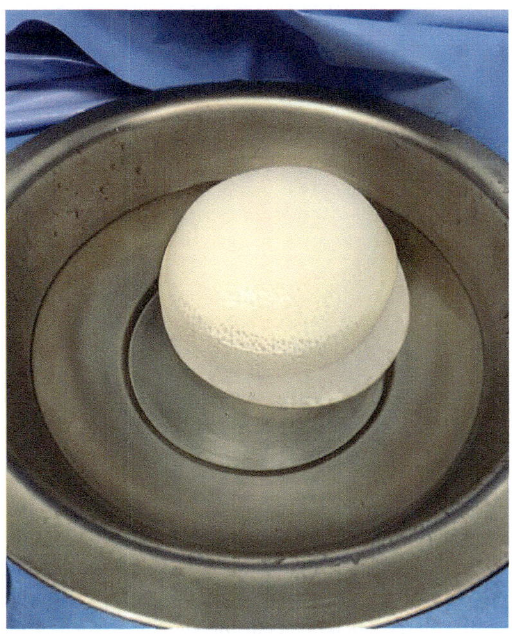

Fig. 18.11 Braxon®Fast hydration in saline solution

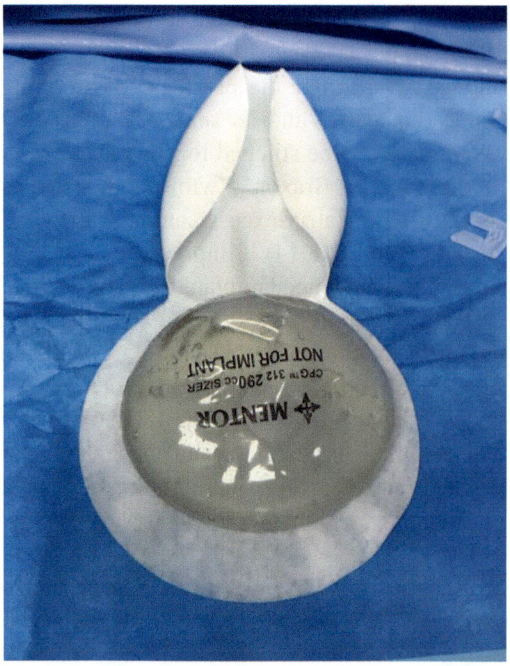

Fig. 18.12 Sizer placement on the ADM. Even in the hydrated state, Braxon®Fast maintains the three-dimensionality of the dome

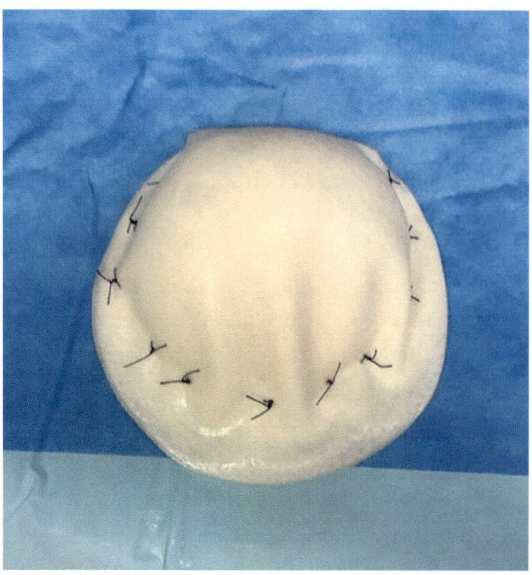

Fig. 18.13 Standardized wrapping technique of Braxon®Fast ADM around the implant. Single stitches are used to join the two flaps and create a snug cover around the implant. Stitches must be placed where the two flaps overlap, so to not create tension on the matrix and to not puncture the prosthesis

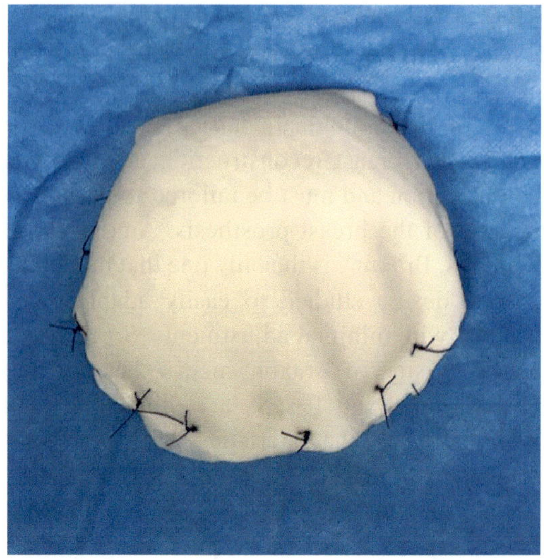

Fig. 18.14 Removal of the matrix excess, leaving enough matrix on the edge for its fixation to the pectoralis major muscle

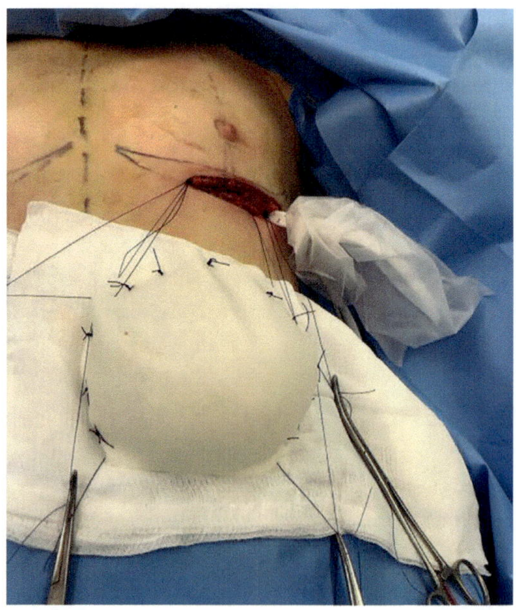

Fig. 18.15 Insertion of the ADM-wrapped implant with parachuting sutures

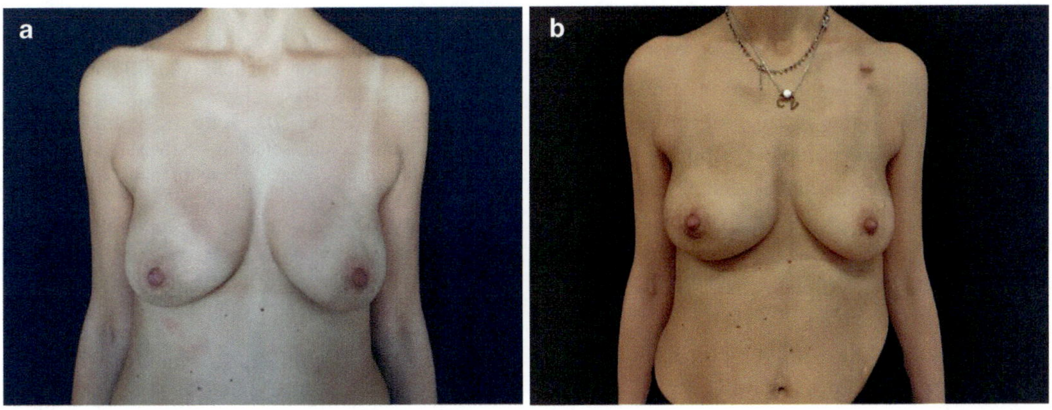

Fig. 18.16 (**a**) Preoperative and (**b**) postoperative pictures of a patients that received Braxon®Fast implants. Natural results with no aesthetic defects can be seen at 2 years follow-up

18.8 New Generation ADMs: Matrices with Adipogenic Stimulus

Research in the biomaterial field is focusing on the development of bioactive matrices that interact with the body's tissues for stimulation of specific biological processes. In breast reconstruction, the aim is to regenerate the subcutaneous breast tissues damaged by the surgery, so to provide the patients a therapeutic treatment that reduces the risk of postoperative complications, and especially capsular contracture. In this scenario, the collagen matrix should be able not only to integrate and create a soft and elastic capsula, but also to sustain the activity of the cells present in breast tissue to restore its structure and composition. Braxon® and Braxon®Fast are the only matrices optimized for breast tissue to specifically perform such regenerative function: they possess adipogenic stimulatory properties specifically intended for the restoration of the breast's adipose component (Adipomatrix® technology).

Adipogenic potential was demonstrated by in vitro and in vivo experiments, comparing different matrices: Braxon®, another ADM commercially available, and a pericardium. It was observed that the three matrices differ for porosity, microscopic structure, and liquid absorption ability. When cultured with human adipose-derived stem cells (ADSCs), only the cells in contact with Braxon® membrane showed lipidic accumulation after 7 days, which increased together with cell proliferation at day 14, indicating successful adipogenic differentiation. Thirty days after implantation in mice, Braxon® was observed to be the only matrix homogeneously colonized by resident cells and with inside well-organized and vascularized deposits of mature adipocytes. The other two membranes showed less (the commercially available ADM) or absent (pericardium) adipogenic stimulation ability in vitro and no adipose tissue was observed after their implantation in vivo [38]. Overall, Braxon® is demonstrated to be the unique adipogenic matrix. Clinical evidence of this biostimulation has not been published yet, however, low rates of capsular contracture have been widely reported with the use of Braxon® [15, 16, 20, 31, 32, 36, 37].

From such study emerges that different origin (dermis or pericardium) and different production technologies lead to different biological results. This should be kept in mind when choosing the material for clinical application.

18.9 Summary with Tips

- The introduction of ADM in implant-based reconstruction has made prepectoral implant placement and complete implant coverage possible, with excellent surgical and aesthetic outcomes
- Braxon® is the only ADM currently available as a preshaped template that allows complete implant coverage ex vivo
- Histological follow-up of prepectoral breast reconstruction shows cellular signs of ADM integration, such as the presence of chronic epithelioid-granulomatous gigantocellular inflammatory infiltration
- Ultrasound follow-up confirms the ADM integration, as the hypoechoic periprosthetic layer of the matrix progressively disappears over time
- Braxon®Fast is the only and most modern ADM optimized for breast reconstruction, given its three-dimensional, pre-curved design and its adipogenic-stimulating properties

References

1. Rebowe RE, Allred LJ, Nahabedian MY. The evolution from subcutaneous to prepectoral prosthetic breast reconstruction. Plast Reconstr Surg Glob Open. 2018;6(6):e1797.
2. Reitsamer R, Peintinger F, Klaassen-Federspiel F, Sir A. Prepectoral direct-to-implant breast reconstruction with complete ADM or synthetic mesh coverage—36-Months follow-up in 200 reconstructed breasts. Breast. 2019;48:32–7.
3. Cemal Y, Albornoz CR, Disa JJ, McCarthy CM, Mehrara BJ, Pusic AL, et al. A paradigm shift in U.S. breast reconstruction: part 2. The influence of changing mastectomy patterns on reconstructive rate and method. Plast Reconstr Surg. 2013;131(3):320e–6e.
4. Jones G, Antony AK. Single stage, direct to implant pre-pectoral breast reconstruction. Gland Surg. 2019;8(1):53–60.
5. Moyer HR, Losken A. Predicting mastectomy skin flap necrosis with indocyanine green angiography: the gray area defined. Plast Reconstr Surg. 2012;129(5):1043–8.
6. Komorowska-Timek E, Gurtner GC. Intraoperative perfusion mapping with laser-assisted indocyanine green imaging can predict and prevent complications in immediate breast reconstruction. Plast Reconstr Surg. 2010;125(4):1065–73.
7. Vidya R, Iqbal FM. A guide to prepectoral breast reconstruction: a new dimension to implant-based breast reconstruction. Clin Breast Cancer. 2017;17(4):266–71.
8. Salibian AA, Frey JD, Karp NS. Strategies and considerations in selecting between subpectoral and prepectoral breast reconstruction. Gland Surg. 2019;8(1):11–8.
9. Sigalove S, Maxwell GP, Sigalove NM, Storm-Dickerson TL, Pope N, Rice J, et al. Prepectoral implant-based breast reconstruction: rationale, indications, and preliminary results. Plast Reconstr Surg. 2017;139(2):287–94.
10. Walia GS, Aston J, Bello R, Mackert GA, Pedreira RA, Cho BH, et al. Prepectoral versus subpectoral tissue expander placement: a clinical and quality of life outcomes study. Plast Reconstr Surg Glob Open. 2018;6(4):e1731.
11. Casella D, Di Taranto G, Marcasciano M, Lo Torto F, Barellini L, Sordi S, et al. Subcutaneous expanders and synthetic mesh for breast reconstruction: long-term and patient-reported BREAST-Q outcomes of a single-center prospective study. J Plast Reconstr Aesthet Surg. 2019;72(5):805–12.
12. Reitsamer R, Peintinger F. Prepectoral implant placement and complete coverage with porcine acellular dermal matrix: a new technique for direct-to-implant breast reconstruction after nipple-sparing mastectomy. J Plast Reconstr Aesthet Surg. 2015;68(2):162–7.
13. Vidya R, Masià J, Cawthorn S, Berna G, Bozza F, Gardetto A, et al. Evaluation of the effectiveness of the prepectoral breast reconstruction with Braxon dermal matrix: first multicenter European report on 100 cases. Breast J. 2017;23(6):670–6.
14. Hester TR, Ghazi BH, Moyer HR, Nahai FR, Wilton M, Stokes L. Use of dermal matrix to prevent capsular contracture in aesthetic breast surgery. Plast Reconstr Surg. 2012;130(5 Suppl 2):126S–36S.
15. Polotto S, Bergamini ML, Pedrazzi G, Arcuri MF, Gussago F, Cattelani L. One-step prepectoral breast reconstruction with porcine dermal matrix-covered implant: a protective technique improving the outcome in post-mastectomy radiation therapy setting. Gland Surg. 2020;9(2):219–28.
16. Onesti MG, Maruccia M, Di Taranto G, Albano A, Soda G, Ballesio L, et al. Clinical, histological, and ultrasound follow-up of breast reconstruction with one-stage muscle-sparing "wrap" technique: a single-center experience. J Plast Reconstr Aesthet Surg. 2017;70(11):1527–36.
17. Maruccia M, Mazzocchi M, Dessy LA, Onesti MG. One-stage breast reconstruction techniques in elderly patients to preserve quality of life. Eur Rev Med Pharmacol Sci. 2016;20(24):5058–66.
18. Maruccia M, Di Taranto G, Onesti MG. One-stage muscle-sparing breast reconstruction in elderly patients: a new tool for retaining excellent quality of life. Breast J. 2018;24(2):180–3.

19. Giudice G, Maruccia M, Nacchiero E, Elia R, Annoscia P, Vestita M. Dual plane breast implant reconstruction in large sized breasts: how to maximise the result following first stage total submuscular expansion. JPRAS Open. 2018;15:74–80.
20. Masià J, iBAG Working Group. The largest multicentre data collection on prepectoral breast reconstruction: the iBAG study. J Surg Oncol. 2020;122(5):848–60.
21. Cattelani L, Polotto S, Arcuri MF, Pedrazzi G, Linguadoca C, Bonati E. One-step prepectoral breast reconstruction with dermal matrix-covered implant compared to submuscular implantation: functional and cost evaluation. Clin Breast Cancer. 2018;18(4):e703–11.
22. Ricci JA, Epstein S, Momoh AO, Lin SJ, Singhal D, Lee BT. A meta-analysis of implant-based breast reconstruction and timing of adjuvant radiation therapy. J Surg Res. 2017;218:108–16.
23. Magill LJ, Robertson FP, Jell G, Mosahebi A, Keshtgar M. Determining the outcomes of post-mastectomy radiation therapy delivered to the definitive implant in patients undergoing one- and two-stage implant-based breast reconstruction: a systematic review and meta-analysis. J Plast Reconstr Aesthet Surg. 2017;70(10):1329–35.
24. Elswick SM, Harless CA, Bishop SN, Schleck CD, Mandrekar J, Reusche RD, et al. Prepectoral implant-based breast reconstruction with postmastectomy radiation therapy. Plast Reconstr Surg. 2018;142(1):1–12.
25. Sinnott CJ, Persing SM, Pronovost M, Hodyl C, McConnell D, Ott Young A. Impact of postmastectomy radiation therapy in prepectoral versus subpectoral implant-based breast reconstruction. Ann Surg Oncol. 2018;25(10):2899–908.
26. Logan Ellis H, Asaolu O, Nebo V, Kasem A. Biological and synthetic mesh use in breast reconstructive surgery: a literature review. World J Surg Oncol. 2016;14:121.
27. Komorowska-Timek E, Oberg KC, Timek TA, Gridley DS, Miles DAG. The effect of AlloDerm envelopes on periprosthetic capsule formation with and without radiation. Plast Reconstr Surg. 2009;123(3):807–16.
28. Basu CB, Leong M, Hicks MJ. Acellular cadaveric dermis decreases the inflammatory response in capsule formation in reconstructive breast surgery. Plast Reconstr Surg. 2010;126(6):1842–7.
29. Koltz PF, Frey JD, Langstein HN. The use of human acellular dermal matrix in the first stage of implant-based breast reconstruction simplifies the exchange procedure. Plast Reconstr Surg. 2013;132(4):691e–2e.
30. Parvizi D, Haas F, Peintinger F, Hubmer M, Rappl T, Koch H, et al. First experience using contrast-enhanced ultrasound to evaluate vascularisation of acellular dermal matrices after implant-based breast reconstruction. Breast J. 2014;20(5):461–7.
31. Berna G, Cawthorn SJ, Papaccio G, Balestrieri N. Evaluation of a novel breast reconstruction technique using the Braxon® acellular dermal matrix: a new muscle-sparing breast reconstruction. ANZ J Surg. 2017;87(6):493–8.
32. Chandarana M, Harries S. Multicentre study of prepectoral breast reconstruction using acellular dermal matrix. BJS Open. 2019;4(1):71–7.
33. Inbal A, Gur E, Lemelman BT, Barsuk D, Menes T, Leshem D, et al. Optimizing patient selection for direct-to-implant immediate breast reconstruction using wise-pattern skin-reducing mastectomy in large and ptotic breasts. Aesthetic Plast Surg. 2017;41(5):1058–67.
34. Caputo GG, Marchetti A, Dalla Pozza E, Vigato E, Domenici L, Cigna E, et al. Skin-reduction breast reconstructions with prepectoral implant. Plast Reconstr Surg. 2016;137(6):1702–5.
35. Thuman J, Freitas AM, Schaeffer C, Campbell CA. Prepectoral wise-pattern staged implant-based breast reconstruction for obese or ptotic patients. Ann Plast Surg. 2019;82(6S Suppl 5):S404–9.
36. Maruccia M, Elia R, Gurrado A, Moschetta M, Nacchiero E, Bolletta A, et al. Skin-reducing mastectomy and pre-pectoral breast reconstruction in large ptotic breasts. Aesthetic Plast Surg. 2020;44(3):664–72.
37. Maruccia M, Elia R, Tedeschi P, Gurrado A, Moschetta M, Testini M, Giudice G. Prepectoral breast reconstruction: an ideal approach to bilateral risk-reducing mastectomy. Gland Surg. 2021;10(10):2997–3006. https://doi.org/10.21037/gs-21-339. PMID: 34804886; PMCID: PMC8575706.
38. Quintero Sierra LA, Busato A, Zingaretti N, et al. Tissue-material integration and biostimulation study of collagen acellular matrices. Tissue Eng Regen Med. 2022;19:477–90. https://doi.org/10.1007/s13770-021-00420-6.

Prepectoral Implants and Radiation Therapy

19

Rashmi Benda, Orit Kaidar-Person, and Philip M. Poortmans

19.1 Introduction

Breast cancer is the most common cancer in women worldwide. It is usually diagnosed at the non-metastatic stage, but up to 30% of women with early breast cancer diagnosis eventually develop metastatic disease in the future [1]. Breast cancer treatment is multidisciplinary, involving surgery, systemic therapy, and radiation therapy (RT), where the most appropriate treatment-sequencing is planned individually [2]. Following the Milan, NSABP, Danish breast Cancer Group, and EORTC trials, patients with early breast cancer were mostly treated with breast-conserving surgery (BCS) and whole breast irradiation (i.e., breast-conserving therapy, BCT). These trials demonstrated an equivalent or a non-inferiority result for BCT compared to mastectomy [3–7]. In 1990, the panel of the National Institutes of Health (NIH) Consensus Development Conference on Treatment of Early-Stage Breast Cancer released a statement that BCT is preferable to total mastectomy because it provides survival equivalence while preserving the breast [8]. A later study even demonstrated that BCT is not just inferior to mastectomy in early-stage breast cancer but may even lead to improved 10-years overall and relative survival compared with mastectomy. These results were suggested to be related to postoperative radiation in the case of BCT, thereby treating subclinical disease by radiation [9]. Nevertheless, a decade after the NIH statement, publications show a trend in the treatment of early-stage breast cancer patients, indicating that more than a third of the patients with early breast cancer who are eligible for breast conservation opt for mastectomy as their primary surgical procedure [10–13].

Additionally, the rates of bilateral mastectomies for unilateral disease for non-hereditary breast cancer increased from 5.4% in 1998 to 29.7% in 2011, with a concurrent increase in reconstructive procedures in this group from 36.9% to 57.2% [14]. These trends are similar to the number of healthy individuals (not breast

R. Benda (✉)
Shore Regional Cancer Center, Requard Radiation Oncology, Easton, MD, USA
e-mail: Rashmi.Benda@umm.edu

O. Kaidar-Person
Breast Cancer Radiation Therapy Unit, Sheba Medical Center, Ramat Gan, Israel

Dept. Radiation Oncology (Maastro), GROW-School for Oncology and Reproduction, Maastricht University Medical Centre+, Maastricht, The Netherlands

P. M. Poortmans
Department of Radiation Oncology, Iridium Netwerk, Wilrijk, Antwerp, Belgium

Faculty of Medicine and Health Sciences, University of Antwerp, Wilrijk, Antwerp, Belgium
e-mail: Philip.poortman@gza.be

© The Author(s), under exclusive license to Springer Nature Switzerland AG 2023
R. Vidya, H. Becker (eds.), *Prepectoral Breast Reconstruction*,
https://doi.org/10.1007/978-3-031-15590-1_19

cancer patients) who seek breast augmentation, as reported on the American Plastic Surgery Website, showing an absolute increase of 41% from 2000 to 2017. These trends indicate the popularity of aesthetic breast procedures in general, but also, the fear of recurrences, fear of RT and the "culture" of breast augmentation and cosmetic surgeries may be an essential factor driving an increase in these procedures for BCT-eligible patients. Although breast conservation continues to be the preferred treatment, supported by several recent studies that suggest better overall survival after BCT compared to mastectomy [9, 15], Mastectomy rates are rising in the United States, from 36.9% in 1998 to 57.2% in 2011, while they were decreasing in the Europe [16]. One of the essential factors to address these trends is to effectively inform patients, surgeons, and other health practitioners about current data, hoping to reverse rising mastectomy rates to optimize survival outcomes and reassure their concerns for recurrence and reluctance to undergo radiation therapy [14, 17].

As opposed to previous years, in-which post-mastectomy irradiation was mainly given to patients with three and more lymph nodes involved, nowadays, with the de-escalation of axillary surgery, the rates of PMRT are increasing in one to three positive nodal group [18, 19]. Additionally, a recent retrospective study reported that local recurrences in early-stage breast cancer, node-negative disease, who underwent immediate reconstruction, were higher if PMRT was omitted. The authors relate these findings to residual breast tissue and possibly residual subclinical disease within the skin [20]. Understanding that the number of patients needing PMRT in immediate reconstruction is growing, ESTRO published delineation guidelines for PMRT in the setting of immediate implant-based reconstruction, aiming to reduce potential complications from PMRT [21]. In order to maintain the progress of breast surgery and reconstructive procedures achieved over the years without compromising oncological outcomes, it is essential to work in a multidisciplinary team and also for radiation oncologists to understand the challenges of mastectomy and reconstruction and similarly for plastic breast/aesthetic surgeons to understand the role of radiation and the challenges in radiation delivery in breast reconstruction.

19.2 Role of Postmastectomy Radiation

In 1997, two studies published in the NEJM looked into using Post-Mastectomy Radiation Therapy (PMRT) in those with T3/4 disease and/or patients with four or more positive lymph nodes [22, 23]. These studies showed a benefit to the comprehensive chest wall and nodal radiation in women with 1–3 positive nodes translating into a Disease-Free Survival (DFS) and overall survival (OS) improvement.

Twenty years later, the European Organisation for Research and Treatment of Cancer (EORTC) 22922–10925 trial, the Canadian-led MA.20 trials, and the Danish population-based DBCG-IMN study confirmed the value of elective nodal irradiation of internal mammary lymph nodes. Eligibility criteria included unilateral histologically confirmed breast adenocarcinoma of stage I, II, or III with a centrally or medially located primary tumor irrespective of axillary involvement and extent of local surgery or an externally located tumor with axillary involvement [24, 25]. All this has expanded the criteria to offer PMRT also to high-risk node-negative patients.

While radiation improves DFS and OS, it is also responsible for cardiac morbidity and mortality when the dose is not considered during treatment planning. After 10-year follow-up, a significantly increased number of deaths were observed among the patients receiving RT before the 90s of last century. The first meta-analysis published on cardiac toxicity by year of treatment reported significantly increased cardiac mortality for left-sided treatment that increased with each 5-year increment [26, 27]. Darby et al. [28] found a risk of cardiac death of 7.4% per 1 Gy of mean heart dose that started at 5 years post-treatment and continued in a linear manner to at least 20 years. While studies showing the higher cardiac toxicity included patients treated with older 2D techniques delivering a much higher dose to the heart, negating the benefit of PMRT with cardiac toxicity, however, increased awareness and gave birth to strategies that significantly reduced cardiac dose, which lead to a sharp decrease in late side effects from RT.

A retrospective analysis of prospectively collected data of 1633 patients treated with mastectomy and adjuvant trastuzumab that participated in the Herceptin Adjuvant (HERA) phase III randomized clinical trial which established the efficacy of trastuzumab in HER-2-positive breast cancer showed PMRT delivery in patients with 1 to 3 positive lymph nodes to decrease locoregional recurrence risk. Although the PMRT benefit was less compared to historical studies, the present findings favor PMRT for HER-2-positive breast cancer patients with 1 to 3 involved nodes. [29] As systemic therapy evolves, with additional targeted drugs such as the anti-HER 2 drugs, we may see a subset of patients that may not need PMRT.

NSABP-B51 is randomized patients with a pathologic complete response to receiving PMRT to the chest wall and regional nodes or observation. While a subset of patients who currently receive PMRT radiation may be able to avoid it in the future, there will always be a need for PMRT [30].

19.3 Radiation Target and Technique

PMRT creates new challenges for breast reconstruction and is targeted to the chest wall, including subcutaneous tissue left behind after mastectomy, including the non-resected part of the axillary lymph node levels I–IV, the interpectoral nodes and the internal mammary nodes (IMN). Extensive radiation of the chest wall and regional nodes increases the complexity of radiation treatment planning. The IMN chain is one of the primary lymphatic drainage pathways of the breast. Anatomic studies based on an extended radical mastectomy series demonstrated that approximately 75% of breast lymphatic drainage is directed to the axilla and 25% to the IMN. Lymphoscintigraphy studies revealed IMN drainage in 28–44% of all patients with breast carcinoma, with an incidence as high as 65% among patients with medial/central tumors. In 1998, Zucali et al. published a 30% increase in distant metastases and a 20% increase in mortality rate among patients with medial/central breast primaries, suggesting that untreated microscopic disease in the IMN may serve as a nidus for DM [31]. The inclusion of IMNs increased the technical challenge for optimizing radiation techniques (see Fig. 19.1).

While ACOSOGZ0011 [32] and AMAROS [33] trials essentially eliminating standard axillary node dissection, this increased the inclusion of radiation to the low axillary nodes. The inclusion of these nodes also results in greater coverage posteriorly in the tangential fields. While some may argue ACOSOGZ0011 did not allow nodal radiation. Therefore, these do not need to be added to the radiation target; radiating to the supraclavicular nodes while ignoring the lower axillary nodes does not follow logic. In addition, although ACOSOGZ0011 did not allow the addition of supraclavicular fields, at least some of the low axillary nodes received partial to full doses. Unfortunately, as ACOSOGZ0011 did not prospectively require the contouring of these nodes with Dose Volume histogram data collection, the study cannot justify the elimination of radiation to these nodes. However, a publication by Monica Murrow and the team showed that even without preoperative axillary imaging or routine use of nodal RT, ALND could be avoided in a large majority of Z0011-eligible patients with excellent regional control [34]. In addition to the British Columbia and Danish trials, more recent data from EORTC and MA20 validate the treatment of extensive nodal radiation.

Chest wall boost radiation is somewhat controversial. Unlike breast boosts in patients who are conserved, there is no randomized trial evaluating the efficacy of a chest wall boost. Mainly in the United States, quite routinely an additional

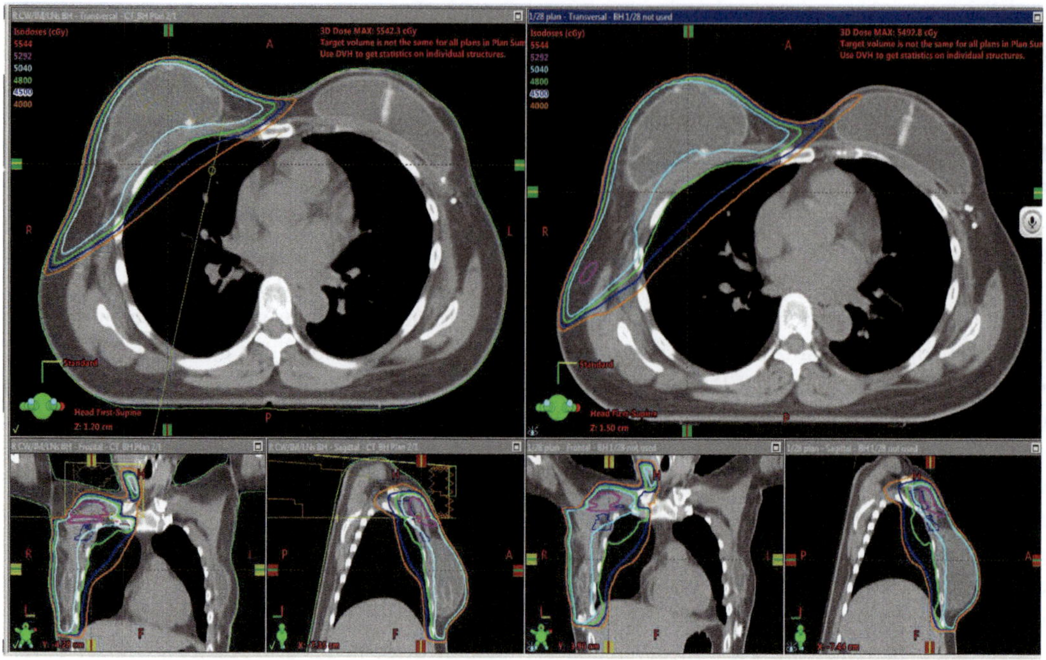

Fig. 19.1 Reduction of the contralateral expander volume allowed for better dosimetry with improved coverage of the target while eliminating the hot spots. Image on the right shows a small volume of 5292 cGy for a prescription dose of 5040 cGy (105% hot spot) while the 4000 cGy line goes into the contralateral breast. The improved beam angle also treats less muscle which may be important in reducing the tightness reported by patients

10 Gy in 5 fractions is applied, usually targeting the 2–3 cm of chest wall skin and subcutaneous tissue surrounding the mastectomy scar which is felt to be at highest risk of recurrence. A higher incidence of implant exposure was reported in patients receiving a boost (7.6%) vs no boost (1.76%) with a p-value of 0.0025, and a 13.4 vs 8.4% rate of capsular contracture with a borderline significance ($p = 0.059$) [35]. Overall implant failure was 35% (boost) vs 19% (no boost) with a p-value <0.0001. In this retrospective review, a chest wall boost did not protect against local failure even in high-risk groups, including young age, positive margins, or with lymphovascular invasion (LVI). Others have shown a decrease in the absolute percentage of local recurrence in patients with high-risk features although not statistically significant [36]. There is no prospective data on this subject, so the clinical practice varies, with most radiation oncologists boosting those with involved margins.

19.4 Radiation Fractionation

Practice patterns vary among countries regarding total dose and fractionation for breast cancer patients who underwent mastectomy with or without reconstruction. The most common RT scheme applied in immediate breast reconstruction is the historical fractionation to a total dose of 50–50.4 Gy in 25–28 fractions [37]. In contrast, an increasing number of countries adopted moderate hypofractionation regimens (e.g., 40 Gy delivered in 15 fractions over 3 weeks) to the chest wall and regional nodes, also in the setting of breast reconstruction. This is based on long-term data from the United Kingdom START A/B trials, showing reduced toxicity of moderate hypofractionation scheme compared to historical fractionation in the intact breast and in PMRT without reconstruction. Even though there is little data from clinical trials specifically evaluating hypofractionation in the setting of immediate breast reconstruction to support its use based on the long-term data of hypofractionation in BCT and long-term use in many European countries such as the UK and the Netherlands, there is no reason to believe that its outcome will be inferior to conventional fractionation [37, 38, 40, 41]. A recent trial by Chen et al. [39] retrospectively evaluated 75 patients treated with postmastectomy radiation in the setting of 2-stage prosthetic breast reconstruction. Patients underwent expander placement at the time of mastectomy with acellular dermis to reinforce the lower pole of the breast. The expansion started 2 weeks after surgery, and the expander was partially deflated before radiation. Expander was exchanged for a permanent implant 3 months after the completion of radiation. Radiation was either 50.4 Gy in 28 fractions or 40.05 Gy in 15 fractions. Bolus material was used in patients at a high risk of skin recurrence. The target volume included the chest wall and regional lymph nodes, including the axillary, internal mammary, and supraclavicular nodes. The median follow-up was 32.5 months. The overall complication rate was 22.7%. The complication rate was lower in patients with hypofractionated RT (14.3%) than those with historical RT (38.5%, $p = 0.017$) and correlation was found between the severity of acute radiation dermatitis and complication rate [dermatitis G0 3/28 (10.7%), G1 5/33 (15.2%), G2 7/10 (70%), and G3 2/4(50%), $p < 0.001$].

A 5-year update of a multi-institution, prospective phase 2 hypofractionated PMRT trial formed the basis for the ongoing randomized RT CHARM trial. Patients were enrolled to receive 3.33 Gy daily to the chest wall (or reconstructed breast), and regional lymphatics in 11 fractions with an optional 4-fraction mastectomy scar boost. The primary endpoint was freedom from grade 3 or higher late non-reconstruction-related radiation toxicities. Secondary endpoints included local and locoregional recurrence rates, cosmesis, and reconstruction complications. Toxicities were scored using Common Terminology Criteria for Adverse Events v4.0. Forty-three patients had plans for breast reconstruction. Of the 43, 40 patients (93%) had pre-RT reconstruction, of which 88% were temporary expanders, 7% were immediate implants, and 5% were prior augmentation implants. Three patients (7%) had post-RT reconstruction. Of the 43 patients, 35% had grade 3 or 4 reconstruction complications attributable to RT. RT-CHARM is a randomized phase 3 trial looking into PMRT patients with implant reconstruction to receive 42.56 Gy in 16 fractions vs 50 Gy in 25 fractions after mastectomy with reconstruction. No boost is allowed in this trial. If results are like those in other breast trials, this will be the new standard fractionation.

19.5 Types of Breast Reconstruction and Radiation

Breast reconstruction following mastectomy is performed using different approaches. Historically, prosthetic breast reconstruction was possible with silicone gel breast implants in the 1960s [42]. The first implant-based reconstructions were performed by placing the implant in the subcutaneous pocket directly underneath the mastectomy skin flap. Although relatively simple, this technique resulted in complications such as implant malposition, rippling, implant exposure, and contracture, which felt to be due to inadequate tissue covering the implant.

The introduction of the acellular dermal matrix (ADM) in 2006 allowed anchoring at the inferior edge of the pectoralis major to the inframammary fold providing a better inferior lateral support and decreasing the inferior lateral displacement. Although, with the introduction of ADM, plastic surgeons are again considering the advantages of prepectoral implant placement. A systematic review [43] examined complication profiles in prepectoral breast reconstruction alone versus prepectoral with ADM or mesh. A review of the PubMed database was performed from inception to March 2017 to identify literature on postmastectomy patients undergoing prepectoral breast reconstruction with and without ADM or mesh. Study characteristics, complication rates, and outcomes were extracted for analysis. Study quality was assessed using the Newcastle-Ottawa Scale, and complication profiles were analyzed using the random-effects model. Twenty-seven studies met the criteria for inclusion out of 550 identified for review. For 1881 total breasts, the complication rate with ADM was 23.4%, while the rate without an additional implant material was 27.5%. The difference in the capsular contracture rate with and without ADM was 2.3% and 12.4%, respectively. The use of ADM in prepectoral breast reconstruction correlated with lower capsular contracture and overall complication rates; however, rates of implant loss, infection, and mastectomy flap necrosis were higher with the use of ADM. Results were variable across studies, and the quality of evidence reported was generally low. Because the methodology for outcome assessment was inconsistent, there is a need for further investigation with comparative studies and standardized outcome reporting.

Retrospective studies have reported objective cosmetic advantages and favorable patient outcomes following prepectoral breast reconstruction compared to subpectoral placement [44–46]. Some have suggested a prepectoral placement of prosthetic devices in the setting of known future radiation therapy [45, 47]. Early outcomes demonstrated less likelihood of superior displacement of prepectoral tissue expanders following radiation therapy than subpectoral tissue expanders. However, in a later study that compared postmastectomy radiation in prepectoral and partial subpectoral tissue expander placement, there was no significant difference in complication rates between the two reconstructive cohorts, including rates of explantation (15.4% vs 19.3%) [48]. More research on breast reconstruction in irradiated patients is needed to determine optimal management in this setting. Mastectomy flap perfusion is a crucial element in achieving a successful prepectoral reconstruction. The nipple is always hypo-perfused after nipple-sparing mastectomy. If the skin perfusion is compromised as well, it is better to stage reconstruction by inserting a tissue expander in the prepectoral plane to allow time for skin flaps to develop better breast perfusion for 2–3 weeks.

In a study [49] evaluating 33 patients with 52 breast reconstructions using the prepectoral technique, 65% of the breasts were irradiated, with two-thirds irradiated with a permanent implant. At a mean follow-up of 25 months, the irradiated breasts had one incidence of seroma and one incidence of wound dehiscence followed by expander removal. There were no capsular contractures in either group.

In a retrospective review, Sinnot [50] reported that subpectoral breast reconstruction had a 52.2% rate of capsular contracture compared to a 16.1% contracture rate in prepectoral breast reconstruction following postmastectomy radiation. Also, 10 of the 12 cases in the capsular contracture grouped in the subpectoral groove were graded 3/4 compared to only two benign cases in the prepectoral group. It has been suggested that the increased surface area coverage of the implant by ADM is protective. Expander migration is also higher in the dual plane than in the prepectoral group during postmastectomy radiation. This is felt due to radiation-induced fibrosis and the pectoralis major muscle contracture causing superior expander displacement. However, critics have questioned the shorter follow-up in the studies with prepectoral implant reconstruction. Importantly, there is a significant concern for the prepectoral position that to create a pocket for the implant, even in the setting of ADM, there is a tendency to leave a thicker skin flap. This may result in more residual breast glandular tissue and potentially subclinical tumor cells within the dermal lymphatics [51].

Becker et al. [52, 53] make a strong case for prepectoral single-stage reconstruction. Prepectoral implants cause less pain related to stretching of the pectoralis muscle during the expansion process as well as reduced term weakness of arm abduction and pain [46, 54]. Others have reported that high-risk patients, such as those with thin skin flaps, high body mass index (BMI), circulatory compromise, prior radiation, and high BMI, are inappropriate for this technique. Becker et al. feel that the prepectoral approach is more attractive and can reduce the risk of vascular compromise and wound healing. They describe a technique using varying volumes of air until desired healing and cosmetic results are achieved when the air is replaced with saline. In their study of 25 patients over 1 year, 3 underwent adjuvant radiation, and 5 had a prior radiation history. Only one patient with prior radiation suffered implant extrusion that required removal in their experience using a technique that utilizes a virtually empty spacer that allows suboptimal skin flaps to recover circulation and avoid ischemic complications. Unlike Wagner et al., their approach did not use ADM. Although, this study is limited to only 25 patients who were all operated on by the same surgeon. A multi-institutional research is needed to see if their results can be translated to a larger population of patients and surgeons.

19.6 Types of Expander and Radiation Therapy

In 2016, the AeroForm device received FDA clearance based on the XPAND trial, which compared the AeroForm to Saline expanders [55]. The patient underwent an expansion in the investigation arm in 10 cc increments up to 30 cc a day of carbon dioxide compared to the periodic bolus of saline by the physician in the control arm. This study concluded the carbon dioxide-based expander was an effective method of tissue expansion with similar overall adverse events compared to saline expanders while providing a more convenient expansion.

Tran et al. noted a significant difference in measured and calculated doses at exit locations in the beam. With the paucity of data on this device, the current recommendation would be to use it cautiously for patients undergoing radiation. While it may be possible to remove the air and replace it with saline, the issue with the metal port affecting the dosimetry is still a concern and needs to be resolved [56]. Advancements in CT acquisition techniques allowing subtraction of the metal density from the treatment planning scan can overcome this issue. Also, a device that helps the patient to easily change the volume is a concern for reproducibility during radiation as once the patient is simulated and a plan generated from that CT scans, it is imperative to keep the anatomy unchanged and a change in implant volume would not allow delivery of the intended dose.

As these techniques evolve, radiation oncologists prefer to remove the air or CO_2 from the expander for treatment. There is concern regarding dose homogeneity at the air or CO_2 interface. This is an area that needs further investigation.

19.7 Types of Mastectomies and Radiation Therapy Timing

National Comprehensive Cancer Network (NCCN) guidelines advise women undergoing implant reconstruction to undergo initial reconstruction with an expander. Integrating breast radiation therapy after mastectomy and reconstruction has become very complex. To achieve satisfactory oncological and cosmetic outcomes, a thorough discussion with the oncologist is essential [57]. With women undergoing autologous reconstruction, this procedure is recommended after completion of radiation therapy to avoid fibrosis resulting in compromised cosmesis. However, no significant differences in complication rates were seen in a study comparing postmastectomy radiation after tissue expander placement with postmastectomy radiation after a permanent implant [58].

In a retrospective study of 113 women who underwent postmastectomy radiation therapy (PMRT) and breast reconstruction, the complication rate was 32% for patients with radiation first and 44% for patients with breast reconstruction first [59]. Early complications were seen more frequently in patients with radiation first, while late complications were more common in patients with breast reconstruction first. Naoum et al. published a retrospective review [60] of 1286 patients who underwent 1814 breast reconstructions between 1997 and 2017. Patients were divided into six groups based on the type of reconstruction and use of postmastectomy radiation. Patients receiving preoperative chemotherapy and those undergoing a mastectomy and reconstruction for local recurrence were excluded. The primary objective was the reconstruction complication defined by surgical re-intervention, such as infection, skin necrosis, and fat necrosis. Implant-related complications such as capsular contracture, implant rupture, exposure, or implant failure were compared between the tissue expander group (TE) and the direct-to-implant (DTI). The secondary objective was to compare the 3-reconstruction types in the setting of immediate reconstruction followed by postmastectomy radiation on multivariate analysis. The median follow-up was 5.8 years. 41.1% of the patients received postmastectomy radiation. In the unirradiated group, complication rates were 11.1%, 12.6%, and 19.5% for the autologous, DTI, and TE reconstruction groups, respectively. In the postmastectomy group, the 5-year incidence was 15.1%, 18.2%, and 36.8%, respectively. Multivariate analysis showed that DTI was associated with a lower complication rate than TE/I, with no significant difference between autologous and DTI groups. They did not find nipple-sparing mastectomy or the use of axillary dissection to influence the complication rate.

BMI and active smoking were significant predictors of complications requiring reoperation, and TE/I was the only predictor of reconstruction failure [61].

Flap thickness is the most crucial factor in predicting outcome. Breast size, likely related to BMI, has also been reported as a significant complication predictor [62].

Preoperative vs adjuvant chemotherapy, TE/I vs Implant, and BMI >30 were significant predictors of overall failure rates, with smoking showing a trend towards significance. PMRT dose, duration, or boost did not predict reconstruction failure or complications.

An open-label, randomized, controlled trial in eight hospitals in the Netherlands [63] where women were assigned to undergo one-stage IBBR with ADM (Strattice, LifeCell, Branchburg, NJ, USA) or two-stage IBBR. The occurrence of adverse outcomes assessed the primary endpoint of quality of life and safety. 142 women were enrolled between 2013 and 2015. 59 (91 breasts) were randomized to DTI with ADM vs TE/I62 (92 breasts). One-stage IBBR with ADM was associated with a significantly higher risk of surgical complications (crude odds ratio 3.81, 95% CI 2.67–5.43, $p < 0.001$), reoperation (3.38, 2.10–5.45, $p < 0.001$), and removal of the implant, ADM, or both (8.80, 8.24–9.40, $p < 0.001$) than two-stage IBBR. Severe (grade 3) adverse events occurred in 26 (29%) of 91 breasts in the one-stage IBBR with ADM group and in five (5%) of 92 in the two-stage IBBR group. The frequency of mild to moderate adverse events was similar in the two groups. The authors cautioned using the single-stage reconstruction. However, this trial included more patients with diabetes, smoking history, and preoperative chemotherapy in the DTI group compared to the TE group.

The timing of reconstruction with respect to radiation therapy remains controversial. The need for PMRT often cannot be determined definitively until the final pathologic evaluation is complete (typically three to 5 days following mastectomy). At our institution, each patient is discussed in a multidisciplinary tumor board after being evaluated by each specialty, but some patients are cN0 but pN+ and the PMRT recommendation cannot be determined before surgery. Also, patients who are cN1 but undergo preoperative chemotherapy may be rendered pN0 and can enroll on NSABP B51 and get randomized to no radiation.

Some have advocated a sentinel lymph node (SLN) biopsy before mastectomy [64]. If the SLNs are tumor free, then the likelihood that PMRT will be needed is low in patients with tumors <5 cm, and immediate reconstruction can be considered. Although, this approach subjects the patient to a second anesthesia.

The positioning and volume of the implant can influence the homogeneity of radiation dose delivered as well as can result in a lower volume of lung irradiated.

Some believe that an over-expanded tissue expander compromises skin integrity which may compromise perfusion and final cosmetic outcome. In addition, as radiation relies on oxygenation, poor vascularity could also compromise the efficacy of radiation.

19.8 Conclusion

While the criteria for PMRT evolves as the pendulum swings from treating only those with four or more lymph nodes to including 1–3 lymph nodes and perhaps in the future excluding those with a pathologic complete response after chemotherapy, there will always be patients who will benefit from PMRT. Many of these women will undergo reconstruction. For optimal results, these patients must be evaluated and discussed by a multidisciplinary team (Figs. 19.1 and 19.2) The data shows several factors, such as patients' BMI and other comorbidities, might influence the ideal reconstruction. Her disease extent will impact the use of preoperative chemotherapy, the extent of surgery as well as the need for PMRT and, in those with more advanced disease, perhaps a radiation boost as well. The data suggests the chest wall boost increases the risk of implant exposure and, in most cases, may not improve local control and, therefore, can be avoided. In a patient with a large tumor or dermal invasion where a boost is considered, a prepectoral implant may not be appropriate for both cosmesis and disease control. As the high-risk tissue surrounds the implant, an electron boost will no longer be feasible, and a photon boost would increase the dose to the lung and possibly the heart in left-sided patients.

When there is uncertainty, it is best to use a tissue expander or an adjustable implant to adjust the volume for the treatment. Although the CO_2 expander offers a convenient and perhaps more comfortable approach to expansion, giving the patient control over their expansion could result in inter-fraction changes in the implant's contour affecting the radiation dosimetry and the outcome; therefore, radiation should not be delivered with these expanders. Prepectoral vs retro pectoral placement should be determined by the extent of disease, the patient's comorbidities, anatomy, and available radiation techniques. The patient's age may also influence the reconstruction decision. While the plastic surgeon might be more motivated to give a younger patient the reconstruction with the best cosmetic outcome, radiation technique is equally important in these patients as they are more likely to have a worse disease and a higher likelihood of late cardiac

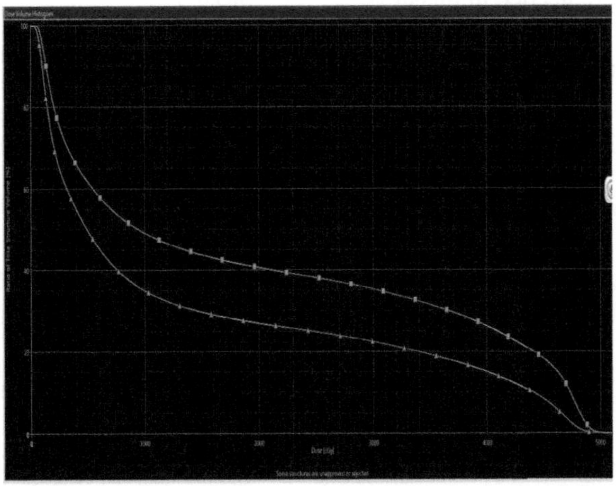

Fig. 19.2 Lung DVH prior to implant deflation (□) vs post deflation lung DVH (Δ). Dose Volume Histogram (DVH) for the lung also significantly decreased by decreasing the volume of the expander. Volume of lung irradiated correlates with the risk of radiation pneumonitis. This demonstrates the importance of a multidisciplinary approach to reconstruction as by reducing the expander volume the radiation dosimetry improved with better coverage while minimizing dose to the normal structures

toxicity well as contralateral breast cancer. Ongoing communication between the plastic surgeon and radiation oncologist is crucial to offer the patient her best chance at local control and survival while reconstruction can improve their quality of life. An adjustable expander/implant allows the plastic surgeon to expand and stretch the tissue while the patient is waiting for radiation. Patients receiving chemotherapy can remain expanded during chemotherapy for several months allowing adequate skin stretching but may need to have the implant volume reduced for radiation to optimize dose delivery to the target and minimize normal tissue dose and, therefore, toxicity (Figs. 19.1 and 19.2).

Physical exams have been felt to be adequate following postmastectomy. While a retro pectoral implant allows a small recurrence to be easily palpable, a prepectoral implant fills the space between the pectoralis muscle and the skin, where any residual breast tissue would be found and, therefore, the area at risk for recurrence. Perhaps, prepectoral implants should be avoided in women at high risk of recurrence. If a prepectoral implant is felt ideal in a high-risk patient, an annual MRI and routine physical exams should allow earlier detection of a recurrence. Additional quality-of-life studies are needed in this area.

While the radiation oncology community continues to improve radiation techniques and doses to improve efficacy and decrease toxicity, the plastic surgery community also continues to improve these patients' cosmetic outcomes, which is very important in the well-being of cancer survivors [62].

References

1. O'Shaughnessy J. Extending survival with chemotherapy in metastatic breast cancer. Oncologist. 2005;10(Suppl 3):20–9.
2. Cardoso F, Costa A, Senkus E, Aapro M, André F, Barrios CH, Bergh J, Bhattacharyya G, Biganzoli L, Cardoso MJ, Carey L, Corneliussen-James D, Curigliano G, Dieras V, El Saghir N, Eniu A, Fallowfield L, Fenech D, Francis P, Gelmon K, Gennari A, Harbeck N, Hudis C, Kaufman B, Krop I, Mayer M, Meijer H, Mertz S, Ohno S, Pagani O, Papadopoulos E, Peccatori F, Penault-Llorca F, Piccart MJ, Pierga JY, Rugo H, Shockney L, Sledge G, Swain S, Thomssen C, Tutt A, Vorobiof D, Xu B, Norton L, Winer E. 3rd ESO-ESMO international consensus guidelines for advanced breast cancer (ABC 3). Ann Oncol. 2017;28(12):3111. https://doi.org/10.1093/annonc/mdx036. Erratum for: Ann Oncol. 2017 Jan 1;28(1):16-33. PMID: 28327998; PMCID: PMC5834023
3. Christiansen P, Carstensen SL, Ejlertsen B, Kroman N, Offersen B, Bodilsen A, Jensen MB. Breast conserving surgery versus mastectomy: overall and relative survival-a population based study by the Danish breast cancer cooperative group (DBCG). Acta Oncol. 2018;57(1):19–25. https://doi.org/10.1080/0284186X.2017.1403042. Epub 2017 Nov 23
4. Fisher B, Jeong J-H, Anderson S, Bryant J, Fisher ER, Wolmark N. Twenty-five-year follow-up of a randomized trial comparing radical mastectomy, total mastectomy, and total mastectomy followed by irradiation. N Engl J Med. 2002;347:567–75.
5. Fisher B, Bauer M, Margolese R, et al. Five-year results of a randomized clinical trial comparing total mastectomy and segmental mastectomy with or without radiation in the treatment of breast cancer. N Engl J Med. 1985;312:665–73.
6. Early Breast Cancer Trialists' Collaborative Group. Effects of radiotherapy and surgery in early breast cancer: an overview of the randomized trials. N Engl J Med. 1995;333:1444–55. [Erratum, N Engl J Med 1996;334:1003.]
7. Veronesi U, Saccozzi R, Del Vecchio M, et al. Comparing radical mastectomy with quadrantectomy, axillary dissection, and radiotherapy in patients with small cancers of the breast. N Engl J Med. 1981; 305:6–11.
8. NIH Consensus Conference. Treatment of early-stage breast cancer. JAMA. 1991;265:391–5.
9. Van Maaren MC, de Munck L, de Bock GH, Jobsen JJ, van Dalen T, Linn SC, Poortmans P, Strobbe LJA, Siesling S. 10 year survival after breast-conserving surgery plus radiotherapy compared with mastectomy in early breast cancer in The Netherlands: a population-based study. Lancet Oncol. 2016;17(8):1158–70.
10. Pesce CE, Liederbach E, Czechura T, Winchester DJ, Yao K. Changing surgical trends in young patients with early stage breast cancer, 2003 to 2010: a report from the National Cancer Data Base. J Am Coll Surg. 2014;219(1):19–28. https://doi.org/10.1016/j.jamcollsurg.2014.03.043. Epub 2014 Apr 1
11. Sinnadurai S, Kwong A, Hartman M, Tan EY, Bhoo-Pathy NT, Dahlui M, See MH, Yip CH, Taib NA, Bhoo-Pathy N. Breast-conserving surgery versus mastectomy in young women with breast cancer in Asian settings. BJS Open. 2018;3(1):48–55. https://doi.org/10.1002/bjs5.50111. PMID: 30734015; PMCID: PMC6354186
12. Mahmood U, Hanlon AL, Koshy M, Buras R, Chumsri S, Tkaczuk KH, Cheston SB, Regine WF, Feigenberg SJ. Increasing national mastectomy rates for the treatment of early stage breast cancer. Ann Surg

Oncol. 2013;20(5):1436–43. https://doi.org/10.1245/s10434-012-2732-5. Epub 2012 Nov 8
13. Yang B, Ren G, Song E, Pan D, Zhang J, Wang Y, Liao N, Tang J, Wang X, Cui S, Jin F, Geng C, Sun Q, Li H, Fan Z, Cao X, Wang H, Wang S, Shao Z, Wu J. Current status and factors influencing surgical options for breast cancer in China: a nationwide cross-sectional survey of 110 hospitals. Oncologist. 2020;25(10):e1473–80. https://doi.org/10.1634/theoncologist.2020-0001. Epub 2020 May 13. PMID: 32333626; PMCID: PMC7543333
14. Kummerow KL, Du L, Penson DF, Shyr Y, Hooks MA. Nationwide trends in mastectomy for early-stage breast cancer. JAMA Surg. 2015;150:9–16.
15. Lagendijk M, van Maaren MC, Saadatmand S, Strobbe LJA, Poortmans PMP, Koppert LB, Tilanus-Linthorst MMA, Siesling S. Breast conserving therapy and mastectomy revisited: breast cancer-specific survival and the influence of prognostic factors in 129,692 patients. Int J Cancer. 2018;142(1):165–75. https://doi.org/10.1002/ijc.31034. Epub 2017 Sep 18
16. Garcia-Etienne CA, Tomatis M, Heil J, Danaei M, Rageth CJ, Marotti L, Rosselli Del Turco M, Ponti A. Fluctuating mastectomy rates across time and geography. Ann Surg Oncol. 2013;20(7):2114–6. https://doi.org/10.1245/s10434-013-2982-x.
17. Albornoz CR, Matros E, Lee CN, et al. Bilateral mastectomy versus breast-conserving surgery for early-stage breast cancer: the role of breast reconstruction. Plast Reconstr Surg. 2015;135:1518–26.
18. EBCTCG (Early Breast Cancer Trialists' Collaborative Group), McGale P, Taylor C, Correa C, Cutter D, Duane F, Ewertz M, Gray R, Mannu G, Peto R, Whelan T, Wang Y, Wang Z, Darby S. Effect of radiotherapy after mastectomy and axillary surgery on 10-year recurrence and 20-year breast cancer mortality: meta-analysis of individual patient data for 8135 women in 22 randomized trials. Lancet. 2014;383(9935):2127–35. https://doi.org/10.1016/S0140-6736(14)60488-8. Epub 2014 Mar 19. Erratum in: Lancet. 2014 Nov 22;384(9957):1848. PMID: 24656685; PMCID: PMC5015598
19. Donker M, Slaets L, van Tienhoven G, Rutgers EJ. Okselklierdissectie versus okselbestraling bij borstkankerpatiënten met een positieve schildwachtklier: de EORTC 10981 AMAROS-studie [Axillary lymph node dissection versus axillary radiotherapy in patients with a positive sentinel node: the AMAROS trial]. Ned Tijdschr Geneeskd. 2015;159:A9302. Dutch
20. Bernstein-Molho R, Laitman Y, Galper S, Jacobson G, Boursi B, Gal-Yam EN, Kaufman B, Friedman E, Kaidar-Person O. Locoregional treatments and ipsilateral breast cancer recurrence rates in BRCA1/2 mutation carriers. Int J Radiat Oncol Biol Phys. 2021;109(5):1332–40. https://doi.org/10.1016/j.ijrobp.2020.11.058. Epub 2020 Nov 28
21. Kaidar-Person O, Vrou Offersen B, Hol S, Arenas M, Aristei C, Bourgier C, Cardoso MJ, Chua B, Coles CE, Engberg Damsgaard T, Gabrys D, Jagsi R, Jimenez R, Kirby AM, Kirkove C, Kirova Y, Kouloulias V, Marinko T, Meattini I, Mjaaland I, Nader Marta G, Witt Nystrom P, Senkus E, Skyttä T, Tvedskov TF, Verhoeven K, Poortmans P. ESTRO ACROP consensus guideline for target volume delineation in the setting of postmastectomy radiation therapy after implant-based immediate reconstruction for early stage breast cancer. Radiother Oncol. 2019;137:159–66. https://doi.org/10.1016/j.radonc.2019.04.010. Epub 2019 May 17
22. Ragaz J, Jackson SM, Le N, Plenderleith IH, Spinelli JJ, Basco VE, Wilson KS, Knowling MA, Coppin CM, Paradis M, Coldman AJ, Olivotto IA. Adjuvant radiotherapy and chemotherapy in node-positive premenopausal women with breast cancer. N Engl J Med. 1997;337(14):956–62. https://doi.org/10.1056/NEJM199710023371402.
23. Overgaard M, Hansen PS, Overgaard J, Rose C, Andersson M, Bach F, Kjaer M, Gadeberg CC, Mouridsen HT, Jensen MB, Zedeler K. Postoperative radiotherapy in high-risk premenopausal women with breast cancer who receive adjuvant chemotherapy. Danish breast cancer cooperative group 82b trial. N Engl J Med. 1997;337(14):949–55. https://doi.org/10.1056/NEJM199710023371401.
24. Poortmans PM, Weltens C, Fortpied C, Kirkove C, Peignaux-Casasnovas K, Budach V, van der Leij F, Vonk E, Weidner N, Rivera S, van Tienhoven G, Fourquet A, Noel G, Valli M, Guckenberger M, Koiter E, Racadot S, Abdah-Bortnyak R, Van Limbergen EF, Engelen A, De Brouwer P, Struikmans H, Bartelink H, European Organisation for Research and Treatment of Cancer Radiation Oncology and Breast Cancer Groups. Internal mammary and medial supraclavicular lymph node chain irradiation in stage I-III breast cancer (EORTC 22922/10925): 15-year results of a randomized, phase 3 trial. Lancet Oncol. 2020;21(12):1602–10. https://doi.org/10.1016/S1470-2045(20)30472-1. Epub 2020 Nov 2. Erratum in: Lancet Oncol. 2021 Jan;22(1):e5
25. Thorsen LBJ, Overgaard J, Matthiessen LW, Berg M, Stenbygaard L, Pedersen AN, Nielsen MH, Overgaard M, Offersen BV, DBCG Radiotherapy Committee. Internal mammary node irradiation in patients with node-positive early breast cancer: fifteen-year results from the Danish breast cancer group internal mammary node study. J Clin Oncol. 2022;40(36):4198–206. https://doi.org/10.1200/JCO.22.00044. Epub 2022 Apr 8
26. Cuzick J, Stewart H, Peto R, et al. Overview of randomized trials of postoperative adjuvant radiotherapy in breast cancer. Cancer Treat Rep. 1987;71(1):15–29.
27. Henson KE, et al. Radiation-related mortality from heart disease and lung cancer more than 20 years after radiotherapy for breast cancer. Br J Cancer. 2013;108:179–82.
28. Darby SC. Risk of ischemic heart disease in women after radiotherapy for breast cancer. NEJM. 2013;368:987–98.
29. Abi Jaouadi J, de Azambuja E, Maki M, Tamim H, Thayil A, Geara F, Piccart M, Poortmans P, Zeidan

YH. Post-mastectomy radiation therapy in human epidermal growth factor receptor 2 positive breast cancer patients: analysis of the HERA trial. Int J Radiat Oncol Biol Phys. 2020;106(3):503–10. https://doi.org/10.1016/j.ijrobp.2019.10.022. Epub 2019 Oct 22
30. Mamounas EP, Bandos H, White JR, et al. NRG Oncology/NSABP B-51/RTOG 1304: Phase III trial to determine if chest wall and regional nodal radiotherapy (CWRNRT) post mastectomy (Mx) or the addition of RNRT to breast RT post breast-conserving surgery (BCS) reduces invasive breast cancer recurrence free interval (IBCRFI) in patients (pts) with positive axillary (PAx) nodes who are ypN0 after neoadjuvant chemotherapy (NC). J Clin Oncol. 2019, 2019:37.
31. Zucali R. Early breast cancer: evaluation of the prognostic role of the site the primary tumor. J Clin Oncol. 1998;16:1363–6.
32. Giuliano AE, Ballman K, McCall L, Beitsch P, Whitworth PW, Blumencranz P, Leitch AM, Saha S, Morrow M, Hunt KK. Locoregional recurrence after sentinel lymph node dissection with or without axillary dissection in patients with sentinel lymph node metastases: long-term follow-up from the American College of Surgeons oncology group (Alliance) ACOSOG Z0011 randomized trial. Ann Surg. 2016;264(3):413–20. https://doi.org/10.1097/SLA.0000000000001863. PMID: 27513155; PMCID: PMC5070540
33. Donker M, van Tienhoven G, Straver ME, Meijnen P, van de Velde CJ, Mansel RE, Cataliotti L, Westenberg AH, Klinkenbijl JH, Orzalesi L, Bouma WH, van der Mijle HC, Nieuwenhuijzen GA, Veltkamp SC, Slaets L, Duez NJ, de Graaf PW, van Dalen T, Marinelli A, Rijna H, Snoj M, Bundred NJ, Merkus JW, Belkacemi Y, Petignat P, Schinagl DA, Coens C, Messina CG, Bogaerts J, Rutgers EJ. Radiotherapy or surgery of the axilla after a positive sentinel node in breast cancer (EORTC 10981-22023 AMAROS): a randomized, multicentre, open-label, phase 3 non-inferiority trial. Lancet Oncol. 2014;15(12):1303–10. https://doi.org/10.1016/S1470-2045(14)70460-7. Epub 2014 Oct 15. PMID: 25439688; PMCID: PMC4291166
34. Morrow M, Van Zee KJ, Patil S, Petruolo O, Mamtani A, Barrio AV, Capko D, El-Tamer M, Gemignani ML, Heerdt AS, Kirstein L, Pilewskie M, Plitas G, Sacchini VS, Sclafani LM, Ho A, Cody HS. Axillary dissection and nodal irradiation can be avoided for Most node-positive Z0011-eligible breast cancers: a prospective validation study of 793 patients. Ann Surg. 2017;266(3):457–62. https://doi.org/10.1097/SLA.0000000000002354. PMID: 28650355; PMCID: PMC5649371
35. Naoum GE. Single stage direct to implant breast reconstruction has lower complication rates than tissue expander and implant and comparable rates to autologous reconstruction in patients receiving postmastectomy radiation. Int J Radiat Oncol Biol Phys. 2020;106:514–24.
36. Albert A, et al. The impact of a postmastectomy chest wall scar boost on local recurrence-free survival in high-risk patients. Clin Breast Cancer. 2019;19(5):363–9.
37. Marta GN, Coles C, Kaidar-Person O, Meattini I, Hijal T, Zissiadis Y, Pignol JP, Ramiah D, Ho AY, Cheng SH, Sancho G, Offersen BV, Poortmans P. The use of moderately hypofractionated post-operative radiation therapy for breast cancer in clinical practice: a critical review. Crit Rev Oncol Hematol. 2020;156:103090.
38. Haviland JS, Owen JR, Dewar JA, Agrawal RK, Barrett J, Barrett-Lee PJ, Dobbs HJ, Hopwood P, Lawton PA, Magee BJ, Mills J, Simmons S, Sydenham MA, Venables K, Bliss JM, Yarnold JR. The UK standardization of breast radiotherapy (START) trials of radiotherapy hypofractionation for treatment of early breast cancer: 10-year follow-up results of two randomized controlled trials. Lancet Oncol. 2013;14(11):1086–94.
39. Chen JS. Influence of radiation dose to reconstructive breast following mastectomy and complication in breast cancer patients undergoing 2 stage prosthetic breast reconstruction. Front Oncol. 2019;9:243.
40. Offersen B, Nielsen HM, Jacobsen EH, et al. Hypo- vs normofractionated radiation of early breast cancer in the randomized DBCG HYPO trial. Radiother Oncol. 2018;127:S312.
41. Wang SL, Fang H, Song YW, et al. Hypofractionated versus conventional fractionated postmastectomy radiotherapy for patients with high-risk breast cancer: a randomized, non-inferiority, open-label, phase 3 trial. Lancet Oncol. 2019;20:352–60.
42. Snyderman RK, Guthrie RH. Reconstruction of the female breast following radical mastectomy. Plast Reconstr Surg. 1971 Jun;47(6):565–7. https://doi.org/10.1097/00006534-197106000-00008.
43. Wagner RD, Braun TL, Zhu H, Winocour S. A systematic review of complications in prepectoral breast reconstruction. J Plast Reconstr Aesthet Surg. 2019;72(7):1051–9.
44. Bernini M. Subcutaneous direct-to-implant breast reconstruction: surgical, functional, and aesthetic results after long-term follow-up. Plast Reconstr Surg Glob Open. 2016;3(12):e574.
45. Nahabedian MY, Cocilovo C. Two-stage prosthetic breast reconstruction: a comparison between prepectoral and partial subpectoral techniques, plastic and reconstructive surgery. Plast Reconstr Surg. 2017;140(6S):22S–30S.
46. Walia GS, Aston J, Bello R, et al. Prepectoral versus subpectoral tissue expander placement: a clinical and quality of life outcomes study. Plast Reconstr Surg Glob Open. 2018;6(4):e1731.
47. Sigalove S. Prepectoral implant-based breast reconstruction and postmastectomy radiotherapy: short-term outcomes. Plast Reconstr Surg Glob Open. 2017:1–7.
48. Sbitany H, Gomez-Sanchez C, Piper M, Lentz R. Prepectoral breast reconstruction in the setting of postmastectomy radiation therapy: an assessment of clinical outcomes and benefits. Plast Reconstr Surg. 2019;143(1):10–20.

49. Sigalove S, Maxwell GP, Sigalove NM, et al. Prepectoral implant-based breast reconstruction and postmastectomy radiotherapy: short-term outcomes. Plast Reconstr Surg Glob Open. 2017;5(12):e1631.
50. Sinnott CJ, Persing SM, Pronovost M, Hodyl C, McConnell D, Ott YA. Impact of postmastectomy radiation therapy in prepectoral versus subpectoral implant-based breast reconstruction. Ann Surg Oncol. 2018;25(10):2899–908.
51. Kaidar-Person O, Vrou Offersen B, Hol S, et al. ESTRO ACROP consensus guideline for target volume delineation in the setting of postmastectomy radiation therapy after implant-based immediate reconstruction for early stage breast cancer. Radiother Oncol. 2019;137:159–66.
52. Becker H, et al. Immediate prepectoral breast reconstruction in suboptimal patients using an air-filled spacer. Plast Reconstr Surg Glob Open. 2019;7:e2470.
53. Becker H, et al. Tissue contraction---a new paradigm in breast reconstruction. Plast Reconstr Surg Glob Open. 2018;6:e1865.
54. Sigalove S, Maxwell GP, Sigalove NM, et al. Prepectoral implant-based breast reconstruction: rationale, indications, and preliminary results. Plast Reconstr Surg. 2017;139:287–94.
55. Ascherman JA, Zeidler K, Morrison KA, et al. Carbon dioxide-based versus saline tissue expansion for breast reconstruction: results of the XPAND prospective, randomized clinical trial. Plast Reconstr Surg. 2016;138(6):1161–70.
56. Moni J, Saleeby J, Bannon E, Lo Y-C, Fitzgerald TJ. Dosimetric impact of the AeroForm tissue expander in postmastectomy radiation therapy: an ex vivo analysis. Pract Radiat Oncol. 2015;5(1):e1–8.
57. Ho AY, Hu ZI, Mehrara BJ, Wilkins EG. Radiotherapy in the setting of breast reconstruction: types, techniques, and timing. Lancet Oncol. 2017;18(12):e742–53. https://doi.org/10.1016/S1470-2045(17)30617-4.
58. Santosa KB. Postmastectomy radiation therapy and two-stage implant-based breast reconstruction: is there a better time to irradiate? Plast Reconstr Surg. 2016;138:761–9.
59. Adesiyun TA, Lee BT, Yueh JH, et al. Impact of sequencing of postmastectomy radiotherapy and breast reconstruction on timing and rate of complications and patient satisfaction. Int J Radiat Oncol Biol Phys. 2011;80(2):392–7.
60. Naoum GE. The impact of chest wall boost on reconstruction complications and local control in patients treated for breast cancer. Int J Radiat Oncol Biol Phys. 2019;105:155–64.
61. Manyam M, et al. Comparing 10 year outcomes in radiated patients with breast autologous reconstruction or tissue expander/implant based reconstruction. Int J Radiat Oncol Biol Phys. 2018;102:S45.
62. Negenborn VL. Quality of life and patient satisfaction after one-stage implant-based breast reconstruction with an acellular dermal matrix versus two-stage breast reconstruction (BRIOS): primary outcome of a randomized, controlled trial. Lancet. 2018;19:1205–14.
63. Dikmans REG, et al. Two-stage implant-based breast reconstruction compared with immediate one-stage implant-based breast reconstruction augmented with an acellular dermal matrix: an open-label, phase 4, multicentre, randomized, controlled trial. Lancet Oncol. 2017;18:251–8.
64. Schrenk P, et al. The use of sentinel node biopsy in breast cancer patients undergoing skin sparing mastectomy and immediate autologous reconstruction. Plast Reconstr Surg. 2005;116(5):1278.

20 Planning Pre-pectoral Implant-Based Breast Reconstruction When Confronted with XRT

Yoav Gronovich, Merav Ben-David, and Michael Scheflan

20.1 Introduction

Implant-based reconstruction is the most common form of breast reconstruction. In the wake of technological advancements and further understanding of the pathophysiology of the various breast tumors, the number of patients requiring radiation therapy as part of the overall treatment program of breast cancer has increased. In many instances, the radiation follows lumpectomy and hence precedes mastectomy for recurrent cancer and reconstruction. In many others, adjuvant radiation therapy follows mastectomy and immediate implant-based breast reconstruction. In the distant past, it was common to avoid reconstruction with implants in irradiated tissues or in patients who are likely to receive radiation therapy in the future. Advancements in reconstructive methods including usage of acellular dermal matrices (ADM), pre-pectoral implant placement, and autologous fat transfer (AFT) enable us to widen the indications for implant-based breast reconstruction without exposing the patient to higher risk for complications. Despite the greater likelihood of complications with implant-based reconstruction in irradiated tissues and the suboptimal or poor results in some, implant-based breast reconstruction is still the most common form of reconstruction in the setting of either postmastectomy radiation therapy or with a remote history of radiation therapy to the breast following lumpectomy.

The chapter is dedicated to Dr. Michael Scheflan, a brilliant pioneer plastic surgeon.

Y. Gronovich (✉)
Head, Plastic and Reconstructive Surgery Department, Shaare Zedek Medical Center, Faculty of Medicine, Hebrew University of Jerusalem, Jerusalem, Israel
e-mail: yoavg@szmc.org.il

M. Ben-David · M. Scheflan
Assuta Medical Center, Tel Aviv, Israel

Faculty of Health Science, Ben Gurion University, Be'er Sheva, Israel
e-mail: Meravak@assuta.co.il; michael@scheflan.co.il

20.2 Radiotherapy (XRT)

20.2.1 The Need

Radiation therapy is considered to be an important part of the combined treatment of many tumors. For breast cancer, radiation treatment has proved to be efficient for invasive ductal and lobular carcinoma, ductal carcinoma in situ (DCIS), and other subtypes. In women with lymph node positive breast cancer, postmastectomy radiation therapy reduces the risk of recurrence and improves overall survival [1].

© The Author(s), under exclusive license to Springer Nature Switzerland AG 2023
R. Vidya, H. Becker (eds.), *Prepectoral Breast Reconstruction*,
https://doi.org/10.1007/978-3-031-15590-1_20

The indications for postmastectomy radiation therapy (PMRT) are on the increase. The American College of Radiology currently recommends radiation for tumors greater than 5 cm or >4 involved lymph nodes. However, PMRT is often applied more broadly, taking into account its benefit in preventing local recurrence [2–4], especially if we adopt the National Comprehensive Cancer Network's recommendation to expand PMRT to patients with tumors 5 cm or smaller and 1–3 positive nodes [5]. Because the indications for postmastectomy radiotherapy have been widened to include not only locally advanced but also intermediate tumor stages, the proportion of patients with immediate breast reconstruction receiving postmastectomy radiotherapy has increased over time [6–10]. It is important to remember that radiation protocols vary greatly from one institution to another. The protocols often differ in terms of fraction number, daily doses, and total radiation dose, resulting in complicated comparison between institutions, as radiation has highly dose/protocol dependent effects [11].

20.2.2 Improvements of Radiation Throughout the Years

Concern about adverse events caused by postmastectomy radiotherapy seems less intense nowadays than in past decades, because of advancements in radiation techniques that have improved treatment tolerability [12]. Data in the literature strongly support a causal relation between better outcomes and improved radiotherapy techniques. Changes in radiotherapy practice over the years include recognition of the importance of fraction size, fraction number, total dose, overall time for both tumor and normal tissue reactions, and the introduction of conservative therapy [13]. Breast radiation protocols and dosing vary greatly by institution, and differences in radiation timing exist even within standard institutional protocols depending on the nature of the cancer and neoadjuvant therapy that has been initiated [14]. Radiation oncology continues to evolve with trials and utilization of more focused radiation delivery instead of simply whole breast radiation [15]. In an effort to streamline reconstruction in the setting of PMRT, many institutions follow an algorithmic approach [16–19].

20.2.3 Classification of Tissue Damage

It is of great importance to identify the variations in intrinsic (cellular) radiosensitivity and extrinsic factors that are associated with a change in the risk of morbidity. It has yet to be determined whether intrinsic cell radiosensitivity or extrinsic factors have greater influence on individual differences in damage expression [20–23]. The known factors influencing normal tissue response account for only 30% of interpatient variability in breast cancer patients under well-controlled conditions, leading to the hypothesis that most of the variability in the severity of these complications is due to differences in cellular radiosensitivity as determined by genetic or epigenetic mechanisms [20, 23]. Identification of the causes of this variability in radiation sensitivity could have important implications for cancer therapy. Evidence of a possible genetic basis for these differences has been provided by reports of increased cellular and tissue radiosensitivity in certain genetic syndromes [24] and of an association among the relative radiosensitivities of different normal cell types in the same individual [25]. This evidence also verifies that cellular radiosensitivity may be related to tissue response. Current radiobiological research efforts are aimed at identifying patients with abnormal radiosensitivity who are at risk for acute and late adverse effects of radiotherapy [26, 27] and at detecting molecules that increase the antitumor effects of radiotherapy [28]. Radiation exposure produces fibrosis, elastosis, and vascular intimal thickening of the skin and subcutaneous tissues. Radiation therapy induces tissue injury that can be categorized as acute or early and chronic or late [29]. The spectrum of acute injury includes erythema, edema, desquamation, hyperpigmentation, and ulceration [30], ranging from mild to severe.

Early effects such as erythema and desquamation usually appear during or immediately after radiotherapy. Acute, grade I radiation dermatitis occurs in up to 85% of irradiated breast cancer patients [30]. Chronic injury involves skin atrophy, dryness, telangiectasia, dyspigmentation, and dyschromia [31]. In the breast, it leads to chronic fibrosis of the skin and subcutaneous tissues [11]. Full manifestation of the chronic changes caused by radiation can take from months to years [32]. The course of radiation sequelae follows a distinct clinical pattern. An erythematous rash can develop on the skin of treated patients within a few hours of exposure and can persist or slowly worsen until the end of radiotherapy treatment. This situation is transient in nature. In severe, rare cases, subepidermal blisters and ulcers may develop. Most of the injuries heal within a timeframe of 10–20 days following last radiation fraction. Late damage becomes more severe, progresses with time, and cannot usually be arrested or reversed [33]. The damage to the surrounding tissue can be classified according to degrees, depending on the appearance of the skin itself and the subdermal quality of elasticity and flexibility, using scores based on the absolute side effect scale proposed by the Radiation Therapy Oncology Group/European Organization for Research and Treatment of Cancer [22], or by alternative nomenclature as proposed by Burnet et al. [34]. For patients undergoing implant-based reconstruction, radiotherapy can lead to increased scarring, capsular contracture, greater risk of infection and skin necrosis, delayed wound healing and pain [35–39]. Autologous reconstruction, when exposed to radiotherapy, is also subject to radiotherapy related complications, including flap atrophy and contracture, fibrosis, and fat necrosis [35, 40, 41]. However, from the patient's perspective, radiotherapy has been shown to adversely affect satisfaction among women receiving implant based, but not autologous reconstruction [42, 43]. Radiation exposure is also associated with higher risk for reconstruction failure. This risk can escalate to as much as three times that found among non-radiated patients [44]. Ongoing collaborative studies between plastic surgeons and radiation oncologists will provide a better understanding of how differences in the delivery of radiation therapy affect outcomes after reconstruction [45].

20.2.4 XRT Before Reconstruction

Previous radiation introduces a significant risk for immediate or delayed implant reconstructive failure and complications, although the reported incidence varies widely among institutions. A pooled analysis indicates approximately 14% incidence of reconstructive failure [11]. Use of autologous tissue from the latissimus dorsi muscle (LD) with implant significantly reduces the incidence of reconstructive failure in previously irradiated fields (72% decreased risk) [46]. Patients who have had previous radiation and present for reconstruction generally fit into two main categories: failed breast conserving therapy (BCT) requiring mastectomy and prompting immediate breast reconstruction (IBR); or true delayed reconstruction following mastectomy and PMRT [11]. Few studies have evaluated the effects of previous breast conserving therapy and completion with radiation on later reconstruction procedures. While some studies on autologous reconstructions show consistent satisfaction and few complications following radiation, others suggest that a history of breast radiation before immediate implant-based breast reconstruction has significantly more major complications and failures, compared to those who do not undergo radiation therapy [47]. This is consistent with other studies on implant-based reconstruction of irradiated breasts [35–39]. Studies that investigated nipple-sparing mastectomy and immediate reconstruction in patients who had received radiation therapy found a higher rate of complications compared with patients without radiation therapy. However, the majority of the reconstructions were successful [48]. Studies that compared the complication rates between prior radiation therapy and postmastectomy radiation therapy on implant-based reconstruction found no significant differences between these two radiation groups, though there was a trend towards fewer complications among women with previous breast conserving therapy before undergoing mastectomy and reconstruction. Other studies on patients undergoing total skin-sparing mastectomy with immediate tissue expander or implant-based reconstruction found no significant differences between prior radiation therapy and postmastectomy radiation therapy in terms of failure rates [49, 50]. Regarding patients' satisfaction and reported outcomes, the findings are inconsistent as well. While some studies reported that radiation therapy adversely affects patient-reported outcomes in breast reconstruction [42, 51, 52], others found no significant differences in 2-year patient-reported outcomes between previous breast conserving therapy with completion of radiation and nonirradiated patients undergoing immediate implant-based breast reconstruction [50]. In contrast, postmastectomy and implant-based reconstruction radiation therapy were associated with significantly worse patient-reported outcomes, compared with either previous breast conserving therapy or no prior radiation [50].

Improvements in radiation technique along with advancement of ADM's and autologous fat transfer (AFT) have changed the old paradigm of delaying breast reconstruction and enabling either a two-stage reconstruction with tissue expanders in the first stage or direct to implant reconstruction even for pre-radiated patients. AFT may be done before implant insertion as a preparation stage for improvement of the tissue quality, or as an adjunct to the same procedure as described by the first author (Y.G.) [53] (Fig. 20.1). AFT for completion of the reconstruction after implant insertion at a later stage is also a common option to improve tissue quality, correct deformations, and add volume. The authors recommend using ADM in a pre-pectoral approach for implant-based reconstruction in for-

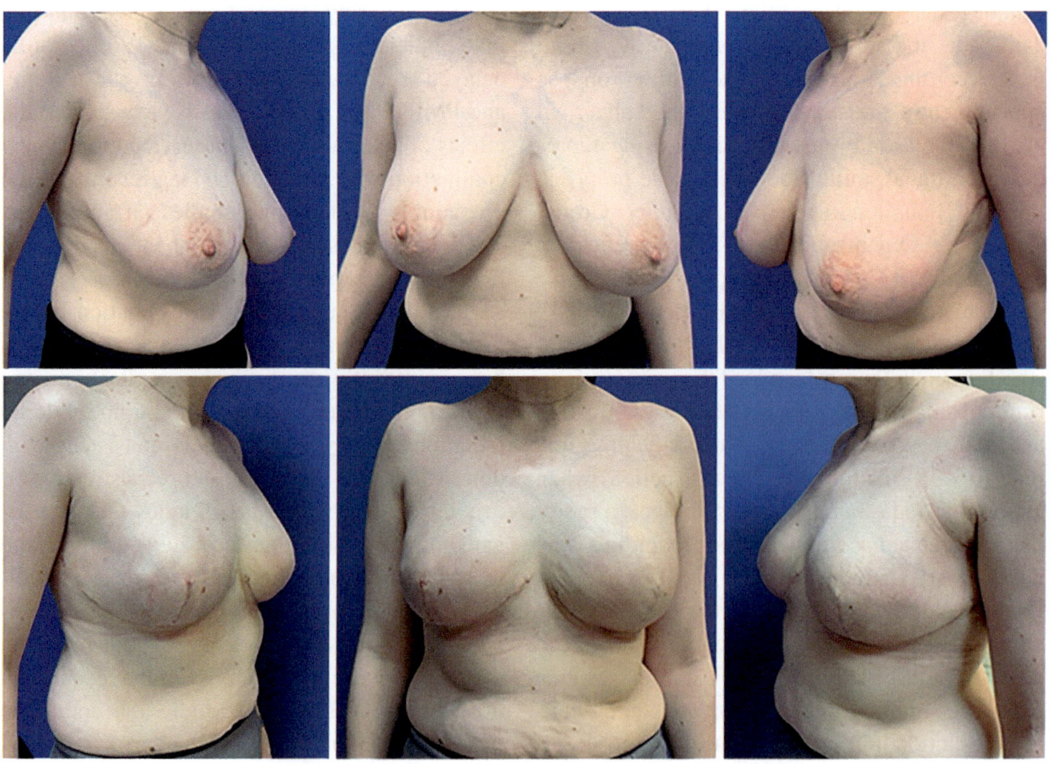

Fig. 20.1 Before reconstruction (above) and 12 months after SSM (wise pattern) and immediate reconstruction of pre-pectoral DTI with Mentor CPG 322 475 cc and Alloderm 8*16 cm plus 6*12 cm and autologous fat of 60 cc per breast (below)

merly irradiated patient. From the author's experience, the degree of tissue damage, following radiation therapy (pigmentation, induration, telangiectasis, atrophy) determines the decision on how to reconstruct the breast. If the tissue is compliant, soft, and elastic with minimal signs of skin damage, as most cases are, then one should feel safe in performing a pre-pectoral reconstruction.

20.3 Pre-pectoral Reconstruction in Face of XRT Before the Reconstruction

20.3.1 Why?

Pre-pectoral reconstruction gained its popularity a few years ago mainly for its simplicity, non-inferiority, and high grade of patients and surgeon's satisfaction. From the author's experience, it is recommended to cover at least the anterior surface of the implant with an ADM in any pre-pectoral reconstruction. The pre-pectoral approach shortens the procedure, eases the recovery of the patient, necessitates less use of narcotics, and creates comparable aesthetic results to partial retro-muscular reconstruction. The contraindications for the pre-pectoral method include: a breast tumor that is located within 5 mm of the pectoralis major muscle, a medical background of high BMI (more than 30), smoking, diabetes mellitus with an HbA1C level of >7.5, or an immunocompromised state. It also cannot be used in the case of badly perfused flaps after mastectomy as measured by clinical evaluation or by one of the advanced technologies. While thick subcutaneous fat is necessary, perfusion is more important than thickness and pre-pectoral immediate reconstruction is recommended even in thin flaps of 0.5 cm of subcutaneous fat, as long as they appear healthy, vascularized, and untraumatized. It is however recommended that patients with very thin flaps undergo a two-stage tissue expander rather than direct to implant approach reconstruction.

20.3.2 Advantages as Compared with Sub-pectoral

Potential aesthetic disadvantages of the sub-pectoral approach such as double bubble, animation deformity, or upward displacement of the implant are eliminated. In patients with ptotic breast who are unwilling to undergo mastopexy on the contralateral breast, the pre-pectoral approach can give a good symmetric shape that may not be achieved by a sub-pectoral approach (Fig. 20.2).

Irradiated patients requesting delayed reconstruction are advised to wait 4–6 months after conclusion of the radiation therapy, in order to allow the inflammatory phase to subside. Fat grafting in these patients during the inflammatory phase at 2 months following the completion of radiation therapy can be done in order to reduce scarring during the fibrotic phase. Tissue quality, including skin tone, pinch, elasticity, and thickness are all taken into account in the final decision on the timing and type of reconstruction. If the tissue has been damaged, with clinical evidence of pigmentation, induration, telangiectasis, and atrophy, then the recommended approach is for autologous tissue reconstruction. Alternatively, a preparatory independent stage of autologous fat transfer (AFT) is indicated before TE or implant is inserted. The first author (YG) recommends the use of an external expansion device (BRAVA) prior to surgery (Fig. 20.3). After a few rounds of BRAVA and AFT and when the quality of the tissue has improved, it will be possible to conclude the reconstruction with a pre-pectoral implant if desired by the patient.

In other patients, whereas the quality of the tissue following radiation therapy is reasonable and adequate for reconstruction, then one needs to decide between a tissue expander and a definitive implant. In patients with a flat tight chest, a two-stage approach is recommended. A tissue expander is inserted and covered by ADM in a pre-pectoral plane to be replaced by a permanent implant in a second stage (Fig. 20.4). Less commonly in a

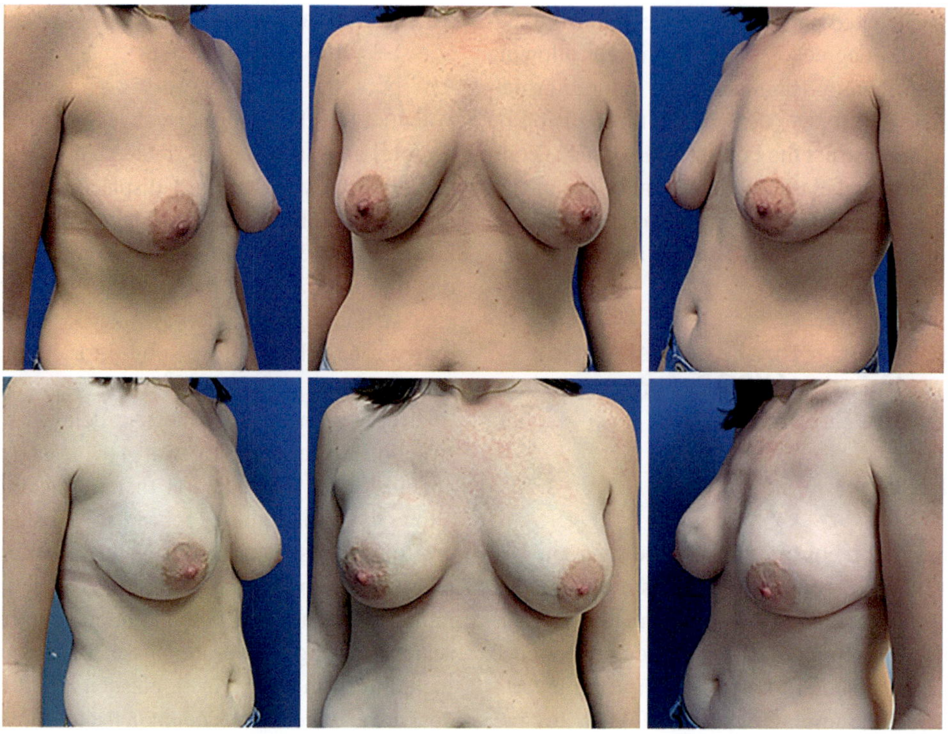

Fig. 20.2 Before reconstruction of bilateral breast (above) and 3 months after NSM (IMF incision) and immediate reconstruction of pre-pectoral DTI with Mentor CPG323 390 cc and Alloderm 8 × 16 cm plus 6 × 12 cm (below)

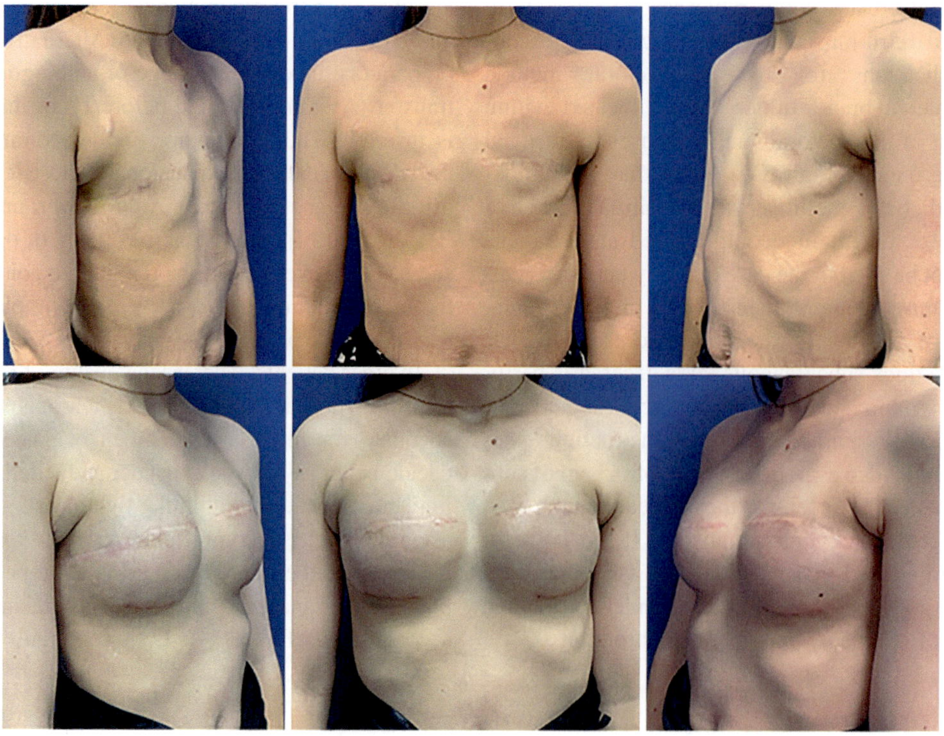

Fig. 20.3 After bilateral mastectomy and left PMRT (6 years) (above) and 3 months after reconstruction of pre-pectoral tissue expander with Mentor CPX4 250 cc and Alloderm 8 × 16 cm plus 6 × 12 cm (IMF incision) (below)

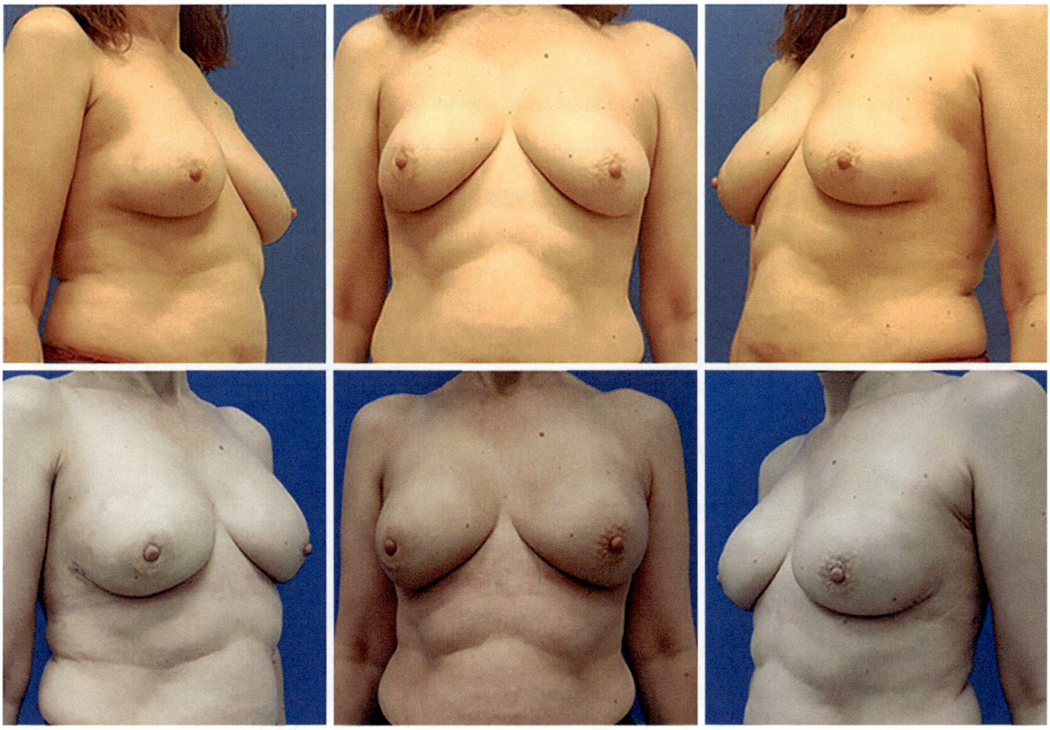

Fig. 20.4 After bilateral lumpectomy and radiation therapy (3 years) (above) and 6 months after NSM (IMF incision) and immediate reconstruction of pre-pectoral DTI with Mentor CPG 321 280 cc and Alloderm 8 × 16 cm plus 6 × 12 cm (below)

patient with loose, pliable soft tissues, it is possible to reconstruct the breast using a permanent implant in the initial stage (DTI). The third author's (MS) practice has been to fat graft all previously irradiated patients undergoing delayed reconstruction, in a separate session 3–4 months before inserting a TE or permanent implant, regardless on the condition of their tissues.

Summary of the author's approach is given in the detailed algorithm below.

Algorithm for delayed reconstruction of previously irradiated breast:

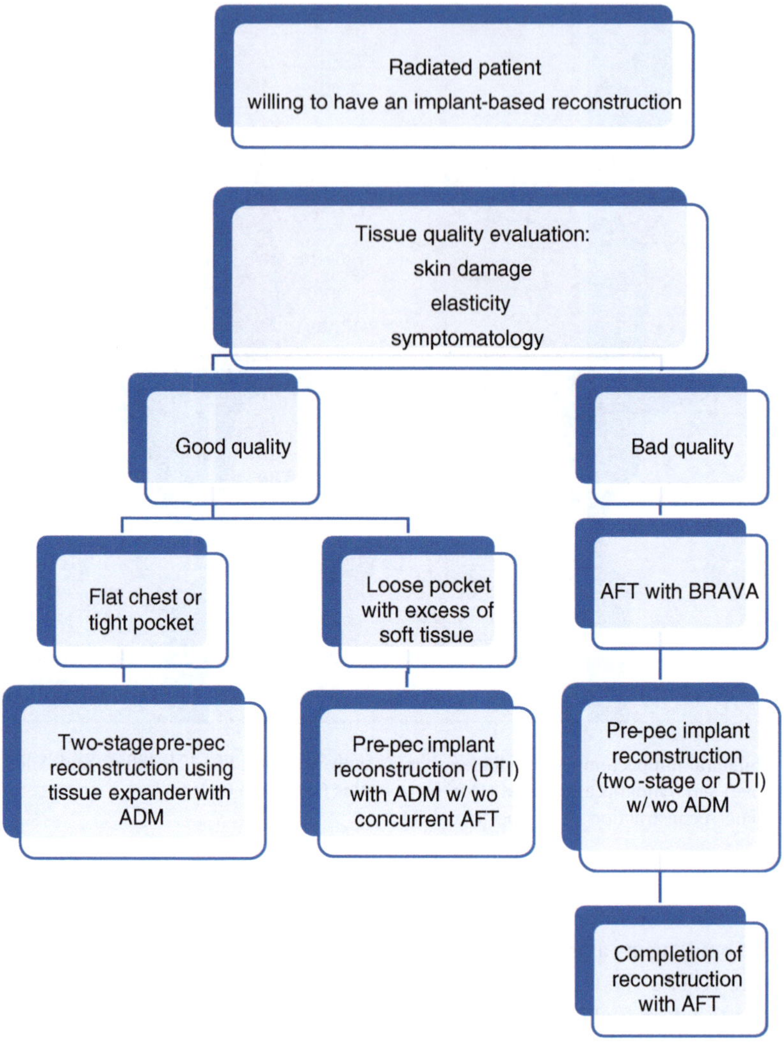

For immediate reconstructions of patients who previously underwent lumpectomy and radiation therapy and who are now faced with breast cancer on the same side, a pre-mastectomy evaluation is needed to decide if the patient is in fact a candidate for implant-based breast reconstruction. Additional risk factors such as smoking, obesity, large pendulous breasts, stretch marks, thin skin, and a layer of subcutaneous fat should be noted. Poor candidates should be consulted on reducing risk factors, or possibly undergo autologous reconstruction. For patients who have no or little clinical evidence of radiation damage, the next assessment should be done after completion of mastectomy. A good reconstruction begins with a good mastectomy (non-traumatized, well perfused flaps). The flaps should be examined by clinical evaluation or using one of the specialized devices. If the quality of the flaps is poor, then the authors recommend that the plan for immediate pre-pectoral reconstruction is aborted and a delayed primary or two-stage approach in a sub-pectoral plane should be considered. In good quality flaps, a pre-pectoral approach is recommended, using a DTI or two-stage procedure, depending on the surgeon's preferences and the patient's wishes as regards breast size (Fig. 20.5).

Summary of the author's approach is given in the detailed algorithm below.

Algorithm for immediate reconstruction of previously irradiated breast:

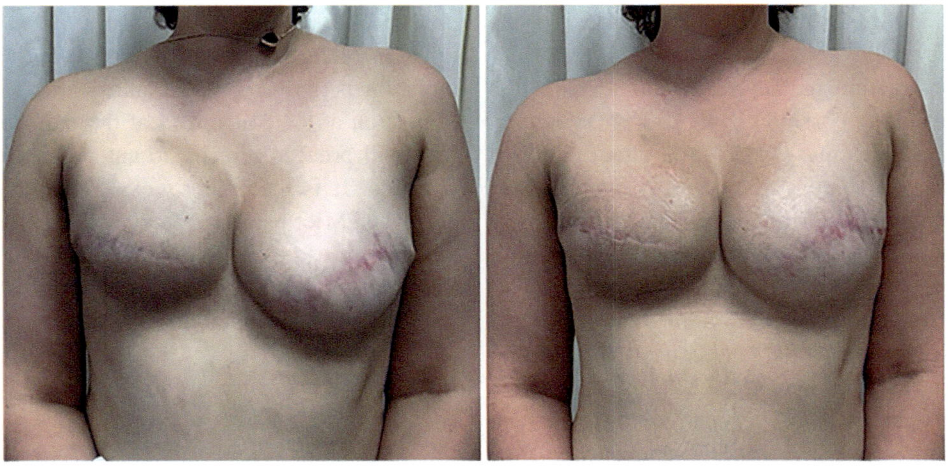

Fig. 20.5 PMRT after Sub-pectoral reconstruction DTI with Allergan 410MF 420 g and Alloderm 8*16 cm (left) and after change of implant to pre-pectoral plane (right)

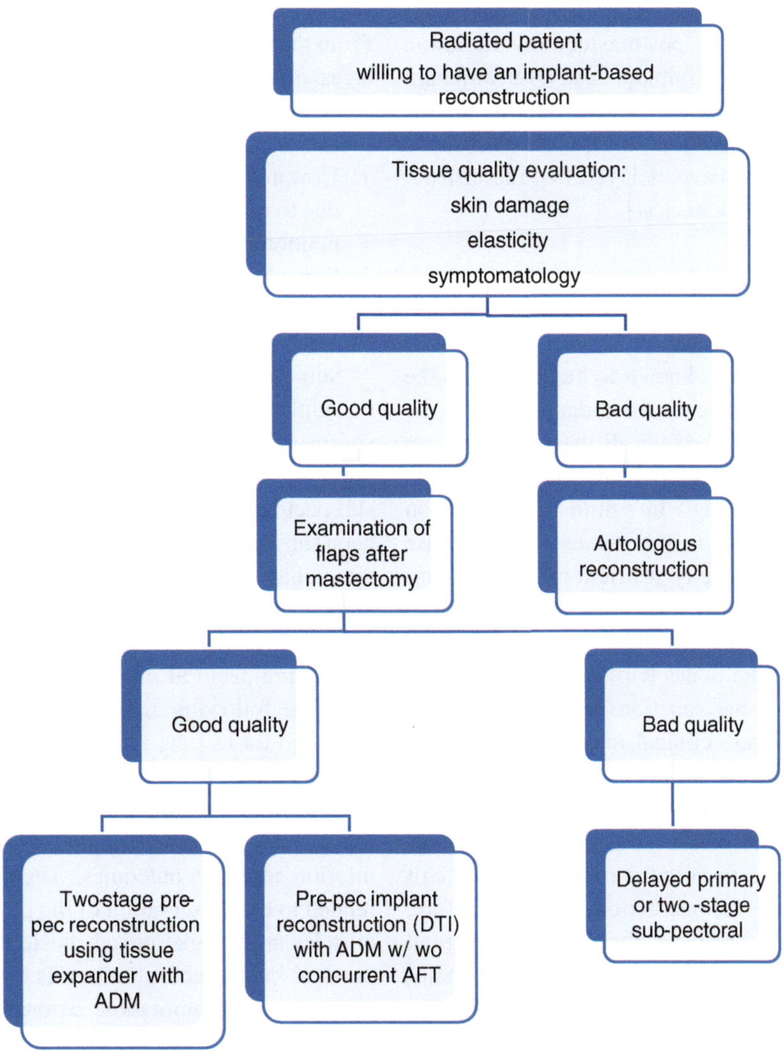

20.3.3 XRT After Reconstruction

Reconstruction of the breast should take into account the possibility of post mastectomy radiation therapy (PMRT) in about 35% of patients. In some of the cases, it is not immediately clear if PMRT is indicated, as the final decision is made only after permanent pathology results of lymph nodes and the breast specimen. Radiation following immediate prosthetic breast reconstruction can occur at two general time points—following the placement of a tissue expander before exchange to permanent implant or following the final exchange to a definitive device. Meta-analyses and recent prospective studies suggest no significant difference in the timing of radiation, though many other studies exist that exhibit contrary findings [11]. Although postmastectomy radiation doubles the risk of implant loss over adjuvant chemotherapy alone, implant-based breast reconstruction is still an acceptable alternative to the more expensive, delayed flap reconstruction for many patients [54].

20.3.4 Influence on the Tissues

Radiation therapy is known to be harmful to the tissues. The beam can cause damage from the skin to the bones through all the soft tissues in between. The skin suffers from mild to moderate dermatitis resulting in mild pigmentation changes, however, in rare cases it may cause hardness and elasticity restrictions due to damaged collagen fibers. The muscles can undergo fibrosis that shrinks the fibers and restricts their activity; even the bones (ribs) suffer damage by impairment of the function of the osteoblasts, however with rare clinical manifestation. When an implant comes within the radiation area, the capsule around it also suffers radiation damage which facilitates contracture. For these reasons, PMRT is known to raise the complication rate of implant-based reconstruction and therefore, many practitioners have changed their original decisions for expected PMRT patients by abstaining from DTI reconstruction. They will then either opt for two-stage reconstruction, where inflation of the expander is stopped during the radiation period and is continued after patient evaluation at the conclusion of the radiation; or they will proceed directly to autologous reconstruction. It is the author's experience that for expected PMRT patients, pre-pectoral DTI reconstruction is a safe alternative with short recovery time and long lasting, stable aesthetic results, and from the oncology point of view, the radiation is administered in close proximity to the surgery (usually 6 weeks) without further delay.

20.3.5 Pre-pectoral Reconstruction in the Face of Expected XRT After Reconstruction

From the author's experience, the main disadvantages of sub-pectoral reconstruction in patients receiving radiation therapy are:

1. Upward lateral displacement of the implant due to fibrosis and shortening of the pectoralis major muscle because of the radiation.
2. Capsular contracture due to radiation damage and its influence on the capsule itself.

Sub-pectoral implant placement may lead to unsightly animation deformity and muscle spasms. Both disadvantages and complications are minimized in the pre-pectoral approach. If a sub-pectoral approach was initially chosen, it has been shown that all these disadvantages improved after changing the implant to the pre-pectoral plane [55–57]. This is the practice of the authors as well (Fig. 20.6).

The pre-pectoral implant-based breast reconstruction following radiation therapy has been evaluated for its long-term results. Advantages of pre-pectoral implant-based breast reconstruction include a natural appearance, shorter operative times, reduced postoperative pain, and non-inferior aesthetic outcomes. These are directly related to the preservation of the pectoralis major muscle in its anatomical position [58]. Pre-pectoral breast reconstruction is associated with elimination of animation deformity and high

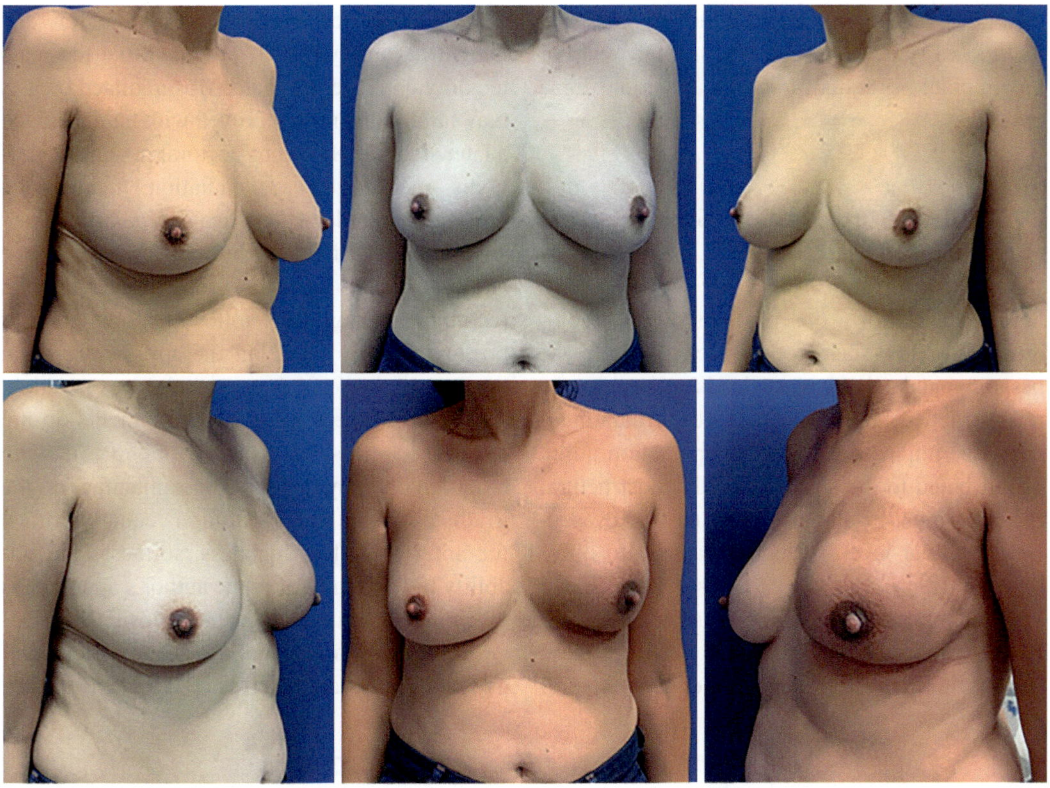

Fig. 20.6 Before reconstruction of the left breast (above) and 6 months after NSM (IMF incision) and immediate reconstruction of pre-pectoral DTI with Mentor smooth round moderate plus, 400 cc and Alloderm 8 × 16 cm plus 6 × 12 cm and AFT of 80 cc, and 3 months after PMRT to the left breast and AFT of 120 cc (below)

patient satisfaction rates [59–61]. Studies comparing sub-pectoral to pre-pectoral expander placement have also demonstrated less pain and capsular contracture, improved rates of expansion, and improved aesthetic outcomes. Few data are available on the impact of radiotherapy on pre-pectoral implants, periprosthetic capsule, and on the pectoralis major muscle [62, 63]. While most of the studies show a stable aesthetic result even after PMRT, they demonstrate slightly higher rates of overall complications in irradiated versus nonirradiated breasts following pre-pectoral implant-based breast reconstruction, although this was not statistically significant. The most notable difference is higher rates of surgical-site infection in irradiated breasts [58]. The use of ADM helps minimize capsular contracture with or without radiation. It supports the implant, offloads the weight of the implant from the soft tissue envelope, and helps to strengthen the skin itself, by incorporation and thickening of the dermal layer. It has a protective effect and reduces implant extrusion and encapsulation rates relative to complete submuscular reconstruction [64–66]. The ADM also serves as a barrier that absorbs some of the radiation, thereby preventing it from penetrating the capsule, implant, and the deeper tissues. Studies showed that irradiated ADM, nonirradiated ADM, and native capsules all exhibited a similar number of blood vessels. Irradiated ADM showed less peri-implant inflammation and nonvascular alpha-smooth actin than irradiated native capsules [67]. Recent studies show that pre-pectoral reconstruction is an effective technique for patients undergoing postmastectomy radiation therapy, with morbidity rates similar to those experienced with complete submuscular or dual-plane implant position with postmastectomy radiation therapy [51]. It is still too early to determine whether full wrap of the implant is better than just anterior dome coverage.

20.3.6 Two-Stage vs. One-Stage Reconstruction

Studies have shown that postmastectomy radiotherapy for two-stage reconstruction where the tissue expander is in place leads more often to reconstructive failure as compared irradiating a definitive implant. A possible explanation might be attributed to the structural and ultrastructural radiation-induced alterations at the microvascular or cellular level, including damage to fibroblasts and fibroblast stem cells, so that repeated surgical procedures could act as an additional factor for worsening local injury [12]. For these reasons, it is the author's recommendation to prefer DTI pre-pectoral reconstruction for any patient requiring PMRT, provided that the mastectomy flaps are adequate. Most radiated breasts may be significantly improved with fat grafting at a later stage. In those pre-pectoral patients undergoing postmastectomy radiation therapy, fat grafting may reduce the effects of radiation fibrosis, soften and thicken the soft-tissue envelope and mastectomy skin flaps [66]. Hence, authors recommend fat grafting following completion of postmastectomy radiation therapy, before or at the time of the second-stage exchange operation. Although pre-pectoral irradiated patients do not experience the same risk of rippling following radiation therapy because of tightening of the irradiated skin, the fat grafting is equally critical for improving skin thickness, softness, and pliability [54]. Summary of the author's approach is given in the detailed algorithm below.

Algorithm for immediate reconstruction of expected irradiated breast (PMRT):

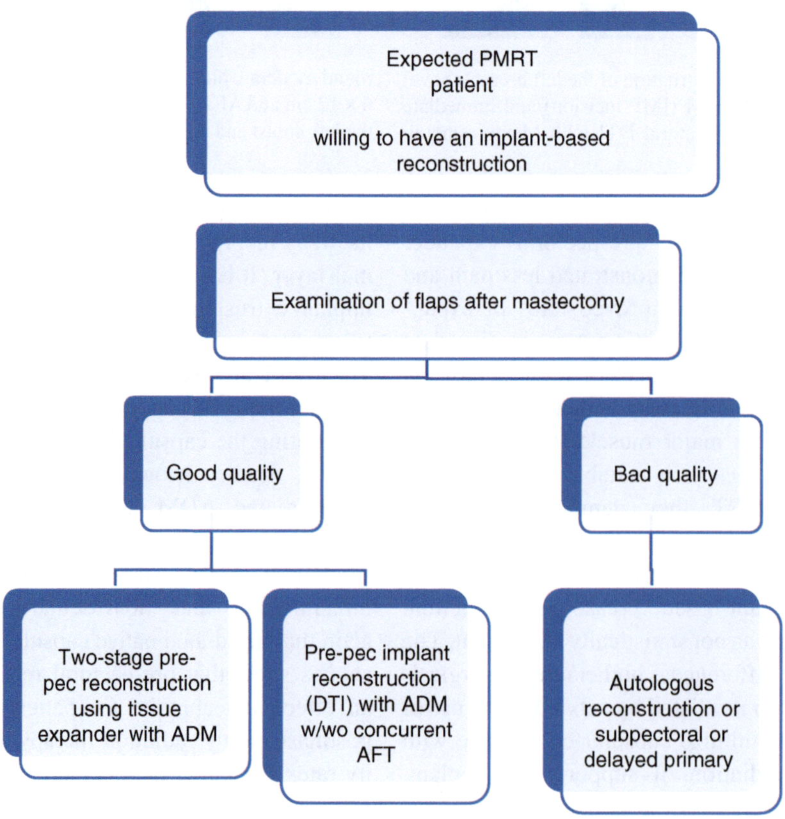

20.4 Summary

Implant-based reconstruction is the most common form of breast reconstruction. Although this has been considered questionable in the face of radiation therapy, advancements both in radiation technology and the use of ADM and fat grafting have made the pre-pectoral approach in one or two stages a safe reconstructive procedure in radiation setting. In previously irradiated patients requesting reconstruction, the decision as to whether implant-based reconstruction is feasible depends on thorough examination of their tissues for clinical signs of radiation damage. In the era of AFT, implant-based reconstruction may be performed even in patients whose tissues have been damaged by radiation therapy, by first regeneration the tissue with fat grafting and then, inserting an implant or tissue expander for completion of the reconstruction process.

20.5 Review of Short Literature to Date Summary with Tips

20.5.1 Tips

Patients who had XRT before reconstruction

- *If the tissue has been damaged, then the recommended approach is for autologous tissue reconstruction. For patients who are willing for autologous fat reconstruction, use of an external expansion device prior to autologous fat transfer (AFT) is essential.*
- *If the tissue is compliant, soft, and elastic with minimal signs of skin damage, as most cases are, then one should feel safe in performing a pre-pectoral reconstruction.*
- *Autologous fat transfer (AFT) may be done before implant insertion as a preparation stage for improvement of the tissue quality*
- *Autologous fat transfer (AFT) can be added as an adjunct to the reconstruction at the same procedure.*
- *Autologous fat transfer (AFT) can be done for completion of the reconstruction after implant insertion at a later stage.*

Patients who had XRT after reconstruction:

- *It is recommended to prefer DTI pre-pectoral reconstruction for any patient requiring PMRT, provided that the mastectomy flaps are adequate.*
- *Autologous fat transfer (AFT) is recommended following completion of postmastectomy radiation therapy, before or at the time of the second-stage exchange operation.*

References

1. Recht A, Comen EA, Fine RE, et al. Postmastectomy radiotherapy: an American Society of Clinical Oncology, American Society for Radiation Oncology, and Society of Surgical Oncology Focused Guideline Update. Ann Surg Oncol. 2017;24:38–51.
2. Taylor ME, Haffty BG, Rabinovitch R, et al. ACR appropriateness criteria on postmastectomy radiotherapy expert panel on radiation oncology-breast. Int J Radiat Oncol Biol Phys. 2009;73:997–1002.
3. Horst KC, Haffty BG, Harris EE, et al. Expert panel on radiation oncology—breast. ACR Appropriateness Criteria® Postmastectomy Radiotherapy. Reston: American College of Radiology (ACR); 2012.
4. Clarke M, Collins R, Darby S, et al. Early Breast Cancer Trialists' Collaborative Group (EBCTCG). Effects of radiotherapy and of differences in the extent of surgery for early breast cancer on local recurrence and 15-year survival: an overview of the randomized trials. Lancet. 2005;366:2087–106.
5. Overgaard M, Hansen PS, Overgaard J, et al. Postoperative radiotherapy in high-risk premenopausal women with breast cancer who receive adjuvant chemotherapy: Danish Breast Cancer Cooperative Group 82b Trial. N Engl J Med. 1997;337:949–55. https://www.nccn.org/store/login/login.aspx?ReturnURL=https://www.nccn.org/professionals/physician_gls/pdf/breast.pdf.
6. Overgaard M, Jensen MB, Overgaard J, et al. Postoperative radiotherapy in high-risk postmenopausal breast-cancer patients given adjuvant tamoxifen: Danish Breast Cancer Cooperative Group DBCG 82c randomized trial. Lancet. 1999;353:1641–8.
7. Ragaz J, Jackson SM, Le N, et al. Adjuvant radiotherapy and chemotherapy in node-positive premenopausal women with breast cancer. N Engl J Med. 1997;337:956–62.
8. McGale P, Taylor C, Correa C, et al. Effect of radiotherapy after mastectomy and axillary surgery on 10-year recurrence and 20-year breast cancer mortality: meta-analysis of individual patient data for 8135 women in 22 randomized trials. Lancet. 2014;383:2127–35.

9. Kummerow KL, Du L, Penson DF, Shyr Y, Hooks MA. Nationwide trends in mastectomy for early-stage breast cancer. JAMA Surg. 2015;150:9–16.
10. Nelson JA, Disa JJ. Breast reconstruction and radiation therapy: an update. Plast Reconstr Surg. 2017;140:60s–8s.
11. Dicuonzo S, Leonardi MC, Radice D, et al. Long-term results and reconstruction failure in patients receiving postmastectomy radiation therapy with a temporary expander or permanent implant in place. Plast Reconstr Surg. 2020;145:317–27.
12. López E, Guerrero R, Núñez MI, et al. Early and late skin reactions to radiotherapy for breast cancer and their correlation with radiation-induced DNA damage in lymphocytes. Breast Cancer Res. 2005;7:690–8.
13. Muresan H, Lam G, Cooper BT, et al. Impact of evolving radiation therapy techniques on implant-based breast reconstruction. Plast Reconstr Surg. 2017;139:1232e–9e.
14. Speers C, Pierce LJ. Postoperative radiotherapy after breast conserving surgery for early-stage breast cancer: a review. JAMA Oncol. 2016;2:1075–82.
15. El-Sabawi B, Carey JN, Hagopian TM, et al. Radiation and breast reconstruction: algorithmic approach and evidence based outcomes. J Surg Oncol. 2016;113:906–12.
16. Patel KM, Albino F, Fan KL, et al. Microvascular autologous breast reconstruction in the context of radiation therapy: comparing two reconstructive algorithms. Plast Reconstr Surg. 2013;132:251–7.
17. Cordeiro PG, Albornoz CR, McCormick B, et al. The impact of postmastectomy radiotherapy on two-stage implant breast reconstruction: an analysis of long-term surgical outcomes, aesthetic results, and satisfaction over 13 years. Plast Reconstr Surg. 2014;134:588–95.
18. Ben-David MA, Granot H, Gelernter I, Scheflan M. Immediate breast reconstruction with anatomical implants following mastectomy: the radiation perspective. Med Dosim. 2016;41(2):142–7.
19. Turesson I, Nyman J, Holmberg E, Oden A. Prognostic factors for acute and late skin reactions in radiotherapy patients. Int J Radiat Oncol Biol Phys. 1996;36:1065–75.
20. Barber JB, Burrill W, Spreadborough AR, Levine E, Warren C, Kiltie AE, Roberts SA, Scott D. Relationship between in vitro chromosomal radiosensitivity of peripheral blood lymphocytes and the expression of normal tissue damage following radiotherapy for breast cancer. Radiother Oncol. 2000;55:179–86.
21. López E, Núñez MI, Guerrero MR, del Moral R, de Dios Luna J, del Mar Rodríguez MM, Valenzuela MT, Villalobos M, Ruiz de Almodóvar JM. Breast cancer acute morbidity evaluated by different scoring systems. Breast Cancer Res Treat. 2002;73:127–34.
22. Peacock JH, Ashton A, Bliss J, Bush C, Eady J, Jackson C, Owen R, Regan J, Yarnold J. Cellular radiosensitivity and complication risk after curative radiotherapy. Radiother Oncol. 2000;55:173–8.
23. Gatti RA. The inherited basis of human radiosensitivity. Acta Oncol. 2001;40:702–11.
24. Núñez MI, Guerrero R, López E, del Moral R, Valenzuela MT, Siles E, Villalobos M, Pedraza V, Peacock JH, Ruiz de Almodóvar JM. DNA damage and prediction of radiation response in lymphocytes and epidermal skin cells. Int J Cancer. 1998;76:354–61.
25. Ruiz de Almodóvar JM, Guirado D, Núñez MI, López E, Guerrero R, Valenzuela MT, Villalobos M, Ruiz de Almodóvar JM. Individualization of radiotherapy in breast cancer patients: possible usefulness of a DNA damage assay to measure normal cell radiosensitivity. Radiother Oncol. 2002;62:327–33.
26. Carlomagno F, Burnet NG, Turesson I, Nyman J, Peacock JH, Dunning AH, Ponder BA, Jackson SP. Comparison of DNA repair protein expression and activities between human fibroblast cell lines with different radio sensitivities. Int J Cancer. 2000;85:845–9.
27. Krause M, Hessel F, Szips D, Hilberg F, Baumann M. Adjuvant inhibition of the epidermal growth factor receptor after fractionated irradiation of FaDu human squamous cell carcinoma. Radiother Oncol. 2004;72:95–101.
28. Haubner F, Ohmann E, Pohl F, et al. Wound healing after radiation therapy: review of the literature. Radiat Oncol. 2012;7:162.
29. Salvo N, Barnes E, van Draanen J, et al. Prophylaxis and management of acute radiation-induced skin reactions: a systematic review of the literature. Curr Oncol. 2010;17:94–112.
30. El-Sabawi B, Carey JN, Hagopian TM, et al. Radiation and breast reconstruction: algorithmic approach and evidenced based outcomes. J Surg Oncol. 2016;113:906–12.
31. Bentzen SM, Thames HD, Overgaard M. Latent-time estimation for late cutaneous and subcutaneous radiation reactions in a single-follow-up clinical study. Radiother Oncol. 1989;15:267–74.
32. Johansson S, Svensson H, Denenkamp J. Timescale of evolution of late radiation injury after postoperative radiotherapy of breast cancer patients. Int J Radiat Oncol Biol Phys. 2000;48:745–50.
33. Burnet NG, Johansen J, Turesson I, Nyman J, Peacock JH. Describing patients' normal tissue reactions: concerning the possibility of individualizing radiotherapy dose prescriptions based on potential predictive assays of normal tissue radiosensitivity. Steering Committee of the BioMed 2 European Union Concerted Action Program on the Development of Predictive Tests of Normal Tissue Response to Radiation Therapy. Int J Cancer. 1998;79:606–13.
34. Jagsi R, Jiang J, Momoh AO, et al. Complications after mastectomy and immediate breast reconstruction for breast cancer: a claims-based analysis. Ann Surg. 2016;263:219–27.
35. Krueger EA, Wilkins EG, Strawderman M, et al. Complications and patient satisfaction following expander/implant breast reconstruction with and

without radiotherapy. Int J Radiat Oncol Biol Phys. 2001;49:713–21.
36. Contant CM, van Geel AN, van der Holt B, Griep C, Tjong Joe Wai R, Wiggers T. Morbidity of immediate breast reconstruction (IBR) after mastectomy by a sub pectorally placed silicone prosthesis: the adverse effect of radiotherapy. Eur J Surg Oncol. 2000;26:344–50.
37. Tallet AV, Salem N, Moutardier V, et al. Radiotherapy and immediate two-stage breast reconstruction with a tissue expander and implant: complications and esthetic results. Int J Radiat Oncol Biol Phys. 2003;57:136–42.
38. Ascherman JA, Hanasono MM, Newman MI, Hughes DB. Implant reconstruction in breast cancer patients treated with radiation therapy. Plast Reconstr Surg. 2006;117:359–65.
39. Williams JK, Carlson GW, Bostwick J III, Bried JT, Mackay G. The effects of radiation treatment after TRAM flap breast reconstruction. Plast Reconstr Surg. 1997;100:1153–60.
40. Rogers NE, Allen RJ. Radiation effects on breast reconstruction with the deep inferior epigastric perforator flap. Plast Reconstr Surg. 2002;109:1919–24; discussion 1925–6.
41. Chetta MD, Aliu O, Zhong L, et al. Reconstruction of the irradiated breast: a national claims-based assessment of postoperative morbidity. Plast Reconstr Surg. 2017;139:783–92.
42. Hu ES, Pusic AL, Waljee JF, et al. Patient-reported aesthetic satisfaction with breast reconstruction during the long-term survivorship period. Plast Reconstr Surg. 2009;124:1–8.
43. Ho AY, Hu ZI, Mehrara BJ, Wilkins EG. Radiotherapy in the setting of breast reconstruction: types, techniques, and timing. Lancet Oncol. 2017;18:e742–53.
44. Muresan H, Lam G, Cooper BT, et al. Impact of evolving radiation therapy techniques on implant-based breast reconstruction. Plast Reconstr Surg. 2017;139:1232–9.
45. Lee KT, Mun GH. Prosthetic breast reconstruction in previously irradiated breasts: a meta-analysis. J Surg Oncol. 2015;112:468–75.
46. Khansa I, Colakoglu S, Curtis MS, et al. Postmastectomy breast reconstruction after previous lumpectomy and radiation therapy: analysis of complications and satisfaction. Ann Plast Surg. 2011;66:444–51.
47. Reish RG, Lin A, Phillips NA, et al. Breast reconstruction outcomes after nipple sparing mastectomy and radiation therapy. Plast Reconstr Surg. 2015;135:959–66.
48. Peled AW, Sears M, Wang F, et al. Complications after total skin-sparing mastectomy and expander-implant reconstruction: effects of radiation therapy on the stages of reconstruction. Ann Plast Surg. 2018;80:10–3.
49. Olinger TA, Berlin NL, Qi J, et al. Outcomes of immediate implant-based mastectomy reconstruction in women with previous breast radiotherapy. Plast Reconstr Surg. 2020;145:1029–35.
50. Albornoz CR, Matros E, McCarthy CM, et al. Implant breast reconstruction and radiation: a multicenter analysis of long-term health-related quality of life and satisfaction. Ann Surg Oncol. 2014;21:2159–64.
51. Behranwala KA, Dua RS, Ross GM, Ward A, A'hern R, Gui GP. The influence of radiotherapy on capsule formation and aesthetic outcome after immediate breast reconstruction using biodimensional anatomical expander implants. J Plast Reconstr Aesthet Surg. 2006;59:1043–51.
52. Lam TC, Borotkanics R, Hsieh F, et al. Immediate two-stage prosthetic breast reconstruction failure: radiation is not the only culprit. Plast Reconstr Surg. 2018;141:1315–24.
53. Gronovich Y, Winder G, Maisel-Lotan A, et al. Hybrid Prepectoral Direct-to-Implant and Autologous Fat Graft Simultaneously in Immediate Breast Reconstruction: A Single Surgeon's Experience with 25 Breasts in 15 Consecutive Cases. Plast Reconstr Surg. 2022;149(3):386–91.
54. Sigalove S, Maxwell GP, Sigalove NM, et al. Prepectoral implant-based breast reconstruction: rationale, indications, and preliminary results. Plast Reconstr Surg. 2017;139:287–94.
55. Spear SL, Schwartz J, Dayan JH, Clemens MW. Outcome assessment of breast distortion following submuscular breast augmentation. Aesthet Plast Surg. 2009;33:44–8.
56. Hammond DC, Schmitt WP, O'Connor EA. Treatment of breast animation deformity in implant-based reconstruction with pocket change to the subcutaneous position. Plast Reconstr Surg. 2015;135:1540–4.
57. Elswick SM, Harless CA, Bishop SN. Prepectoral implant-based breast reconstruction with postmastectomy radiation therapy. Plast Reconstr Surg. 2018;142:1–12.
58. Sbitany H. Important considerations for performing prepectoral breast reconstruction. Plast Reconstr Surg. 2017;140(6S Prepectoral Breast Reconstruction):7S–13S.
59. Gabriel A, Maxwell GP. Prepectoral breast reconstruction in challenging patients. Plast Reconstr Surg. 2017;140(6S Prepectoral Breast Reconstruction):14S–21S.
60. Nahabedian MY, Cocilovo C. Two-stage prosthetic breast reconstruction: a comparison between prepectoral and partial subpectoral techniques. Plast Reconstr Surg. 2017;140(6S Prepectoral Breast Reconstruction):22S–30S.
61. Zhu L, Mohan AT, Abdelsattar JM, et al. Comparison of subcutaneous versus submuscular expander placement in the first stage of immediate breast reconstruction. J Plast Reconstr Aesthet Surg. 2016;69:e77–86.
62. Bernini M, Calabrese C, Cecconi L, et al. Subcutaneous direct-to-implant breast reconstruction: surgical, functional, and aesthetic results after long-term follow-up. Plast Reconstr Surg Glob Open. 2015;3:e574.

63. Sbitany H, Wang F, Peled AW, et al. Immediate implant based breast reconstruction following total skin-sparing mastectomy: defining the risk of preoperative and postoperative radiation therapy for surgical outcomes. Plast Reconstr Surg. 2014;134:396–404.
64. Seth AK, Hirsch EM, Fine NA, Kim JY. Utility of acellular dermis-assisted breast reconstruction in the setting of radiation: a comparative analysis. Plast Reconstr Surg. 2012;130:750–8.
65. Spear SL, Seruya M, Rao SS, et al. Two-stage prosthetic breast reconstruction using AlloDerm including outcomes of different timings of radiotherapy. Plast Reconstr Surg. 2012;130:1–9.
66. Moyer HR, Pinell-White X, Losken A. The effect of radiation on acellular dermal matrix and capsule formation in breast reconstruction: clinical outcomes and histologic analysis. Plast Reconstr Surg. 2014;133:214–21.
67. Sbitany H, Gomez-Sanchez C, Piper M, et al. Prepectoral breast reconstruction in the setting of postmastectomy radiation therapy: an assessment of clinical outcomes and benefits. Plast Reconstr Surg. 2019;143:10–20.

21 Fat Grafting for Volume Augmentation in Prepectoral Breast Reconstruction

William R. Moritz, Halley Darrach, Hayden Schott, Michael Finnan, Sarah Chiang, Annahita Fotouhi, Franca Kraenzlin, Nima Khavanin, Karan Chopra, and Justin M. Sacks

21.1 Introduction

Prosthetic breast reconstruction remains the most common method of post-mastectomy breast reconstruction [1]. However, variation exists within this procedure. Surgeons can choose to perform reconstruction immediately after mastectomy or delay reconstruction. Furthermore, implants can be placed above or below the pectoralis major and serratus anterior. Currently, delayed reconstruction is the most popular in the United States [2].

Since the introduction of silicone breast implants in the 1960s, the location of implant placement has varied, largely dependent on the available technology and techniques of the time. Early on, implants were placed superficial to pectoralis major in the subcutaneous plane [3]. However, this method produced unacceptably high rates of skin flap necrosis, capsular contracture, and implant migration due to insufficient soft tissue support [4, 5]. Surgeons mitigated these complications by moving the implant into the submuscular plane [4]. However, this method resulted in loss of shoulder mobility [6], pain [7], and animation deformity [8]. Acellular dermal matrices were introduced in 2001, allowing for coverage and support to the implant at the lower pole where coverage could not be achieved with the pectoralis major. This new technology mitigated the morbidity precluding previous attempts at subcutaneous reconstruction [9]. Aided by the proliferation of skin perfusion assessment technologies, prepectoral implant placement has become the standard for prosthetic breast reconstruction.

With the use of acellular dermal matrices, rates of skin flap necrosis and explantation are now similar in prepectoral and submuscular reconstruction [10]. Prepectoral reconstruction has a number of benefits over submuscular reconstruction, including improved shoulder mobility, reduced post-operative pain, and greater satisfaction with breast shape [6]. However, this technique creates unique challenges. Unlike submuscular or partial subpectoral placement, prepectoral placement results in an obvious step-off between the implant and chest wall. This is especially obvious at the upper pole, where there is a noticeable loss of the breast's "tear-drop" shape. Furthermore, relatively thin skin flaps are less

W. R. Moritz · H. Schott · M. Finnan · S. Chiang · A. Fotouhi · J. M. Sacks (✉)
Division of Plastic and Reconstructive Surgery, Department of Surgery, School of Medicine, Washington University, St. Louis, MO, USA
e-mail: moritzwr@wustl.edu; jmsacks@wustl.edu

H. Darrach · F. Kraenzlin · N. Khavanin · K. Chopra
Department of Plastic and Reconstructive Surgery, The Johns Hopkins University School of Medicine, Baltimore, MD, USA

© The Author(s), under exclusive license to Springer Nature Switzerland AG 2023
R. Vidya, H. Becker (eds.), *Prepectoral Breast Reconstruction*,
https://doi.org/10.1007/978-3-031-15590-1_21

adept at hiding contour irregularities and implant rippling [8]. Fat grafting remains the primary means for correcting these deformities. In 2016, autologous fat grafting was performed in 30% of all breast reconstructions over 30,000 patients [11]. While widely used and easy to perform, fat grafting has a high rate of complications, including high resorption rates, oil cyst formation, and fat necrosis/calcification [12]. Losken et al. [13] found that these complications were significantly more common in implant-based reconstruction than all other breast reconstructions. Postoperative volume retention rates at 140 days lie at 25–50% for small and large volume grafts, respectively [14].

Given the low rates of volume retention after autologous fat grafting, many patients require more than one attempt at fat grafting to correct deformities. However, the amount of available fat for grafting is limited, especially in thin patients [15]. For this reason, careful preoperative assessment and surgical planning are required before pursuing prepectoral alloplastic breast reconstruction.

21.2 Operative Technique

Autologous fat grafting has three goals: First, to correct contour irregularities created during mastectomy; second, to mask implant rippling visible through relatively thin tissue flaps; and third, to create a natural breast shape through volume augmentation (Fig. 21.1). Due to low volume retention rates, it is important to note that one procedure might not be adequate to correct all deformities. In our experience, patients receiving prepectoral reconstruction require greater volumes of grafted fat to correct deformities compared with those receiving submuscular or partial subpectoral reconstruction. Patients should be counseled that several procedures might be required to achieve their desired aesthetic results.

When offering prepectoral reconstruction, the first decision a surgeon must consider is the timing of autologous fat grafting. While it can be provided during initial tissue expander placement, many surgeons advocate a conservative approach, waiting until final volume is achieved and permanent implants are placed. This is for

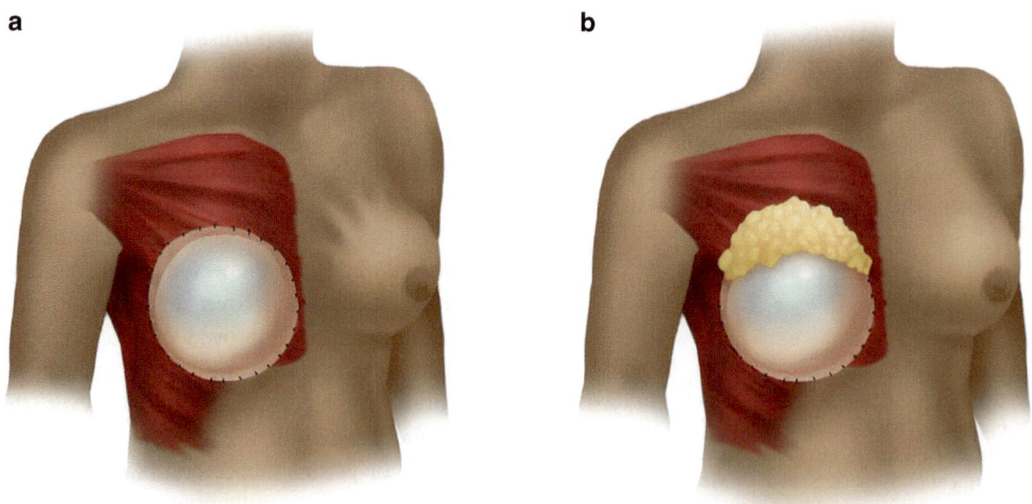

Fig. 21.1 (**a**) Prepectoral implant placement demonstrating "rippling" deformity. (**b**) Fat grafting to the superior pole can correct rippling deformity [60]. Reproduced with permission from AME publishing group

multiple reasons. First, it allows for definitive pathology to return after mastectomy. This will ensure that negative margins have been achieved, and a patient's treatment plan has been decided. Furthermore, delaying fat grafting until after permanent implant placement will allow for the patient to reach their ideal volume, revealing contour irregularities and areas of thin skin that must be corrected with volume augmentation. Finally, delaying fat grafting will avoid further compromise of the relatively thin tissue flaps for prepectoral reconstruction. In our preferred technique, upper pole contour irregularities are corrected first, while rippling deformities are corrected in secondary fat grafting procedures (Fig. 21.2). At our institution, we choose to perform initial fat grafting at the time of permanent implant placement. However, other surgeons may choose to delay the procedure even longer [16].

Proper evaluation of the patient is required to achieve the optimal aesthetic outcomes. In our experience, the contour irregularities following mastectomy are most apparent when the patient is standing. Preoperative marking of the patient should be performed while the patient is in the standing position, identifying areas in need of volume augmentation. Compared with submuscular and partial subpectoral reconstruction, we typically find that patients who have received prepectoral reconstruction require greater volume augmentation at the upper pole. Secondary goals should be considered when marking the patient. Additional fat can be harvested to augment certain areas of the breast, for instance, to build cleavage or improve projection at the intended nipple position. However, it is necessary that the aesthetic goals of the patient always guide these decisions. Implant rippling is typically addressed in secondary fat grafting procedures.

Preoperative planning also includes selection of lipoaspiration sites. Previous studies have found that the harvest location does not affect graft take or complications [17–19]. However, Ullman et al. [18] found that fat harvested from the thigh has greater structural integrity while fat taken from the abdomen demonstrates greater vascularity. Careful selection is necessary to avoid the creation of contour irregularities at the harvest site. At our institution, we typically select the flanks, abdomen, and thighs, depending on the available fat for harvest and patient preference, taking care to avoid reharvesting from previous lipoaspiration sites. Contour irregularities can be avoided by taking care to not excessively harvest from the superficial layer of fat and avoiding areas with high subcutaneous adherence, including the lateral gluteal depression, gluteal crease, distal posterior thigh, mid-medial thigh, and inferolateral iliotibial tract [20].

When infiltrating harvested fat, greater care must be taken in cases of prepectoral reconstruction. Thin tissue flaps offer limited protection to the implant and place it at risk for rupture by the

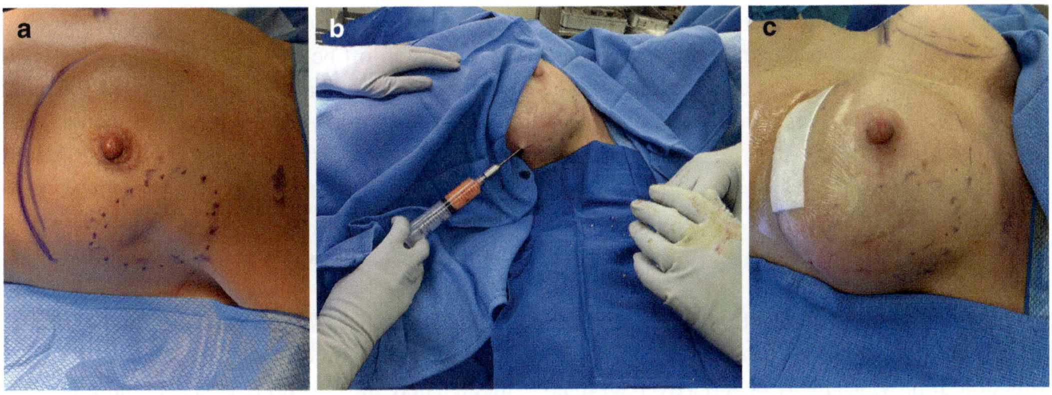

Fig. 21.2 (**a**) A patient exhibits contour irregularities at the time of permanent implant placement. (**b**, **c**) Fat is harvested from the abdomen and infiltrated at the upper pole, correcting the deformity and creating a natural breast shape

cannula or seeding from skin flora. It is our preference to use a second hand to protect the implant while placing harvested fat in the subcutaneous plane. It can also be tempting to account for high fat resorption rates and overcorrect deformities. However, we recommend against this. The thin skin flaps of prepectoral reconstruction are particularly sensitive to pressure necrosis, and excessive volume augmentation could place them at risk of complication. Further, overfilling can overload the native vasculature and result in significant or total graft loss [21].

The methods of fat harvesting and processing are an important consideration and have been areas of research for several years. Studies have found that the method of harvesting can impact cell viability. Hand-held syringe aspiration, suction-assisted lipectomy, and ultrasound-assisted lipectomy have all been found to result in varying rates of cellular survival [22–28]. Improving the number of stromal vascular fraction cells and adipose stem cells might improve graft survival and volume retention [29]. Recent animal studies have shown that processing fat on Telfa gauze might improve outcomes compared with centrifugation [30]. However, this technique might not be feasible in large volumes of lipoaspirate, and these findings have not been replicated in human trials [22, 29, 31, 32]. Mixing harvested fat with platelet-rich plasma has been studied with varying results. Salgarello et al. [33] found that use of platelet-rich plasma did not lead to a significant improvement in clinical outcomes among breast reconstruction patients. However, Gentile et al. [34] noted in 2013 that mixing transplanted fat and platelet-rich plasma resulted in an improvement of breast contour and volume retention after 1 year when compared with standard fat grafting.

21.3 Discussion

Prepectoral breast reconstruction has emerged as the most popular method of implant-based reconstruction. It provides many benefits over submuscular or partial subpectoral implant placement [5, 35–38]. It requires shorter operative times and is less invasive [39]. Further, without manipulation of pectoralis major, patients report less post-operative pain and muscle spasms [7, 38, 39]. Furthermore, the pectoralis major remains in its anatomical position, avoiding the loss of shoulder mobility [6] and animation deformity [40] associated with submuscular reconstruction.

Prepectoral reconstruction is not a new invention. Early alloplastic reconstruction relied on placement of the implants in the subcutaneous plane. However, without proper soft tissue support of the implant, patients experienced high rates of complications, including capsular contracture, skin flap necrosis, and implant descent and migration, requiring explantation. However, the development of acellular dermal matrices, new tissue expanders, and technologies for intraoperative flap perfusion assessment has provided surgeons with the tools to avoid these complications [39, 41–45].

Fat grafting is an important adjunct to all breast reconstruction. However, it is especially important in prepectoral reconstruction [37, 46]. Acellular dermal matrices typically serve as an internal corset in this technique, supporting the weight of the implant while also providing additional coverage to implant surface irregularities. While some surgeons may extend ADM coverage to encompass the entire implant [47], we prefer to limit coverage to the inferior pole, minimizing material cost and decreasing risk of capsular contracture. However, the relatively thin tissue flaps utilized in this technique poorly camouflage implant irregularities not covered by the ADM. Furthermore, patients will commonly notice a step-off between implant and chest wall. These aesthetic challenges can present a source of distress for many patients. Patients who receive prepectoral reconstruction report higher dissatisfaction with rippling deformity than those who receive subpectoral reconstruction [48]. However, concerns can be addressed with autologous fat grafting.

We typically offer all patients autologous fat grafting at the time of tissue expander replacement. There are several reasons behind this decision. First, it allows for negative margins to be verified by pathology. Second, it allows areas of thin skin and contour irregularities to declare themselves after the patient's ideal size has been achieved. Unfortunately, the thin tissue flaps utilized for prepectoral reconstruction limit the volume of fat that can be transferred at one time. For the majority of patients undergoing two-stage implant-based reconstruction, a single round of fat grafting is required. Only 15–18% of patients will require subsequent fat grafting procedures to correct irregularities [12, 37, 44]. However, patients who previously received radiotherapy may be more likely to require additional procedures [13]. At our institution, we always advise our patients that they might require multiple rounds of fat grafting to achieve their aesthetic goals.

Technical considerations to reduce the incidence of rippling in breast reconstruction have been reported [35, 39]. One such technique is underfilling the tissue expander so that the implant is placed in a tight pocket without excess skin [49]. Furthermore, careful selection of the implant could reduce the incidence of these defects; implants should be closely matched with the native breast width and filled to the outer shell's capacity [35]. Form stable gel implants may also reduce the incidence of rippling [35, 50–53] while overfilling saline implants might have a similar effect [49]. However, many patients may still require volume augmentation of the upper pole even in the absence of rippling.

Previously, fat grafting for alloplastic reconstruction was hindered by concerns that it could potentially interfere with early detection of cancer recurrence [54]. However, recent studies support that fat grafting is safe in this cohort. Petit et al. [12] found no evidence to suggest that lipofilling procedures can interfere with radiographic breast cancer detection. Delay et al. [55] reported similar findings after 10 years of follow-up of 734 procedures. Furthermore, Seth et al. [16] found that cancer recurrence and overall survival did not differ between patients who receive fat grafts and those who did not at long-term follow-up. However, fat grafting is associated with a number of complications and may require reoperation due to liponecrosis or oil cyst formation [12, 16, 55], particularly if patients receive regional radiotherapy [56].

Cosmesis and patient satisfaction are important outcomes for autologous fat grafting in cancer reconstruction. de Blacam et al. [57] reported improvement in volume, contour, placement, and superomedial fullness at a mean follow-up of 10.8 months. However, harvested fat is subject to a high degree of fat resorption. Choi et al. [14] reported that volume retention for large and small grafts after 140 days was 52 and 27%, respectively. For this reason, short-term cosmetic results may be impermanent, and long-term follow-up studies are required to adequately evaluate outcomes in this cohort. Long-term outcomes of fat grafting have yet to be widely studied in prepectoral breast reconstruction [35, 37–40, 43, 44, 47, 58]. However, recent studies appear to indicate good aesthetic results at long-term follow-up. Fat grafting was significantly associated with a reduction of rippling deformity in prepectoral reconstruction 1–3.5 years after reconstruction [53]. Furthermore, patients who receive autologous fat grafting report higher psychosocial and sexual well-being after implant-based reconstruction at a mean follow-up of 42 months [59]. However, no study to date has evaluated the complication rates within this cohort, and it is still unknown if thinner flaps result in different rates of graft survival, cyst formation, or fat necrosis. Nonetheless, autologous fat grafting remains an important adjunct to prepectoral breast reconstruction, allowing patients to achieve their optimum aesthetic outcomes.

21.4 Summary

- In prepectoral breast reconstruction, fat grafting can be used to correct contour irregularities, mask implant rippling, and create a natural breast shape.
- Post-operative volume retention rates at 140 days lie at 25–50% for small and large volume grafts, respectively. Several fat grafting procedures may be required to achieve desired aesthetic outcomes.

- We prefer to perform fat grafting at the time of permanent implant placement.
- Preoperative evaluation should occur with the patient standing, which allows contour irregularities to be most pronounced.
- Initial grafting procedures should address upper pole fullness, with secondary procedures to address implant rippling, cleavage building, and nipple projection.
- Flanks, abdomen, and thighs are ideal lipoaspiration sites. Surgeons should avoid the lateral gluteal depression, gluteal crease, distal posterior thigh, mid-medial thigh, and inferolateral iliotibial tract. Sites of previous lipoaspiration should also be avoided. Avoid extensively harvesting from the superficial layer of fat.
- Protect the implant with a second hand when infiltrating at the recipient site. This will help the surgeon avoid implant rupture.
- Avoid overfilling to improve fat volume retention. This can put the skin flaps at risk of pressure necrosis.
- Methods of fat processing is an ongoing area of research, although mixing lipoaspirated fat with platelet-rich plasma may improve volume retention rates.
- Future studies evaluating long-term aesthetic outcomes in fat grafting for breast reconstruction are necessary.

References

1. Albornoz CR, Bach PB, Mehrara BJ, et al. A paradigm shift in U.S. Breast reconstruction: increasing implant rates. Plast Reconstr Surg. 2013;131(1):15–23. https://doi.org/10.1097/PRS.0b013e3182729cde.
2. American Society of Plastics Surgeons. Plastic surgery statistics report. American Society of Plastic Surgeons; 2020. Published online 2020:1–26. http://scholar.google.com/scholar?hl=en&btnG=Search&q=intitle:Plastic+Surgery+Statistics+Report#1.
3. Nahabedian MY, Glasberg SB, Maxwell GP. Introduction to "prepectoral breast reconstruction". Plast Reconstr Surg. 2017;140(6S):4S–5S. https://doi.org/10.1097/PRS.0000000000004066.
4. Gruber RP, Kahn RA, Lash H, Master MR, Apfelberg D, Laub DR. Breast reconstruction following mastectomy: a comparison of submuscular and subcutaneous techniques. Plast Reconstr Surg. 1981;67(3):312–7.
5. Highton L, Johnson R, Kirwan C, Murphy J. Prepectoral implant-based breast reconstruction. Plast Reconstr Surg Glob Open. 2017;5(9):1–9. https://doi.org/10.1097/GOX.0000000000001488.
6. Caputo GG, Zingaretti N, Kiprianidis I, et al. Quality of life and early functional evaluation in direct-to-implant breast reconstruction after mastectomy: a comparative study between prepectoral versus dual-plane reconstruction. Clin Breast Cancer. 2021;21(4):344–51. https://doi.org/10.1016/j.clbc.2020.11.013.
7. Wallace MS, Wallace AM, Lee J, Dobke MK. Pain after breast surgery: a survey of 282 women. Pain. 1996;66(2):195–205. https://journals.lww.com/pain/Fulltext/1996/08000/Pain_after_breast_surgery__a_survey_of_282_women.12.aspx.
8. King CA, Bartholomew AJ, Sosin M, et al. A critical appraisal of late complications of prepectoral versus subpectoral breast reconstruction following nipple-sparing mastectomy. Ann Surg Oncol. 2021;28(13):9150–8. https://doi.org/10.1245/s10434-021-10085-z.
9. Basu CB, Leong M, Hicks MJ. Acellular cadaveric dermis decreases the inflammatory response in capsule formation in reconstructive breast surgery. Plast Reconstr Surg. 2010;126(6):1842–7. https://doi.org/10.1097/PRS.0b013e3181f44674.
10. Manrique OJ, Banuelos J, Abu-Ghname A, et al. Surgical outcomes of prepectoral versus subpectoral implant-based breast reconstruction in young women. Plast Reconstr Surg Glob Open. 2019;7(3):1–5. https://doi.org/10.1097/GOX.0000000000002119.
11. American Society of Plastic Surgeons. Plastic surgery statistics report. American Society of Plastic Surgeons; 2016. Published online 2016:1–25. https://www.plasticsurgery.org/documents/News/Statistics/2016/plastic-surgery-statistics-full-report-2016.pdf.
12. Petit JY, Lohsiriwat V, Clough KB, et al. The oncologic outcome and immediate surgical complications of lipofilling in breast cancer patients: a multicenter study-Milan-Paris-Lyon experience of 646 lipofilling procedures. Plastic Surgery Complete: The Clinical Masters of PRS-Breast Reconstruction. Published online 2015:14–19. https://doi.org/10.1097/PRS.0b013e31821e713c.
13. Losken A, Pinell XA, Sikoro K, Yezhelyev MV, Anderson E, Carlson GW. Autologous fat grafting in secondary breast reconstruction. Ann Plast Surg. 2011;66(5):518–22. https://doi.org/10.1097/SAP.0b013e3181fe9334.
14. Choi M, Small K, Levovitz C, Lee C, Fadl A, Karp NS. The volumetric analysis of fat graft survival in breast reconstruction. Plast Reconstr Surg. 2013;131(2):185–91. https://doi.org/10.1097/PRS.0b013e3182789b13.
15. Weichman KE, Broer PN, Thanik VD, et al. Patient-reported satisfaction and quality of life following breast reconstruction in thin patients: a comparison between microsurgical and prosthetic implant recipients. Plast Reconstr Surg. 2015;136(2):213–20. https://doi.org/10.1097/PRS.0000000000001418.

16. Seth AK, Hirsch EM, Kim JYS, Fine NA. Long-term outcomes following fat grafting in prosthetic breast reconstruction: a comparative analysis. Plast Reconstr Surg. 2012;130(5):984–90. https://doi.org/10.1097/PRS.0b013e318267d34d.
17. Small K, Choi M, Petruolo O, Lee C, Karp N. Is there an ideal donor site of fat for secondary breast reconstruction? Aesthet Surg J. 2014;34(4):545–50. https://doi.org/10.1177/1090820X14526751.
18. Ullmann Y, Shoshani O, Fodor A, et al. Searching for the favorable donor site for fat injection: in vivo study using the nude mice model. Dermatol Surg. 2005;31(10):1304–7. https://doi.org/10.1097/00042728-200510000-00007.
19. Li K, Gao J, Zhang Z, et al. Selection of donor site for fat grafting and cell isolation. Aesthet Plast Surg. 2013;37(1):153–8. https://doi.org/10.1007/s00266-012-9991-1.
20. Rohrich RJ, Smith PD, Marcantonio DR, Kenkel JM. The zones of adherence: role in minimizing and preventing contour deformities in liposuction. Plast Reconstr Surg. 2001;107(6):1562.
21. del Vecchio DA, del Vecchio SJ. The graft-to-capacity ratio: volumetric planning in large-volume fat transplantation. Plast Reconstr Surg. 2014;133(3):561–9. https://doi.org/10.1097/01.prs.0000438471.23249.6e.
22. Fisher C, Grahovac TL, Schafer ME, Shippert RD, Marra KG, Peter RJ. Comparison of harvest and processing techniques for fat grafting and adipose stem cell isolation. Plast Reconstr Surg. 2013;132(2):351–61. https://doi.org/10.1097/PRS.0b013e3182958796.
23. Smith P, Adams WP, Lipschitz AH, et al. Autologous human fat grafting: effect of harvesting and preparation techniques on adipocyte graft survival. Plast Reconstr Surg. 2006;117(6):1836–44. https://doi.org/10.1097/01.prs.0000218825.77014.78.
24. Keck M, Kober J, Riedl O, et al. Power assisted liposuction to obtain adipose-derived stem cells: impact on viability and differentiation to adipocytes in comparison to manual aspiration. J Plast Reconstr Aesthet Surg. 2014;67(1):e1. https://doi.org/10.1016/j.bjps.2013.08.019.
25. Lee JH, Kirkham JC, McCormack MC, Nicholls AM, Randolph MA, Austen WG. The effect of pressure and shear on autologous fat grafting. Plast Reconstr Surg. 2013;131(5):1125–36. https://doi.org/10.1097/PRS.0b013e3182879f4a.
26. Pu LLQ, Coleman SR, Cui X, Ferguson REH, Vasconez HC. Autologous fat grafts harvested and refined by the Coleman technique: a comparative study. Plast Reconstr Surg. 2008;122(3):932–7. https://doi.org/10.1097/PRS.0b013e3181811ff0.
27. Ochoa O, Robinson J, Beran SJ. Cosmetic comparative lipoplasty analysis of in vivo-treated adipose tissue. Plast Reconstr Surg. 2000;105:2152–8.
28. Crawford JL, Hubbard BA, Colbert SH, Puckett CL. Fine tuning lipoaspirate viability for fat grafting. Plast Reconstr Surg. 2010;126(4):1342–8. https://doi.org/10.1097/PRS.0b013e3181ea44a9.
29. Strong AL, Cederna PS, Rubin JP, Coleman SR, Levi B. The current state of fat grafting. Plast Reconstr Surg. 2015;136(4):897–912. https://doi.org/10.1097/prs.0000000000001590.
30. Canizares O, Thomson JE, Allen RJ, et al. The effect of processing technique on fat graft survival. Plast Reconstr Surg. 2017;140(5):933–43. https://doi.org/10.1097/PRS.0000000000003812.
31. Tuin AJ, Domerchie PN, Schepers RH, et al. What is the current optimal fat grafting processing technique? A systematic review. J Craniomaxillofac Surg. 2016;44(1):45–55. https://doi.org/10.1016/j.jcms.2015.10.021.
32. Cleveland EC, Albano NJ, Hazen A. Roll, spin, wash, or filter? Processing of lipoaspirate for autologous fat grafting: an updated, evidence-based review of the literature. Plast Reconstr Surg. 2015;136(4):706–13. https://doi.org/10.1097/PRS.0000000000001581.
33. Salgarello M, Visconti G, Rusciani A. Breast fat grafting with platelet-rich plasma: a comparative clinical study and current state of the art. Plast Reconstr Surg. 2011;127(6):2176–85. https://doi.org/10.1097/PRS.0b013e3182139fe7.
34. Gentile P, di Pasquali C, Bocchini I, et al. Breast reconstruction with autologous fat graft mixed with platelet-rich plasma. Surg Innov. 2013;20(4):370–6. https://doi.org/10.1177/1553350612458544.
35. Sbitany H. Important considerations for performing prepectoral breast reconstruction. Plast Reconstr Surg. 2017;140(6S):7S–13S. https://doi.org/10.1097/PRS.0000000000004045.
36. Snyderman RK, Guthrie RH. Reconstruction of the female breast following radical mastectomy. Plast Reconstr Surg. 1971;47(6):565–7.
37. Sbitany H, Piper M, Lentz R. Prepectoral breast reconstruction: a safe alternative to submuscular prosthetic reconstruction following nipple-sparing mastectomy. Plast Reconstr Surg. 2017;140(3):432–43. https://doi.org/10.1097/PRS.0000000000003627.
38. ter Louw RP, Nahabedian MY. Prepectoral breast reconstruction. Plast Reconstr Surg. 2017;140(5S):51S–9S. https://doi.org/10.1097/PRS.0000000000003942.
39. Sigalove S, Maxwell GP, Sigalove NM, et al. Prepectoral implant-based breast reconstruction: rationale, indications, and preliminary results. Plast Reconstr Surg. 2017;139(2):287–94. https://doi.org/10.1097/PRS.0000000000002950.
40. Jones G, Yoo A, King V, et al. Prepectoral immediate direct-to-implant breast reconstruction with anterior AlloDerm coverage. Plast Reconstr Surg. 2017;140(6S):31S–8S. https://doi.org/10.1097/PRS.0000000000004048.
41. Nahabedian MY. What are the long-term aesthetic issues in prepectoral breast reconstruction? Aesthet Surg J. 2020;40:S29–37. https://doi.org/10.1093/ASJ/SJAA164.
42. Wagner RD, Braun TL, Zhu H, Winocour S. A systematic review of complications in prepectoral

breast reconstruction. J Plast Reconstr Aesthet Surg. 2019;72(7):1051–9. https://doi.org/10.1016/j.bjps.2019.04.005.
43. Khavanin N, Gust MJ, Grant DW, Nguyen KT, Kim JYS. Tabbed tissue expanders improve breast symmetry scores in breast reconstruction. Arch Plast Surg. 2014;41(1):57–62. https://doi.org/10.5999/aps.2014.41.1.57.
44. Elswick SM, Harless CA, Bishop SN, et al. Prepectoral implant-based breast reconstruction with postmastectomy radiation therapy. Plast Reconstr Surg. 2018;142(1):1–12. https://doi.org/10.1097/PRS.0000000000004453.
45. Jordan SW, Khavanin N, Fine NA, Kim JYS. An algorithmic approach for selective acellular dermal matrix use in immediate two-stage breast reconstruction: indications and outcomes. Plast Reconstr Surg. 2014;134(2):178–88. https://doi.org/10.1097/PRS.0000000000000366.
46. Delay E, Guerid S. The role of fat grafting in breast reconstruction. Clin Plast Surg. 2015;42(3):315–23. https://doi.org/10.1016/j.cps.2015.03.003.
47. Reitsamer R, Peintinger F. Prepectoral implant placement and complete coverage with porcine acellular dermal matrix: a new technique for direct-to-implant breast reconstruction after nipple-sparing mastectomy. J Plast Reconstr Aesthet Surg. 2015;68(2):162–7. https://doi.org/10.1016/j.bjps.2014.10.012.
48. Baker BG, Irri R, Maccallum V, Chattopadhyay R, Murphy J, Harvey JR. A prospective comparison of short-term outcomes of subpectoral and prepectoral Strattice-based immediate breast reconstruction. Plast Reconstr Surg. 2018;141(5):1077–84. https://doi.org/10.1097/PRS.0000000000004270.
49. Graziano FD, Henderson PW, Jacobs J, Salzberg CA, Sbitany H. How to optimize prepectoral breast reconstruction. Aesthet Surg J. 2020;40:S22–8. https://doi.org/10.1093/asj/sjaa214.
50. Panettiere P, Marchetti L, Accorsi D. Soft cohesive silicone gel breast prostheses: a comparative prospective study of aesthetic results versus lower cohesivity silicone gel prostheses. J Plast Reconstr Aesthet Surg. 2007;60(5):482–9. https://doi.org/10.1016/j.bjps.2006.04.020.
51. Brown MH, Shenker R, Silver SA. Cohesive silicone gel breast implants in aesthetic and reconstructive breast surgery. Plast Reconstr Surg. 2005;116(3):768–79. https://doi.org/10.1097/01.prs.0000176259.66948.e7.
52. Cordeiro PG, McGuire P, Murphy DK. Natrelle 410 extra-full projection silicone breast implants: 2-year results from two prospective studies. Plast Reconstr Surg. 2015;136(4):638–46. https://doi.org/10.1097/PRS.0000000000001636.
53. Belmonte BM, Campbell CA. Safety profile and predictors of aesthetic outcomes after prepectoral breast reconstruction with meshed acellular dermal matrix. Ann Plast Surg. 2021;86(6S Suppl 5):S585–92. https://doi.org/10.1097/SAP.0000000000002764.
54. Riggio E, Bordoni D, Nava MB. Oncologic surveillance of breast cancer patients after lipofilling. Aesthet Plast Surg. 2013;37(4):728–35. https://doi.org/10.1007/s00266-013-0166-5.
55. Delay E, Garson S, Tousson G, Sinna R. Fat injection to the breast: technique, results, and indications based on 880 procedures over 10 years. Aesthet Surg J. 2009;29(5):360–76. https://doi.org/10.1016/j.asj.2009.08.010.
56. Rietjens M, de Lorenzi F, Rossetto F, et al. Safety of fat grafting in secondary breast reconstruction after cancer. J Plast Reconstr Aesthet Surg. 2011;64(4):477–83. https://doi.org/10.1016/j.bjps.2010.06.024.
57. de Blacam C, Momoh AO, Colakoglu S, Tobias AM, Lee BT. Evaluation of clinical outcomes and aesthetic results after autologous fat grafting for contour deformities of the reconstructed breast. Plast Reconstr Surg. 2011;128(5):411–8. https://doi.org/10.1097/PRS.0b013e31822b669f.
58. Hudson DA. Optimizing aesthetics with prosthetic prepectoral breast reconstruction. Plast Reconstr Surg. 2018;141(4):611e–2e. https://doi.org/10.1097/PRS.0000000000004206.
59. Le NK, Persing S, Dinis J, et al. A comparison of BREAST-Q scores between prepectoral and subpectoral direct-to-implant breast reconstruction. Plast Reconstr Surg. 2021;148(5):708e–14e. https://doi.org/10.1097/prs.0000000000008410.
60. Darrach H, Kraenzlin F, Khavanin N, Chopra K, Sacks JM. The role of fat grafting in prepectoral breast reconstruction. Gland Surg. 2019;8(1):61–6. https://doi.org/10.21037/gs.2018.10.09.

22 The LOTUS Pre-pectoral Breast Reconstruction

M. Asher Schusterman II and Robert D. Rehnke

22.1 Introduction

Breast reconstruction remains a primary competency for plastic surgeons. Over the last 50 years, the pendulum has swung from silicone implant-based reconstructions to autologous flaps (both pedicled and free tissue transplants), back to primarily implant-based approaches. This return has been motivated by limited financial resources and the recent evolution towards less destructive mastectomies—emphasizing preservation of the nipple-areola and soft tissue envelope. This evolution in mastectomy techniques has enabled significant improvement in implant-based reconstruction in the pre-pectoral plane. Our focus, for over 25 years, has been on understanding the anatomy of the superficial fascia system (SFS) [1]. It forms the boundaries of the corpus mammae, or breast gland, and guides a mastectomy aimed at removing the tissue containing all the lobular and ductal elements of ectodermal origin which are the source of breast carcinomas. This strategy achieves negative tumor margins while maintaining as much of the skin envelope and superficial fascia system (SFS) as is oncologically prudent. This journey has seen more precise mastectomy resections, rendered safe due to the importance of modern adjuvant therapies, such as radiation, hormonal therapy, cytotoxic chemotherapy, and targeted chemotherapy. We experienced a breakthrough, however, when we began reconstructing the circummammary ligament (CML) immediately following the mastectomy using an internal purse string suture. This significantly decreased the volume of tissue that needed to be replaced, which enabled primary reconstruction with autologous fat grafting alone. Immediate fat grafting, however, is limited by the surgical dead space left by removing the corpus mammae. In addition, it is difficult to achieve breast projection with fat grafting alone. We solved this problem by constructing a novel three-dimensional scaffold, composed of absorbable mesh, to fill the space and stent it against contracting/scaring forces. The biologic mesh becomes integrated into the patient's cellular and extracellular healing matrix during the next several weeks and months. Under microscopic H&E observation, the mesh becomes an engineered fascia of high cellularity consisting of fibroblasts, macrophages, dense collagen, and capillaries (Fig. 22.1). This then becomes the structural support and blood supply that supports adipogenesis and tissue ingrowth between the mesh subsegments, which are fostered by serial fat grafting sessions (Fig. 22.2). The place-

M. Asher Schusterman II
Institute for Reconstructive Surgery, Houston Methodist Willowbrook Hospital, Houston, TX, USA
e-mail: maschustermanii@houstonmethodist.org

R. D. Rehnke (✉)
Private Practice Plastic Surgery, St. Petersburg, FL, USA

The Center for Surgical Excellence, St. Petersburg, FL, USA

© The Author(s), under exclusive license to Springer Nature Switzerland AG 2023

R. Vidya, H. Becker (eds.), *Prepectoral Breast Reconstruction*,
https://doi.org/10.1007/978-3-031-15590-1_22

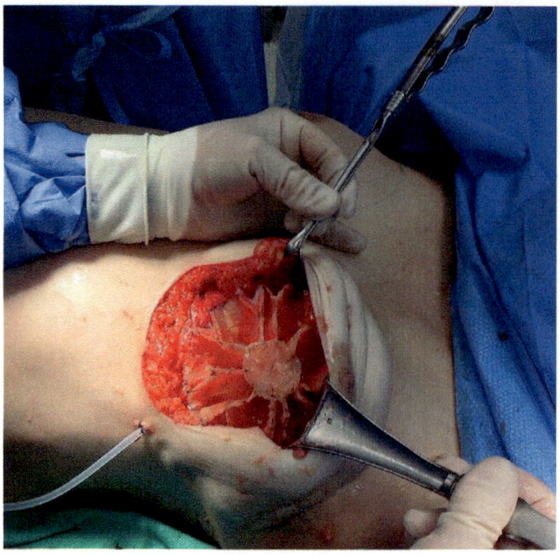

Fig. 22.1 Insertion of a 3-D, absorbable mesh scaffold, for immediate reconstruction of a skin and nipple-sparing mastectomy. The implant fills the dead space, created by the removal of the corpus mammae, and provides surface area for sequential fat grafting sessions, as it turns into an "engineered fascia" that provides projection to the reconstructed breast

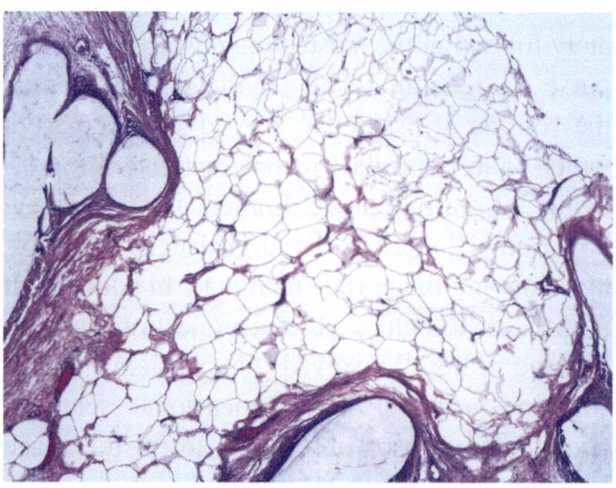

Fig. 22.2 H&E stain of a biopsy of a reconstructed breast, taken at 10 months post-implantation, showing a cellular ingrowth of fibroblast, collagen, and capillaries around the P4HB monofilaments, with mature adipose tissue between the segments of mesh

ment of the absorbable mesh implant, named the LOTUS and described in our 2020 paper [2], provides surface area, projection, and maintains a low tissue tension space—all of which is ideal for creating an in vivo bioengineering zone mimicking multiple geometrically designed modified tissue engineering chambers, which are fractal variants of the body's own SFS lobular fat units (Fig. 22.3). The tissue engineering chamber concept was described by Doldere, et al. in 2011 [3].

The clinical success we have experienced with the over 118 cases in the last 6 years promises to bring the quality of an autologous reconstruction, with the simplicity and low morbidity, of an implant reconstruction. This should make breast reconstruction, once again, a procedure performed by nearly all plastic surgeons, making access to quality care universal.

22.1.1 Minimally Invasive Mastectomy

For over 25 years, we have performed immediate breast reconstructions as a team comprised of general surgeon and plastic surgeon. The mastectomies began as skin-sparing mastectomy, with the peripheral borders of the dissection stopping at the fusion of the superficial fascia with the deep fascia of the chest wall, or circummammary ligament (Fig. 22.4). The three-dimensional corpus mammae, which again contains the lobular and ductal elements responsible for carcinomas of the breast, exists within this corpus lamina which is midway between the anterior and posterior superficial fascia layers. During puberty, breast development expands the corpus mammae and compresses the corpus lamina into an anterior capsule and posterior capsule of the corpus mammae. At the periphery of the breast gland, the corpus lamina fuses with the anterior and posterior layers, where it abruptly becomes a two-dimensional layer of fascia, within the circummammary ligament. Over the last five and a half years, we have refined our anatomically driven mastectomy technique, removing the gross anatomic breast gland with an intact capsule while preserving as much of the surrounding superficial fascia system as is possible.

This technique, which we have called a minimally invasive mastectomy, conceptually divides the breast dissection into two phases. Phase one is the resection of the sub-quadrant involved with the tumor, roughly 12.5–25% of the entire breast. In this sub-quadrant, we use any method neces-

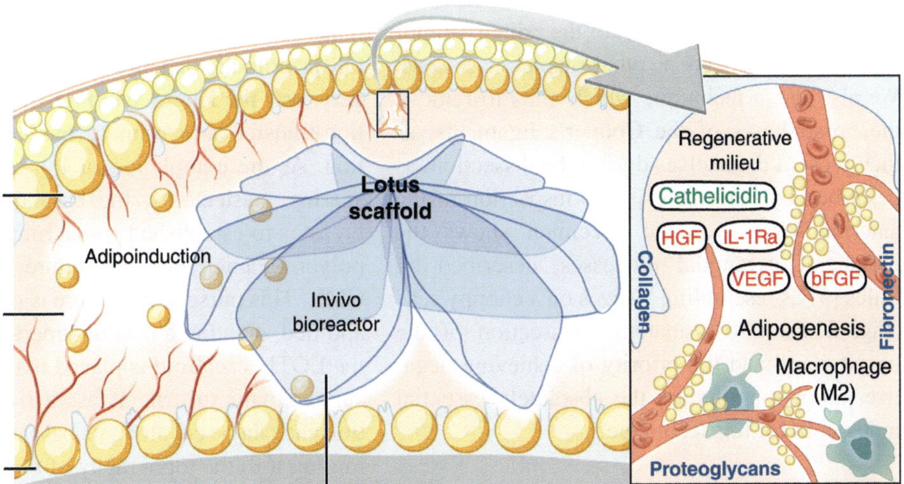

Fig. 22.3 Illustration of the multisegmented, open tissue engineering chambers, which are fanned out around central axis. The LOTUS implant is placed in the dead space created by removal of the corpus mammae and comes in direct contact with the remnants of the superficial fascia, whose capillary termini are the location of active adipogenesis. The inset shows growth factors that have been identified in the mesh peri-prosthetic fluid

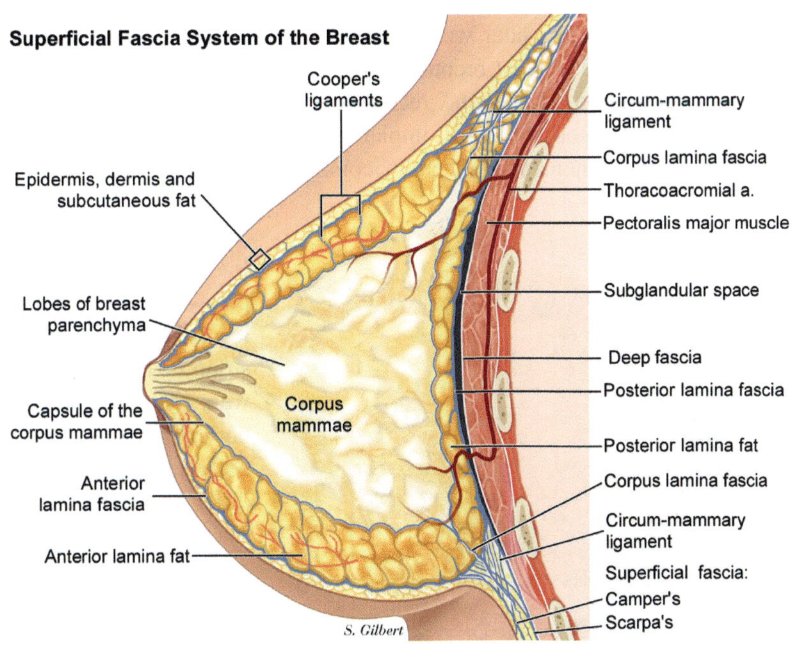

Fig. 22.4 Sagittal view of the breast illustrating the fusion of the superficial fascia layers to the deep fascia and chest wall in a zone of fascial fusion that make up the borders of the breast, which we have called the circummammary ligament

sary to achieve negative margins. For example, if the tumor is superficial, the overlying skin may be removed. If it is deep, a portion of the muscle below may be removed, and if the tumor is peripherally located, part of the circummammary ligament may be removed. Then, in phase two, which encompasses the remaining 75–87.5% of the breast, the intact corpus mammae is removed, sparing skin, muscle, nipple, and the superficial fascia system.

Preoperative imaging, including 3-D mammograms, ultrasound, and MRI, are essential in locating the sub-quadrant of the primary tumor and assuring there are no other suspicious lesions. We also use a technique which aims to remove the broad bases of the Cooper's ligaments, as they present themselves during the dissection, as described by Salibian [4]. The inspection of the anterior surface of the specimen shows the peripheral pyramidal processes, described by Stiles [5] as resembling "waves on a choppy sea" (Fig. 22.5). Gross anatomic dissection of the breast gland and the priority of achieving negative tumor margins are the absolutely essential motivators for this technique.

22.1.2 LOTUS Breast Reconstruction

In early 2015, we began using a bio-absorbable mesh scaffold, in place of silicone breast implants, for pre-pectoral immediate breast reconstructions following a minimally invasive mastectomy. Two years later we performed our first *delayed* LOTUS breast reconstructions following explantation of silicone reconstruction implants. These absorbable mesh implants were made from two-dimensional sheets of commercially available mesh. Our novel construction of a three-dimensional device from two-dimensional materials, made under sterile conditions in the OR prior to the patient entering the room for surgery, was the key to avoiding silicone and using lipo-transfer as a primary mode of reconstruction. At the completion of the skin- or nipple-sparing mastectomy, the base diameter of the breast is re-established with a running permanent polypropylene barbed suture through the CML. This purse string suture is placed, cinched, and tied, creating a nest of superficial fascia that the LOTUS scaffold is placed in (Fig. 22.6). It is sutured to the superficial fascia to anchor its position and can be cut along its base to facilitate contouring it to the topography of the chest wall. As opposed to silicone implants, which have no integration potential, the LOTUS attains complete cellular integration within the first 1–2 months post op. The mesh implants remain stiff but soften over time as the mesh dissolves. They are typically difficult to palpate after 3 years have passed.

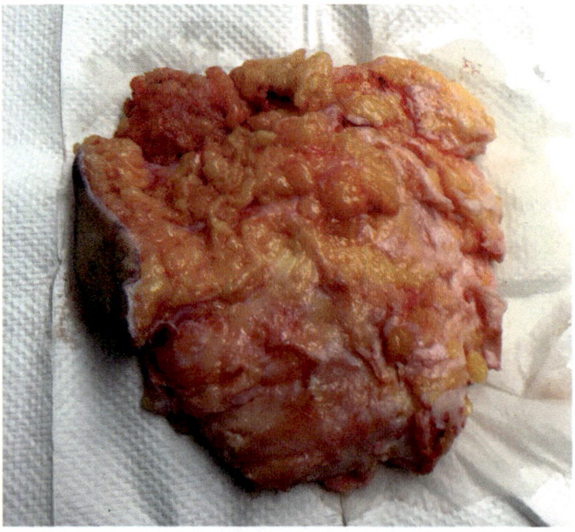

Fig. 22.5 Anterior view of a nipple-sparing mastectomy specimen, with skin of the upper outer quadrant, which overlies the tumor. Note the peripheral pyramidal processes at the surface, which are large vertical retinaculum or Cooper's ligaments

The implants are assembled from four or five 15 × 20-cm sheets of absorbable mesh, depending on the custom design for each breast. We have used three different products, TIGR Surgical Mesh (Novus Scientific PTE. Ltd., Singapore), SERI Surgical Scaffold (Allergan, Inc., Medford, Mass.), and Phasix Mesh (C.R. Bard, Inc./Davol Inc., Warwick, R.I.), which is fabricated from poly-4-hydroxybutyrate (P4HB), a biologically fermented product of a genetically modified strain of E. coli bacteria. The first three patients were reconstructed with TIGR and SERI mesh, but every patient since has had the P4HB product, which has been chosen for its superior handling characteristics and bio-compatibility [1]. The construction of the implants starts with assessment of the volume of the corpus mammae to be replaced, and the dimensions of the base diameter and projection of the breast in question. Mastectomy unhinges the tensegrity unit of the SFS, but the purse string placed through the CML re-establishes the tension of the skin and fascia system, which also exerts compression on the LOTUS. A smaller mesh implant can now be relied on to support the skin envelope and nipple-

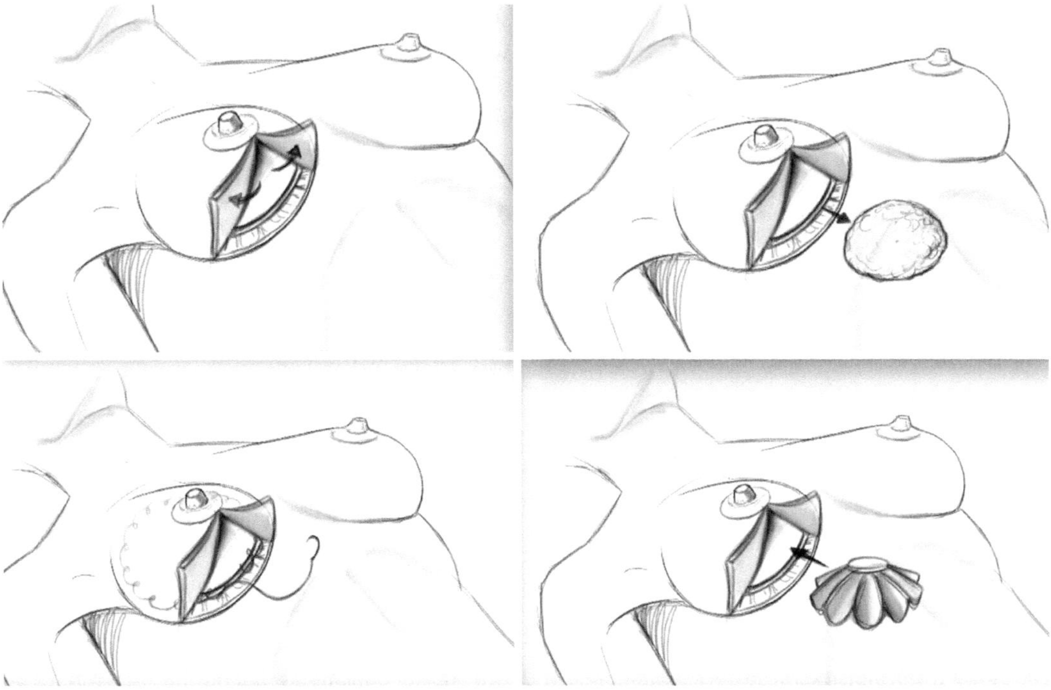

Fig. 22.6 Steps in an immediate LOTUS breast reconstruction: nipple-sparing mastectomy, through an inverted "T" or inframammary incision; purse string suture to cinch the circum-mammary ligament; insertion of a long-term absorbable mesh scaffold

areola complex as sequential fat grafting sessions are performed.

The construction of the three-dimensional pleated mesh surfaces are united by a stitch at the core; the segments of mesh fan out radially in the 12 positions of a clock, anchored peripherally to the circular base sheet of mesh, that is the diameter of the footprint of the breast. A smaller apical circular mesh sheet acts to anchor these segments, which radiate around this anterior dial, and is placed directly beneath the nipple-areola. The bi-polar cautery is used sterile, in a saline bath, to fuse adjacent mesh segments into multiple subsegments, thus creating a tensioned network of mesh similar to bubble wrap. The mesh provides the network of tension, and the spaces between the subsegments (which eventually fill with fat) are a discontinuous group of compressive elements. This classic tensegrity system is similar to the natural engineering of the superficial fascia system. The first month post-implantation shows rapid ingrowth of fibroblast, creating a cast of collagen fibers, macrophages, and lymphocytes, along with capillary vascularization which resembles native facia. The open segments between the mesh have ingrowth of adipose tissue, which is believed to come from the terminus of the capillaries supplying the SFS fat preserved at minimally invasive mastectomy [6]. Autologous fat grafting pushes this process forward as it is injected into this environment of in vivo bioreactors (Fig. 22.7). The mesh subsegments are multiple, partially open, tissue engineering chambers that are arranged radially around a central core. In the planning stages, one can estimate the volume the implant will generate from the equation for the volume of a hemisphere: $\frac{\frac{4}{3}\pi r^3}{2}$.

Fat grafting of autologous lipoaspirate is begun at 3–4 weeks post-implantation of the LOTUS scaffold, once cellular ingrowth has

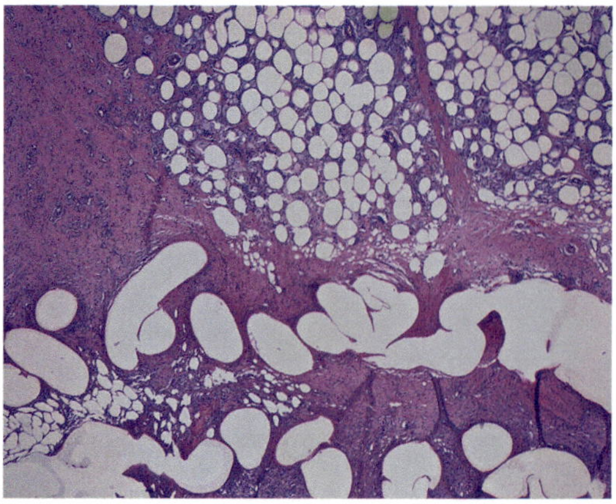

Fig. 22.7 H&E stains of LOTUS reconstruction showing fat grafted at the surface of the mesh scaffold has arranged itself into small lobules supported by small fascial septa

developed vascularity. Typically, a smaller volume of grafted fat is injected during the first session: subcutaneously, beneath the device along the chest wall, and finally into the segments of the implant. Larger volumes of fat grafting are anticipated at subsequent sessions, spaced 3–4 months apart, until the desired volume of healthy tissue is obtained. The typical patient has required two fat grafting procedures, in addition to the implantation of the LOTUS device at the time of mastectomy [2].

Pitfalls can develop if the skin envelope is too large and redundant or, conversely, too small and tight. The size and dimensions of the LOTUS implant should be chosen to prevent excessive soft tissue envelope contracture, which could lead to tight vertical retinaculum fibers and limit soft tissue envelope expansion during fat grafting. Tight vertical retinaculum can be treated with Rigottomy releases, using percutaneous, large-bore needles (14 g) to break up these attachments. Overly aggressive releases, however, can lead to bleeding and post-grafting fluid collections or seromas in the resulting dead space. Choosing the appropriate size implant and performing the first fat grafting session within the first 3–4 weeks after implantation avoid excessive contracture and and the need for excessive releases. On the other end of the spectrum, smaller skin/fascia envelopes, which are tight to begin with, need to be stented with a larger, more stable scaffold to prevent wound contracture that would make it difficult to expand with fat grafting. Again, reliable projection is virtually impossible to obtain with fat grafting alone.

22.2 Results

Since our first LOTUS absorbable mesh implant reconstruction, in February of 2015, we have 50 patients who had reconstruction following complete mastectomy for cancer (37 immediate and 13 delayed). 50 breasts had therapeutic mastectomies while 19 breasts were high risk for cancer development and underwent prophylactic mastectomies. This gave a total of 69 LOTUS reconstructions following mastectomy in 50 patients over a mean follow-up of 26 months.

The most serious adverse events were three local recurrence of cancer in the subcutaneous soft tissue envelope, diagnosed on follow-up physical exams in the clinic. This represents a 6% local regional recurrence (3/50 therapeutic mastectomies = 6%), with a mean follow-up time of 2 years and 2 months. Our clinic's historical reference (2008–2015), made up of 39 therapeutic skin and nipple-sparing mastectomies and immediate reconstruction using silicone implants, instead of absorbable mesh and fat grafting, was 7.69% local regional recurrence and mean follow-up of 7 years. This is similar to Gerber's reported experience with nipple-sparing mastectomy and traditional autologous flap reconstructions reported in 2009, where 60 index cases had a local recurrence rate of 11.7% at a mean follow-up of 8.4 years [7]. The higher recurrence rate of our historical series and Gerber's, compared to our LOTUS reconstruction experience, makes sense as the mean follow-up time was greater in these two groups. All three cases of recurrence, in our LOTUS reconstruction series, were in patients with high-risk cancers where, for various reasons, adjuvant therapy was not administered. Therefore, these cases were not totally unexpected events (Table 22.1).

The next most important adverse events were palpable masses found after fat grafting. A total of 11 breasts had palpable masses, all found on

Table 22.1 Local recurrence

Patient	Time to recurrence	Stage	Tumor	Adjuvant therapy			Nipple recurrence	Misc. information
				Chemo Rx	Hormone	Radiation		
5	1 year	Stage IA T1Nx	IDC Her2 Neu+	–	–	–	(–)	The index cancer was after bilateral lumpectomy and Radiation Rx. No adjuvant Herceptin prior to recurrence
23	1 year	Stage IA T1cNo	IDC ER+ 2 synchronous tumors at DX	–	+/–	–	(–)	ASA 3 BMI 40. Aborted attempt at Chemo. Stopped Hormone Rx prior to recurence
38	0.5 year	Stage IIB T2N0	IDC Triple-Neg Grade 3	–	–	–	(–)	Refused adjuvant Chemo and Radiation Rx. Had niece in her 30s who died of the same cancer

physical exam, which turned out to be oil cysts in 6 cases (8.7%) and fat necrosis in the remaining 5 cases (7.2%). Radiologic surveillance detected another 16 clinically silent oil cysts (23.2%) and 7 lesions determined radiologically to be fat necrosis (10.1%). All lesions were benign. A total of ten biopsies were performed (six open excisional biopsies in the office and four ultrasound guided biopsies in the radiology suite) for a biopsy rate of 14.5%. All ten biopsies showed benign findings, and the remaining lesions were deemed benign using radiologic criteria and then followed to establish stability. Of the breasts mentioned above, four (5.8%) had *macroscopic oil cysts* mixed with fat necrosis, which were each several centimeters in size and easily palpated on physical exam, but not visible to the naked eye. Three out of four were in the difficult situation of salvage of failed silicone reconstructions or post-op radiation. All other instances, of post-operative masses, were noticeable only on careful breast exam.

Other significant adverse events included post-op fluid collections in eight breasts (11.6%). Four of these occurred following minimally invasive mastectomy and LOTUS implantation and four were following subsequent fat grafting sessions. Three of these cases did not have drains placed at the time of mastectomy (we had explored the utility of allowing post-surgical exudate to come and go on its own without standard post-operative drains, since protein growth factors and anti-microbial proteins are known to be present in peri-prosthetic fluid). Six of the eight breasts had bacterial contamination of the seroma fluid as determined by cultures taken at the time of fluid drainage (only two breasts had clinical signs of cellulitis). All cases resolved with oral antibiotics. A seventh patient had a minor superficial infection/cellulitis of a fat injection site that resolved with oral antibiotics. Therefore, our rate of minor infection (resolving with oral antibiotics) was approximately 10% (7 of 69 breasts). There were no cases of major infection, or infection requiring readmission or intra-venous antibiotics.

There were two cases of partial nipple-areolar loss due to ischemia (both had simultaneous skin reduction procedures for ptosis), and a third due to resection for cancer involvement, for a rate of 4.3%. Of the six breasts that received radiation therapy, only one breast complication developed: chronic post-radiation telangiectasia. Anecdotally, radiation therapy made accumulation of fat more difficult, with radiation cases requiring twice as many sequential fat grafting sessions.

There were no instances of hematoma, mesh migration, capsular contracture, extrusion, mastectomy flap necrosis, explantation of the implant, or chronic pain associated with the LOTUS.

22.2.1 Recommended Post Reconstruction Surveillance

In this early experience with a new technique for breast reconstruction, oil cysts and fat necrosis were common complications, but only 6% of patients had cancer recurrence, all found on physical exam and diagnosed by excisional biopsy in the office. Ultrasound was best at diagnosing deeper masses suspected of being benign oil cysts or fat necrosis. As mentioned above, in four instances radiologic exams were equivocal, requiring needle biopsy.

22.2.2 Reconstruction Outcome Grading

We have only recently started using Breast Q surveys in the last year. Until more of this patient-oriented outcome data is available, we have had to rely on subjective grading. The four members of our office staff and the operating plastic surgeon, all familiar with the patients in the LOTUS series, evaluated the cosmetic outcomes. Of the 69 breasts reconstructed, one was lost to follow-up and 8 had not yet completed reconstruction. The remaining 60 were assigned a grade (A, B, C, D, F) to each outcome, and the results were tabulated and averaged. A grade of "A" was defined as a result where you could not tell that the operated breast from the unoperated breast, or in case of bilateral reconstructions you could not tell that the patient had any surgery. "B" grades were given to excellent results, but it was detectable that the patient had reconstruction. A "C" grade went to patients that would look good in clothes but did not have natural results without clothes. "D" grades went to poor, but acceptable reconstructive results. Patients who would have done better with no reconstruction and an external prothesis were given an "F". To help offset the inherent bias in a self-evaluation, we combine our results into three groups: (A + B), C, and (D + F). It is unlikely that any observer would confuse a result between A/B and D/F, but bias could assign more A grades and fewer F grades. It should also be noted that staff members were charged to be brutally honest in their grading, as the object of the exercise was to determine who got great results and who did not, so as to learn why and evolve the technique. (It turned out that the staff members were stricter graders than the operating surgeon). The resulting grade scores were A/B: 65%; C: 21%; D/F: 14%. This means that roughly 2 of every 3 patients had an excellent result. Most patients with a D/F score could have improved their grade had they opted for an additional fat grafting session.

22.2.3 Conclusions

The history of mastectomy, over the last 100 years, has been one of decreasing deformation and increased precision. This has naturally led to better breast reconstructions and enabled pre-pectoral breast reconstruction techniques. Emerging technologies in fat grafting have produced autologous reconstruction techniques without the morbidity of flap surgery. Our use of absorbable mesh scaffolds has allowed for immediate breast reconstruction, combined with serial fat grafting sessions, to achieve a natural breast, in as few as two fat grafting operations. In our hands this has been absent serious complications. All local recurrence of cancer has been in the immediate sub-dermal tissue and found easily with physical exam. Oil cysts and fat necrosis have been the most common complication, which in the majority of cases can be ruled benign on radiologic criteria; when in doubt, minimally invasive needle biopsy is performed. As the technique evolves, it is anticipated that other less common, but more serious complications of fluid collections and infections can be avoided by the development of best practices. This new technique holds the hope of a breast reconstruction with the natural results of autologous reconstructions and the simplicity of implant reconstructions. In this sense, it is a hybrid technique, using the best of each, in a novel approach.

References

1. Rehnke RD, Groening RM, Van Buskirk ER, Clarke JM. Anatomy of the superficial fascia system of the breast. Plast Reconstr Surg. 2018;142(5):1135–44.
2. Rehnke RD, Schusterman MA, Clarke JM, Price BC, Waheed U, Debski RE, Badylak SF, Rubin JP. Breast reconstruction using a three-dimensional absorbable mesh scaffold and autologous fat grafting. Plast Reconstr Surg. 2020;146(4):409e–13e.
3. Doldere JH, Thompson EW, Slavin J, et al. Long-term stability of adipose tissue generated from a vascularized pedicle fat flap inside a chamber. Plast Reconstr Surg. 2011;127:2283–92.
4. Salibian A, Harness JK, Mowlds DS. Staged suprapectoral expander/implant reconstruction. Plast Reconstr Surg. 2017;139(1):30–9. https://doi.org/10.1097/PRS.0000000002845.
5. Stiles H. The surgical anatomy of the breast and axillary lymphatic gland. Edinburgh: Oliver and Boyd; 1892. https://doi.org/10.1136/bmj.1.2007.1452.
6. Su X, Lyu Y, Wang W, et al. Fascia origin of adipose cells. Stem Cells. 2016;34:1407–19.
7. Gerber B, Krause A, Dieterich M, et al. The oncologic safety of skin sparing mastectomy with conservation of the nipple-areola complex and autologous reconstruction: an extended follow-up study. Ann Surg. 2009;249(3):461–8. https://doi.org/10.1097/sla.0b013e31819a044f.

Endoscopic-Assisted Nipple and Skin Sparing Mastectomy

23

Hung-Wen Lai and Chi Wei Mok

23.1 Introduction

Minimally invasive or minimal access breast surgery essentially described surgical techniques performed with the assistance of endoscopic instruments and more recently robotic surgical platform [1]. Key features of this technique revolve around adequate yet small incision(s) placed in inconspicuous or hidden areas leading to better aesthetic outcomes (Fig. 23.1), while not compromising on safety and allowing for immediate breast reconstruction to be performed through the same incision(s) [2–4]. The use of endoscopic instruments helps to improve visualization through better optics and thereby allowing for oncologic resection to take place through small incisions [5–7]. Endoscopic-assisted mastectomy was first performed and popularized in a few Asian countries [7–10], where the clear advantage seemed to be improved aesthetic outcomes for women with small breasts in whom a breast conserving surgery results in poor aesthetic outcomes as well as the risk of inadequate resection or margin involvement. There were multiple studies reporting on the technical feasibility, aesthetic and safety outcomes of the technique over the years [7, 8, 11–15] but it has yet to become the mainstream or standard in the surgical management of breast cancer. Possible reason for this includes the lack of long-term follow-up data to establish oncologic safety in terms of loco-regional and distant recurrence as well as disease survival outcomes data. In addition, patient selection and suitability may be another factor on why endoscopic-assisted surgery was not routinely offered and established as standard of care. This chapter aims to shed some light on the technique of endoscopic-assisted nipple or skin sparing mastectomy in the management of breast cancer. Figure 23.1 illustrated various photos and graphic illustrations for nipple sparing mastectomies (NSM), including conventional, endoscopic, and robotic assisted NSM.

H.-W. Lai (✉)
Endoscopic and Oncoplastic Breast Surgery Center, Changhua, Taiwan

Comprehensive Breast Cancer Center, Changhua, Taiwan

Minimal Invasive Surgery Research Center, Changhua Christian Hospital, Changhua, Taiwan

Kaohsiung Medical University, Kaohsiung, Taiwan
e-mail: 143809@cch.org.tw

C. W. Mok
Division of Breast Surgery, Department of Surgery, Changi General Hospital, Singapore, Singapore

Singhealth Duke-NUS Breast Centre, Singapore, Singapore
e-mail: mok.chi.wei@singhealth.com.sg

© The Author(s), under exclusive license to Springer Nature Switzerland AG 2023

R. Vidya, H. Becker (eds.), *Prepectoral Breast Reconstruction*,
https://doi.org/10.1007/978-3-031-15590-1_23

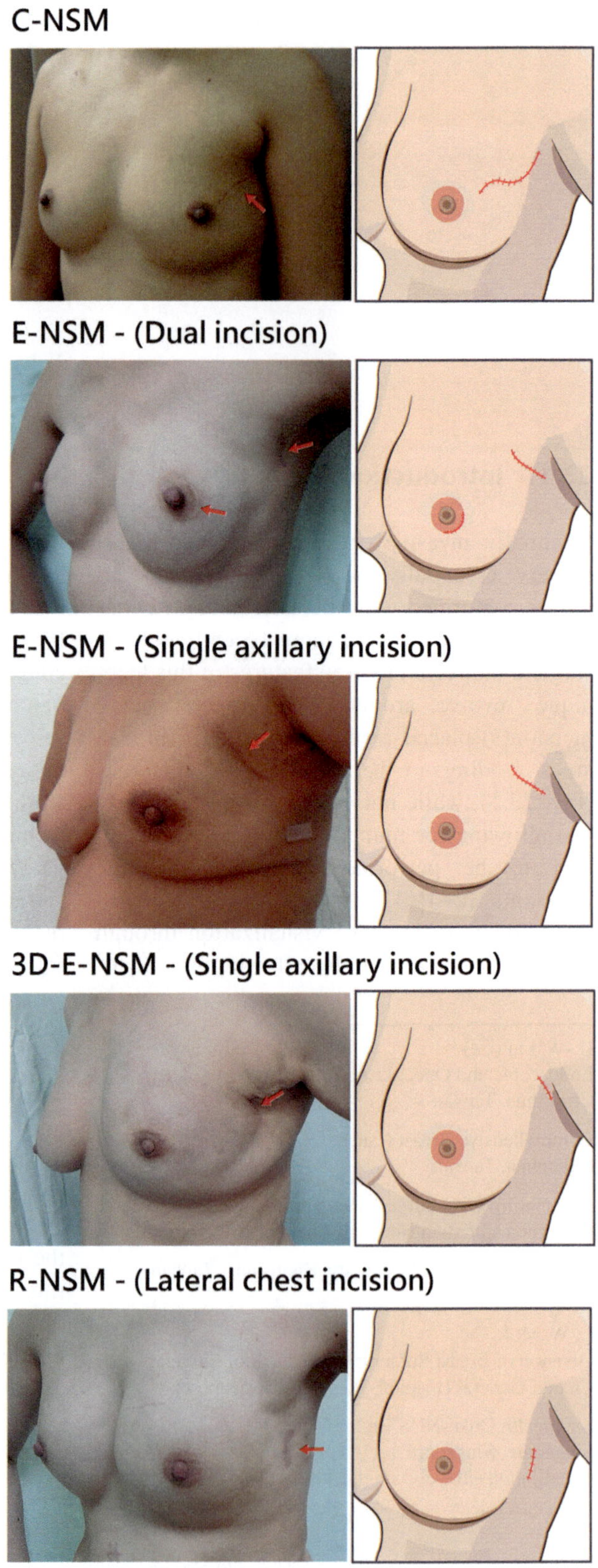

Fig. 23.1 Different operations methods and related wound incisions. *C-NSM* conventional nipple sparing mastectomy, *E-NSM* endoscopic-assisted nipple sparing mastectomy, *3D-E-NSM* single port 3-dimensional videoscope assisted endoscopic nipple sparing mastectomy, *R-NSM* robotic-assisted nipple sparing mastectomy

23.2 Detailed Technique Description [16]

23.2.1 Positioning and Sentinel Lymph Node Biopsy

Positioning of patients was done in a supine position with ipsilateral arms placed at 90° out on an arm board. In patients requiring sentinel lymph node biopsy (SLNB), single or dual modality utilizing Tc99m and/or methylene blue dye could be used. A small amount (2–3 mCi) of radioisotope Tc99m was injected intradermally before operation (either on the day or 1 day prior). After injection of the blue dye, a handheld gamma probe was used to identify any hot spots and thereafter the location of the hottest nodes were then marked. In cases where dual modality is used, approximately 2–3 mL of diluted 1% methylene blue (Merck, Darmstadt, Germany) was injected into areolar region (subdermal plane) in equally divided aliquot.

23.2.2 Skin Incision for E-NSM

In terms of skin incision, placement can be in the axilla or lateral chest wall as a single or dual incision depending on the nature of op and need for axillary staging procedure. Dual axillary-areolar or axillary-inframammary incision could be alternative choices (Fig. 23.2). Incision length was usually 3–6 cm, and this was determined by the size of the breast. After axillary incision, axillary staging procedure was performed as indicated and complete axillary lymph node dissection (ALND) up to level II could be done before or after mastectomy in the event of positive frozen section analysis.

23.2.3 Posterior Plane Dissection

After completion of axillary staging procedure, dissection started out from the lateral border of the pectoralis major muscle. The margin between pectoralis muscle and parenchyma was clearly identified. With the use of an endoscopic Ultra Retractor vein harvester (Karl Storz or Johnson & Johnson KK, Fig. 23.3), the pectoral muscle fascia was dissected off posterior portion of breast parenchyma. Adequate hemostasis was ensured with electrocauterization or other energy devices (bipolar scissor or harmonic scalpel). In order to create adequate working space, counter traction was applied by retracting surrounding tissue with the Ultra Retractor under endoscopic guidance and a suction tube can be used to evacuate mist and smoke. Common instruments used in endoscopic-assisted breast surgeries were shown in Fig. 23.3.

23.2.4 Skin Flap Dissection

A solution containing lidocaine 0.05% and epinephrine 1:1,000,000 was injected subcutaneously into the whole breast to help with analgesia, hemostasis, and plane dissection. An approximately 3–5 mm thick skin flap was created via skin flap tunnelling method from axillary or lateral chest wound. When dual incisions were used, a semi-circular peri-areolar skin incision or inframammary incision (3–4 cm) was made depending on surgeon's preference. Skin flap tunnelling method can be performed with an optical trocar Xcel (Johnson & Johnson, Tokyo, Japan, Fig. 23.3) under endoscopic guidance or palpation guided with a Metzenbaum scissor. Operation techniques were illustrated in Fig. 23.4.

23.2.5 Single Port Air Inflation or Retraction Type E-NSM

In retraction type E-NSM, the septa between skin flap and parenchyma was dissected and taken off under endoscopic guidance using endoscissors, bipolar scissors, or a harmonic scalpel. In inflation type E-NSM, a single port was inserted from

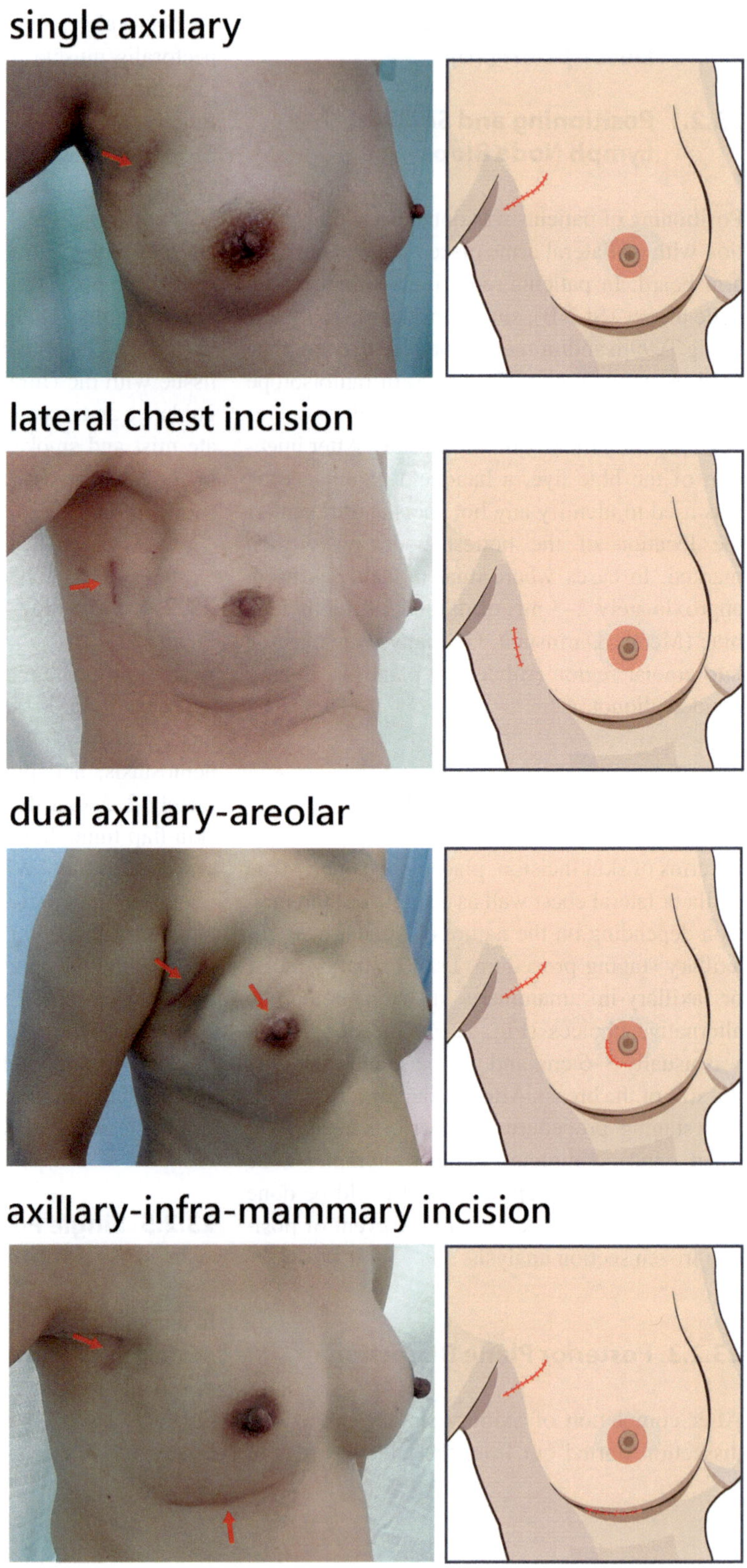

Fig. 23.2 Different incisions used for endoscopic-assisted nipple sparing mastectomies

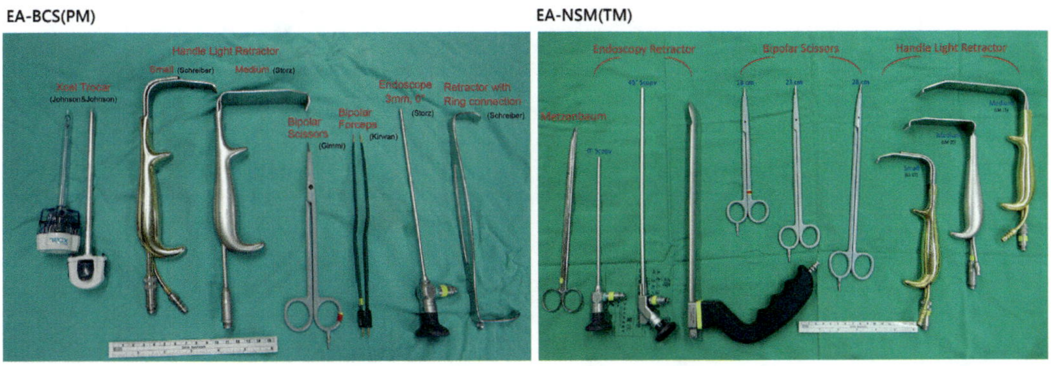

Fig. 23.3 Common instruments used for endoscopic-assisted breast surgeries. *EA-BCS* endoscopic-assisted breast conserving surgery, *PM* partial mastectomy, *EA-NSM* endoscopic-assisted nipple sparing mastectomy, *TM* total mastectomy

the axillary or lateral chest wound. Thereafter, carbon dioxide inflation was performed with the pressure set at 8–10 mmHg (Fig. 23.5). Single port air inflation would provide more space for dissection and facilitate the NSM procedure. 3D videoscope could be used to enhance the depth perception and the authors found it to be valuable in endoscopic-assisted nipple sparing mastectomy [16]. Figure 23.5 illustrated operations techniques of single port 3D E-NSM.

23.2.6 Sub-nipple Biopsy

Following skin flap development, a sub-nipple biopsy and fresh frozen section analysis could be performed in case of nipple sparing mastectomy (Fig. 23.4). If cancer involvement was found in the sub-nipple area, the nipple was removed and conversion to a skin sparing mastectomy was performed instead. After completion of skin flap development as well as detaching the breast off the pectoralis major fascia and peripheral attachment, the entire breast specimen could be removed via the axillary or peri-areolar incisions (Fig. 23.4).

23.2.7 Subpectoral Prothesis Breast Reconstruction

Following removal of the specimen, copious irrigation of the mastectomy pocket was performed with saline or iodine. Subsequently, the lateral border of the pectoralis major muscle was raised for submuscular pocket dissection. Dissection was performed medially towards the sternal border, taking care not to injure the perforator vessels. Inferiorly, the dissection was carried out beyond the inframammary fold over the lateral aspect, below which the muscle was released to continue the dissection to the subcutaneous plane thus allowing for a more natural placement of the implant (Fig. 23.4). In the lateral border, the superficial fascia of the serratus anterior muscle was dissected posteriorly such that it was just enough to accommodate the lateral border of the implant. Prothesis implant was then placed and followed with drains placement in both submuscular and subcutaneous planes. Care was taken when tagging the free muscle edges laterally to ensure adequate implant coverage.

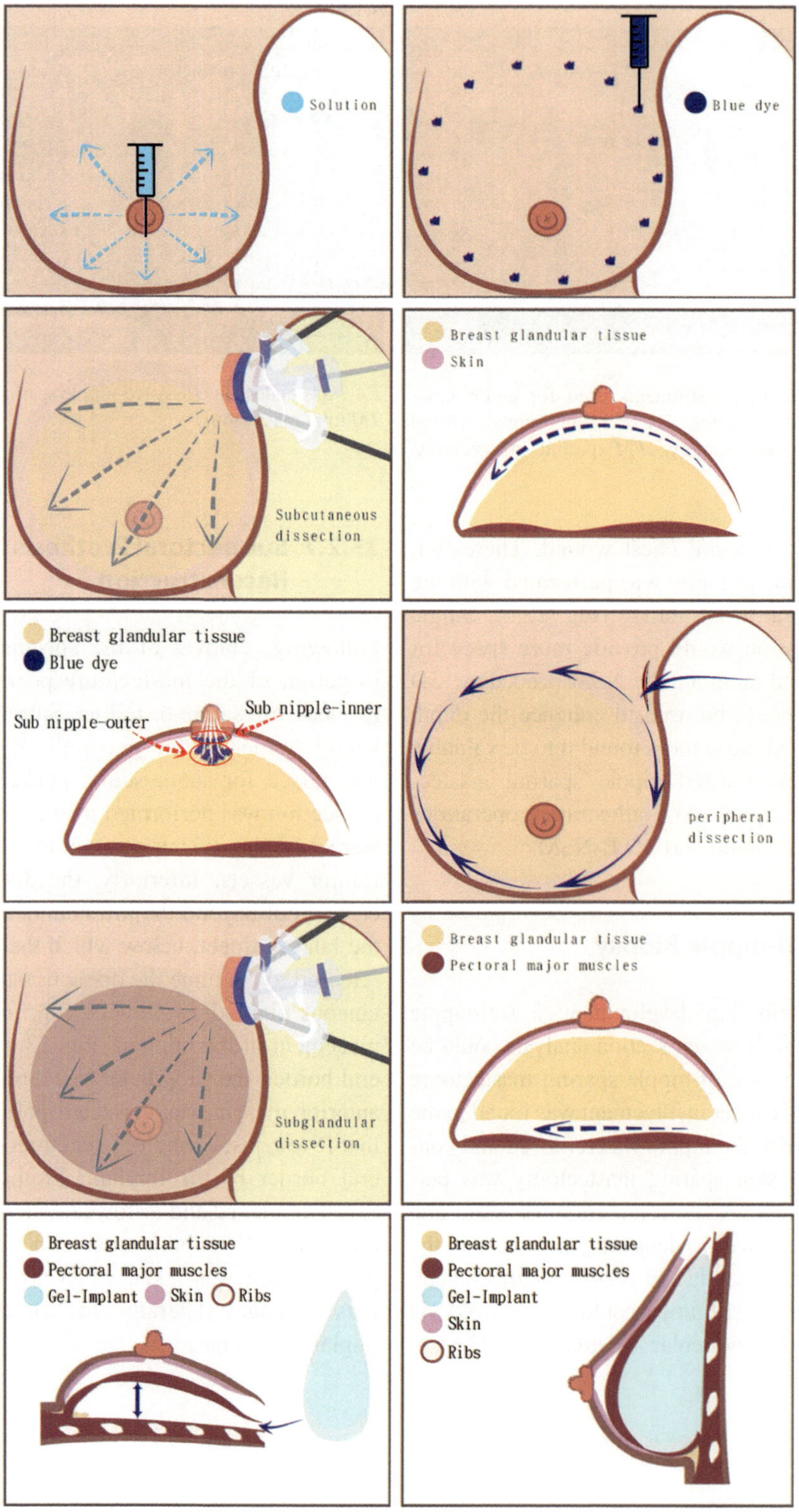

Fig. 23.4 Operative techniques of single axillary incision endoscopic-assisted nipple sparing mastectomy with immediate gel implant reconstruction were illustrated with cartoons

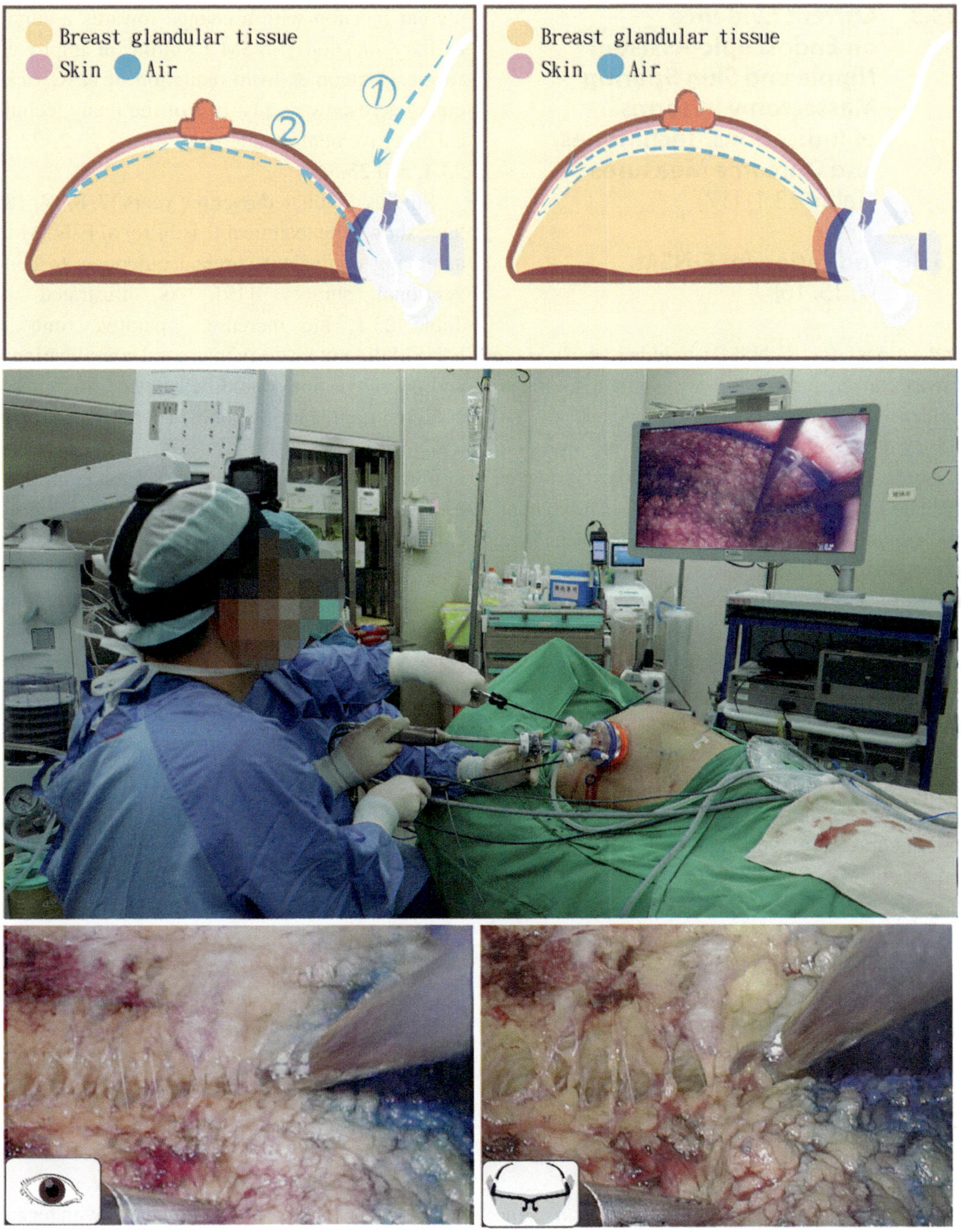

Fig. 23.5 Concepts and operative procedures of single port 3-dimensional videoscope assisted endoscopic nipple sparing mastectomy (3D-E-NSM) were illustrated with photos and cartoons

23.3 Current Evidence on Endoscopic-Assisted Nipple and Skin Sparing Mastectomy in Terms of Indications, Techniques, and Outcome Measures (Table 23.1) [17]

23.3.1 Indication for E-NSM [7, 15, 16]

Indications for E-NSM included early-stage breast cancer, tumor size of less than 5 cm, no evidence of multiple lymph node metastases, and no evidence of skin or chest wall invasion. Patients for whom E-NSM was contraindicated included those with apparent NAC involvement, inflammatory breast cancer, breast cancer with chest wall or skin invasion, locally advanced breast cancer, breast cancer with extensive axillary lymph node metastasis (stage IIIB or later), and patients with severe co-morbid conditions, such as heart disease, renal failure, liver dysfunction, and poor performance status.

With regard to breast size and shape, the ideal candidates were patients with small to medium size, none to mildly ptotic breast. In terms of breast cup size, recommendations were made for breast cup size C and below. Women with breast cup size larger than E or breast mastectomy weight >600 g and ptotic breast were not good candidates for E-NSM and immediate gel implant breast reconstruction due to technical difficulty and sub-optimal cosmetic outcomes.

23.3.2 Technique Refinements of E-NSM

Over the years, changes in techniques such as the use of insufflation in place of retraction for improved visualization and sparing of peri-areolar incision with a change towards a single axillary incision E-NSM resulting in improved surgical outcomes from reduction of NAC ischemia/necrosis were just two of the many technical improvements made (Figs. 23.1, 23.2, 23.3, 23.4, and 23.5).

Studies conducted over the years [7, 8, 14, 18] have shown the technical feasibility of E-NSM in achieving equivalent surgical outcomes to conventional surgery [19]. As illustrated in Table 23.1, the increased operative time in E-NSM did not result in increased complications, and operative time could be reduced after overcoming initial learning curve. There was not clinically or statistically significant increase in terms of intra-operative blood loss. Common complications associated with E-NSM were similar to conventional techniques and include skin flap or nipple necrosis and this could be attributed to the skin flap thickness and therefore blood supply to the flap especially in cases where the dermis was exposed. Studies using tumescent for skin flap reported ease of dissection and maintenance of adequate skin flap thickness.

23.3.3 Aesthetic Outcome

In terms of aesthetic outcomes and patient satisfaction assessment, most patients were regarded as being satisfied with the cosmesis especially in terms of scar placement and length of skin incision (Figs. 23.1 and 23.2). However, most of the assessments were done at about 3–6 months after operation and perhaps a repeat assessment should be performed at approximately 2–3 years after the initial operation such that remodelling of breast parenchyma would have been completed and in cases where adjuvant radiotherapy is required. Details on each of the studies especially with regard to recurrence, conversion or complications rate had previously been reported in a review article [20].

Table 23.1 Current evidence of cohort studies and selected case series on endoscopic-assisted vs conventional nipple sparing mastectomy

No	Author	Year of publication	Number of patients/ breasts treated	Operative method	Average operation time (minutes, range or ± SD)	Intra-operative blood loss (mL or g)	Margin positive, *n* (%)	Complications, *n* (%)	Follow up (months)	Local recurrence	Distant metastases	Death
1	Kitamura et al [11]	2002	20/21	E-NSM	237 ± 60	356 ± 286 g	1 (4.8)	Prosthesis related complications: 1(4.8)	19.2 ± 9.8 (5.8–35.2)	No data	No data	0%
			24/25	C-NSM	176 ± 32	189 ± 72 g	2 (8.0)	Prosthesis related complications: 3(12.0)	No data	No data	No data	0%
2	Fan et al [12]	2009	43	E-NSM	168 ± 32	115 ± 44	0%	Nipple or skin flap necrosis: 5 (11.6)	16.9 ± 11.2	0%	0%	0%
			54	C-BCS	139 ± 37	102 ± 48	0%	Seroma: 6 (11.1)	20.1 ± 11.9	5.9%	0%	1.9%
3	Wang et al [8]	2016	24	E-NSM	BCS + SNB: 102.38 ± 28.8; BCS + Ax: 122.49 ± 40.5	No data	10.6% (85/681)	No data	12	0.3% (2/681)	No data	No data
			25	C-NSM	69 [55–104]	45 [10–80]	28.3% (17/60)	Mesh infection: 11.7% (7/60)	No data	No data	No data	No data
4	Wang et al [13]	2017	30	E-NSM		No data	No data	No data	27.77 ± 20.43	No data	No data	No data
			30	C-NSM		No data	No data	No data	43.22 ± 19.80	No data	No data	No data
5	Du et al [14]	2017	157	E-NSM	197	95 mL	No data	Infection: 5 (3.18); Skin edge necrosis: 11 (7.01); Lymphedema: 15 (9.55)	74 (52–111)	0%	4.5%	3.2%
			189	C-BCS	165	83 mL	No data	Infection: 8 (4.23); Skin edge necrosis: 16 (8.46); Lymphedema: 23 (12.16)	No data	3.2%	1.6%	3.2%
6	Lai et al [15]	2016	269	E-NSM/ E-SSM	282 ± 161 (65–1310)	104.5 ± 74.9 (20–650)	1.1% (3/269)	Overall: 15.2% (48/315)	26.8 (3.3–68.6)	1.1% (3/269)	No data	0.4% (1/269)
7	Lai et al [16]	2018	50	E-NSM	244.3 ± 82.8 (138–425)	74.5 ± 47.7 (25–250)	0%	6% (3/50: Nipple partial ischemia: 2%, Seroma formation: 4%)	21.6 ± 11.3 (1–42.4)	0%	0%	0%

E-NSM Endoscopic assisted nipple sparing mastectomy, *E-SSM* Endoscopic assisted skin sparing mastectomy, *C-NSM* Conventional nipple sparing mastectomy, *C-BCS* Conventional breast conserving surgery, *BCS* Breast conserving surgery, *SNB* Sentinel lymph node biopsy, *Ax* axillary lymph node dissection

23.4 Discussion

23.4.1 Dual Incision

Since the first case report in 2001 [2], endoscopic breast surgery has evolved and new techniques or advancement have been made over the last 20 years. Conventional endoscopic nipple sparing mastectomy (E-NSM) techniques started with two separate small incisions over the axilla and peri-areolar region (Fig. 23.2). The axilla incision is used for axillary staging procedure and endoscopic vein retractor harvesting, dissection, and separation of breast parenchyma from pectoralis muscle fascia. After complete dissection at the posterior aspect, a small peri-areolar wound is then created for dissection of septa between the breast parenchyma and skin flap. Mastectomy specimen is then removed from either the peri-areolar or axillary incision. The resulting scar will normally be fairly inconspicuous as they are hidden in the axilla or peri-areolar region. However, one of the commonly seen complications resulting from the peri-areolar incision would be NAC ischemia or necrosis which can be devastating, especially in cases of implant reconstruction whereby any secondary infection could be disastrous leading to possible implant removal.

23.4.2 Single Axillary Incision Hybrid E-NSM [15]

To reduce the risk of NAC ischemia/necrosis, the authors developed a new technique which utilized a single axillary incision and demonstrated improved outcome in terms of NAC ischemia or necrosis (Figs. 23.2 and 23.4). This technique paved the way for a new trend of single axillary incision endoscopic mastectomy. To prevent surgical margin involvement and inadequate tumor resection, patient selection for single axillary incision hybrid E-NSM is favored in selected patients with tumors located in the upper outer quadrant and at an adequate distance from the skin. In large and ptotic breast, dual axillary-inframammary fold (IMF) incisions might be a good alternative whereby the scar is normally well hidden in the IMF (Fig. 23.2). The authors recommend a single axillary incision endoscopic hybrid technique NSM for women diagnosed with early-stage, clinically node-negative breast cancer indicated for mastectomy, with small to medium-sized breast and minimal ptosis.

23.4.3 Insufflation Technique [6, 15, 16]

Single axillary incision hybrid E-NSM was promising especially with regard to the lower risk of NAC necrosis. It was, however, technically challenging and demanding to perform the surgery with limited space and visualization. Once again, the authors drew from their vast experience in gasless endoscopic breast surgery to find yet another solution to this problem with insufflation. The use of insufflation in endoscopic breast surgery marked another milestone in terms of technique development as insufflation greatly increased the operative space as well as visualization (Fig. 23.5). In addition, insufflation also helped with plane dissection and hemostasis.

23.4.4 3-Dimensional (3D) Imaging [16]

3D imaging, which was a technical innovation in endoscopic and laparoscopic surgery, had been shown to enhance depth perception and thereby facilitate operations. We found that the adoption of a single port air insufflation system and 3D videoscope (Fig. 23.5) decreased the technical difficulty of conventional 2D single incision/access E-NSM. Our preliminary experience with this technique has shown promising results with excellent aesthetic outcomes and short learning curve.

23.4.5 Other Advancements in Endoscopic-Assisted Breast Surgery: Robotic-Assisted Nipple Sparing Mastectomy

Other than 3D imaging, the next revolutionary and potential practice changing advancements in endoscopic breast surgery would be the advent of robotic-assisted mastectomy. Robotic-assisted surgery, on the other hand, incorporated 3-dimensional imaging system and offered the flexibility of robotic arms as well as instruments with high degree of motion had been increasingly used in different field of surgeries. Robotic-assisted nipple sparing mastectomy (R-NSM), which introduced the da Vinci surgical platform through a small axillary wound for the conduct of NSM with (or without) immediate prothesis breast reconstructions (Fig. 23.6) was reported to have the potential to overcome the technical difficulty of E-NSM and showed promising aesthetic outcomes [21–24]. In addition, there were also a few studies exploring the use of robotic platform in immediate autologous breast reconstruction [24–26]. The advantages reported in all the studies were similar and that include better visualization with 3-dimensional (3D) optics and improved ergonomics from instruments with high degree of freedom of movement. The three main disadvantages of this technique were attributed to prolonged operative time, increased cost as well as availability of robotic surgical platform [27, 28]. A consensus statement of robotic mastectomy had been published recently from pioneers of robotic breast surgeries [29], and the indications, contraindications, technique, and cautions for the use of R-NSM were clearly described.

23.4.6 Implant Reconstruction with Endoscopic-Assisted Mastectomy: Subpectoral vs Pre-pectoral Implant Placement

In almost all studies of endoscopic-assisted mastectomy, the main modality of choice for immediate reconstruction would be the use of implant/breast prothesis. Subpectoral pocket placement of implant (Figs. 23.4 and 23.6) remained the most common method with or without the use of acellular dermal matrix (ADM) to provide additional implant coverage over the inferolateral aspect. There has been increasing number of studies exploring the use of pre-pectoral implant placement with a few utilizing ADM/synthetic mesh as a complete wrap [30, 31]. This technique is promising as it is postulated to significantly reduce the operative time if compared to subpectoral pocket placement without compromise to implant exposure/infection should there be skin flap necrosis. E-NSM or R-NSM has the potential for pre-pectoral prothesis breast reconstruction as the single axillary or lateral chest incisions of E-NSM or R-NSM were associated with low skin flap and NAC ischemia/necrosis. Pre-pectoral direct to implant breast reconstruction in E-NSM and R-NSM would be the next step of evolution in the development of minimal access mastectomy [32–34].

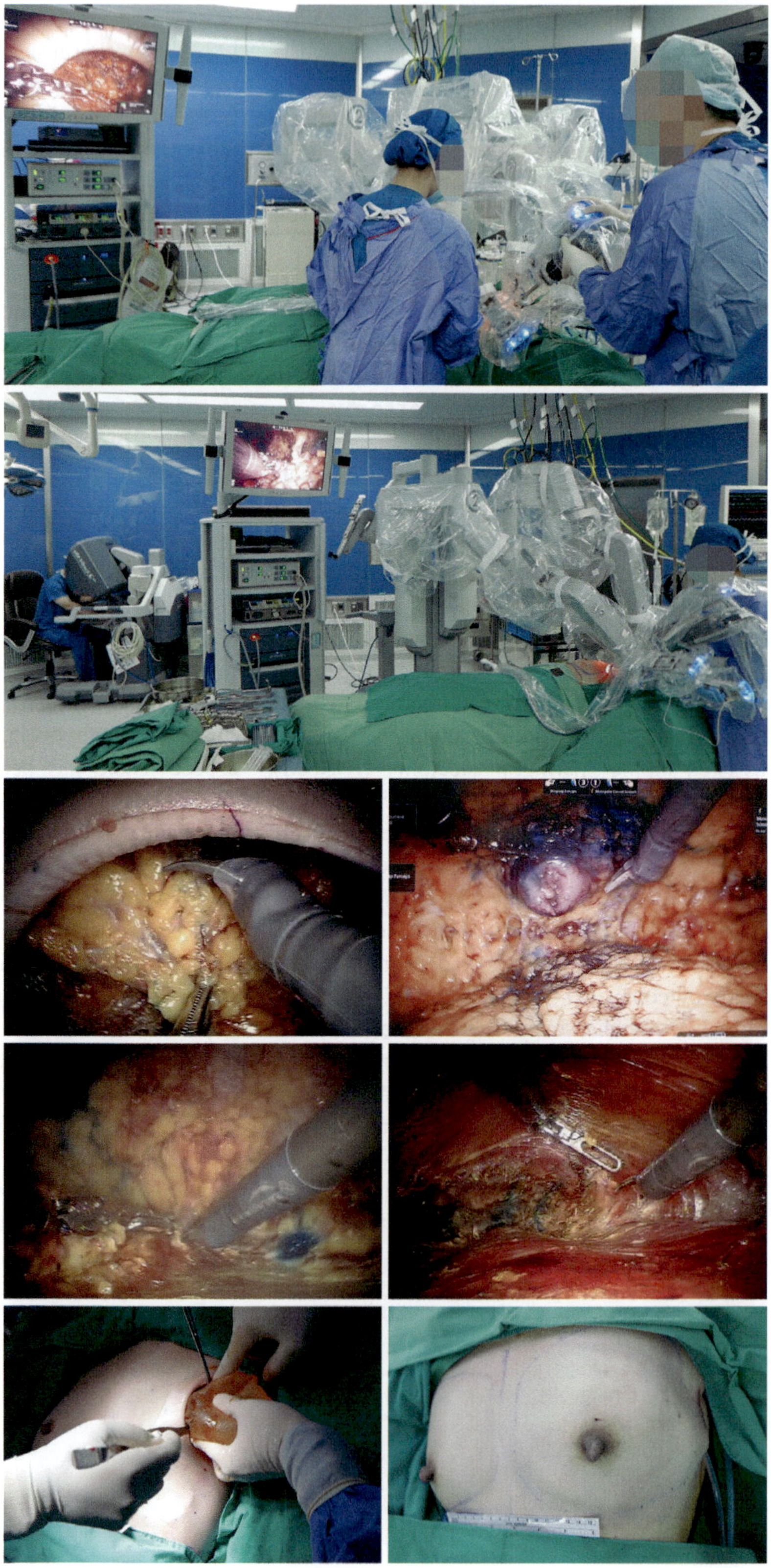

Fig. 23.6 Photos illustrated the operative procedures of robotic-assisted nipple sparing mastectomy (R-NSM) with da Vinci Si for patient with breast cancer. Immediate gel implant breast reconstruction was performed at the same time

23.5 Conclusion

With the advent of improved technology and better surgical techniques, minimally invasive and minimal access breast surgery is likely to stay for the next decade or so. Continued development of technique and improved outcomes will increase the likelihood of this surgical option being placed as the standard of care in the management of breast cancer. Future directions in terms of international multi-centers' collaborations and a structured training system for endoscopic- and/or robotic-assisted breast surgery are of paramount importance while the long-term oncologic outcomes as well as cost-effectiveness analyses are much anticipated in the near future to further consolidate the use of endoscopic-assisted techniques in the surgical management of breast cancer.

References

1. Mok CW, Lai HW. Evolution of minimal access breast surgery. Gland Surg. 2019;8(6):784–93. https://doi.org/10.21037/gs.2019.11.16. PMID: 32042687; PMCID: PMC6989909.
2. Tamaki Y, Sakita I, Miyoshi Y, Sekimoto M, Takiguchi S, Monden M, Noguchi S. Transareolar endoscopy-assisted partial mastectomy: a preliminary report of six cases. Surg Laparosc Endosc Percutan Tech. 2001;11(6):356–62. https://doi.org/10.1097/00129689-200112000-00003. PMID: 11822858.
3. Ozaki S, Ohara M, Shigematsu H, Sasada T, Emi A, Masumoto N, Kadoya T, Murakami S, Kataoka T, Fujii M, Arihiro K, Okada M. Technical feasibility and cosmetic advantage of hybrid endoscopy-assisted breast-conserving surgery for breast cancer patients. J Laparoendosc Adv Surg Tech A. 2013;23(2):91–9. https://doi.org/10.1089/lap.2012.0224. Epub 2012 Dec 28. PMID: 23272727.
4. Leff DR, Vashisht R, Yongue G, Keshtgar M, Yang GZ, Darzi A. Endoscopic breast surgery: where are we now and what might the future hold for video-assisted breast surgery? Breast Cancer Res Treat. 2011;125(3):607–25. https://doi.org/10.1007/s10549-010-1258-4. Epub 2010 Dec 3. PMID: 21128113.
5. Fukuma E. [Endoscopic breast surgery for breast cancer]. Nihon Geka Gakkai Zasshi. 2006;107(2):64–8. Japanese. PMID: 16613205.
6. Tukenmez M, Ozden BC, Agcaoglu O, Kecer M, Ozmen V, Muslumanoglu M, Igci A. Videoendoscopic single-port nipple-sparing mastectomy and immediate reconstruction. J Laparoendosc Adv Surg Tech A. 2014;24(2):77–82. https://doi.org/10.1089/lap.2013.0172. Epub 2014 Jan 8. PMID: 24401140; PMCID: PMC3935461.
7. Lai HW, Chen ST, Chen DR, Chen SL, Chang TW, Kuo SJ, Kuo YL, Hung CS. Current trends in and indications for endoscopy-assisted breast surgery for breast cancer: results from a six-year study conducted by the Taiwan endoscopic breast surgery cooperative group. PLoS One. 2016;11(3):e0150310. https://doi.org/10.1371/journal.pone.0150310. PMID: 26950469; PMCID: PMC4780808.
8. Wang ZH, Qu X, Teng CS, Ge ZC, Zhang HM, Yuan Z, Gao YG, Lu C, Yu JA, Zhang ZT. Preliminary results for treatment of early stage breast cancer with endoscopic subcutaneous mastectomy combined with endoscopic sentinel lymph node biopsy in China. J Surg Oncol. 2016;113(6):616–20. https://doi.org/10.1002/jso.24199. Epub 2016 Apr 4. PMID: 27040619.
9. Ho WS, Ying SY, Chan AC. Endoscopic-assisted subcutaneous mastectomy and axillary dissection with immediate mammary prosthesis reconstruction for early breast cancer. Surg Endosc. 2002;16(2):302–6. https://doi.org/10.1007/s004640000203. Epub 2001 Nov 16. PMID: 11967683.
10. Nakajima H, Sakaguchi K, Mizuta N, Hachimine T, Ohe S, Sawai K. Video-assisted total glandectomy and immediate reconstruction for breast cancer. Biomed Pharmacother. 2002;56(Suppl 1):205s–8s. https://doi.org/10.1016/s0753-3322(02)00281-0. PMID: 12487283.
11. Kitamura K, Ishida M, Inoue H, Kinoshita J, Hashizume M, Sugimachi K. Early results of an endoscope-assisted subcutaneous mastectomy and reconstruction for breast cancer. Surgery. 2002;131(1 Suppl):S324–9. https://doi.org/10.1067/msy.2002.120120. PMID: 11821832.
12. Fan LJ, Jiang J, Yang XH, Zhang Y, Li XG, Chen XC, Zhong L. A prospective study comparing endoscopic subcutaneous mastectomy plus immediate reconstruction with implants and breast conserving surgery for breast cancer. Chin Med J (Engl). 2009;122(24):2945–50. PMID: 20137479.
13. Wang Y, Wu JX, Guan S. A technique of endoscopic nipple-sparing mastectomy for breast cancer. JSLS. 2017;21(2):e2017.00028. https://doi.org/10.4293/JSLS.2017.00028. PMID: 28684896; PMCID: PMC5482913.
14. Du J, Liang Q, Qi X, Ming J, Liu J, Zhong L, Fan L, Jiang J. Endoscopic nipple sparing mastectomy with immediate implant-based reconstruction versus breast conserving surgery: a long-term study. Sci Rep. 2017;7:45636. https://doi.org/10.1038/srep45636. PMID: 28361955; PMCID: PMC5374499.
15. Lai HW, Lin SL, Chen ST, Kuok KM, Chen SL, Lin YL, Chen DR, Kuo SJ. Single-axillary-incision endoscopic-assisted hybrid technique for nipple-sparing

mastectomy: technique, preliminary results, and patient-reported cosmetic outcome from preliminary 50 procedures. Ann Surg Oncol. 2018;25(5):1340–9. https://doi.org/10.1245/s10434-018-6383-z. Epub 2018 Feb 26. PMID: 29484564.
16. Lai HW, Mok CW. Endoscopic mastectomy with immediate implant reconstruction. In: Minimally invasive (endoscopic & robotic) breast surgery. Elsevier; 2020. p. 79–112. https://doi.org/10.1016/b978-0-323-73405-9.00005-4.
17. Mok CW, Lai HW. Endoscopic-assisted surgery in the management of breast cancer: 20 years review of trend, techniques and outcomes. Breast. 2019;46:144–56. https://doi.org/10.1016/j.breast.2019.05.013. Epub 2019 May 20. PMID: 31176887.
18. Lai HW, Chen ST, Mok CW, Lin SL, Tai CM, Chen DR, Kuo SJ. Single-port 3-dimensional videoscope-assisted endoscopic nipple-sparing mastectomy in the management of breast cancer. Plast Reconstr Surg Glob Open. 2019;7(8):e2367. https://doi.org/10.1097/GOX.0000000000002367. PMID: 31592384; PMCID: PMC6756665.
19. Sakamoto N, Fukuma E, Higa K, Ozaki S, Sakamoto M, Abe S, Kurihara T, Tozaki M. Early results of an endoscopic nipple-sparing mastectomy for breast cancer. Ann Surg Oncol. 2009;16(12):3406–13. https://doi.org/10.1245/s10434-009-0661-8. PMID: 19662457.
20. Frey JD, Salibian AA, Lee J, Harris K, Axelrod DM, Guth AA, Shapiro RL, Schnabel FR, Karp NS, Choi M. Oncologic trends, outcomes, and risk factors for locoregional recurrence: an analysis of tumor-to-nipple distance and critical factors in therapeutic nipple-sparing mastectomy. Plast Reconstr Surg. 2019;143(6):1575–85. https://doi.org/10.1097/PRS.0000000000005600. PMID: 30907805.
21. Toesca A, Peradze N, Manconi A, Galimberti V, Intra M, Colleoni M, Bonanni B, Curigliano G, Rietjens M, Viale G, Sacchini V, Veronesi P. Robotic nipple-sparing mastectomy for the treatment of breast cancer: feasibility and safety study. Breast. 2017;31:51–6. https://doi.org/10.1016/j.breast.2016.10.009. Epub 2016 Nov 2. PMID: 27810700; PMCID: PMC5278881.
22. Sarfati B, Struk S, Leymarie N, Honart JF, Alkhashnam H, Tran de Fremicourt K, Conversano A, Rimareix F, Simon M, Michiels S, Kolb F. Robotic prophylactic nipple-sparing mastectomy with immediate prosthetic breast reconstruction: a prospective study. Ann Surg Oncol. 2018;25(9):2579–86. https://doi.org/10.1245/s10434-018-6555-x. Epub 2018 Jun 29. PMID: 29959612.
23. Lai HW, Chen ST, Lin SL, Chen CJ, Lin YL, Pai SH, Chen DR, Kuo SJ. Robotic nipple-sparing mastectomy and immediate breast reconstruction with gel implant: technique, preliminary results and patient-reported cosmetic outcome. Ann Surg Oncol. 2019;26(1):42–52. https://doi.org/10.1245/s10434-018-6704-2. Epub 2018 Aug 14. PMID: 30109537.
24. Park HS, Lee J, Lee DW, Song SY, Lew DH, Kim SI, Cho YU. Robot-assisted nipple-sparing mastectomy with immediate breast reconstruction: an initial experience. Sci Rep. 2019;9(1):15669. https://doi.org/10.1038/s41598-019-51744-2. Erratum in: Sci Rep. 2020;10(1):7602. PMID: 31666551; PMCID: PMC6821761.
25. Houvenaeghel G, Bannier M, Rua S, Barrou J, Heinemann M, Knight S, Lambaudie E, Cohen M. Robotic breast and reconstructive surgery: 100 procedures in 2-years for 80 patients. Surg Oncol. 2019;31:38–45. https://doi.org/10.1016/j.suronc.2019.09.005. Epub 2019 Sep 10. PMID: 31526915.
26. Lai HW, Lin SL, Chen ST, Lin YL, Chen DR, Pai SS, Kuo SJ. Robotic nipple sparing mastectomy and immediate breast reconstruction with robotic latissimus Dorsi flap harvest—technique and preliminary results. J Plast Reconstr Aesthet Surg. 2018;71(10):e59–61. https://doi.org/10.1016/j.bjps.2018.07.006. Epub 2018 Aug 2. PMID: 30122600.
27. Kuo WL, Huang JJ, Huang YT, Chueh LF, Lee JT, Tsai HP, Chen SC. Robot-assisted mastectomy followed by immediate autologous microsurgical free flap reconstruction: techniques and feasibility in three different breast cancer surgical scenarios. Clin Breast Cancer. 2020;20(1):e1–8. https://doi.org/10.1016/j.clbc.2019.06.018. Epub 2019 Sep 4. PMID: 31780382.
28. Lai HW, Chen ST, Tai CM, Lin SL, Lin YJ, Huang RH, Mok CW, Chen DR, Kuo SJ. Robotic- versus endoscopic-assisted nipple-sparing mastectomy with immediate prosthesis breast reconstruction in the management of breast cancer: a case-control comparison study with analysis of clinical outcomes, learning curve, patient-reported aesthetic results, and medical cost. Ann Surg Oncol. 2020;27(7):2255–68. https://doi.org/10.1245/s10434-020-08223-0. Epub 2020 Feb 3. PMID: 32016631.
29. Lai HW, Chen ST, Mok CW, Lin YJ, Wu HK, Lin SL, Chen DR, Kuo SJ. Robotic versus conventional nipple sparing mastectomy and immediate gel implant breast reconstruction in the management of breast cancer—a case control comparison study with analysis of clinical outcome, medical cost, and patient-reported cosmetic results. J Plast Reconstr Aesthet Surg. 2020;73(8):1514–25. https://doi.org/10.1016/j.bjps.2020.02.021. Epub 2020 Feb 18. PMID: 32238306.
30. Lai HW, Toesca A, Sarfati B, Park HS, Houvenaeghel G, Selber JC, Cheng FT, Kuo WL, Peradze N, Song SY, Mok CW. Consensus statement on robotic mastectomy-expert panel from international endoscopic and robotic breast surgery symposium (IERBS) 2019. Ann Surg. 2020;271(6):1005–12. https://doi.org/10.1097/SLA.0000000000003789. PMID: 31977514.
31. Jones G, Yoo A, King V, Jao B, Wang H, Rammos C, Elwood E. Prepectoral immediate direct-to-implant

breast reconstruction with anterior AlloDerm coverage. Plast Reconstr Surg. 2017;140(6S Prepectoral Breast Reconstruction):31S–8S. https://doi.org/10.1097/PRS.0000000000004048. PMID: 29166345.

32. Casella D, Di Taranto G, Marcasciano M, Sordi S, Kothari A, Kovacs T, Lo Torto F, Cigna E, Calabrese C, Ribuffo D. Evaluation of prepectoral implant placement and complete coverage with TiLoop bra mesh for breast reconstruction: a prospective study on long-term and patient-reported BREAST-Q outcomes. Plast Reconstr Surg. 2019;143(1):1e–9e. https://doi.org/10.1097/PRS.0000000000005078. PMID: 30303929.
33. Rathat G, Herlin C, Bonnel C, Captier G, Duraes M. Endoscopic nipple-sparing mastectomy with immediate prepectoral implant-based reconstruction: a case report. Am J Case Rep. 2019;20:1812–6. https://doi.org/10.12659/AJCR.919669. PMID: 31801936; PMCID: PMC6913238.
34. Parcells A, Spiro S. Exploration of robotic direct to implant breast reconstruction. Plast Reconstr Surg Glob Open. 2020;8(1):e2619. https://doi.org/10.1097/GOX.0000000000002619. PMID: 32095418; PMCID: PMC7015590.

The Functional and Cost-Effectiveness of Prepectoral Breast Reconstruction

24

L. Cattelani and S. Polotto

24.1 Functional Evaluation of Prepectoral ADM-Assisted Breast Reconstruction

24.1.1 Introduction

Nowadays, reconstructive procedures are considered a cornerstone of breast cancer treatment [1]. Patients are often characterized by younger age and good prognoses and therefore, they expect good aesthetic results and an optimal functional restoration. Patients' quality of life (QoL) should be a national health system priority and for this reason, science and technology advancements should improve short- and long-term reconstructive surgical results. As postoperative impairment of upper limb function (ULF) leads to a significant QoL detriment, directly related to chronic pain, an accurate evaluation of the functional impact of each reconstructive technique should be mandatory [2].

Upper limb performances can be assessed by both objective and subjective tests. Standardized methods can measure precisely muscular function, whereas subjective ones refer to patients' personal sensations and experiences.

24.1.2 Background of Breast Reconstruction

After the first pioneering attempts of breast reconstruction in the 1960s, the need to provide an adequate implant coverage led to the use of the subpectoral technique. However, creating an unnatural space for the implant beneath muscles tightly adherent to the thoracic wall (pectoralis major, serratus anterior) requires their partial detachment and the consequent functional decline.

Then, the unpleasant results of pure subpectoral technique (insufficient lower pole expansion, poor breast ptosis, difficult placement implants bigger than 300 cc) led to the development of dual-plane procedure that equally causes a remarkable loss of muscular function, as the pectoralis major (PM) is wholly detached from its lower origin to cover only the implant's upper pole, whereas the lower pole is positioned subcutaneously.

In early 2000s, ADMs were introduced to cover implants' inferolateral portion but, until recently, a variable degree of muscular sacrifice was considered an unavoidable tribute to implant breast reconstruction.

Lastly, the application of ADMs allowing an anterior or even a full-coverage of the implant led to the birth of the prepectoral breast reconstruction (PPBR). In this way, the breast is recon-

L. Cattelani (✉) · S. Polotto
Department of Breast Surgery, University Hospital of Parma, Parma, Italy

© The Author(s), under exclusive license to Springer Nature Switzerland AG 2023

R. Vidya, H. Becker (eds.), *Prepectoral Breast Reconstruction*,
https://doi.org/10.1007/978-3-031-15590-1_24

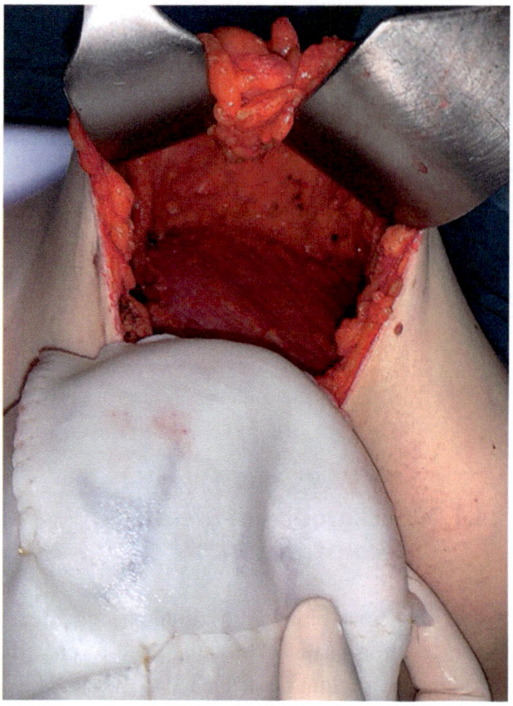

Fig. 24.1 Prepectoral ADM-wrapped implant positioning with an intact PM fascial plane. *ADM* acellular dermal matrix, *PM* pectoralis major

structed in its original position, anteriorly to the PM and without any muscular damage (Fig. 24.1).

Microsurgical techniques, in particular DIEP reconstruction, represent another optimal typology of breast reconstruction, as the abdomen represents the best donor site for the quality and amount of tissue. Unfortunately, not all patients are suitable for this kind of surgery and free-flap surgery requires skilled surgeons with a wide experience.

Finally, latissimus dorsi (LD) flap still represents a suitable autologous immediate breast reconstruction in selected patients when it is designed as an "extended" flap or associated with lipofilling [3, 4].

24.1.3 Notes of Chest Wall Area Functional Anatomy

The PM, which significantly contributes to shoulder stability, represents the most important muscle for the adduction, internal rotation, and flexion of the humerus. Moreover, it extends the humerus when the arm is hyper flexed; when it is fixed, the muscle lifts the trunk, which can be helpful in climbing or during inspiration. PM disinsertion causes a significant impairment of shoulder stability and of upper limb strength [5].

The primary function of the serratus anterior muscle is the abduction and external rotation of the scapula, essential for upper limb anteversion; moreover, the muscle pulls the scapula towards the thorax and acts as accessory inspiration muscle.

Finally, LD's primary functions are shoulder intra-rotation, adduction and extension of the arm and its depression when raised; it assists in holding the scapula against the thorax during upper limb movements. With the arms fixed above the head, it can raise the trunk upwards. It is an important muscle in rowing and swimming.

24.1.4 Subjective Validated Tests to Evaluate Upper Limb Function

Subjective tests are fundamental to assess upper limb impairment after reconstructive surgery. Even if this kind of evaluations could not detect some functional deficit as precisely as objective tests do, they show the impact of the surgery on patients' everyday routine.

– *BREAST-Q* (Memorial Sloan Kettering Cancer Center and the University of British Columbia) is nowadays one of the most used to evaluate patients' QoL after breast reconstructive surgery. The "Physical well-being: chest" section for subpectoral or prepectoral reconstruction, and the "Physical well-being: back and shoulder" section for LD flap reconstruction are of particular interest for postoperative functional evaluation.

Other tests include:

- *Disabilities of the Arm, Shoulder, and Hand questionnaire (DASH)* and its short form *(quickDASH)*
- *Shoulder Pain and Disability Index (SPADI)*
- *American Shoulder and Elbow Surgeons (ASES) Society Standardized Shoulder Assessment Form*
- *Western Ontario Shoulder Instability index (WOSI)*
- *Manual muscle test (MMT)*
- Postoperative pain evaluation, through the *Brief Pain Inventory*, either in its complete or short-form

24.1.5 Objective Validated Tests to Evaluate Upper Limb Function

Objective tests provide raw data to accurately assess postoperative ULF and their trend throughout the follow-up period.

- *Isokinetic tests* such as isokinetic dynamometry are considered the gold standard methods to measure strength and endurance of muscles that govern joint movements [6]. *Maximal voluntary isometric muscular contraction* (MVIC) is a simple standardized test to measure muscle strength using a strain gauge tensiometer, *maximal isokinetic peak torque* (MIPT) examines shoulder internal and external rotation, and *isokinetic muscle performance* (IMPT) provides information about muscle strength and function.
- *Shoulder passive and active range of motion (ROM)* can be objectively assessed using a goniometer or a digital inclinometer.
- *One-repetition maximum (1RM) test* aims to measure maximal muscle strength.
- *Maximum voluntary contraction test (MVC)*
- *Surface or intramuscular electromyography (EMG)*
- *Constant Murley Score (CS)*

24.1.6 Functional Impact of Breast and Reconstructive Surgery

Before evaluating the functional impact of breast reconstruction, morbidities related to *mastectomy* should be considered, being that these surgeries inextricably connected. After oncologic breast surgery, from 20 to 65% of patients experience different kinds of long-lasting postoperative pain, gathered as post-mastectomy pain syndrome [7]. Common symptoms associated with this kind of surgery include pectoralis tightness, myofascial pain syndrome, rotator cuff disease, and adhesive capsulitis. Moreover, a significant percentage of patients show a continuous ULF decline in the long-term follow-up, which reflects the importance of a rehabilitation therapy integrated in the postoperative period to diminish patients' QoL impairment [8].

Whereas *sentinel lymph node biopsy (SLNB)* is rarely associated with long-term functional issues, *axillary lymph node dissection (ALND)* involves a high rate of postoperative ULF impairment. In fact, patients undergone ALND report a significant elevation and abduction deficit at 6 and even at 12 postoperative month (POM), limited shoulder ROM in abduction and flexion up to 2 POM, and about 30% of patients complain a postoperative ULF worsening [9–11]. Some authors report a myofascial pain syndrome, which affects 44.8% of patients undergone breast surgery associated with ALND and involving LD (25.9%), serratus anterior (24.0%), PM (20.7%), infraspinatus (19.0%), and trapezius (13.8%), clearly demonstrating that trigger points activation factors are mainly related to muscle manipulation, but can also extend to areas untouched by surgery [7].

Subpectoral breast reconstruction, both direct-to-implant (DTI) and two-step tissue expander/implant (TE/I), causes surgical damage of chest wall muscles (namely, PM, serratus anterior, and sometimes even the upper portion of the rectus abdominis fascia) with a significant loss of their function and impairment of shoulder stability.

Leonardis et al. reported that two-step TE/I subpectoral reconstruction compromises shoulder joint functional structure, thus diminishing upper limb strength and stability. An unstable shoulder joint severely affects usual activities of daily living, representing a common patients complaint [12]. In addition, they demonstrate that even the function of the intact PM region (clavicular portion) results strongly affected in the postoperative period. Compensatory mechanisms might not be effective enough in ULF restoration, that sometimes remain permanently impaired [13].

In a further study, the same author examined subpectoral and LD flap reconstruction suggesting that the preservation of shoulder function should be fundamental in the decision-making process of reconstructive technique. In fact, PM and LD represent the two main contributors to shoulder stability, and their combined damage can hardly be compensated [14].

Kim et al. reported that mastectomy associated with implant subpectoral positioning significantly affects shoulder ROM. Flexion and abduction seem to be more impaired than shoulder rotation; however, early postoperative rehabilitation may lead to short-term shoulder ROM complete recovery [10]. On the other hand, no significant functional difference was evidenced between three different reconstructive methods (TE/I, LD flap, free TRAM flap) at three POM; in fact the ULF appear to be equally impaired by the different kinds of reconstruction, whereas at 6 POM LD group showed a higher deficit in arm adduction and internal rotation [15].

In addition, De Haan et al. evidenced a significant objective decrease in torque strength at the side of the subpectoral reconstruction [5].

In the immediate postoperative period, muscular fibers are stretched by the underlying implant or expander, and for this reason the patients might experience an acute feeling of tension in the breast area, which may also evolve into a chronic discomfort [13].

The direct contact of the PM with the subcutaneous tissue entails fixed adhesions worsened by PM movements, leading to the so-called *animation deformity*. Moreover, a small percentage of patients experience an intractable and involuntary PM spasms, provoked by a medial and lateral pectoral nerve surgical damage that, once established, tend to chronicize. In these cases, the shift of the implant pocket to prepectoral plane may not solve these symptoms, which could require PM denervation and even its disinsertion from the humerus [16].

A certain percentage of patients with these disabling postoperative drawbacks finally decided to have their implants removed, or asked for a complete autologous reconstruction, thus requiring a challenging revisional surgery. Recently, an increasing number of surgeons choose to reposition an unsatisfying subpectoral implant in the prepectoral space, with relevant functional and aesthetical improvement (Figs. 24.2 and 24.3).

The decreased viability of the muscles can also be assessed instrumentally. The ultrasound imaging can show the fibrotic changes and the decreased volume of muscles involved in subpectoral pocket (thinned of about 50% of their original volume), and the Doppler probes highlight the decreased muscles perfusion [17].

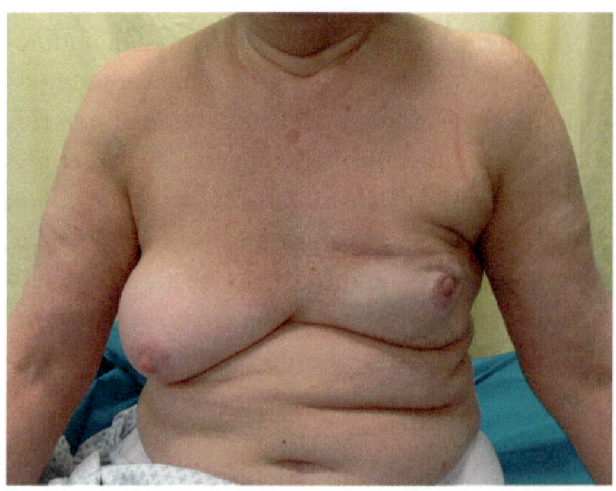

Fig. 24.2 Left subpectoral reconstruction with definitive implant and associated painful animation deformity and capsular contracture

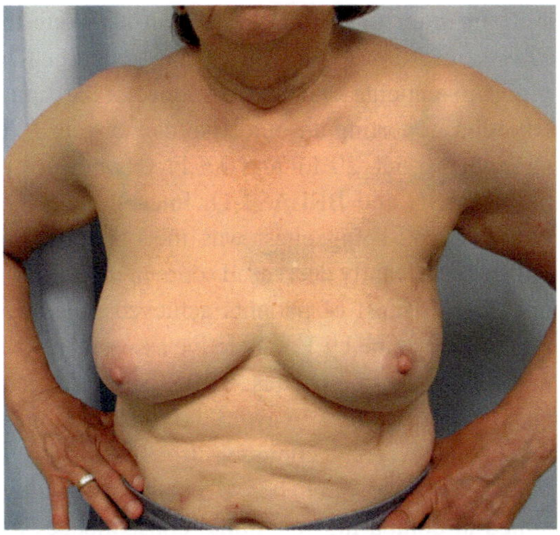

Fig. 24.3 Complete resolution of aesthetic and functional issues after implant repositioning in the prepectoral plane

Table 24.1 Most frequent complications related to submuscular breast reconstruction

Longer duration of surgery
Longer recovery time
More post-operative pain and need for opioids
Increased costs
Pectoralis major muscle tightness
Myofascial pain syndrome
Rotator cuff disease
Adhesive capsulitis
Loss of shoulder ROM
Diminished upper limb strength
Unstable shoulder joint
Intractable and involuntary muscle spasms
Animation deformity
Atrophy and fibrotic changes in the muscle and weakness
Permanent objective impairment of upper limb function
Chronic subjective patient' discomfort
Unsatisfying aesthetic result

Most frequent complications related to submuscular reconstruction have been listed in Table 24.1; surprisingly, patients usually accept these problems as normal and rarely complain about them. As further explained in the specific paragraph, most symptoms can be resolved by repositioning the implant in the prepectoral space or simply prevented choosing the prepectoral technique.

Lee et al. performed a systematic review about functional morbidity after breast reconstruction performed with different *LD flap* techniques, revealing that a vast percentage of patients (41%) reported subjective ULF impairment. The results of DASH questionnaire in daily and working activities evidenced a slight impairment in daily activities, whereas more significant problems in sport and art sections were reported. Moreover, whereas some authors found a significant shoulder ROM limitation and strength impairment in the early postoperative follow-up period, an almost complete ULF recovery may be reached within 1 year after surgery (up to 90–95% of baseline function) [3, 18, 19].

DIEP flap reconstructive techniques could involve donor site functional morbidity, as slight trunk flexion and extension impairment, that might also not completely return to baseline [20, 21]. Moreover, Alba et al. evidenced that patients undergone autologous reconstruction reported significantly higher upper limb postoperative pain, when compared with those undergone subpectoral reconstruction. Also ULF is impaired by DIEP flap positioning, as shoulder ROM is decreased of about 28.6% and MMT ranges are consistent with this percentage [22].

24.1.7 Pro-active Physiotherapist Approach

Considering the persistent ULF impairment caused by breast surgery and its impact on patients' QoL, nowadays a great importance is given to a pro-active physiotherapist approach, in order to prevent and reduce this unpleasant drawback [23].

Early shoulder mobilization should be allowed in the immediate postoperative period, within

1 week after surgery if reconstruction has not been performed and within 2 weeks if patients have undergone breast reconstruction. Long-term shoulder joint immobilization seems to provoke shoulder dysfunction. On the contrary, early upper limb mobilization improves shoulder abduction and flexion ROM since the first post-operative month [10].

Moreover, Phillips et al. underline how a precocious physiotherapeutic program aimed to improve patients' physical health status significantly reduces work-loss problems, being also cost-effective [24].

24.1.8 Functional Advantages of Prepectoral Breast Reconstruction

At present, there is still a paucity of literature assessing the functional outcome of PPBR; however, some authors have begun to objectivize functional advantages of this technique.

Schaeffer et al. compared two-stage PPBR and immediate ADM-assisted subpectoral implant positioning. The functional outcome was measured through the number of days necessary until the reach of a full pre-operatory shoulder ROM. Interestingly, PPBR patients experienced significantly lower pain scores, requiring fewer opioids in the postoperative period; finally, they were able to return to full active shoulder ROM in half time than patients of subpectoral group (11.8 Vs 24.2 days) [25].

Leonardis et al., after ascertaining shoulder function impairment due to submuscular techniques, suggest considering PPBR whenever possible in order to avoid ULF impairment due to PM disinsertion [14]. Patel et al. examined a group of patients undergone subpectoral reconstruction, reporting an objective decrease in PM strength (about 20%) and ULF, examined by QuickDASH and BREAST-Q. Interestingly, the physical well-being chest was the only section with a significantly decreased score in the follow-up. Even if most of patients achieved objective return to baseline ULF, subjective assessment did not reflect this trend. Thus, PPBR is encouraged also by these authors to avoid the functional burden of subpectoral technique [26].

In 2018, we published a perspective study aimed at comparing functional consequences of subpectoral and prepectoral breast reconstruction [27]. Our results significantly increased the evidence suggested by the above-mentioned studies; in fact, whereas only 26.7% of patients undergone submuscular reconstruction were analgesic consumption-free after one postoperative week, 76.9% of PPBR patients were out of therapy at the same time point, as shown in Table 24.2.

Recently, we published another study about PPBR, examining retrospectively the subgroup of reconstructed patients undergone post-mastectomy adjuvant radiation therapy (RT). Surprisingly, even in irradiated PPBR, BREAST-Q Physical well-being-Chest section did not demonstrate a significant ULF impairment (94.0% no RT VS 92.9% RT *p*-value = <0.001) [14, 28].

Based on our results, it may be affirmed that PPBR does not significantly impair ULF, allowing a complete function recovery within one postoperative month, and a fast return to usual activity, sport, and life routine.

Table 24.2 Results of functional and satisfaction tests (*BPI* brief pain inventory, *CM* Constant Murley score)

	Group 1 (PPBR)				Group 2 (submuscular)				*p*-value
Symmetry after first operation (monolateral)	81.25%				10.81%				<0.001
	Mean	95% CI	Median	Std. deviation	Mean	95% CI	Median	Std. deviation	
Length of operation (monolateral) (min)	165.00			56.27	168.22			66.33	0.928
BPI day 1	17.56	12.53–22.60	16.00	15.52	44.11	39.36–48.87	45.00	15.83	<0.001
BPI day 7	8.23	3.24–13.22	1.00	15.39	21.96	16.37–27.54	20.00	18.59	<0.001
CM day 7	65.67	62.65–68.69	69.00	9.31	52.36	48.68–56.03	53.00	12.23	<0.001
CM day 1	71.62	68.74–74.49	75.00	8.87	60.36	57.19–63.52	62.00	10.54	<0.001
Dash	9.92	4.13–15.72	00.00.00	17.87	29.18	24.10–34.26	29.00	16.91	<0.001
Breast Q	92.21	89.28–95.13	94.00	9.03	76.07	71.70–80.44	79.00	14.55	<0.001
Return to usual work (days)	34.56	27.76–41.37	30.00	21.00	57.31	45.96–68.66	45.00	37.77	<0.001
	Paracetamol	Ketoprofen	Opioids	No	Paracetamol	Ketoprofen	Opioids	No	*p*-value
Analgesic consumption day 1	30.8%	61.5%	7.7%	0%	8.9%	66.7%	24.4%	0%	0.012
Analgesic consumption day 7	12.8%	10.3%	0%	76.9%	48.9%	24.4%	0%	26.7%	<0.001

24.2 Economic Evaluation of Prepectoral ADM-Assisted Breast Reconstruction

24.2.1 Introduction

Many concomitant factors are determining an increase in the rate of mastectomies in local treatment and risk-reduction of breast cancer. Parallel to this trend, nipple- and skin-sparing techniques have spread allowing immediate definitive breast reconstruction (BR) in most cases. Recommended quality standards of breast care in Europe consider as a satisfactory rate of immediate reconstruction after mastectomy higher than 70% for patients under 70 of age.

In reality, despite the various deliberative acts of politics, very few countries and centers, both inside and outside Europe, come close to these numbers (Table 24.3).

The reasons for such failure are extremely complex, also in relation to the variety of inspiring criteria of public health systems. Even more disappointing is that, among the quality indicators of centers dedicated to breast surgery, there is no adequate evaluation of the aesthetic and functional results of the interventions.

Although it is not our intention to analyze in depth all the variables that influence the aptitude to perform the reconstruction, we would like to emphasize some of them in order to acquire a modern *forma mentis* that the breast surgeon should adopt in the decision-making process, avoiding passively suffering contradictory distortions determined by tendentious economic evaluations.

24.2.2 Causes of a Suboptimal Rate of Breast Reconstruction

24.2.2.1 Availability of Various Approaches to Breast Reconstruction

Delayed breast reconstructions involve, in the majority of cases, autologous free-flap transfer with microvascular anastomosis. These techniques require a considerably longer duration of the intervention and lead to a prolonged recovery time compared to implant-based reconstructions. The technical knowledge and experience for autologous reconstructions can only be acquired and maintained in dedicated centers for excellence with relevant caseload. Necessarily, these centers cannot be numerically widespread and, as a consequence, the waiting time for complex autologous reconstructions in many areas is calculated in years. This could be a strong disincentive factor for the choice of BR by the patient. Furthermore, distance from reconstruction center represents a proven disheartening element for the woman [29, 30].

Some attempts to perform a cost/utility evaluation of BR, in addition to the fragility of using a retrospective method, did not obtain a satisfactory quotation of the numerous advantages obtained with the prepectoral technique compared to other modalities, as they limit themselves to using only patients-reported questionnaires mainly representative of the subjective satisfaction with regard to the reconstructed breast [31].

It is a matter of fact that access to BR, although slowly rising, remains limited, characterized by a

Table 24.3 Approximate percentage of breast reconstruction after mastectomy in some countries

Country	% Breast reconstruction	Year of publication
Australia	18%	2014
France	27.4%	2012
England	21.5%	2017
USA	43.3%	2014
Canada	16%	2012
Italy	55%	2017
Sweden	9.3%	2013
Denmark	14%	2010

wide national and international variability, despite its undeniable impact on the QoL of the patients [32, 33]. Older women, unfavorable socioeconomic level, low-volume hospitals are independent factors of lower probability to be reconstructed. Differences in plastic surgeon density may partially explain regional variations in BR rate and different types of technical approach [34].

The immediate BR, although it may be considered the ideal choice, in practice suffers from considerable difficulties; everyone has had experience of how complicated it can be to organize a joint operation between breast and plastic surgeons. Many logistic barriers, concerns about the quality of the skin flaps after mastectomy, suboptimal planning about the duration of the operation, and even a disharmonious distribution of responsibilities in post-surgical surveillance come up in many cases. Probably, despite their initial specialization, without hesitation, more plastic surgeons and breast surgeons should become oncoplastic surgeons, so as to be able to offer a better availability of immediate BR.

Through an accurate patient selection, direct-to-implant reconstruction, particularly the prepectoral one, represents an easy-to-learn technique available to be performed in most breast units. By adopting this reconstructive approach, more than 70% of BR will not need complex surgery or contralateral interventions aimed at achieving symmetry [27]. ADM-assisted prepectoral reconstruction is becoming a kind of disclosure revolution in breast reconstruction, with a low rate of postoperative complications (about 6.4%) [28].

24.2.2.2 Acceptability of Breast Reconstruction

Low rates of BR in many countries could be related to a dissatisfactory process of the acceptability of the procedure by the patient. More than 80% of patients after mastectomy would consider BR when they are correctly informed of the choice [33]. Some physicians do not even mention the option of BR to the patient, others consider BR to be only a possibility; the lesser part of them explains that mastectomy and reconstruction are the usual surgical approach to breast cancer that cannot be applied to conservative treatment. It is easy to understand that only a surgeon enthusiastic about the reconstruction can be convincing for the patient so that she can reach a correct acceptance probability.

Undoubtedly women increase their hesitation when any delayed additional intervention involves a further significant suspension of their ability to normal life along with other risks (e.g., 7% risk of blood transfusion). In particular, patients over 60 years of age would rarely agree to return to the operating room for a delayed reconstruction, fearing that this option is unlikely to be considered anything but an explicit tribute to female vanity. They believe that a specific new, long-lasting, reconstructive intervention is not proportionate to obtain a simple cosmetic improvement [33].

On the other hand, the satisfaction perceived by the BR shows no age-related differences [35, 36] (Figs. 24.4 and 24.5).

Precisely because of this complex psychological context of women, breast and plastic surgeons play a fundamental role in the acceptance of reconstruction, presenting the most compatible reconstructive modality for the single patient.

Whenever possible, the opportunity to have their breasts reconstructed during the same mastectomy operation, without any substantial additional burden of inactivity, pain, or scarring, could represent a significant contribution to the path of acceptability. Moreover, one-step BR strongly contributes to the concept that reconstruction is an essential component of the oncologic treatment, rather than an optional possibility.

24.2.3 Bases of the Economical Evaluation

The limited public resources make it necessary for surgeons to have a cost analysis when they want to introduce a new technique and in fact this type of evaluation has become quite common. However, in most cases, when we undertake a pure assessment of intra-hospital costs, we find a

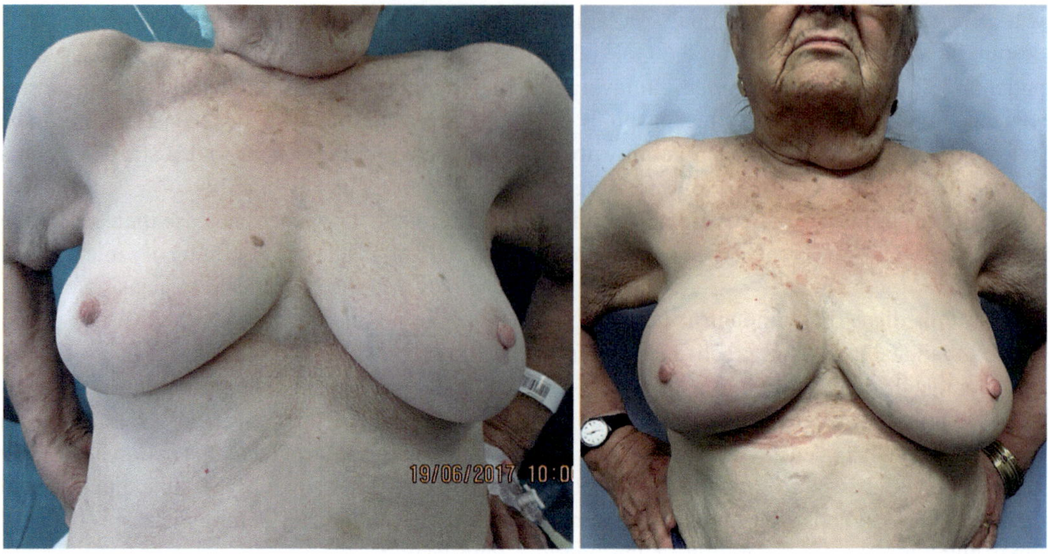

Figs. 24.4 and 24.5 A 82-year-old patient strongly requesting reconstruction: before (Fig. 24.4) and 6 months (Fig. 24.5) after right PPBR DTI with ADM. Despite the slight asymmetry, the patient reported high degree of satisfaction with the reconstructed breast. *PPBR* prepectoral breast reconstruction, *DTI* direct-to-implant, *ADM* acellular dermal matrix

particularly insidious terrain. Current cost-evaluation has left aside value in health care and pure cost-containment resulted in sometimes counterproductive.

In fact, while every single hospital tends to pay the utmost attention to its own budget, it is easy to understand that all the physical and psychological consequences that follow a certain intervention, after discharge will weigh on the economic resources of the state.

Moreover, we must keep in mind that the mission of a national public health system, beyond any effort to contain costs, is to generate adequate social wellness in terms of the consequences of a widely prevalent disease. Performance metrics in health tend to focus principally on inputs and outputs, but they are silent on a range of other consequences valued by patients, including pain, function, and quality of live (QoL) as well as the experience of care itself. When evaluating a BR, we should not refer to the size of the reimbursements, as in many countries they are not proportional to the real costs. In addition, two-step procedures are inappropriately more profitable for hospitals, as they receive in that eventuality two distinct reimbursements.

Therefore, a correct evaluation setting should be based on the cost/value ratio. In fact, the most frequent occurrence is that a new surgical procedure, regarding direct costs, is more expensive than the traditional one. Some methods aimed at cost/effectiveness evaluation have appeared in the literature, however the perception remains that they are inadequate as regards to the monetary rating of the extra-hospital utilities. Although uneasy to do, we should pay paramount attention to the consequences of interventions that fall outside the health care sector (e.g., economic production, sickness work-absence insurance, social services, rehabilitation) [37].

When taking both the patient's and the payer perspective, the comparison between various reconstruction modalities requires analyzing longitudinally every single advantage/disadvantage connected with the innovative technique and rating all services and activities necessary for a complete care cycle, in order to set up the more accurate value rating [38]. Below, we try to perform an outcomes measurement and their rating through the Health Technology Assessment of our experience with implant-based reconstructions, whether sub- or prepectoral, and the data of recent literature regarding autologous reconstruction [39–44].

24.2.3.1 Operative Time

Including the mastectomy, free-flap reconstruction lasts more than 360 min, while subpectoral BR requires at least 210 min overall when considering two-steps TE/I, while 150 min on average in the eventuality of direct prosthesis. Taking in account that, for prepectoral BR, the total wrapping of the implant with ADM can be prepared in a table aside while mastectomy is completed and sutured any axillary incision and moreover there is no need to harvest the muscular pocket, the operation lasts 90 min. Savings are both for operative room resource and for the patient who are spared anesthetic drugs. The hourly cost of the operating room, including staff, is 823 Euros.

24.2.3.2 Duration of Hospitalization

According to the recent literature, the mean hospital-stay for free-flap autologous reconstruction ranged from 3.9 to 4.8 days, while for implant-based subpectoral is of 2.1 days. For one-step prepectoral reconstruction, the hospitalization is less than 24 h. Therefore, the innovative technique allows you to save from 1 to 3.5 days of hospitalization in comparison with the subpectoral implant or autologous reconstruction, respectively, at the unit cost of 400 Euros per day.

24.2.3.3 Pain and the Need for Analgesics

Prepectoral reconstruction is a substantially painless procedure, and patients do not report a traumatizing experience, requiring in most cases only the intake of paracetamol; they do not require analgesics to be taken within a week after the operation. This characteristic allows the extreme reduction in hospitalization, generally in overnight setting.

Unlike other methods, the use of analgesic-narcotics is never necessary, thus alleviating both early side effects of such substances and the risk of possible morphine-derivative drug dependence, a problem that has generated concerns in recent years.

We ascertained that the prepectoral method achieves 60% savings for analgesic drugs compared to the subpectoral. Treatment-related discomfort caused by high degree of pain should be considered a relevant drawback for the value of more complex reconstructive procedures which is reflected in the psychological experience and recovery time [45].

24.2.3.4 Physical and Functional Integrity

Nowadays, with the same effectiveness of different treatments in the resolution of a disease, the maintenance of the integrity of the body structures is of primary importance, even comparable to the survival itself. The preservation of a dynamic lifestyle for the patient, both in the work context and not, requires extreme attention to the consequences of each therapeutic maneuver, particularly in the surgical field.

If we can offer timely breast reconstruction without trauma to the muscle structures, unlike subpectoral implantation, it means leaving the arm function intact, as previously outlined.

Otherwise, autologous reconstruction can involve significant alterations at the level of the donor site such as the presence of additional scars, the possible weakening of the abdominal wall, together with the risk of disfiguring complications in sites other than the district of the primary disease. New health problems generated as a consequence of a surgical procedure are strongly detrimental for the whole value of any treatment. When a new illness occurs, all outcomes must be remeasured. Seeking ways to minimize these drawbacks is an essential goal of reconstructive innovation. Prepectoral reconstruction can be considered potentially immune from any care-induced adjunctive burden. In addition, a conservative reconstruction preserves the body structures which remain available should a different mode of reconstruction become necessary in the future. Maybe, if possible, it is time to overcome the medieval custom of recovering from an illness by paying the price of a new disability.

24.2.3.5 Normal Activity Recovery Time

Time required to achieve recovery and return to normal function after completion of all steps of reconstructive process represents a critical outcome for patients and deserves high consideration in determining the value of a reconstructive approach. A muscle-sparing reconstruction allows a prompt mobility of the arm with a reduction almost to zero in the need of rehabilitation. Subpectoral implants have a 50% probability of postoperative physiotherapy treatment, while an autologous reconstruction of 25%. The cost of a physiotherapy cycle, including the physychiatric evaluation, can be estimated at 700 Euros.

For the one-step prepectoral reconstruction, the mean recovery time for the return to normal activity is 30 days, for the direct-to-implant subpectoral it is 55, for the 2 step TE/I an additional 25 days must be considered for the second step, while for autologous reconstruction is 65 days. The cost of 1 day out of work is estimated at 62.5 Euros.

Therefore, direct-to implant prepectoral BR leads to additional financial savings in comparison to other methods both due to reduced absence from work and lack of need for physical therapy. Fewer outpatient visits (45 € each) allow further savings.

24.2.3.6 Stability of the Reconstructed Breast and Need for Revision Surgery

One of the most important outcomes to evaluate, when comparing different approaches to BR, is the likelihood of ongoing interventions aimed to correcting functional or aesthetic changes in reconstructive result over time. We are therefore referring to the stability of the reconstructed breast as obtained early, as well as its long-term acceptability.

Until recent years, there was no doubt about the superiority of the autologous reconstruction with regard to the stable softness and naturalness of the shape compared to the BR obtained with subpectoral implants. In fact, the latter method is burdened by a significant percentage of deleterious modifications such as severe animation deformity, capsular contracture III and IV Baker grade, superomedial dislocation of the implant, onset of chronic pain of the upper body. Because of this, the rate of unexpected revision operations approaches 30% [46]. A prudential estimate of the average cost for each revision surgery is around 3400 Euros. Autologous reconstruction generally achieve, out of the setting of post-mastectomy radiotherapy, a high degree of stability over time, although flap revision for shaping may be necessary in over 40% of cases. In our experience of 480 breasts rebuilt with prepectoral one-step reconstruction, during 5 years of follow-up, the rate of unplanned surgical revisions was only 3.3%, mainly related to post-radiotherapy deleterious modifications. In not radiated patients, no capsular contracture, animation deformity, or dislocation of the implant was registered. The initial softness and natural shaping of the reconstructed breast resulted perfectly stable for nearly all women (Figs. 24.6 and 24.7).

Implant removal for late infection or extrusion/skin necrosis occurred in four cases. Revisions were due to impending extrusion of the implant or capsular contracture after radiation in three cases and in two cases to a progressive unacceptable increase of the ptosis. Seven lipomodeling for correction of rippling are included in this percentage.

24.2.3.7 Aesthetic Outcome and Patient Satisfaction

There are validated tool measures used to assess aesthetic satisfaction and quality of live related to reconstruction by patient's questionnaires. The BREAST-Q (Memorial Sloan Kettering Cancer Center and University of British Columbia, 2006) has been used in a prospective trial comparing one-step PPBR with ADM and subpectoral implant, whether DTI or 2-step TE/I. The results, reported in Table 24.4, were statistically better for patients who underwent PPBR ($P < .001$). Of note, regarding unilateral mastectomies, the achievement of satisfactory symmetry was 81.25% for prepectoral versus 10.81% for subpectoral ($P < .001$) [27].

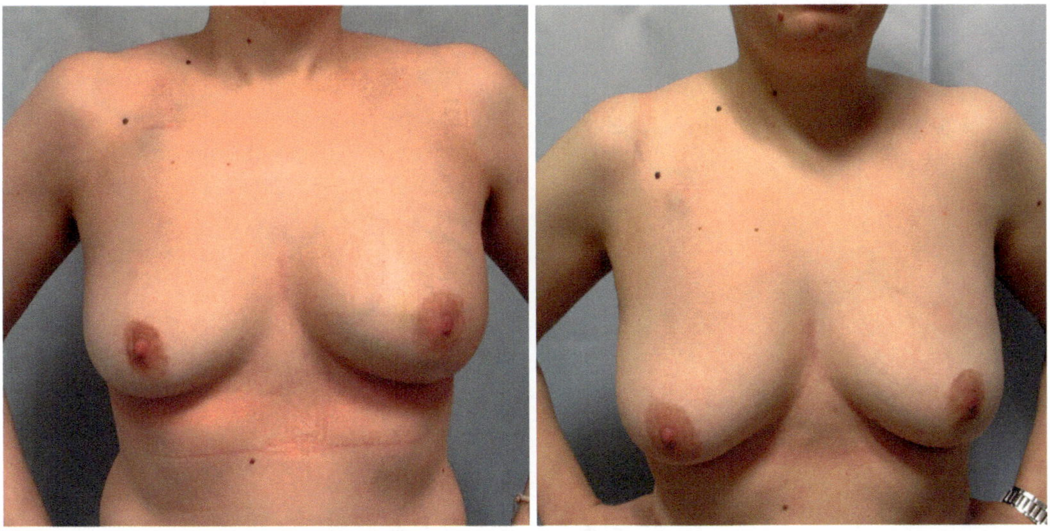

Figs. 24.6 and 24.7 51-year-old patients 27 days (Fig. 24.6) and 3 years (Fig. 24.7) after left PPBR DTI with ADM. Softness and shape of reconstruction perfectly stable over time. *PPBR* prepectoral breast reconstruction, *DTI* direct-to-implant, *ADM* acellular dermal matrix

Table 24.4 BREAST-Q™ results: higher scores reflect a better outcome

BREAST-Q™ reconstruction module post-operative (mean scores ± standard deviation)	PPBR (39 pat.)	Subpectoral BR (45 pat.)	*p*-value
Satisfaction with breasts	90. 1 ± 4.5	73.5 ± 9.7	<0.001
Psychosocial well-being	94.3 ± 2.7	79.4 ± 8.4	<0.001
Physical well-being chest	95.1 ± 4.7	68.1 ± 7.5	<0.001
Sexual well-being	79.7 ± 14.9	64.9 ± 18.7	<0.001
Satisfaction with implants	7.1 ± 0.7	3.4 ± 1.5	<0.001

PPBR prepectoral breast reconstruction, *BR* breast reconstruction, *pat.* patients

24.2.4 In-Hospital Costs

In-hospital costs have been summarized in Table 24.5.

24.2.5 Monetary Evaluation of Outcomes

Monetary evaluation of outcomes have been summarized in Table 24.6.

The total costs shown in Table 24.5 must be added to those in Table 24.6 to obtain a reliable economic comparison between the various reconstructive methods (Table 24.7).

At the end of our examination of the economic aspects, some relevant advantages of prepectoral one-step PPBR over other methods remain monetary unrated such as physical integrity, pain experience, and aesthetic satisfaction. Despite their economic non-convertibility, clearly they can further increase both the conve-

Table 24.5 In-hospital costs for completion of the planned reconstruction, expressed in euros (Fiscal year 2018)

	1st outpatient visit + preoperative tests	Operating room + staff (823 €/hour)	Implanted materials	Hospital stay (400 €/day)	Outpatient visits/ medications (45 € each)	Total
One-step PPBR + ADM (complete coverage)	**97.5**	**1234**	(Prosthesis 550 + ADM 3000) **3550**	**400**	**135**	**5416**
Subpectoral DTI (no ADM)	**97.5**	**2057**	**550**	**840**	**135**	**3679**
2-step subpectoral TE/I (no ADM)	(97.5 × 2) **195**	(2057 + 1234) **3291**	(Expander 550 + Prosthesis 550) **1100**	(1st step 840 + 2nd step 600) **1440**	(1st step 360 + 2nd step 135) **495**	**6521**
Autologous free flap	**300**	**4938**	**0**	**1740**	**225**	**7203**

PPBR prepectoral breast reconstruction, *ADM* acellular dermal matrix, *DTI* direct-to-implant, *TE/I* tissue expander/implant

Table 24.6 Extra-hospital + unplanned (early and late) surgical revision + symmetrization costs expressed in euros (Fiscal year 2018)

	Days out of work for completed reconstruction (€ 62/day)	Physiotherapy (€ 700/1 cycle)	Early reoperative complications (average cost € 2170)	Symmetrization [after unilateral mastectomy] (average cost € 2845)	Late revision/remodeling surgery (average cost € 3482)	Total
One-step PPBR + ADM (total wrapping)	**1875**	Probability 0% **0**	Probability 3.2% **68.4**	Probability 18.7% **532**	Probability 3.3% (including lipomodeling) **114.9**	**2590**
Subpectoral DTI (no ADM)	**3457**	Probability 50% **350**	Probability 17.1% [47] **371**	Probability 89.2% **2537**	Probability 30% **1044**	**7759**
2-step subpectoral TE/I (no ADM)	**5312**	Probability 50% **350**	Probability 11.4% **247.4**	Probability 89.2% **2537**	Probability 30% **1044**	**9517**
Autologous free flap	**4062**	Probability 25% **175**	Probability 5.8% [48] **125.9**	Probability 39% **1109**	Probability 17% **592**	**6064**

PPBR prepectoral breast reconstruction, *ADM* acellular dermal matrix, *DTI* direct-to-implant, *TE/I* tissue expander/implant

Table 24.7 Total cost of different reconstructions including intra-hospital, extra-hospital, and social security costs, based on a follow-up of at least 4 years

One-step PPBR + ADM (total wrapping)	€ 8006
Subpectoral DTI (no ADM)	€ 11,438
2-step subpectoral TE/I (no ADM)	€ 16,038
Autologous free flap	€ 13,267

PPBR prepectoral breast reconstruction, *ADM* acellular dermal matrix, *DTI* direct-to-implant, *TE/I* tissue expander/implant

nience and acceptability of this modern reconstructive procedure.

24.3 Conclusion

Evidence emerged of the substantial superiority of PPBR over other implant-based breast reconstruction methods with regard to the functional outcome for patients.

Consequently, this muscle-sparing technique, when feasible, deserves a primary consideration in breast restoring plan after mastectomy.

By incorporating the PPBR, without hesitation, into the knowledge base of each team dedicated to oncoplastic breast surgery, in the near future it will be possible to avoid unnecessary permanent damages to the performance status of most patients by also adding an incomparable value to the path of the best conservative treatment of breast cancer.

The systematic evaluation of the functional outcomes of all breast reconstructions is highly recommended for continuous feedback on the effectiveness of surgical procedures.

The conservativeness, timeliness, and stability of the reconstructive approach must be among the driving factors of the decision analysis according to an overall vision of the results. This orientation will be an expression of the values and expectations that society considers to be priorities.

Prepectoral immediate BR, despite the non-negligible cost of the ADM, when feasible, should be considered, after a cost/value analysis, a dominant option in comparison to the traditional interventions. It can significantly contribute to an ethical improvement in the availability and acceptability of BR. The surgeons dedicated to breast reconstruction will be called, in the near future, to the difficult role of mediating between different interests of the various economic actors in order to create the best option for the patient.

24.4 Summary with Tips

- Quality of Life of patients undergone mastectomy and immediate breast reconstruction is directly related to postoperative upper limb function.
- Oncoplastic surgeons should evaluate the functional impact of reconstructive surgery, utilizing both objective and subjective validated tests.
- Prepectoral breast reconstruction preserves upper limb function and shoulder stability, thus significantly decreasing postoperative pain and allowing patients' to promptly return to their regular life.
- Quality standard of breast cancer care in Europe recommend over 70% immediate reconstruction for patients under 70 years.
- A correct cost-effectiveness evaluation of breast reconstruction should consider not only direct costs of surgical procedure and but also a longitudinal economic evaluation of extra-hospital expenses and costs related to the instability of reconstruction. Physical integrity need to be seriously considered.
- In this perspective, prepectoral breast reconstruction appears to be a dominant procedure for most patients, due to its optimal and stable results, also confirmed by long-term follow-up.

References

1. Albornoz CR, Bach PB, Mehrara BJ, et al. A paradigm shift in U.S. Breast reconstruction: increasing implant rates. Plast Reconstr Surg. 2013;131(1):15–23.
2. Ness KK, Wall MM, Oakes JM, et al. Physical performance limitations and participation restrictions among cancer survivors: a population-based study. Ann Epidemiol. 2006;16:197–205.

3. Cattelani L, Spotti A, Pedrazzi G, et al. Latissimus dorsi myocutaneous flap in immediate reconstruction after salvage mastectomy post-lumpectomy and radiation therapy. Plast Reconstr Surg Glob Open. 2019;7(7):e2296.
4. Sood R, Easow JM, Konopka G, et al. Latissimus dorsi flap in breast reconstruction: recent innovations in the workhorse flap. Cancer Control. 2018;25(1):1073274817744638.
5. de Haan A, Toor A, Hage JJ, et al. Function of the pectoralis major muscle after combined skin-sparing mastectomy and immediate reconstruction by subpectoral implantation of a prosthesis. Ann Plast Surg. 2007;59(6):605–10.
6. Meldrum D, Cahalane E, Conroy R, et al. Maximum voluntary isometric contraction: reference values and clinical application [published correction appears in Amyotroph Lateral Scler. 2008;9(1):63]. Amyotroph Lateral Scler. 2007;8(1):47–55.
7. Torres Lacomba M, Mayoral del Moral O, Coperias Zazo JL, et al. Incidence of myofascial pain syndrome in breast cancer surgery: a prospective study. Clin J Pain. 2010;26(4):320–5.
8. Hayes SC, Rye S, Battistutta D, et al. Upper-body morbidity following breast cancer treatment is common, may persist longer-term and adversely influences quality of life. Health Qual Life Outcomes. 2010;8:92.
9. Helms G, Kühn T, Moser L, et al. Shoulder-arm morbidity in patients with sentinel node biopsy and complete axillary dissection—data from a prospective randomised trial. Eur J Surg Oncol. 2009;35(7):696–701.
10. Kim KH, Yeo SM, Cheong IY, et al. Early rehabilitation after total mastectomy and immediate reconstruction with tissue expander insertion in breast cancer patients: a retrospective case-control study. J Breast Cancer. 2019;22(3):472–83.
11. Sagen A, Kaaresen R, Sandvik L, et al. Upper limb physical function and adverse effects after breast cancer surgery: a prospective 2.5-year follow-up study and preoperative measures. Arch Phys Med Rehabil. 2014;95(5):875–81.
12. Rancourt D, Hogan N. Stability in force-production tasks. J Mot Behav. 2001;33(2):193–204.
13. Leonardis JM, Lyons DA, Giladi AM, et al. Functional integrity of the shoulder joint and pectoralis major following subpectoral implant breast reconstruction. J Orthop Res. 2019;37(7):1610–9.
14. Leonardis JM, Diefenbach BJ, Lyons DA, et al. The influence of reconstruction choice and inclusion of radiation therapy on functional shoulder biomechanics in women undergoing mastectomy for breast cancer. Breast Cancer Res Treat. 2019;173(2):447–53.
15. Myung Y, Choi B, Kwon H, et al. Quantitative analysis of shoulder function and strength after breast reconstruction: a retrospective cohort study. Medicine (Baltimore). 2018;97(24):e10979.
16. Govshievich A, Kirkham K, Brull R, et al. Novel approach to intractable pectoralis major muscle spasms following submuscular expander-implant breast reconstruction. Plast Surg Case Studies. 2015;1(3):68–70.
17. Roxo AC, Nahas FX, Pinheiro Rodrigues NC, et al. Functional and volumetric analysis of the pectoralis major muscle after submuscular breast augmentation. Aesthet Surg J. 2017;37(6):654–61.
18. Lee KT, Mun GH. A systematic review of functional donor-site morbidity after Latissimus dorsi muscle transfer. Plast Reconstr Surg. 2014;134(2):303–14.
19. de Oliveira RR, do Nascimento SL, Derchain SF, et al. Immediate breast reconstruction with a Latissimus dorsi flap has no detrimental effects on shoulder motion or postsurgical complications up to 1 year after surgery. Plast Reconstr Surg. 2013;131(5):673e–80e.
20. Atisha D, Alderman AK. A systematic review of abdominal wall function following abdominal flaps for postmastectomy breast reconstruction. Ann Plast Surg. 2009;63(2):222–30.
21. Lee KT, Park JW, Mun GH. Impact of rectus muscle injury during perforator dissection on functional donor morbidity after deep inferior epigastric perforator flap breast reconstruction. Plast Reconstr Surg Glob Open. 2019;7(10):e2484.
22. Alba B, Schultz B, Qin LA, et al. Postoperative upper extremity function in implant and autologous breast reconstruction. J Reconstr Microsurg. 2020;36(2):151–6. https://doi.org/10.1055/s-0039-1698439.
23. Ballal H, Hunt C, Bharat C, et al. Arm morbidity of axillary dissection with sentinel node biopsy versus delayed axillary dissection. ANZ J Surg. 2018;88(9):917–21.
24. Phillips CJ, Phillips R, Main CJ, et al. The cost effectiveness of NHS physiotherapy support for occupational health (OH) services. BMC Musculoskelet Disord. 2012;13:29.
25. Schaeffer CV, Dassoulas KR, Thuman J, et al. Early functional outcomes after prepectoral breast reconstruction: a case-matched cohort study. Ann Plast Surg. 2019;82(6S Suppl 5):S399–403.
26. Patel AU, Day SJ, Pencek M, et al. Functional return after implant-based breast reconstruction: a prospective study of objective and patient-reported outcomes. J Plast Reconstr Aesthet Surg. 2020;73(5):850–5.
27. Cattelani L, Polotto S, Arcuri MF, et al. One-step prepectoral breast reconstruction with dermal matrix-covered implant compared to submuscular implantation: functional and cost evaluation. Clin Breast Cancer. 2018;18(4):e703–11.
28. Polotto S, Bergamini ML, Pedrazzi G, et al. One-step prepectoral breast reconstruction with porcine dermal matrix-covered implant: a protective technique improving the outcome in post-mastectomy radiation therapy setting. Gland Surg. 2020;9(2):219–28.
29. Albornoz CR, Cohen WA, Razdan SN, et al. The impact of travel distance on breast reconstruction in the United States. Plast Reconstr Surg. 2016;137(1):12–8.

30. Roughton MC, Di Egidio P, Zhou L, et al. Distance to a plastic surgeon and type of insurance plan are independently predictive of postmastectomy breast reconstruction. Plast Reconstr Surg. 2016;138(2):203e–11e.
31. Cattelani L, Polotto S. The economics of prepectoral breast reconstruction. Plast Reconstr Surg. 2018;142(3):415e–7e.
32. Ilonzo N, Tsang A, Tsantes S, et al. Breast reconstruction after mastectomy: a ten-year analysis of trends and immediate postoperative outcomes. Breast. 2017;32:7–12.
33. Retrouvey H, Zhong T, Gagliardi AR, et al. How patient acceptability affects access to breast reconstruction: a qualitative study. BMJ Open. 2019;9(9):e029048.
34. Régis C, Le J, Chauvet MP, et al. Variations in the breast reconstruction rate in France: a nationwide study of 19,466 patients based on the French medico-administrative database. Breast. 2018;42:74–80.
35. Sisco M, Johnson DB, Wang C, et al. The quality-of-life benefits of breast reconstruction do not diminish with age. J Surg Oncol. 2015;111(6):663–8.
36. Johnson DB, Lapin B, Wang C, et al. Advanced age does not worsen recovery or long-term morbidity after postmastectomy breast reconstruction. Ann Plast Surg. 2016;76(2):164–9.
37. Porter ME. What is value in health care? N Engl J Med. 2010;363(26):2477–81.
38. Glasberg SB. The economics of prepectoral breast reconstruction. Plast Reconstr Surg. 2017;140(6S Prepectoral Breast Reconstruction):49S–52S.
39. Momeni A, Ramesh NK, Wan D, et al. Postoperative analgesia after microsurgical breast reconstruction using liposomal bupivacaine (Exparel). Breast J. 2019;25(5):903–7.
40. Thacoor A, van den Bosch P, Akhavani MA. Surgical management of cosmetic surgery tourism-related complications: current trends and cost analysis study of the financial impact on the UK National Health Service (NHS). Aesthet Surg J. 2019;39(7):786–91.
41. Nguyen PD, Herrera FA, Roostaeian J, et al. Career satisfaction and burnout in the reconstructive microsurgeon in the United States. Microsurgery. 2015;35(1):1–5.
42. Highton L, Johnson R, Kirwan C, et al. Prepectoral implant-based breast reconstruction. Plast Reconstr Surg Glob Open. 2017;5(9):e1488.
43. Frey JD, Salibian AA, Karp NS, et al. Examining length of hospital stay after microsurgical breast reconstruction: evaluation in a case-control study. Plast Reconstr Surg Glob Open. 2017;5(12):e1588.
44. Liu C, Momeni A, Zhuang Y, et al. Outcome analysis of expander/implant versus microsurgical abdominal flap breast reconstruction: a critical study of 254 cases. Ann Surg Oncol. 2014;21(6):2074–82.
45. Roth RS, Qi J, Hamill JB, et al. Is chronic postsurgical pain surgery-induced? A study of persistent postoperative pain following breast reconstruction. Breast. 2018;37:119–25.
46. Becker H, Fregosi N. The impact of animation deformity on quality of life in post-mastectomy reconstruction patients. Aesthet Surg J. 2017;37(5):531–6.
47. Bennett KG, Qi J, Kim HM, et al. Comparison of 2-year complication rates among common techniques for postmastectomy breast reconstruction. JAMA Surg. 2018;153(10):901–8.
48. Fischer JP, Nelson JA, Au A, et al. Complications and morbidity following breast reconstruction—a review of 16,063 cases from the 2005–2010 NSQIP datasets. J Plast Surg Hand Surg. 2014;48(2):104–14.

25 Prepectoral Breast Reconstruction Using a Bio-Synthetic Scaffold

Hilton Becker

25.1 Introduction

The elevation of the pectoral muscle is being performed much less frequently. The negative effects of elevating the muscle include increased surgical time, a more invasive procedure, opening new tissue planes, increased post-operative pain, a longer recovery, animation deformity, chronic discomfort, pain, and shoulder dysfunction. The primary advantage of elevating the muscle is to provide more coverage of the implant, especially in the upper pole [1–3]. In order to compensate for the extra coverage, the use of biological matrices, synthetic meshes, and fat grafting has been partially effective. The use of matrices in combination with tissue expanders has become increasingly common in implant-based immediate breast reconstruction [4]. Utilization of matrices in revision breast surgery was first reported in 2003 [5], and its use in breast reconstruction was introduced in 2005 [6].

Biological matrices offer additional support but are extremely expensive and have other complications such as failure to integrate and infection. Synthetic meshes made from knitted absorbable or permanent fibers used as an internal bra have also been used with some success [7, 8]. Permanent meshes are too rigid, and absorbable meshes are very thin and eventually absorb. Therefore, we have resorted to using multiple layers of long-term absorbable meshes and noticed improved results. Fat grafting is of significant benefit if the flap is thick enough to incorporate the graft. Lining the flap with a mesh results in the "sandwich effect" which greatly facilitates fat grafting and adding more layers of mesh thickens the flap even further (Fig. 25.1).

In an effort to improve the functionality of a DuraSorb (Surgical Innovation Associates) long-term absorbable mesh, we initially soaked the mesh

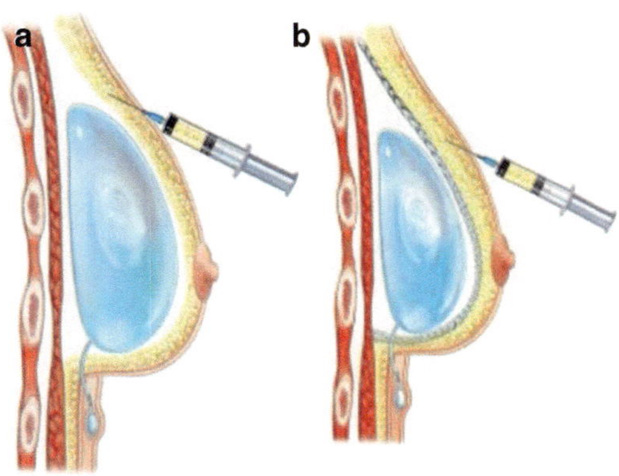

Fig. 25.1 (**a**) The volume of fat that can be injected into a skin flap is limited. (**b**) When a skin flap is lined with mesh a sandwich effect is created, enabling larger volumes of fat to be injected

H. Becker (✉)
Department of Surgery, Charles E. Schmidt College of Medicine, Boca Raton, FL, USA

Florida Atlantic University, Boca Raton, FL, USA
e-mail: Hilton@beckermd.com

© The Author(s), under exclusive license to Springer Nature Switzerland AG 2023

R. Vidya, H. Becker (eds.), *Prepectoral Breast Reconstruction*,
https://doi.org/10.1007/978-3-031-15590-1_25

in platelet-rich plasma (PRP); however, the ability of the mesh to retain the PRP was poor (Fig. 25.2). We then created a three-dimensional mesh and coated it with fat. When PRP was applied to this mesh, it adhered and formed a bio-synthetic scaffold which softens over time and retains the fat graft (Fig. 25.3). We present a technique where PRP is incorporated into a synthetic mesh enhanced with fat to promote healing and aesthetic outcomes in prepectoral breast reconstruction.

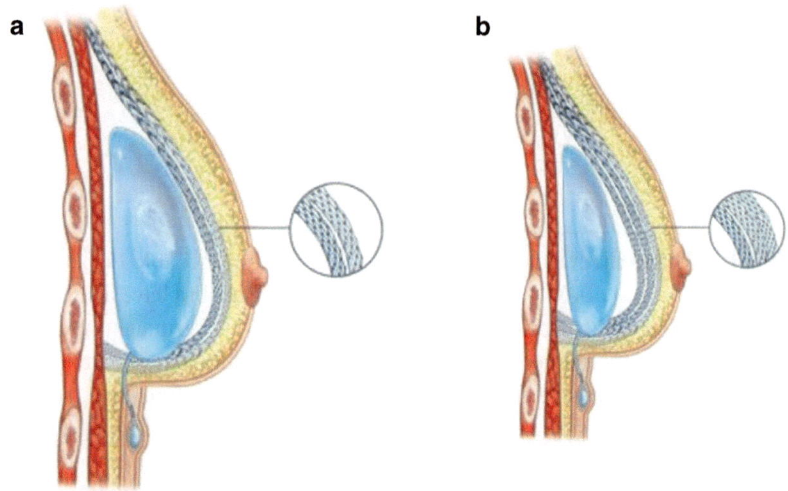

Fig. 25.2 Two layers of mesh. Three layers of mesh

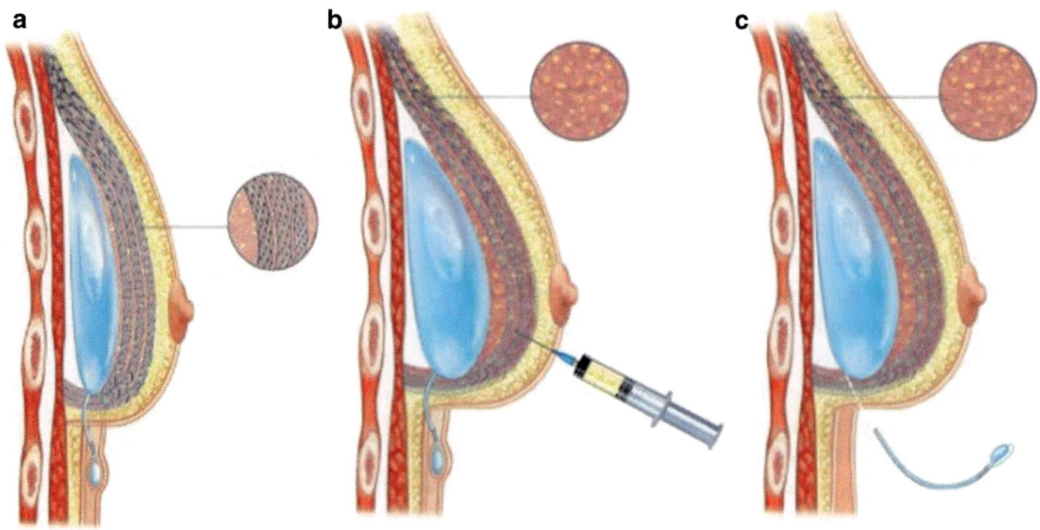

Fig. 25.3 (**a**) Biomesh (PRP and fat impregnated) placed above the implant. (**b**) Fat injected into the biomesh 2–3 months later. (**c**) Injection port removed

25.2 Procedure

Informed consent is obtained from the patients where the procedure is outlined in detail, and the alternatives, benefits, and risks are discussed. The bio-synthetic scaffold is created with multiple layers of DuraSorb (polydioxanone) or Galaflex (poly-4-hydroxybutyrate mesh) or fashioned into constructs.

The donor site is infiltrated with dilute ropivacaine and epinephrine, and fat grafting is harvested with a 4 or 5-mm cutting cannula to maximize stromal vascular fraction (SVF) [9]. The fat is irrigated and strained to remove the oil and then placed on the mesh or in the mesh bag. The fat and mesh are then supplemented with PRP combined with calcium and thrombin [10–12]. Alternatively, individual pyramidal structures can be created by folding 6 × 6 sheets and suturing them with PDS sutures (Figs. 25.4 and 25.5). These can be used to fill in defects (e.g., following lumpectomy or in place of a small implant in immediate or revision reconstruction). Closed suction drains are placed through long subcutaneous tunnels and sutured to the skin. The skin incisions are then closed in layers using 3-0 interrupted Vicryl to the deep tissues and two rows of 4-0 Monocryl (Ethicon) to the skin. The breast is taped into position.

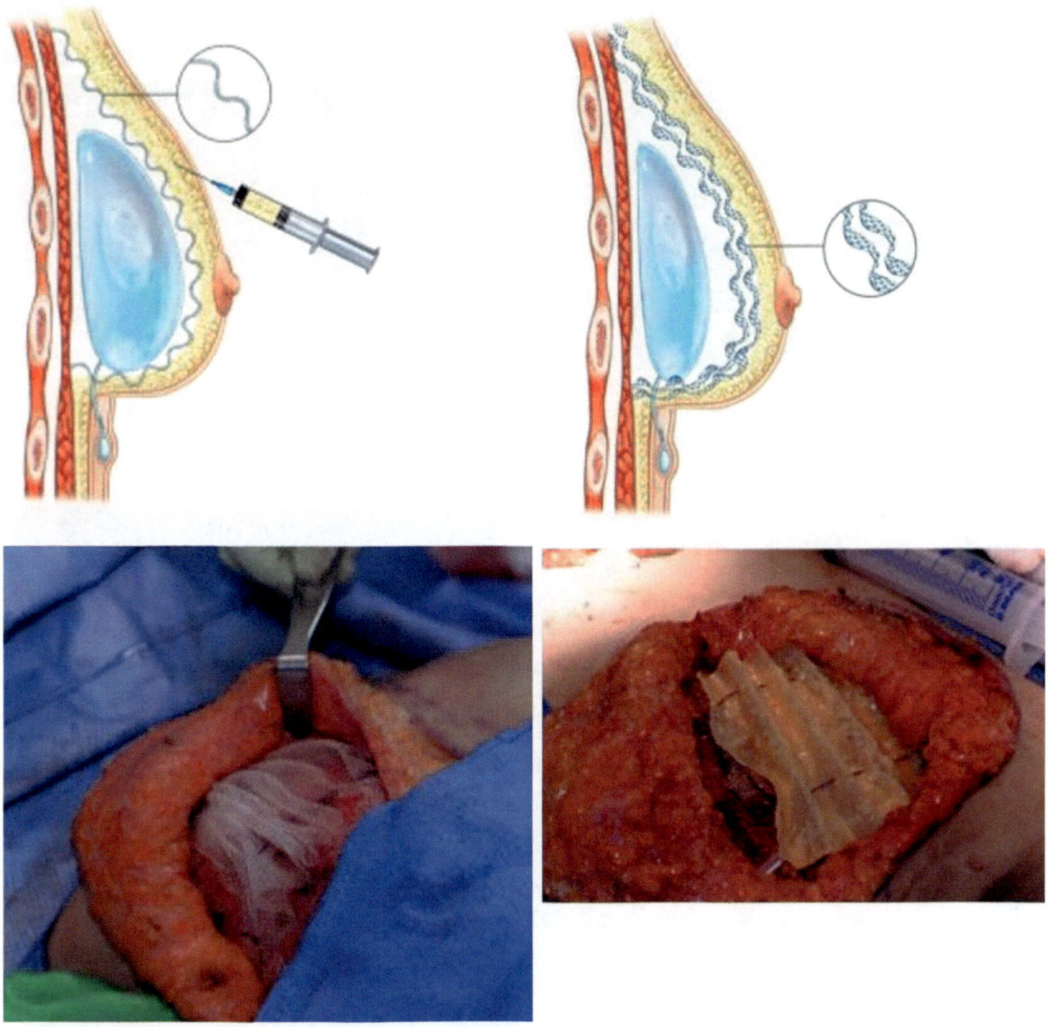

Fig. 25.4 Corrugated mesh

In patients undergoing immediate prepectoral breast reconstruction, our standard approach is to use an adjustable implant. The implant is placed underfilled with air to prevent flap compromise [13]. A layer of biomesh is placed over the implant, a smaller implant is used as the mesh containing considerable volume.

Further volume will be added later. When the correct size is achieved, the injection port is removed leaving the patient with a small, well-padded implant. If sufficient fat can be grafted post-operatively, the implant is removed leaving the patient with a totally autologous implant. External volume enhancement is used to keep the scaffold expanded and stimulate tissue ingrowth. Further fat can be grafted into the scaffold as soon as 2 months.

In selected patients, multiple layers of biomesh are used without an implant. The layers of biomesh can be formed to the desired shape of the breast. Further fat grafting can be done 1–2 months following the initial surgery (Figs. 25.6, 25.7, 25.8, 25.9, and 25.10).

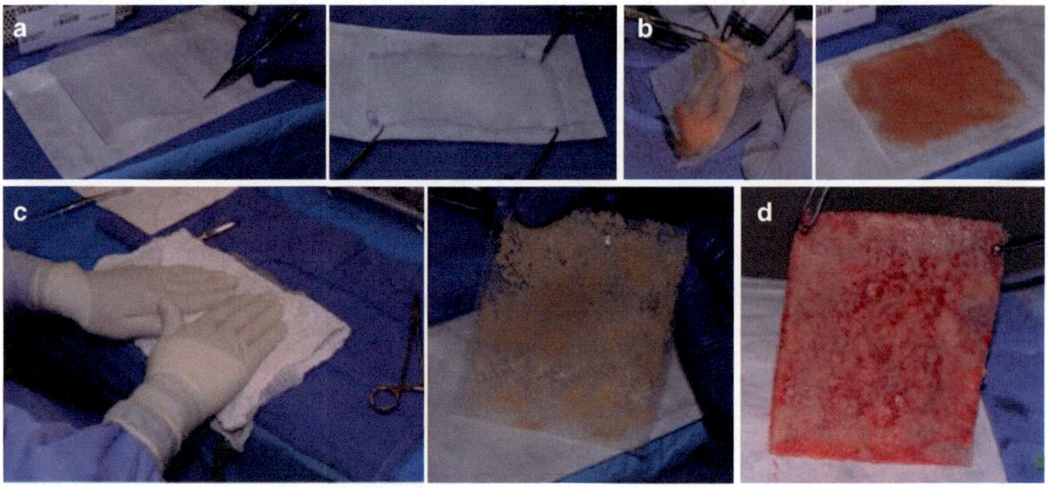

Fig. 25.5 Biomesh Preparation. (**a**) Double layer of mesh sutured to form a bag. (**b**) Mesh impregnated with fat. (**c**) Mesh patted dry to remove free oil. (**d**) PRP added

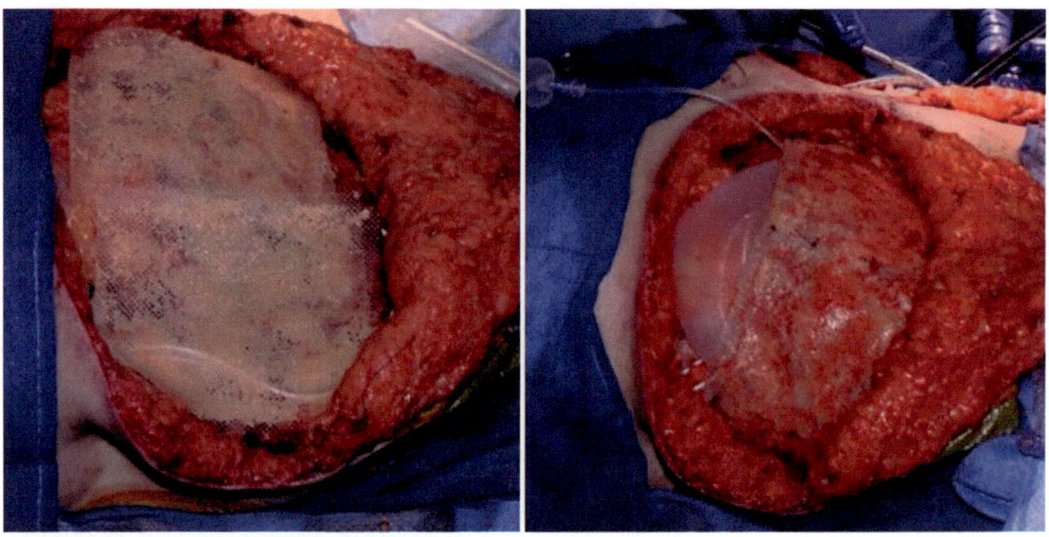

Fig. 25.6 Mesh with fat inserted PRP applied prior to closure

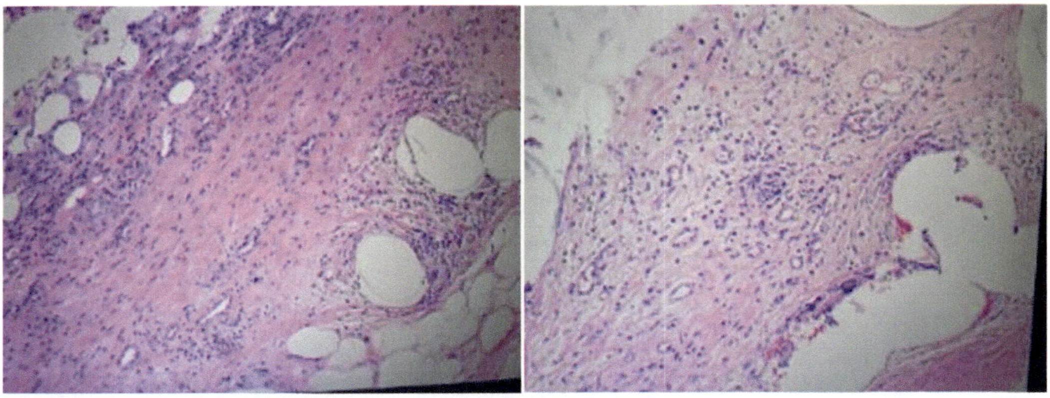

Fig. 25.7 Histology a 6 weeks. Angiogenesis, collagen and fat deposition seen

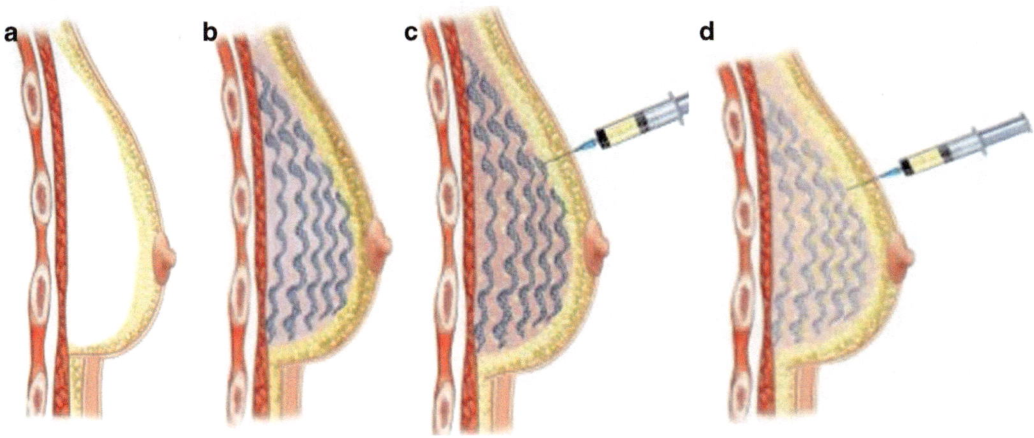

Fig. 25.8 Creating a scaffold for enhanced volume. (**a**) Following mastectomy. (**b**) Biologic scaffold inserted. (**c**) Fat grafting. (**d**) Further fat grafting. Mesh dissolving

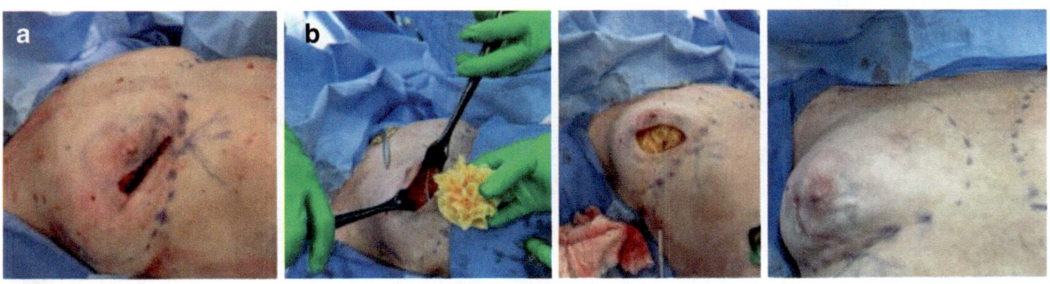

Fig. 25.9 Following Lumpectomy. (**a**) Following lumpectomy. (**b**) Biomesh prepared and inserted

25.2.1 Results

Over a 1-year period, (over 30) cases using biomesh have been performed.

Cases include:

1. Lumpectomy defects (F 9)
2. Immediate breast reconstruction with an adjustable saline implant (Fig. 25.3)
3. Immediate breast reconstruction without implants (Fig. 25.11)
4. Revision reconstruction (Fig. 25.10)

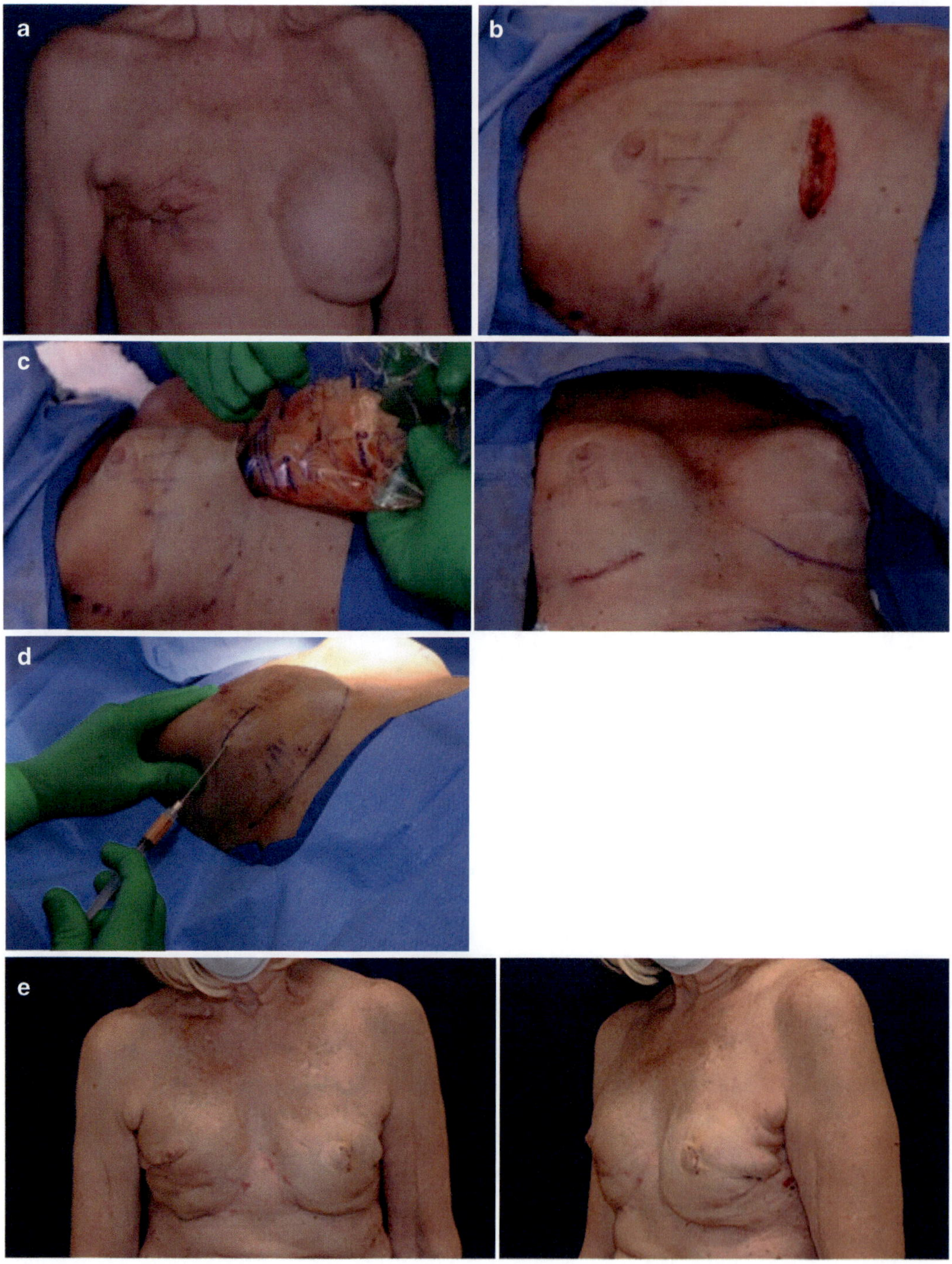

Fig. 25.10 Delayed reconstruction. (**a**) Following mastectomy and radiation loss of expander on the right breast. (**b**) Pocket created. (**c**) Biomesh inserted with a Keller funnel. (**d**) Fat grafting into the bio mesh 2 months. (**e**) Final result

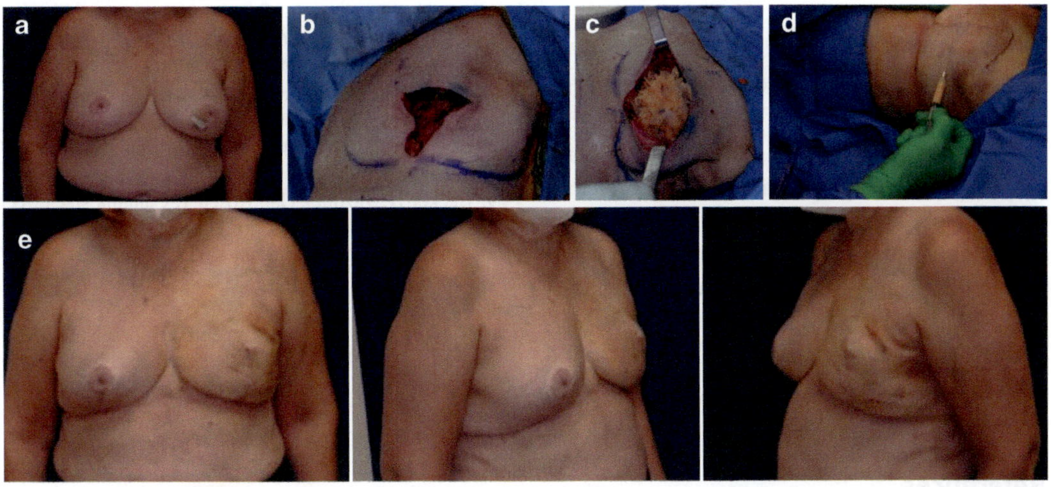

Fig. 25.11 Immediate reconstruction. (**a**) Patient with carcinoma of the left breast. (**b**) Following left mastectomy. (**c**) Insertion of biomesh. (**d**) Fat grafting a 6 weeks. (**e**) Result at 2 months

Good retention of the scaffold has been noted and there has only been one cases of infection in a radiated patient. We continue to follow the patients regularly and inquire about their satisfaction, monitor for complications, and document cosmetic outcomes with photography.

25.3 Discussion

This technique has arisen from our prior work on tendon healing. It was long believed that tendons had no intrinsic healing ability [14]. In our studies we showed that a tendon placed in tissue culture with a hole cut out will only produce a thin layer of fibroblasts on the perimeter of the hole. However, if PRP is placed in the hole, fibroblasts rapidly migrate into the PRP matrix and lay down collagen. When tension is applied to the tendon, the fibroblasts become more robust and align along the lines of tension [15]. We believe that a bio-synthetic scaffold will behave in a similar fashion.

The use of PRP promotes tissue integration and enhances wound healing. PRP is commonly used as a method of introducing concentrated growth factors to surgical sites.

Regenerative tissue engineering is becoming increasingly utilized in surgical procedures. Rehnke [16] described a three-dimensional construct to reconstruct the breast.

By implanting a three-dimensional SVF-coated scaffold containing PRP in the mesh spaces, surrounding tissue and fat can be allowed to grow into the scaffold creating autologous tissue that can later be fat grafted. Techniques of coating mesh with fat have been described and utilized successfully for breast reconstruction; however, it is unlikely that fat that is not in direct contact with a blood supply will survive, especially if the spaces in the mesh are large. Therefore, we resorted to a spongy-like mesh coated with SVF. This has significant collagen and cellular content which can survive in the tissue fluid and the space in the mesh containing PRP which acts as substrate for cellular ingrowth (Fig. 25.7).

25.4 Conclusion

Prepectoral breast reconstruction with a bio-synthetic mesh is an ideal option for enhancing the skin flap following mastectomy, particularly the upper pole to compensate for the muscle.

The bio-synthetic mesh can also be used to repair lumpectomy defects and to reconstruct the breast following mastectomy without a flap or implant.

Further volume can be added to the scaffold, with fat grafting at a later stage.

References

1. Becker H, Fregosi N. The impact of animation deformity on quality of life in post-mastectomy reconstruction patients. Aesthet Surg J. 2017;37(5):531–6. https://doi.org/10.1093/asj/sjw264. PMID: 28158447.
2. Gabriel A, Sigalove S, Sigalove NM, Storm-Dickerson TL, Rice J, Pope N, Maxwell GP. Prepectoral revision breast reconstruction for treatment of implant-associated animation deformity: a review of 102 reconstructions. Aesthet Surg J. 2018;38(5):519–26. https://doi.org/10.1093/asj/sjx261. PMID: 29365064.
3. Campbell CA, Losken A. Understanding the evidence and improving outcomes with implant-based prepectoral breast reconstruction. Plast Reconstr Surg. 2021;148(3):437e–50e. https://doi.org/10.1097/PRS.0000000000008229. PMID: 34432700.
4. Hallberg H, Rafnsdottir S, Selvaggi G, et al. Benefits and risks with acellular dermal matrix (ADM) and mesh support in immediate breast reconstruction: a systematic review and meta-analysis. J Plast Surg Hand Surg. 2018;52(3):130–47. https://doi.org/10.1080/2000656x.2017.1419141.
5. Duncan D. Correction of implant rippling using allograft dermis. Aesthet Surg J. 2001;21(1):81–4. https://doi.org/10.1067/maj.2001.113438.
6. Spear SL, Parikh PM, Reisin E, Menon NG. Acellular dermis-assisted breast reconstruction. Aesthet Plast Surg. 2008;32(3):418–25. https://doi.org/10.1007/s00266-008-9128-8.
7. Becker H, Lind JG II. The use of synthetic mesh in reconstructive, revision, and Cosmetic Breast Surgery. Aesthet Plast Surg. 2013;44(4):1120–7. https://doi.org/10.1007/s00266-020-01822-y.
8. Logan Ellis H, Asaolu O, Nebo V, Kasem A. Biological and synthetic mesh use in breast reconstructive surgery: a literature review. World J Surg Oncol. 2016;14(1):121. https://doi.org/10.1186/s12957-016-0874-9.
9. Becker H, Vazquez OA, Rosen T. Cannula size effect on stromal vascular fraction content of fat grafts. Plast Reconstr Surg Glob Open. 2021;9(3):e3471. https://doi.org/10.1097/GOX.0000000000003471. PMID: 33907655; PMCID: PMC8062151.
10. Gabling VLW, Açil Y, Springer IN, Hubert N, Wiltfang J. Platelet-rich plasma and platelet-rich fibrin in 13 human cell culture. Oral Surg Oral Med Oral Pathol Oral Radiol Endod. 2009;108(1):48–55. https://doi.org/10.1016/j.tripleo.2009.02.007.
11. Gentile P, Calabrese C, De Angelis B, et al. Impact of the different preparation methods to obtain autologous non-activated platelet-rich plasma (A-PRP) and activated platelet-rich plasma (AA-PRP) in plastic surgery: wound healing and hair regrowth evaluation. Int J Mol Sci. 2020;21(2):431. https://doi.org/10.3390/ijms21020431.
12. De Angelis B, D'Autilio MF, Orlandi F, et al. Wound healing: in vitro and in vivo evaluation of a bio-functionalized scaffold based on hyaluronic acid and platelet-rich plasma in chronic ulcers. J Clin Med. 2019;8(9):1486. https://doi.org/10.3390/jcm8091486.
13. Becker H, Mathew PJ. Immediate prepectoral breast reconstruction in suboptimal patients using an air-filled spacer. Plast Reconstr Surg Glob Open. 2019;7(10):e2470. https://doi.org/10.1097/GOX.0000000000002470. PMID: 31772895; PMCID: PMC6846304.
14. Becker H, Graham MF, Cohen IK, Diegelmann RF. Intrinsic tendon cell proliferation in tissue culture. J Hand Surg Am. 1981;6(6):616–9. https://doi.org/10.1016/s0363-5023(81)80146-3. PMID: 7310091.
15. Graham MF, Becker H, Cohen IK, Merritt W, Diegelmann RF. Intrinsic tendon fibroplasia: documentation by in vitro studies. J Orthop Res. 1984;1(3):251–6. https://doi.org/10.1002/jor.1100010304. PMID: 6481508.
16. Rehnke RD, Schusterman MA II, Clarke JM. Breast reconstruction using a three-dimensional absorbable mesh scaffold and autologous fat grafting: a composite strategy based on tissue-engineering principles. Plast Reconstr Surg. 2020;146(4):409e–13e.

Correction to: Evolution of Pre-Pectoral Breast Reconstruction

Hilton Becker, Raghavan Vidya,
Oscar Adrian Vazquez, and Simon Cawthorn

Correction to: Chapter 1 in: R. Vidya, H. Becker (eds.), *Prepectoral Breast Reconstruction*, https://doi.org/10.1007/978-3-031-15590-1_1

The original version of Chapter 1 was inadvertently published without the author name "Oscar Adrian Vazquez". The corresponding author is Dr. Vidya. The chapter has been updated.

The updated version of this chapter can be found at
https://doi.org/10.1007/978-3-031-15590-1_1

© The Author(s), under exclusive license to Springer Nature Switzerland AG 2023

R. Vidya, H. Becker (eds.), *Prepectoral Breast Reconstruction*,
https://doi.org/10.1007/978-3-031-15590-1_26

Index

© The Editor(s) (if applicable) and The Author(s), under exclusive license to Springer Nature Switzerland AG 2023
R. Vidya, H. Becker (eds.), *Prepectoral Breast Reconstruction*,
https://doi.org/10.1007/978-3-031-15590-1

GPSR Compliance

The European Union's (EU) General Product Safety Regulation (GPSR) is a set of rules that requires consumer products to be safe and our obligations to ensure this.

If you have any concerns about our products, you can contact us on ProductSafety@springernature.com

In case Publisher is established outside the EU, the EU authorized representative is:

Springer Nature Customer Service Center GmbH
Europaplatz 3
69115 Heidelberg, Germany

Batch number: 10732801

Printed by Printforce, the Netherlands